# A History of Surgery at Cook County Hospital

*Edited by*
*Patrick D. Guinan*
*Kenneth J. Printen*
*James L. Stone*
*James S. T. Yao*

*A History of Surgery at Cook County Hospital*
© Copyright 2015, Patrick D. Guinan, Kenneth J. Printen,
James L. Stone, and James S. T. Yao

All rights reserved. No part of this book may be used or reproduced in any manner whatsoever without written permission from the publisher, except in the case of brief quotations in critical articles and reviews.

First Edition   ISBN 13: 978-1-937484-26-2
AMIKA PRESS   466 Central Ave #23 Northfield IL 60093   847 920 8084
info@amikapress.com   Available for purchase on amikapress.com

# *Dedication*

Robert J. Freeark, MD, was a tireless worker completely dedicated to the teaching of residents and students. He was the heart and soul of the surgical program at Cook County Hospital. His second career after County at Loyola University is just as impressive as the first. He rebuilt the Loyola program to be one of the premier training programs in the country. We, the four editors, are unanimous in dedicating this book in honor of his great contribution to surgical training. In addition to Dr. Freeark, we would like to pay tribute to Dr. Frank Milloy and Ms. Louise Rzeszewski. Dr. Milloy, as Secretary of the Karl Meyer Surgical Society, kept the Surgical Society going with annual cocktail parties at the Congress of the American College of Surgeons in October and a dinner party every third year when the Congress met in Chicago. Without his leadership, we probably would not have an alumni party every year. Sadly, he passed away in March, 2011. He will be missed by all of us. Ms. Louise Rzeszewski, known to everyone as "Miss R.," was an icon in the operating room. She presided over the busiest operating rooms in town and was able to deal with different personalities. She was always fair and firm with special skill in handling those surgical residents who would always want to do one more case.

Finally, we must pay tribute to our patients for placing their trust in a group of young, inexperienced, but eager-to-learn surgeons, and a dedicated voluntary and salaried surgical attending staff.

— *The Editors*

# Table of Contents

**Acknowledgement**
The Editors    vi

**Foreword**
Alon P. Winnie    vii

**Preface**
The Editors    xi

**A Tribute to Robert J. Freeark, MD**
The Editors    xiv

**A Tribute to Frank J. Milloy, Jr., MD**
The Editors    xvi

**A Tribute to Miss R. (Louise Rzeszewski), RN, BSN**
The Editors    xviii

## The Hospital and Surgical Education

**Chapter 1: Cook County Hospital: A Brief History**
Patrick Guinan, Frank J. Milloy    3

**Chapter 2: Surgical Education at Cook County Hospital**
Kenneth Printen, Hernan Reyes    15

## Contribution of Chicago Area Medical Schools to Surgery at CCH

**Chapter 3: Rush Medical College**
Frank J. Milloy    65

**Chapter 4: Northwestern University**
James S.T. Yao, Robert M. Vanecko    83

**Chapter 5: University of Illinois**
Philip E. Donohue, Kenneth Printen    107

**Chapter 6: Loyola University**
Harold Haley, Frank Folk, Kenneth Printen    117

**Chapter 7: Chicago Medical School**
Michael J. Zdon    127

## Prominent Surgical Services at Cook County Hospital

**Chapter 8: Trauma Unit**
David R. Boyd, Kimberly Kay Ormsby Nagy, Kenneth J. Printen, James S.T. Yao    143

**Chapter 9: Evolution of Burn Surgical Service**
Marella L. Hanumadass, Takayoshi Matsuda    185

**Chapter 10: Hand Surgery**
Sidney J. Blair, John Elstrom, James L. Stone    207

# TABLE OF CONTENTS

### Chapter 11: Breast Tumor Service
Frank Folk   221

### Chapter 12: Bernard Fantus and Development of the World's First Blood Bank
James L. Stone, Richard J. Fantus, Henry H. Fantus   229

### Chapter 13: Hektoen Institute for Medical Research
Patrick Guinan   239

## Specialty Surgery at Cook County Hospital

### Chapter 14: Cardio-Thoracic Surgery
Frank Milloy, Milton Weinberg, Walter Barker, Constantine Tatooles   251

### Chapter 15: Evolution of Pediatric Surgery at CCH
Hernan Reyes, Jayant Radhakrishnan   261

### Chapter 16: Neurological Surgery
James L. Stone, George R. Cybulski   285

### Chapter 17: Vascular Surgery
Richard Keen, James S.T. Yao   301

### Chapter 18: Urological Surgery
Patrick Guinan   321

### Chapter 19: Orthopedic Surgery
John A. Elstrom   333

### Chapter 20 : Plastic Surgery
Raymond L. Warpeha   359

### Chapter 21: Otolaryngological Surgery
Kenneth Printen, Hugh Hazenfield   369

### Chapter 22: Oral and Maxillofacial Surgery
John M. Sisto, James L. Stone   377

### Chapter 23: Ophthalmological Surgery
Philip Dray, Alexander Constantaras   381

### Chapter 24 Colon Rectal Surgery
Herand Abcarian   385

## Remembrances

### Chapter 25 Historical Vignettes and Photo Memoir   393

## Appendices

List of Surgical Residents at Cook County Hospital   442

Compendium of Cook County Hospital Trauma Unit (CCHTU)
   Published Literature   446

The Greek's   463

# Acknowledgement

We are honored to have had the late Alon Winnie write the Foreword for this book. Al was a great friend and the distinguished Chair of the Department of Anesthesiology at CCH. Without anesthesia, there would be no surgery. The Department of Anesthesiology under Winnie and also Vincent Collins played an important role in the growth of the Department of Surgery. Dr. Alon Winnie passed away shortly before the printing of this volume, and the editors would like to take this space to pass on our condolences to his family. The broad world of medicine will remember him as an innovator and critical thinking physician most active in the areas of pain management and regional anesthesia. It will also note that he was the Chair of the Department of Anesthesia at the University of Illinois College of Medicine in Chicago for seventeen years, after which he returned to CCH as the Chairman of Anesthesia and Pain Management. History will also record the impressive number of awards he received from his peers that indicated his overall excellence and forward thinking approach to his chosen field.

Those of us who trained in the disciplines of surgery described in this book at the same time that Al was pursuing his residency training will remember the jovial, hard working, and very knowledgeable resident in a wheelchair who eschewed the easy outs of psychiatry or radiology to stay where he wanted to be, in the operating room. It's not easy to do a spinal anesthetic sitting in a wheelchair below a fracture table with the patient awake and suspended just above your head, but All could do it and most often with more dispatch than those who did it in the conventional manner. As surgeons we always felt better for our patients and ourselves with Al on the other side of the ether screen.

Sleep well, friend. You've earned it.

—*The Editors*

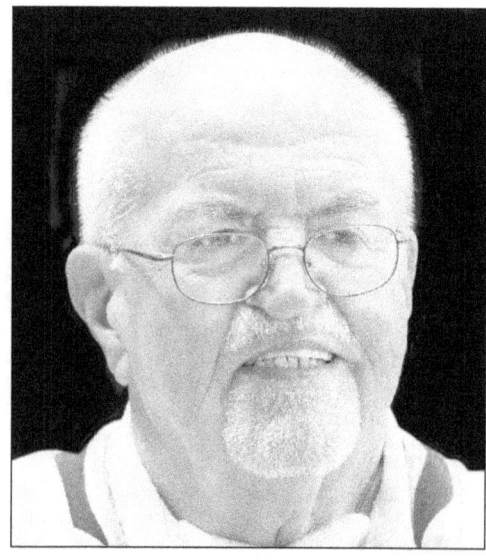

**Alon P. Winnie**

# Foreword

It was in medical school on my first clerkship at Cook County Hospital that I got the bug. I saw and did things there that I had never experienced at the private-university-affiliated hospitals, and I decided then and there that County was the place where I could really become a doctor. My decision was confirmed during the last lecture in medicine in my senior year. The lecture was entitled "Diseases You Will Never See" and was delivered by a famous internist, his renown due to the daily column he wrote in the *Chicago Tribune*. Most significantly, after he finished his laundry list of diseases we would never see, he advised the class not to choose an internship at Cook County Hospital where the educational experience was "See one, do one, teach one," but rather intern at one of the university hospitals where you could learn not just the science but also the art of medicine. After that lecture, I knew I was going to County, which I did, and it was no mistake. Although the working conditions were not ideal, like the majority of my fellow interns, I loved it!

And by the end of my internship (July 1958 to July 1959), I had seen (and treated) the vast majority of "the diseases we would never see." Furthermore, since the house staff, interns, and residents interacted as they were becoming real doctors, there was a "band of brothers" type of camaraderie that made tough, often exhausting work enjoyable. The only problem my internship presented was the fact that I enjoyed every service I was assigned to, making the choice of a specialty very difficult.

That choice suddenly became limited by an unexpected turn of events. While working on the ENT Service, I developed acute bulbospinal poliomyelitis, which first required a tracheotomy performed by Dr. Trier Morch, at that time Chairman of Anesthesia and Dr. Paul O'Brien, the on-call night surgeon. I was then placed on one of the first positive pressure ventilators, which was invented by Dr. Morch. While on the ventilator, which had no monitors or alarms on it, my "band of brothers" took turns sitting with me around the clock in case the ventilator malfunctioned, which it did six times. So I literally owe my life to the County interns and residents who took an extra call to sit with me, in addition to the calls they took on their own services. Unbelievable!

By the time I was discharged seven months later, I had recovered the use of my arms but not my legs, so whatever specialty I entered, I would have to perform it from a wheelchair. Although I was urged by many to consider radiology and psychiatry, I remembered that I had enjoyed anesthesia when I rotated through it as an intern. What appealed to me about the specialty of anesthesiology was not just that it allowed pain-free surgery, but it also enabled management of the medical problems of the surgical patient intraoperatively. I also felt that as an anesthetist, I could provide important psychological support to patients undergoing a very stressful, and sometimes terrifying, experience. However, the real question was, could I perform anesthesia in a wheelchair? Dr. Morch, who by then was no longer Chairman of Anesthesia, suggested that there was no place like County to see if I could do it. He reasoned that since there was no County residency in anesthesia at that time, if I found I could do it, then I could apply to one of the institutions that did have an approved residency program. So I tried it. I found I could do it. And I applied for a position in the programs in the other four large public hospitals in the United States. Interestingly, none of the four would take me. "You can't possibly do anesthesia in a wheelchair" was the reply to one of my applications. But the gods wanted me to do anesthesia, or so it would seem, when Doctor Vincent J. Collins came to Chicago from New York's Bellevue Hospital to set up a residency in anesthesiology at our own Cook County Hospital. About three weeks after his arrival, he called me into his office and told me that upon the recommendation of Drs. Freeark and Baker, he had decided to take me as his first resident. Obviously, I accepted his kind offer, though I must admit, as I left his office, I really wanted to tell him, "If you didn't take me, who the hell would you take?" There certainly wasn't a line of applicants outside his door! However, in fairness, over the next year, he was successful in recruiting some great faculty and residents. The anesthesia program grew rapidly and was approved by the Residency Review Committee on its first review.

Of course, one of the reasons I was particularly pleased to be able to take my residency at County was that I could continue to train with the surgery residents, many of whom were already friends from my internship (and many of whom sat with me when I was on the ventilator). Another reason was that the Department of Anesthesiology, of necessity, worked hand and glove with the Department of Surgery, which was probably the best clinical department in the hospital, and, therefore, attracted excellent residents. So as a result, we all really worked as a team, and the residents on both sides of the ether shield were pleased with their clinical experience. I will admit, however, that there were a few bumps in the road, and that not everything went smoothly. For example, it is best for the patient if the surgeon waits to make the incision until anesthesia is established, so it was infuriating to the surgery resident when the anesthesia resident arrived in the O.R. late. Similarly, anesthesia residents were enraged when a surgery resident brought a patient to the O.R. without essential laboratory studies and/or without appropriate evaluation of obvious clinical problems. These "silly" demands by the anesthesia residents earned for their department the title of "The Department of Preventative Surgery," but ultimately, the preoperative problems were resolved, after which an "uneventful anesthetic" was provided as the essential surgery was carried out. (When asked "What is essential surgery?" Marv Tiesenga, one of the night surgeons, replied, "Every patient needs a surgical procedure. Our job is simply to find out which one.") However, as stated, the bumps were few, and the atmosphere in the O.R. was one of cooperation. Our department carried out many clinical research projects, which not infrequently required the cooperation of the surgeons, none of whom caused us problems in these endeavors. As a matter of fact, the junior surgery residents traditionally spent a three-month rotation on anesthesia, and quite a few of them actually participated in our research projects. In short, the Surgery Department enhanced the growth and development of our department in this and many other ways. After I finished my three years of training, I stayed at County as an attending anesthesiologist for almost nine years, so I continued to work with the surgical residents and faculty and developed many warm and lasting friendships with them over those years.

In all, I spent fourteen years (1958-1972) at Cook County Hospital—as an intern, resident, and attending—and I believe I received the best clinical and academic training in anesthesiology available in this country. I believe my surgical friends and colleagues writing and editing this book are doing so because they feel the same way about their specialties. An index of my belief in the quality of the surgical training is my response when friends, confronted by the need for surgery, ask me "Who do you recommend as a surgeon?" I answer, "If possible, find a surgeon who trained at Cook County Hospital. They are the best." Short of that, I suggest they find out which surgeons the anesthesiologists choose for themselves or their families when they need surgery. They know, better than anyone, who's well trained and who's not.

In closing, let me say that it has been a privilege for me to participate, even in a small way, to this important book, which provides long overdue documentation of the excellence of the Department of Surgery at Cook County Hospital.

*—Alon P. Winnie, MD*
*May 16, 1932–January 18, 2015*

# Preface

In 2002, Cook County Hospital (CCH) moved to a new building and was renamed John H. Stroger, Jr. Hospital of Cook County in honor of John Stroger, President of the Cook County Board of Commissioners. Today, as the old main County Hospital building stands alone and empty, it casts a stark shadow over what used to be a 3,000-bed hospital associated with six medical schools providing free service to a large underprivileged population. From the day it opened its doors in 1866, it became the best known public hospital in Chicago, if not in the world. The richness of pathology found in its patients attracted many to come to County for training. An internship at County was the most sought-after position in the country, and most of the leading physicians and surgeons in Chicago did their training there. At the onset of both world wars, CCH surgical courses were given to surgeons going abroad. By the 1960s, it was said that 20 percent of surgeons in the world had at least some training at CCH or were taught by CCH-trained surgeons.

Many books have been published on Cook County Hospital. Unlike these other titles, however, *A History of Surgery at Cook County Hospital* is a summation of the evolution of surgical training and practice in a public hospital. Special emphasis is placed on the history of surgical practice and education, including all surgical specialties and prominent surgical services at the hospital. We, the four editors and authors of various chapters, all chose County for our surgical training, and we came with one single purpose: "to learn to be a surgeon." We knew CCH was not the Ritz Carlton Hotel, and we were determined not to let a substandard working environment frustrate our intentions to be skillful surgeons with sound surgical judgment. Surgeons need to be independent-minded, and there was no better place than County to develop independent judgment on case management. We have no quarrels with those who wanted to change the political systems of the governing body of the hospital to make it a better place for our patients. However, our first priority remained "to learn to be a surgeon."

Surgery at CCH began with anatomy and pathology. Christian Fenger, the most influential surgeon in Chicago and the first Chair of Surgery at Northwestern University, was a pathologist by training. Under his leadership, the Department of Surgery grew with famous surgeons like Nicolas Senn, John B. Murphy, Karl Meyer, William and Charles Mayo, and others from many regions and countries who came to learn from Fenger and his disciples. Unlike eastern schools where surgical training was centered on producing professors, Cook County-trained surgeons provided care to communities. Thus, it is no surprise that Fenger's students founded the American College of Surgeons. The Fenger training system has been called the Midwestern School of Surgery or in a narrow sense, the Chicago School of Surgery. It soon became apparent that a structured training program was needed to provide better patient care. This concept led to the formation of governing bodies to set standards for the training of surgeons. Credentialing governing bodies such as the Accreditation Council for Graduate Medical Education

(ACGME), American Board of Surgery (ABS), American Board of Medical Specialties (ABMS), and Resident Review Committee (RRC) began to enforce rules and requirements for training programs. At the same time, various specialty boards were established, and each board had its own certifying examination.

The most drastic change came in the late 1950s with the addition of full-time salaried attending staff, beginning with the appointment of Dr. Robert J. Freeark, first as Director of Surgical Education and later as Chairman of Surgery. This transformation was much needed for better accountability of patient care, and most importantly, better supervision and education of surgical residents. Under the leadership of Freeark, a group of full-time salaried surgeons was added to the staff. Like all academic centers, surgical subspecialties began to develop and flourish. With delicate handling, Dr. Freeark was able to maintain a balance of coverage by full-time and voluntary staff. This practice continued until 1980, when the independent Cook County surgical residency program merged with that of the University of Illinois. With the merger, that is, the elimination of the independent Cook County surgical program, the voluntary staff was no longer part of the workforce of the hospital. Looking back at the Northwestern surgical service, the all-voluntary service operated from 1866 to 1978 and provided 113 years of free service to Cook County Hospital. Such a tradition will never be repeated.

The contents of this book comprise 25 chapters, categorized under five sections:

- *The hospital and surgical education*
- *Contribution of Chicago area medical schools to surgery at Cook County Hospital*
- *Prominent surgical services at Cook County Hospital*
- *Specialty surgery at Cook County Hospital*
- *Remembrances*

The Chicago area schools include Rush Medical School, Northwestern University Medical School, University of Illinois, Loyola University, University of Chicago, and Chicago Medical School. All these schools provided attending surgeons without compensation to care for patients at Cook County Hospital. Section IV describes several surgical services that achoeved world renown in the country: the first blood bank in the United States, the hand and burn surgical services, the breast tumor service, the first trauma unit in the United States, the arterial bank during the era of homograft surgery, the Cook County Graduate School, and finally, the Hektoen Institute for Medical Research. Development of specialty surgery was inevitable, and by the 1930s surgical subspecialty services emerged with ophthalmology as the first. Section III shows these specialties, including cardiothoracic, pediatric, neurological, vascular, orthopedic, plastic, urology, otolaryngology, and colon-rectal surgery as they brought expert care to patients. Finally, Section V is a walk down memory lane with a chapter on historical vignettes and a DVD/CD of photo memoirs. The historic vignettes derive from many former trainees who sent in their remembrances of their time at County. Likewise, many old photos were sent in from alumni and collected from the archives of the American College of Surgeons, Galter Library of Feinberg School of Medicine, Northwestern University, and Rush University. These photos were organized in 10 sections in a PowerPoint presentation format. We consider both historical vignettes and photo memoirs to be a unique feature of this book.

Standing alone, not far from the old County Hospital, is the Pasteur statue. More than a century has passed since the opening of Cook County Hospital, but the inscription at the base of the statue remains true for a public hospital:

> *One doesn't ask of one who suffers: What is your country and what is your religion? One merely says, you suffer. This is enough for me. You belong to me and I shall help you.*
>
> —Louis Pasteur

Amid all the outcries about health care reform, these words remind us—the physicians and surgeons—that we have the responsibility of providing care to underprivileged populations. That is what the doctors at the County through the years were, and are, all about.

—The Editors

# A Tribute to Robert J. Freeark, MD (1927–2006)

A *History of Surgery at Cook County Hospital* is a summation of the growth of an institute of learning from the humble beginning in 1866 to the new John Stroger Hospital opening in 2002. During this period, one of the most drastic changes was the transformation to a full-time salaried attending staff in the late 1950s. Such change is needed for better supervision of resident training, and most importantly, for accountability of patient care. Robert Freeark was recognized as someone special, and at the completion of his residency in 1958, he was appointed Director of Surgical Education at County by the legendary Karl Meyer, Chief of Surgery and Medical Superintendant of the Hospital. In this capacity, Robert Freeark was the first full-time employed physician in the Department of Surgery. He was appointed to the Northwestern faculty in 1960 and soon after became the Chief of Surgical Services at County, an appointment that included administrative responsibility for all the surgical specialties. He was also promoted to Professor of Surgery at Northwestern University Medical School.

As Chief of Surgery he upgraded both formal teaching and surgical supervision by supplementing the volunteer attending staff with carefully selected salaried surgeons. The "Two Bobs," Freeark and Baker, expanded the academic and research scope of the institution and together established one of the first modern trauma units in the country. Emergency helicopter transport, the first in Chicago, was established with a heliport directly across Harrison Street from the hospital in Pasteur Park, right next to the Greek's, the favorite watering hole for the numerous young doctors, nurses, and medical and allied health care students who worked and learned in the West Side Medical Center. Dr. Freeark established the Sumner Koch Burn Unit and appointed John Boswick to lead it. He also supported David Boyd in developing the first statewide Trauma System in the United States and appointed John Raffensperger to be the first full-time director of Pediatric Surgery. At the basis of these reforms was the firm belief that the physicians, both salaried and volunteer, who worked at the County—not the bureaucrats, either medical or political—were the best qualified to determine the diagnostic modalities and the treatment options as well as the structure of the system for the patients who presented there for care. This approach energized the medical staff at the attending and resident levels across the board and resulted in Freeark's appointment as Hospital Director in 1968.

Robert Freeark was selected as Hospital Director at a troublesome time, not only for County but also for large city- and county-based hospitals nationwide. Political infighting, financial problems, restive house staffs and resultant public unrest made caring for the medically indigent doubly difficult. Dr. Freeark led an effort to foster cooperation among all the stakeholders, including the County Board and the old-time political guard. Although his efforts did not produce the hoped-for amalgamation of cares, concerns, and solutions, they did produce a spirit of cooperation, frank discussions, and transparent decision-making processes among members of the medical staff, which was to become a hallmark of

# A TRIBUTE TO ROBERT J. FREEARK, MD (1927–2006)

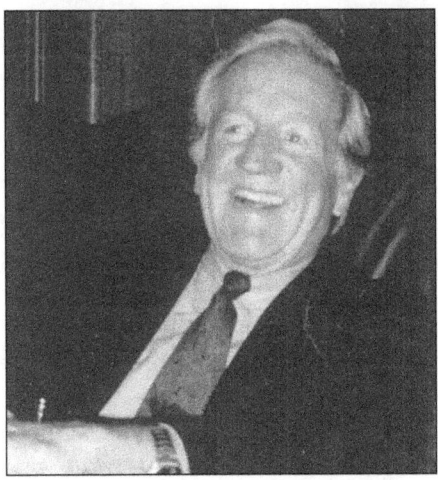

*Robert J. Freeark, MD*

Freeark-directed medical enterprises. In the face of unrelenting bureaucratic opposition, he publically resigned along with several other prominent staff members from other departments in 1970.

In the post-County period of his life, Dr. Freeark continued on the staff of Northwestern in association with his County colleague, Dr. Jim Hines. In 1970, he returned to a leadership role when he accepted the Chairmanship of Surgery at the Loyola Stritch School of Medicine at its new location in the Chicago suburb of Maywood. Freeark developed a full-time surgical faculty for the first time in the school's history. Great cooperative efforts, which emanated from the Chair down to the lowest instructor, soon resulted in an abundance of patients and enhanced the reputation not only of the hospital but also of the educational training program, of the Hines/Loyola surgical residency.

Bob Freeark was a regular guy who accomplished extraordinary things. Gracious and unassuming, he exemplified the best in medicine, wearing effortlessly, it seemed, the "Four Hats" of medicine: clinical practice, teaching, research, and administration. In addition, he was a dedicated family man, loving husband and father, good citizen, supporter of the arts, and mentor and friend to many. Dr. Freeark's *curriculum vita* lists multiple publications, honors, and awards, among them a Chicago Young Man of the Year he shared with the Chicago Cubs' Ernie Banks. He was an active, contributing member of more than a dozen surgical societies, serving as president of half of them. Hundreds of surgeons and medical students benefited from his teaching at Northwestern, Loyola, the County, and his numerous scientific presentations. Dozens of surgeons conducted research, published papers, and progressed in academic life because of his assistance and exhortation. Best of all, he never lost sight of his trainees and colleagues from the most famous of the professors to the most remote rural practitioners. It therefore seems fitting to dedicate this volume to Robert J. Freeark, a surgeon who left his stamp on a generation of County Hospital surgeons, and proudly wielded that stamp so boldly during his time with us. We, the editors, all are better surgeons today because of him.

—*The Editors, written with assistance from Frank Folk*

# A Tribute to Frank Milloy, MD

This book, *A History of Surgery at Cook County Hospital*, is the record of a great institution, and in particular, a major department within that institution: the Department of Surgery. For almost 200 years, that department and that institution, at its several locations, have served the sick poor in the city of Chicago, particularly intheir surgical needs.

In the history ansd development of Cook County Hospital, the house staff and alumni organizations have played an important role. The first such organization was the Cook County Hospital Alumni Association founded in 1910. The object of the Association was stated as follows:

*The object of the Organization shall be the perpetuation of the fraternal spirit engendered in the early association, and the perfection of a large working body which shall have for its object, the advancement of medical science and the betterment of the medical profession.*

In 1916, the Cook County Intern Council was founded to strive for the improvement of the practice, teaching, and general value of the internship. Under an Editorial Committee, the Council published a pamphlet entitled *The County Intern*. This official quarterly publication called attention to critical issues such as legal liability and health insurance for house staff. In the mid-1930s and duing the early 1940s, as World War II raged, several topics on war injuries were published in *The County Intern*.

In 1964, there was renewal of the Cook County Hospital Interns and Residents Alumni Association. Arthur Bernstein was elected as President, Samuel Hoffman as Secretary/Treasurer, and Donald Miller as Vice-President. Under the editorship of Louis Boshes, the Association published a newsletter that highlighted some of the leading surgeons at County. In 1966, the Karl A. Meyer Surgical Society, Surgical Alumni Association of Cook County Hospital, with membership limited to surgical trainees.

Frank Milloy was appointed Secretary of the Karl Meyer Surgical Society. During his more than a half-century of involvement with County, Frank Milloy served in positions that spanned the gamut of his medical career, from student through internship and residency, and finally to attending surgeon in the Division of Thoracic and Cardiovascular Surgery (1983-1998). Always interested in surgery, Dr. Milloy interned at County Hospital from 1947 to 1949, and while assigned to Dr. Egbert Fell's service, assisted him with the first heart operation performed at the hospital in February 1948. He served as Associate Director of Chicago Artery Bank with Dr. Fell as Medical Director. The bank provided homograft for replacement of aorta due to aneurysm formation. Though his training was interrupted by military service during the Korean War (1950-1952), Dr. Milloy completed his training in both general and thoracic surgery by 1958 and embarked on a long career in the private practice of thoracic surgery at several of the major teaching hospitals in Chicago.

We were indeed fortunate to have Frank Milloy as Secretary of the Karl Meyer Surgical Society. Throughout his long association with the Society, he has continued to remind us all of the heritage that those of us who trained at the County inherited. Under his stewardship, an annual reception during the ACS Congress and a dinner party when ACS Congress is in Chicago (every third year) were organized. He conceived the idea for the Society to support an annual resident prize for the Chicago Surgical Society, and finally, the Christian Fenger Surgical Excellence Award, which is annually given to an outstanding member of the Karl Meyer Surgical Society. Milloy also presides over the directors' meeting every September. His letter to the members always captures the changing scene of the six medical schools in Chicago and County Hospital. No one has done more than Frank Milloy to keep the fraternal spirit of interns-residents-alumni alive. We, the editors, would like to thank Frank Milloy for his precision and perseverance in maintaining our institution's history.

—*The Editors*

# Dedication to Miss R. (Louise B. Rzeszewski) RN, BSN

No history of Cook County Hospital could be considered complete without acknowledgement of the enormous debt of gratitude owed to the nursing staff of County, who gave the best of care to our patients. The nursing staff also provided the matrix within which the medical students and house staff could learn and perfect their craft. They were always there teaching us, mostly by suggestion. The longer one spent as a medical student or physician at County, the more evident it became that if you listened to the nurse's advice, you somehow got smarter and your patients usually got better quicker. In the course of time, most of the physicians and nurses learned to live in a symbiotic relationship that worked to the benefit of all concerned and often spilled into the social arena at the Greek's or even more formal arrangements such as matrimony.

Cook County School of Nursing is a unique organization. It was a private operation with its own Board of Directors, which contracted each April with Cook County to employ and provide nursing services for Cook County Hospital. This included all RNs, with the exception of nurse anesthetists, LPNs, nurses' aides, dieticians, and most likely all physical and occupational therapists. In addition, the School of Nursing was responsible for the student nurse affiliation programs for pupils from nursing schools in Illinois, Indiana, Wisconsin, Minnesota, and North Dakota, all of whom rotated through County for experience. All these student nurses and the postgraduate nurses who came to County for specialty training lived in the School of Nursing building located conveniently next to Karl Meyer Hall at the corner of Polk and Wolcott Avenues. This last fact was well known to the medical student and house staff population of the West Side Medical Center.

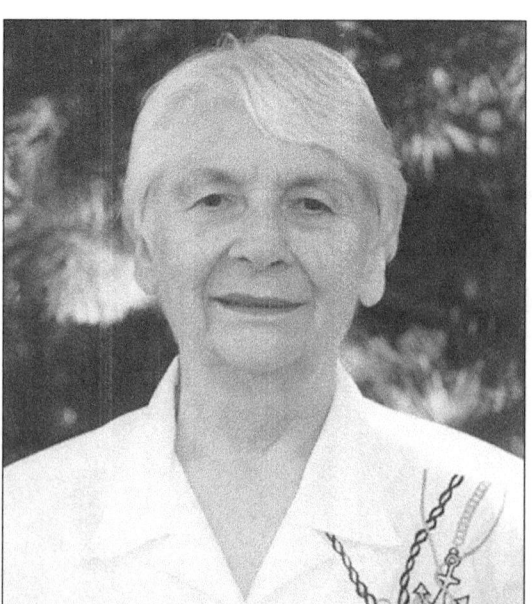

"Miss R"—Louise Rzeszewski, RN

## DEDICATION TO MISS R. (LOUISE B. RZESZEWSKI) RN, BSN

In the midst of surgical training, the one common ground all of us had to traverse was the operating room suite with its curious mix of egos, raging testosterone (although now increasing levels of estrogen), dreams of technical brilliance, fears of judgmental failures, and its very specific and regimented hierarchy. Seated at the top of that hierarchy on the operational side from 1958 to 1981 as the Supervisor of the Main OR was Ms. Louise B. Rzeszewski, RN, BSN, better known as "Miss R." After a four-year stint as a staff and head nurse at County, Miss R. spent a year at Massachusetts General Hospital as a recovery room nurse before returning to County to take over the operation of the Main OR and administrative supervision of all the rest of the operating facilities in the County Medical Center. And operate them she did. In addition, she was scrub nurse for Dr. Karl Meyer for almost four years of Saturday-afternoon surgical clinics held in the surgical amphitheater of the Main OR. With a combination of the wisdom of Solomon and the patient persistence of Job, day after day she saw to it that some 30-odd operating rooms were staffed and ready to go at the appointed hour, adjudicated territorial disputes between angry residents of varying specialties, and prioritized the progression of the myriad of add-on and emergency cases to insure the best use of her strained resources to provide expeditious care for the most seriously ill patients. Miss R. did this for most of us with the patience of an older sister trying to help a younger sibling cut and eat a Thanksgiving meal, but without the eye rolling and multiple deep sighs that usually accompany that exercise. In short, her job entailed, in large measure, taking a group of young, talented gunslingers and turning them into mature surgeons. For all your help in making us a bit more human, we thank you and wish to acknowledge your contributions to the surgeons of Cook County Hospital.

— *The Editors*

# Section I

# The Hospital and Surgical Education

# Cook County Hospital: A Brief History

*Patrick Guinan, MD*
*Frank Milloy, MD*

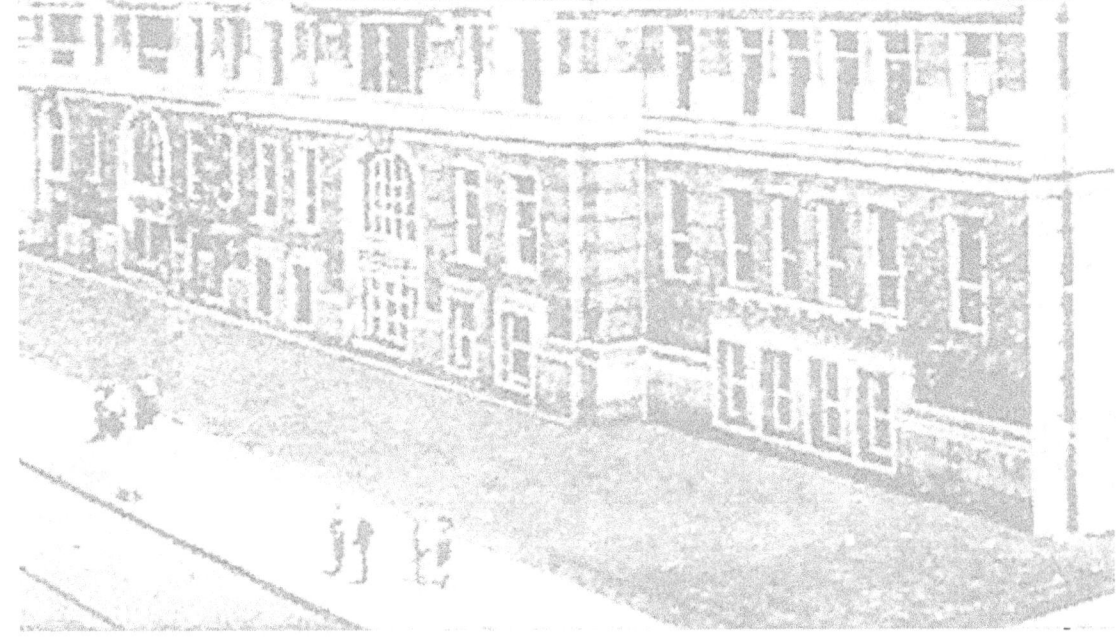

- *Fort Dearborn*
- *Almshouse*
- *Tippecanoe Hall*
- *Mercy Hospital*
- *Jefferson Hospital*
- *18th & LaSalle Street*
- *1825 West Harrison Street (1876)*
- *1825 West Harrison Street (1912)*
- *Louis Pasteur Statue*
- *Contraction*
- *Conclusion*
- *References*

The Cook County Hospital (CCH, Figure 1–1) has had a long and illustrious history. At one time, it was the largest general hospital in the world with a bed capacity of 4,500.[1] It has served the sick and injured of Cook County, Illinois, who were too poor to pay for adequate medical care since the incorporation of the County of Cook in the State of Illinois in 1832. The almost two centuries of inpatient care of the indigent citizens of Cook County make for a complex history, and over the past 180+ years the hospital has had eight different locations. It is currently named the Stroger Hospital of Cook County (Table 1).

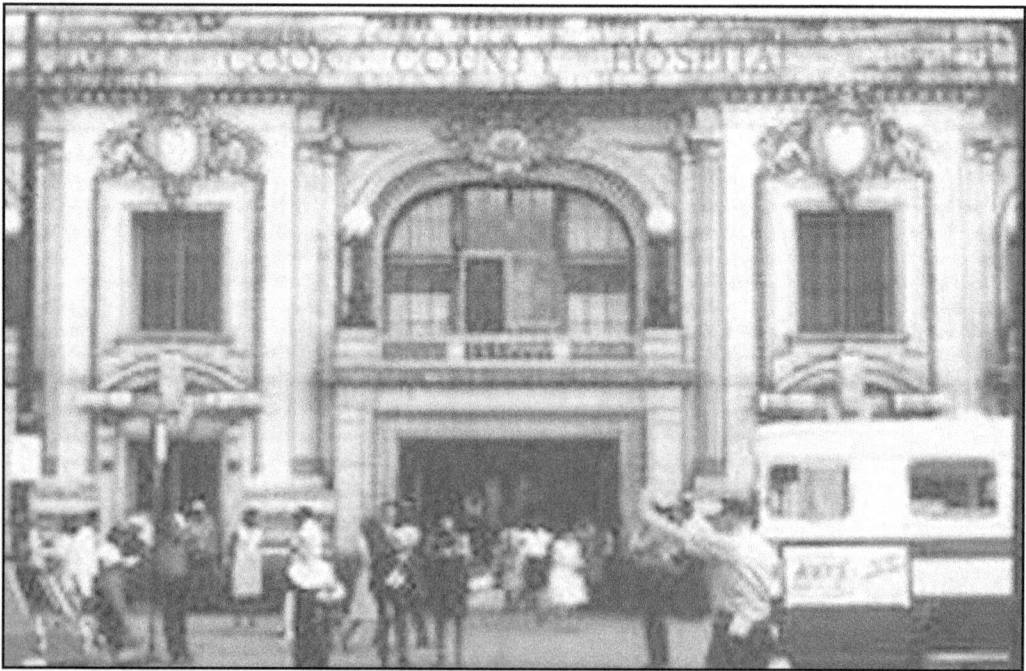

*Figure 1–1  Cook County Hospital*

### TABLE 1—COOK COUNTY HOSPITALS (1803–2002)

|    |                   | Location                             | Dates     | Years |
|----|-------------------|--------------------------------------|-----------|-------|
| 1. | Fort Dearborn     | Michigan Avenue at the Chicago River | 1803–1832 | 19    |
| 2. | Almshouse         | Randolph and Clark                   | 1832–1847 | 15    |
| 3. | Tippecanoe Hall   | Kinzie and State                     | 1847–1851 | 4     |
| 4. | Mercy Hospital    | 2537 S. Prairie                      | 1851–1863 | 12    |
| 5. | Jefferson Hospital| 6500 W. Irving Park Road             | 1863–1866 | 3     |
| 6. | LaSalle Hospital  | 18th & Arnold                        | 1866–1876 | 10    |
| 7. | Cook County Hosp. | 1825 W. Harrison                     | 1876-1912 | 36    |
| 8. | Cook County Hosp. | 1828 W. Harrison (new building)      | 1912-2002 | 90    |
| 9. | Stroger Hospital  | 1828 W. Harrison                     | 2002      |       |

## Fort Dearborn

Fort Dearborn was founded as a trading post at the confluence of the Chicago River and Lake Michigan in the 1770s by Jean Baptiste Point du Sable.[2] It was garrisoned in 1803 by the U.S. Army to provide medical care for the settlement. The first surgeon in Fort Dearborn was William C. Smith and the first recorded surgical procedure was a bilateral leg amputation performed by Dr. Elijah Dewey Harmon in 1832.

## Almshouse

A poorhouse, owned by Cook County, was constructed on the "public square" in 1832 and was the county hospital successor to Fort Dearborn (Figure 1–2). It was

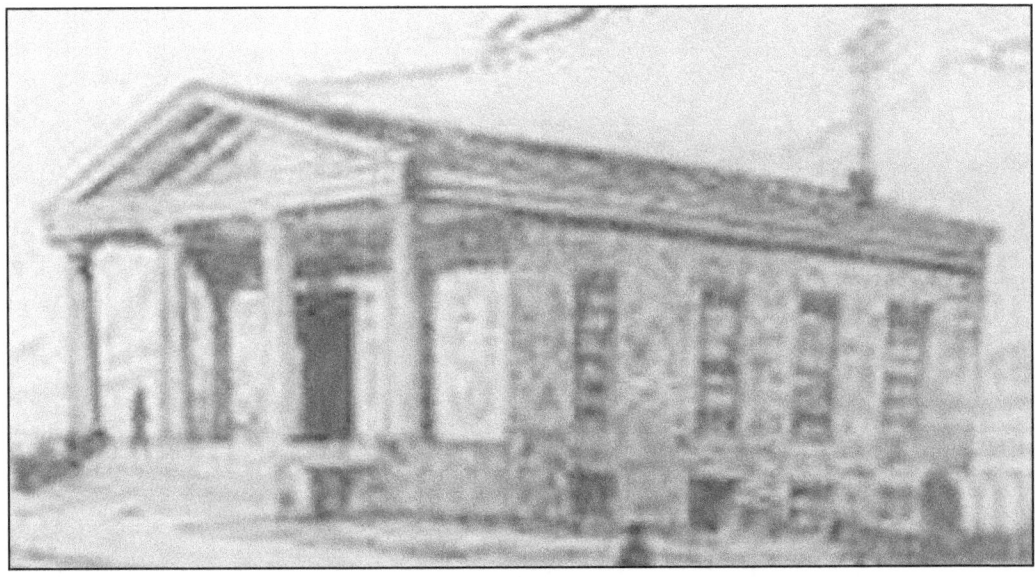

*Figure 1–2 Almshouse*

designed for isolation of patients suffering from cholera. The noteworthy surgical procedure performed at the Almshouse in 1838 was, again, a leg amputation[3] (or possibly a hip disarticulation). As scarlet fever threatened the city, the poorhouse was unable to meet the needs of its patients. In 1847, the county rented Tippencanoe Hall at Kinzie and State Streets.

## Tippecanoe Hall

In an effort to separate the sick from non-ill poor, Cook County officials "rented a building on the north side of the river and put it in order."[4] Tippecanoe Hall, a large warehouse, became the first general hospital in the Chicago area (Figure 1–3). Drs. Daniel Brainard, James Blaney, and James Herrick of Rush Medical College served as the first medical staff of the institution. Since county authorities furnished most of the supplies, the building was known as First Cook County Hospital. For whatever reason, this was a short-lived hospital solution, lasting only four years. In 1850, Tippecanoe Hall closed and another effort was made to solve a growing need when Brainard rented room for 12 beds in the Lake House Hotel on the north bank of the river near the present location of the *Chicago Tribune* building. It also happened that Brainard had befriended a group of Sisters of Mercy nuns, which eventually led to the founding of Mercy Hospital.

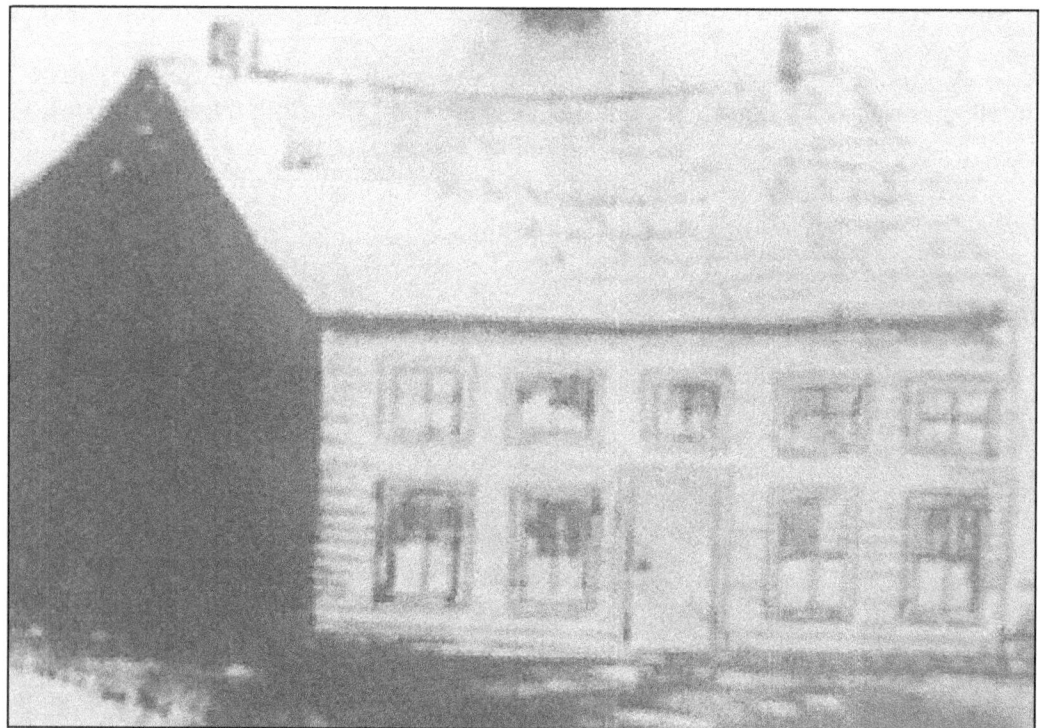

*Figure 1–3 Tippeeanoe Hall*

## Mercy Hospital

In 1850, persuaded by Dr. Brainard, four nuns of the Sisters of Mercy rendered care to patients in the Lake House. By 1853, the nuns built their own hospital at Wabash and Van Buren Streets, which became Chicago's first private hospital with Rush faculty as its staff. For the next 12 years, Cook County cared for its patients at Mercy Hospital. The county paid $3.00 per patient.[5]

## Jefferson Hospital

During the upheaval of the Civil War, the County of Cook had facilities in the township of Jefferson (6500 W. Irving Park Road) and in August 1863 moved its patients from Mercy Hospital to a building on that property.

## 18th & LaSalle Streets

The City of Chicago built a cholera hospital, a frame house, at this site in 1854.[6] The building was demolished and replaced by a substantial brick building in 1857 (Figure 1–4), but its opening was delayed by a conflict between homeopaths and allopaths. Later, citing inadequate care provided by the poor farm, it was recommended that the County procure the city hospital and use it as a

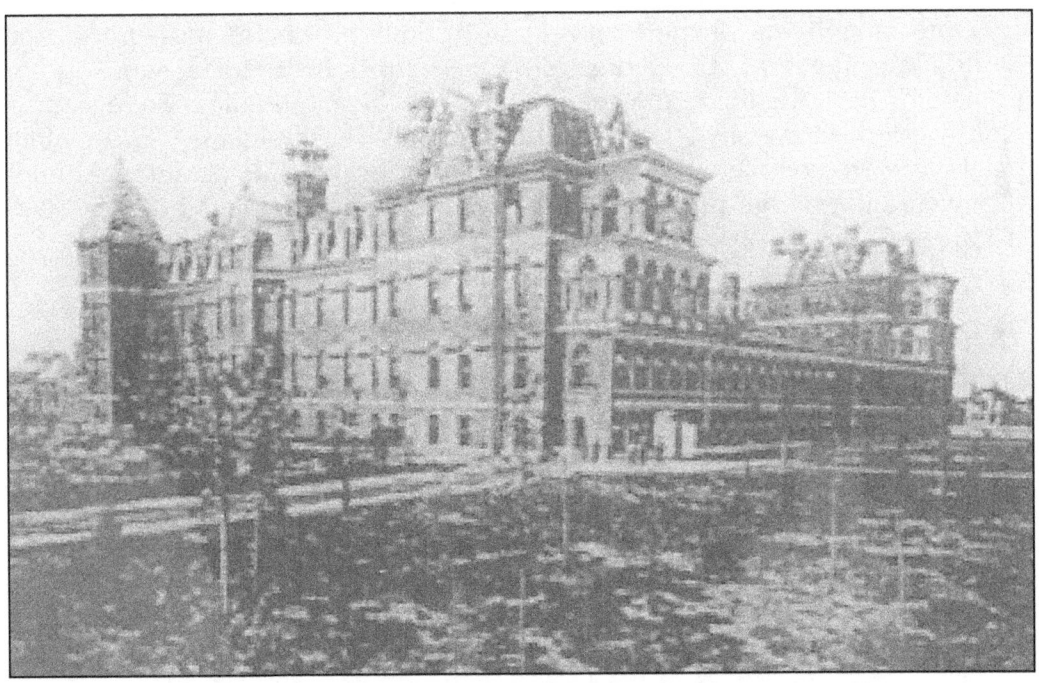

*Figure 1–4 1866: Cook County Hospital at 18th and LaSalle Streets*

facility for indigents. It was subsequently occupied by the U.S. Government during the Civil War[7] and was known as Desmarres Eye and Ear Hospital. In 1862, the U.S. Army discharged its last patient from the hospital and returned it to the county. Even before the hospital had been vacated by the government, Drs. George Amerman and Joseph Ross were engaged in a movement to re-establish it as a charitable institution. Subsequently, Dr. Amerman had himself elected to the Board of Commissioners and was instrumental in the push for the establishment of a county hospital. Dr. Amerman is considered the Father of Cook County Hospital. In 1866, LaSalle Hospital opened in January when patients arrived from the poorhouse and from Mercy Hospital.

The LaSalle Street County Hospital marked a transition from ad hoc medical care to more organized and specialized academic care. The hospital had 130 beds and increased to 220 in 1870. Dr. Nils Quales, a Rush medical student, was appointed the first intern in 1866.

The hospital staff reflected the increasing reputation of its members. These included Dr. H. Wesley Jones, Dr. Henry M. Lyman, Dr. Charles G. Smitt, and Dr. Joseph P. Ross. Dr. Nicholas Senn, an intern, was representative of the quality of the house staff.

## 1825 West Harrison Street (1876)

Because of Chicago's population growth, a larger hospital was required, and for $119,000 the county purchased the block bounded by Harrison, Wood, Polk, and Wolcott Streets. On it was an imposing red brick Victorian structure reminiscent of the Smithsonian Institution "castle" museum on the Mall in Washington, D.C. (Figure 1–5). One-third of the medical staff was appointed by Rush Medical College, one-third by Chicago Medical College (now Northwestern University), and one-third by outside physicians.[8] Two patient pavilions were completed and opened on October 6, 1876. Additional buildings were built on the property until the bed capacity reached 2,000 in 1909 (Figure 1–5).

## 1825 West Harrison Street (1912)

In 1912, the Cook County Board felt that the 1876 buildings were inadequate and began construction (1912–1916) of a large, block-long building facing north on the south side of Harrison Street between Wood and Wolcott Streets (Figure 1–6). The building—designed by Paul Gerhardt and Richard Schmidt, the County Architect—is instantly recognizable by its stunning Beaux Arts façade and its three-story Ionic columns (Figure 1–7).

For years, County Hospital had academic affiliations with Rush Medical College, Northwestern University, Loyola University, Chicago Medical School, and University of Chicago. It has been called an institute of learning—not only for students, interns, and residents—but also for attending staff.

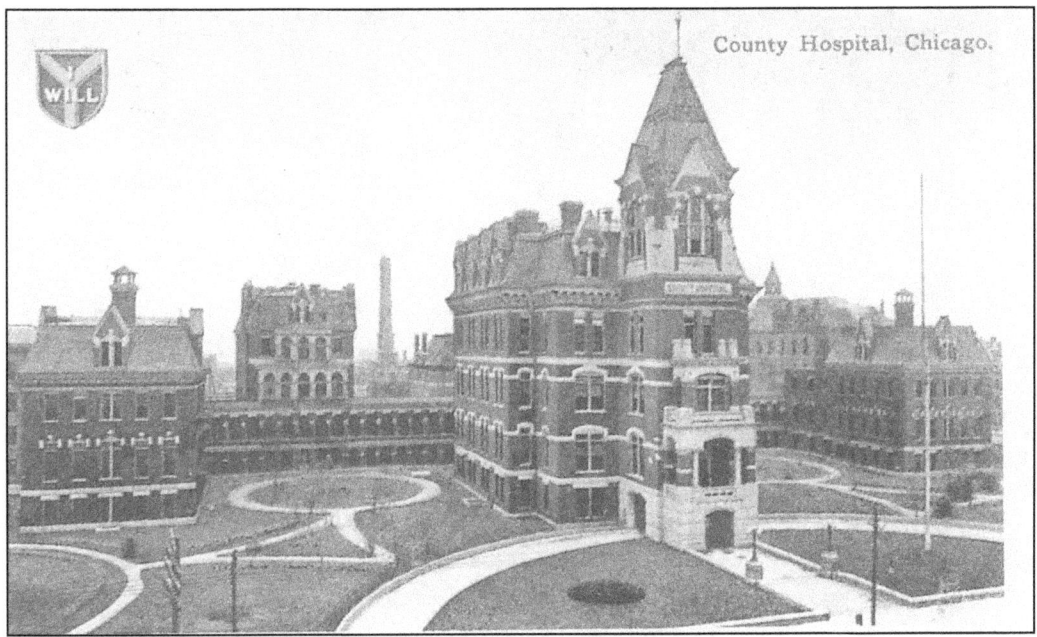

*Figure 1–5  1876: Cook County Hospital at 1825 West Harrison Street*

Karl Meyer joined CCH in 1914 as Medical Superintendant and Attending Surgeon. During his 53-year tenure, many buildings were added to the campus. These include the psychopathic hospital (1914), Building E for Cook County Department of Education (1921), Building A, the Men's Medical Building (1928), the Children's Hospital (1928), the Nurses' Residence (1935), the Laundry (1938), the

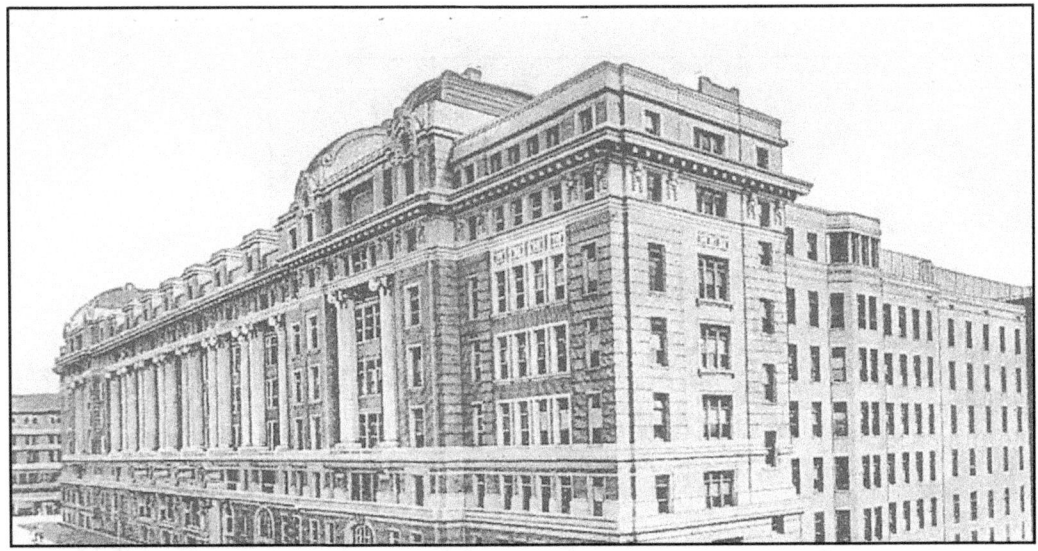

*Figure 1–6  1912 Cook County Hospital at 1825 West Harrison Street*

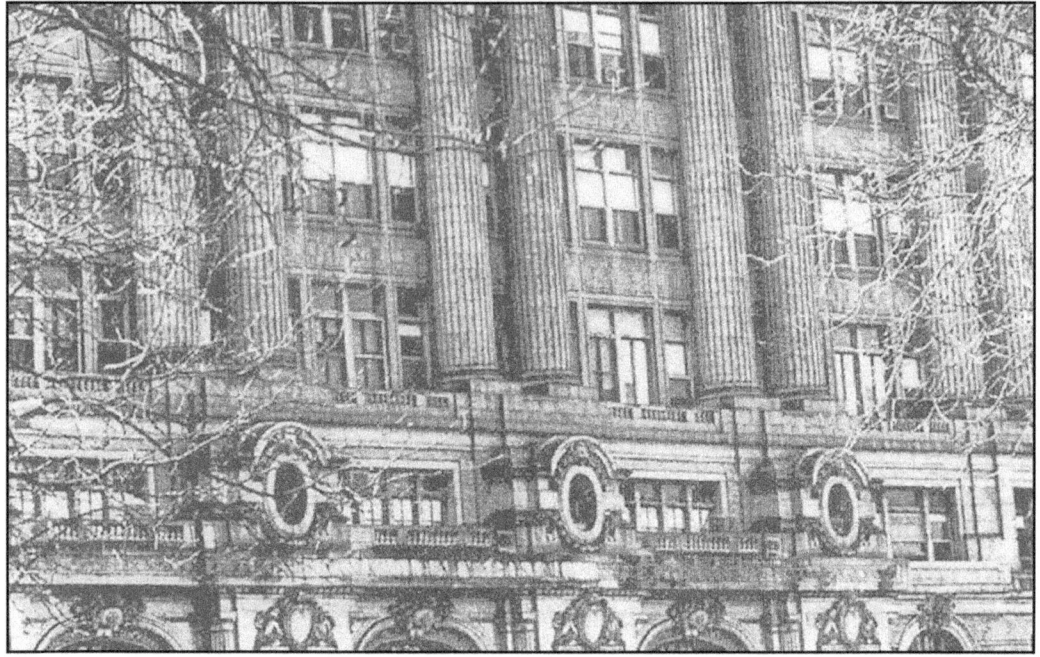

*Figure 1-7  Beaux Arts Facade and its three-story Ionic columns*

Fantus Clinic (1939), Garage and Paint Shop (1950), Radiation Center (1953), Karl Meyer Hall (1953), Warehouse (1958), and the Hektoen Building (1964). A diagram of the buildings in the Cook County Hospital campus is shown in Figure 1-8, and an aerial view of the campus can be seen in Figure 1-9.

The hospital also attracted media attention. *ER*, the Emmy award-winning

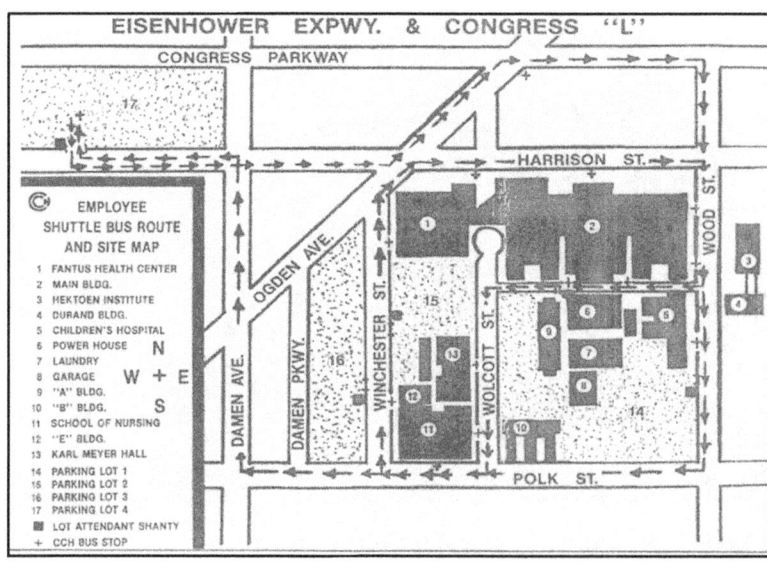

*Figure 1-8 Shuttle Bus Route Map showing the various buildings at the campus of CCH*

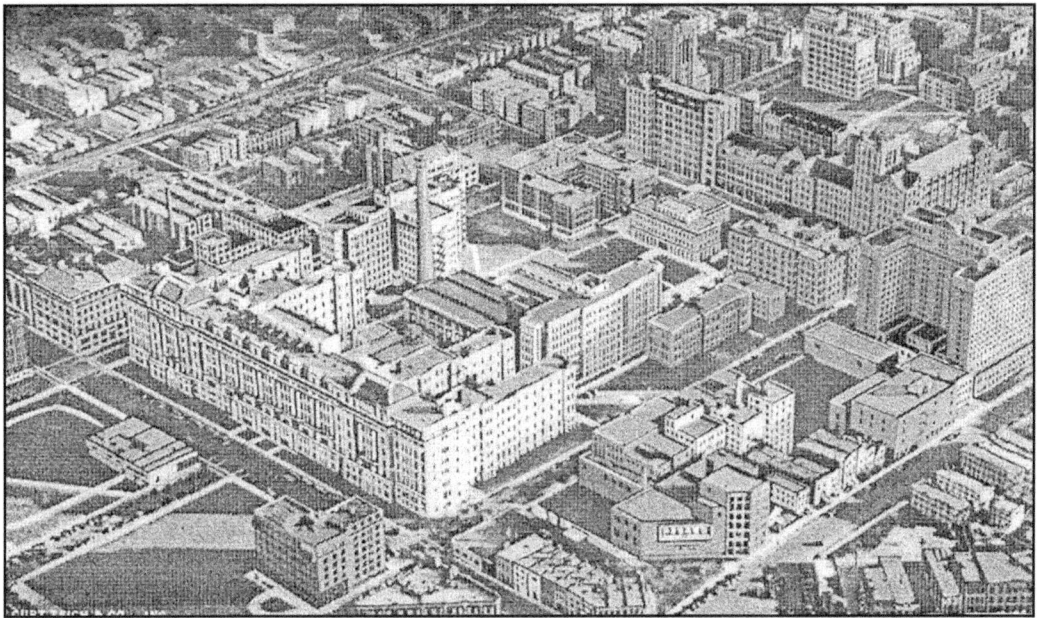

Figure 1–9  Aerial view of the Cook County Hospital campus

American medical drama television series, took notes from the ER at Cook County Hospital. The *ER* series was set primarily in the emergency room of a fictional General Hospital in Chicago, Illinois. In the movie *The Fugitive,* Harrison Ford was shown in front of the hospital (Figure 1–10). In 1996, Diana, Princess of Wales, visited Cook County Hospital.

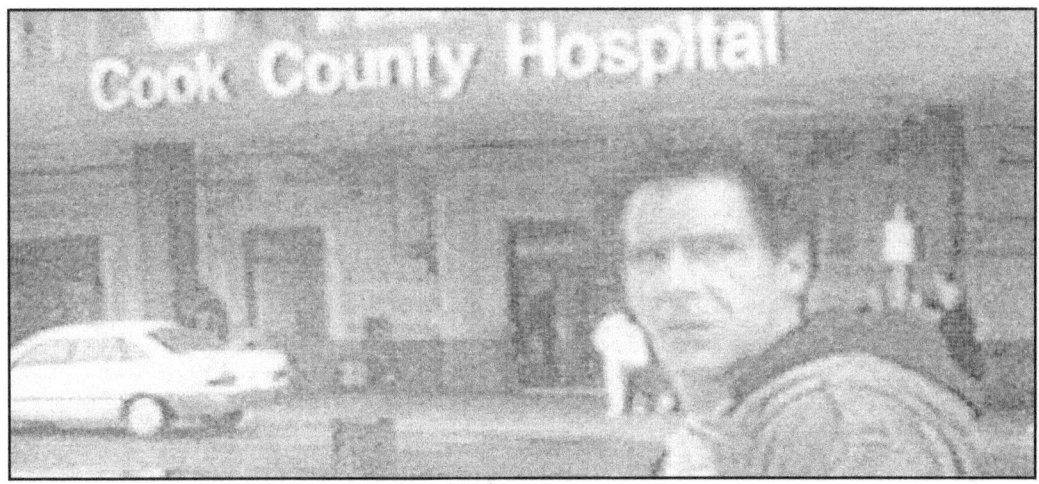

Figure 1–10  In the movie **The Fugitive**, *Harrison Ford is pictured at the front entrance of CCH.*

## Louis Pasteur Statue

Across the street in front of the hospital, there is a small park. The park serves as a serene "front yard" for the sometimes frantic hospital environment. In the center of the park is a statue. A bust of Louis Pasteur, "servant of humanity," sits atop a tall art deco shaft, which rests on a low rectangular base (Figure 1–11). Near the base, a bronze plaque holds an inscription :

*One doesn't ask of one who suffers: What is your country and what is your religion? One merely says, You suffer. That is enough for me. You belong to me and I shall help you.* —Louis Pasteur

The inscription captures the historic spirit of Cook County Hospital.

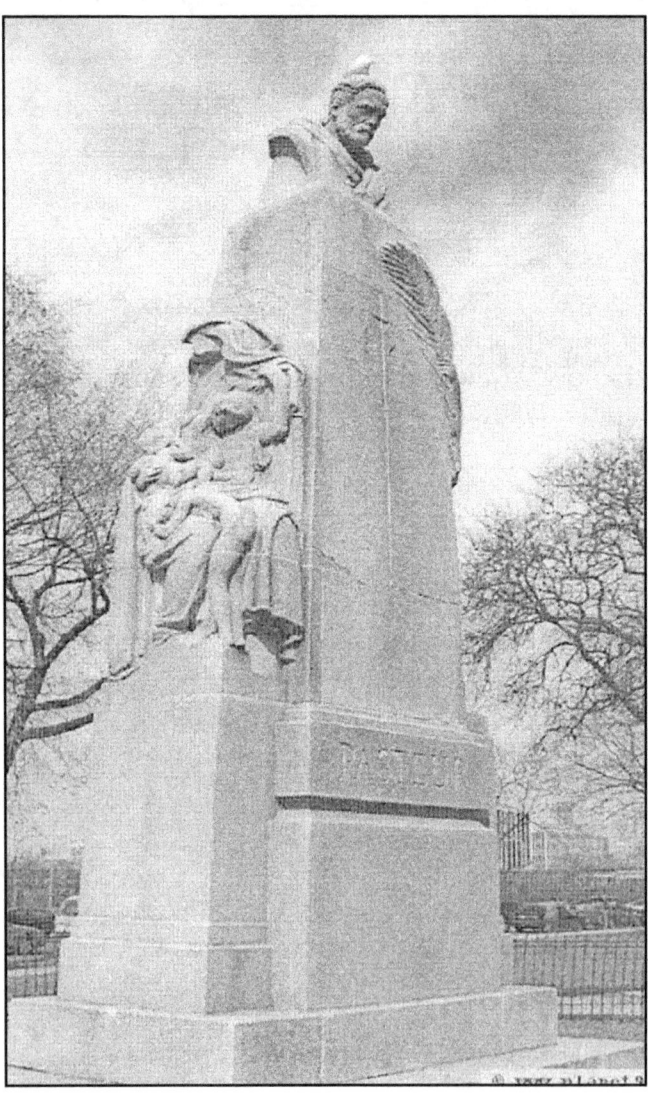

*Figure 1–11 Statue of Louis Pasteur*

In 1928, 33 years after he died, the people of Chicago erected a monument sculpted by Leon Hermant to Louis Pasteur, the "servant of humanity." In 1946, this work of art was moved from Grant Park to a green space across from the old hospital as an inspiration to the medical staff, nurses, and physicians who would train there. These days, Pasteur stands alone facing the hallowed, abandoned, still magnificent legend.

## Contraction

The Cook County Hospital reached its physical high point in 1953 with the construction of the interns' and residents' Karl Meyer Hall and the Hektoen Laboratory Building in 1964. Changes were occurring in medicine including the Medicare and Medicaid Acts in 1965; the Hill Burton Bill, which promoted VA construction; and finally, DRGs in 1982. This legislation resulted in a lessened need for county-supported indigent care facilities as reflected in the decrease of bed capacity that occurred at the Cook County Hospital: from a high of 3,800 beds in 1965 to 600 in 2008.

The changes also are reflected in the gradual decrease in the number of buildings that make up the Cook County Hospital campus: from 21 to the current six. The demolition of buildings included Infectious Diseases, 1970; Psychopathic Hospital, 1972; Morgue, 1974; Female Medicine (B Building), 1980; Male Medicine (A Building), 1984; Karl Meyer Hall, 1998; Pediatrics, 2007; and Main, 2008.

## Conclusion

Certainly an era has ended. The days when county governments were responsible for the care of the indigent sick have passed. Now, with mandated insurance such as Medicare and Medicaid, individuals have more choices for their care and prefer not to go to "County." This is all for the good. Medical education has changed, and medical schools control curricula and do not depend so heavily on county "teaching" materials.

This is not to deny that an incredible amount of compassionate care was given at the CCH. That institution alone contributed enormously to the advancement of medical education and research. This is nowhere more evident than in the field of surgery. It can be argued that the surgical advances developed between 1890 and 1920, and up to the present, would never have occurred without indigent care hospitals, the prototype of which is the Cook County Hospital.

# References

1. Johnson CB. *Growth of Cook County. Vol 1*. Chicago: Board of Commissioners of Cook County; 1960.
2. Cronon W. *Nature's Metropolis: Chicago and the Great West*. New York: WW Norton and Co: New York; 1991.
3. *Medical Chicago: An Historical Sketch of the First Practitioners of Medicine*. Chicago: Fergus Printing Co; 1879.
4. *Westerly Chicago Democrat*. April 16, 1847.
5. Quine W. Early History of Cook County Hospital to 1870. *Bull Soc Med Hist*. 1911;1:15-24.
6. McNealy R. The influence of Cook County Hospital on Medical Education in the United States. *Q Bull NU Med Sch*. 1957; 31:169-173.
7. Meyer K. Historical Background of Cook County Hospital. *Q Bull NU Med Sch*. 1949; 21:271-276.
8. Lyman H. A Bit of the History of the Cook County Hospital. *Bull Soc Med Hist*. 19111:25-36.

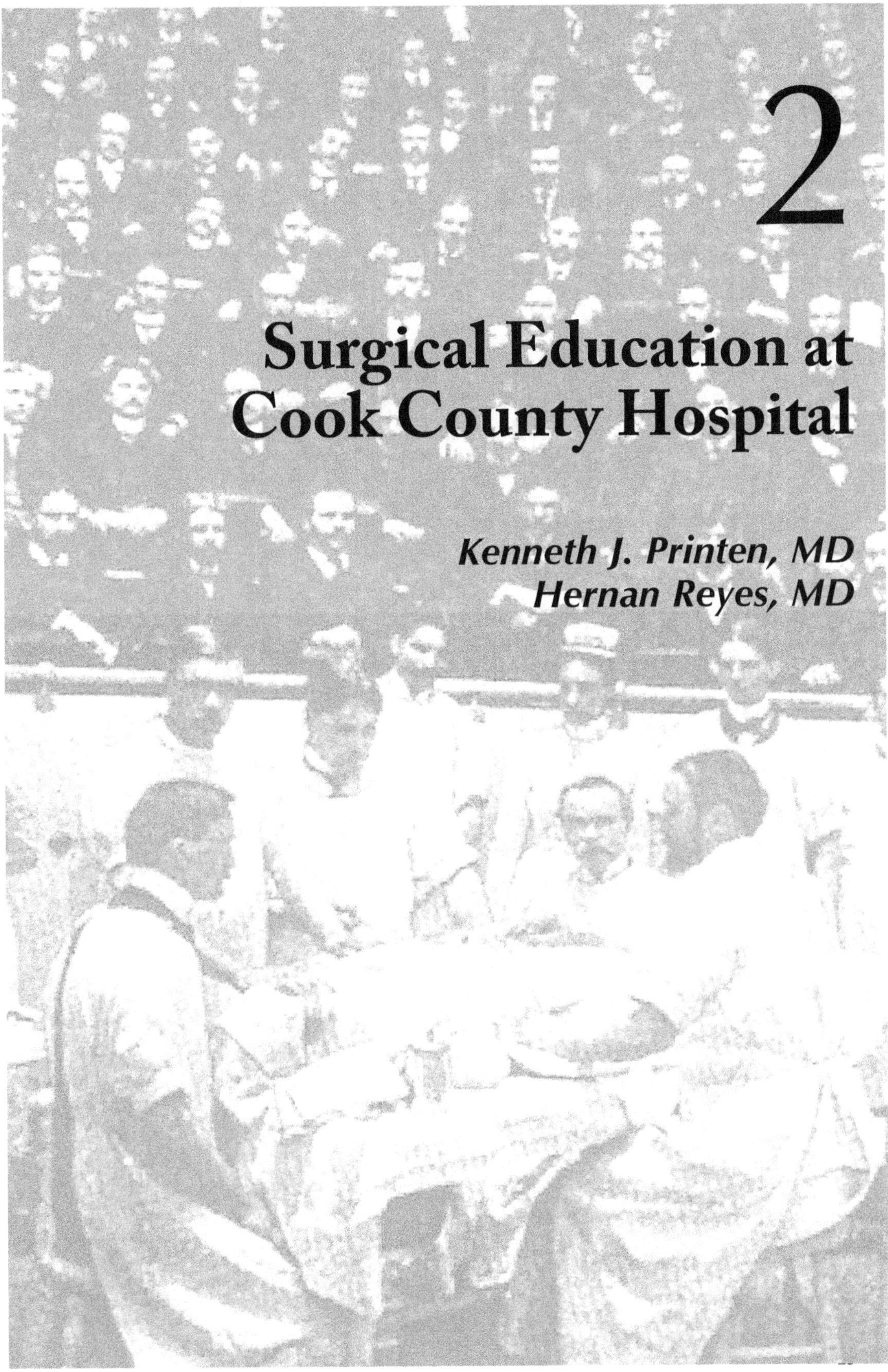

# Surgical Education at Cook County Hospital

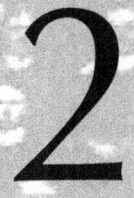

Kenneth J. Printen, MD
Hernan Reyes, MD

- *Introduction*
- *Clinical Practice and Patient Care Activities*
  - *The Beginning*
  - *The Late 1960s and 1970s*
- *The Era of All Voluntary Staff*
  - Attending Surgeons
  - Internship
  - Residency
  - Surgical Amphitheatre Teaching
  - The Night Surgeon
  - The Cook County Graduate School of Medicine
- *The Era of Full-time Salaried Attending Staff*
  - The Freeark Era – 1958-1968
    - Interim Chairs: Robert J. Baker – 1969; Frank Folk – 1970-1972
  - The Moss Era – 1972-1977
    - Interim Chair: Dr. Robert Moody – 1977
  - The Jonasson Era – 1978-1986
    - Interim Chair: Hernand Abcarian – 1986
  - The Reyes Era – 1986-1998
    - Organization
    - Attending Staff
    - Clinical Activity
    - Education
- *The New Cook County Hospital—John H. Stroger, Jr. Hospital – 2000*

## Introduction

With the appointment in January 1866 of the first warden (nonmedical supervisor) of the hospital, Mr. B. F. Chase, and the first matron (Chief of Nursing Service), Mrs. Chase, Dr. George Amerman and Dr. Joseph P. Ross were credited with reactivating Old County Hospital, which had been seized by the government during the Civil War. After the war, in 1865, Drs. Amerman and Ross maneuvered to re-establish the erstwhile City Hospital as a charitable institution. By clever electioneering, they managed to get themselves elected to the Cook County Board of Supervisors and were soon able to have the board take over the hospital. In 1866, the hospital opened as the "Old County Hospital."[1]

While the avowed purpose of the Old County Hospital was really the care of a combination of private and county patients, the matter of education of interns and residents was never far from the minds of those in charge of the hospital. From the very beginning, the wards of the hospital were open to all physicians for teaching purposes. In the *Chicago Medical Journal*, Volume 23, 1866, the following statement appears:

*The ward of the hospital will be open to medical students and regular practitioners of medicine on Tuesday and Friday at half past one.*[2]

There were both medical and surgical clinics and autopsies were performed. The medical journal went on to say:

*We trust a new era has dawned in the medical culture of the northwest. An opportunity for clinical instruction for bedside observation and study to the numerous students of this city has been a desideration greatly needed and now that we have a hospital so perfect and complete, affording an abundance of material and every facility for thorough clinical courses, we hope that those young men preparing to enter the profession will avail themselves of its advantage.*[2]

Patterns in medical care and education in public hospitals has evolved considerably during the last half of the 20th century. At Cook County Hospital there was a house-staff-based system of medical care delivery and education. Supervision was from voluntary attending physicians and unpredictable as a result. This was replaced by a system of full-time attending physician supervision of house-staff-directed care and education. A system of established goals and expectations was gradually implemented. The changes that took place, and which continue to evolve, are the product of a more aggressive and deliberate scrutiny of treatment outcomes and educational programs by regulatory bodies, the public who support these institutions, and the patients who utilize them. Accountability in patient care and the education of future medical practitioners in the various specialties as measured by predictable and quantifiable results have propelled hospital and clinical department administrations to be more focused on their approach and implementation of their mission and goals in order to fulfill expected results.

From the time CCH opened its doors to learning, it played a significant role in the education of Chicago surgeons, especially in the early days.[3] To keep pace with the requirement of a structured surgical education program, staffing of the hospital had to change from an all voluntary staff to a full-time salaried staff to provide broader educational activities, including surgical subspecialty care, and in recent years, minimally invasive surgical procedures. Surgical training is no longer a haphazard apprenticeship, and it must follow the guidelines set by governing bodies. The 80-hour work limit for house staff is an example that the good old days' work habits are no longer with us.

In order to have a better perspective of the changes that have taken place from the time the hospital was established in 1866 up until the mid-1960s, a brief review of the surgical practice and surgical education that took place is immensely valuable in giving us a better understanding of the activities during that period. The era of all voluntary staffs, amphitheatre teaching, the night surgeon, and the Cook County Graduate School of Medicine occupied a unique place in the history of surgical education at Cook County Hospital, and each will be discussed separately.

## Clinical Practice and Patient Care Activities

### The Beginning

Prior to 1965, the surgery wards at Cook County Hospital frequently carried a census of 70 beds. It was 50 beds in the beginning, but this was quickly increased to 70 to accommodate the increase of patients. More often than not, these beds were fully occupied (Figure 2–1), and additional beds were made available for emergency admissions placed in any empty space in the ward. It was not at all unusual to find a row of beds in the center aisle of a ward, or one or more patients in the examining room with a nasogastric tube, or receiving IV fluids or blood transfusion while waiting for a vacant bed. Interns and residents were often reminded to discharge patients early in the morning to accommodate for the previous night's admissions. Wards were segregated by gender, and the only privacy each patient had while undergoing an examination or a procedure was a portable screen. There were a few private rooms with two to four patients receiving more intensive treatment, often with a nasogastric tube, Foley catheter, CVP line, or IV fluid/blood transfusion, and requiring more nursing supervision. These rooms were designed to be closest to the nurses' desk. Typically, the ward was assigned a head nurse, one medication nurse, and several student nurses (primarily during the morning and afternoon shifts). They were assisted by several nurse's aides, one or two practical nurses, and a ward clerk. It was not unusual that a single nurse with a contingent of nurse's aides and practical nurses would be left to staff the entire ward at night. This staffing became especially problematic when several emergency patient admissions occurred, and one or more of

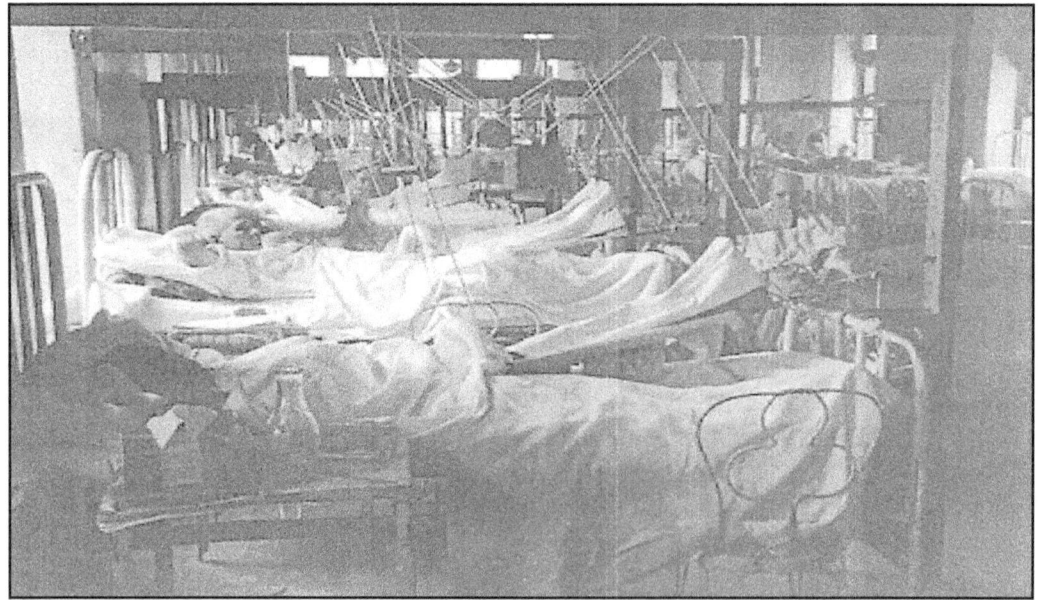

*Figure 2–1  A typical crowded ward at Cook County Hospital*

the patients was taken to the operating room for surgical intervention. Delay in timely administration of medications, re-starting IV fluids, irrigating nasogastric tubes, or changing Foley catheters was often the norm. Despite the dedication of the nursing staff, the sheer volume of patients was simply overwhelming.

The regular ward was divided into three services, color coded for easier identification. Except for routine elective surgical admissions from the outpatient clinics, each surgical ward alternated for the day's admissions from the emergency room. At the time, there were four male wards (including Ward 56, Karl Meyer's service in the Children's Hospital) and two female wards for general surgery. Surgical subspecialties either had their own assigned ward or shared a ward with other specialties. Due to a large volume of patients, orthopedic surgery was assigned two male and one female ward with an overflow fourth ward when needed.

The general surgery wards were staffed with a senior resident, a junior resident, and three rotating interns. There were five medical schools providing attending surgeons and associates for staffing of the ward. Wards 60 and 56 were Northwestern's service, 61 was Loyola's, and University of Illinois and Rush had Wards 62 and 63 respectively. Chicago Medical School also shared Ward 62. Each service was assigned a volunteer senior attending surgeon and his associate, either of whom would come to the hospital to make patient rounds and cover elective surgery once a week. Attending patient rounds were rare, and attending coverage for elective surgery was primarily provided by the associate attending surgeon, some of whom were knowledgeable and conscientious.

In effect, the main responsibility for patient rounds was that of the senior resident (typically on his or her last year of residency). The first round of the day, conducted early in the morning, was basically made in front of the board in the nurses' office where the names of the patients were posted. Decisions were made regarding treatments and diagnostic studies including consultations needed. Only patients with serious problems—those admitted during the night with emergency conditions whether operated on or not, and those scheduled for elective surgery—were seen and evaluated, after which the senior resident and one intern proceeded to the operating room to perform scheduled elective surgery or operate on an emergency patient that was not completed by the on-call surgical team. The junior resident and two interns were left in the ward to perform the assigned tasks for the day, including patient rounds. One or two of the house staff was always available to join the team in the operating room when needed. For the most part, either one intern or the junior resident routinely joined the surgical team in the operating room, especially when the case was to be performed by the junior resident. When all the scheduled operations were completed, the whole team made a full ward patient round. All patients were seen, evaluated, and discussed. This was conducted in almost all cases by the senior resident, who by this time was on his or her last year of training. In theory, any management or diagnostic problems the senior resident may have had were to be discussed with his or her senior attending surgeon or associate. For practical purposes, this discourse took place only on a few occasions. Most of these discussions occurred when the associate attending surgeon, or rarely, the senior attending surgeon came to the hospital to assist in an operation, especially in a major elective surgical procedure.

For the most part, the attending surgeon, when present, served as the teaching assistant, although on a few occasions he would "steal" the case from the resident, which would make the latter extremely unhappy. Emergency cases at night or on weekends and holidays were performed by a team headed by the night surgeon. The night surgeon position was a unique educational experience at County, one that merits a separate discussion later.

Anesthesia for elective and emergency operations was provided by a group of nurse anesthetists. Very few full-time physician anesthesiologists were at the hospital because of the low salary paid by the county. Elective operations requiring regional anesthesia were routinely staffed by the surgical resident assigned on rotation to anesthesia. This type of anesthesia coverage ensured that the scheduled operations were rarely delayed and allowed the surgeon to operate on all cases scheduled that day. The main operating rooms were located on the eighth floor of the main building. There were 14 operating suites (seven large main suites and seven smaller rooms) in addition to a cystoscopy suite. The Amphitheatre was located at the end of the eighth-floor corridor.

The operating suites were designed to have a main suite joined to a smaller operating room serviced by one scrub sink. Access to the adjacent smaller operating room was through the main operating suite, so traffic was a constant problem when both operating rooms were in use. Two wide windows installed in the main operating suites were kept open for the most part to allow cross ventilation, but they also allowed flies to enter the rooms (Figure 2–2). It was only later that window screens were installed. On numerous occasions, the circulating nurse

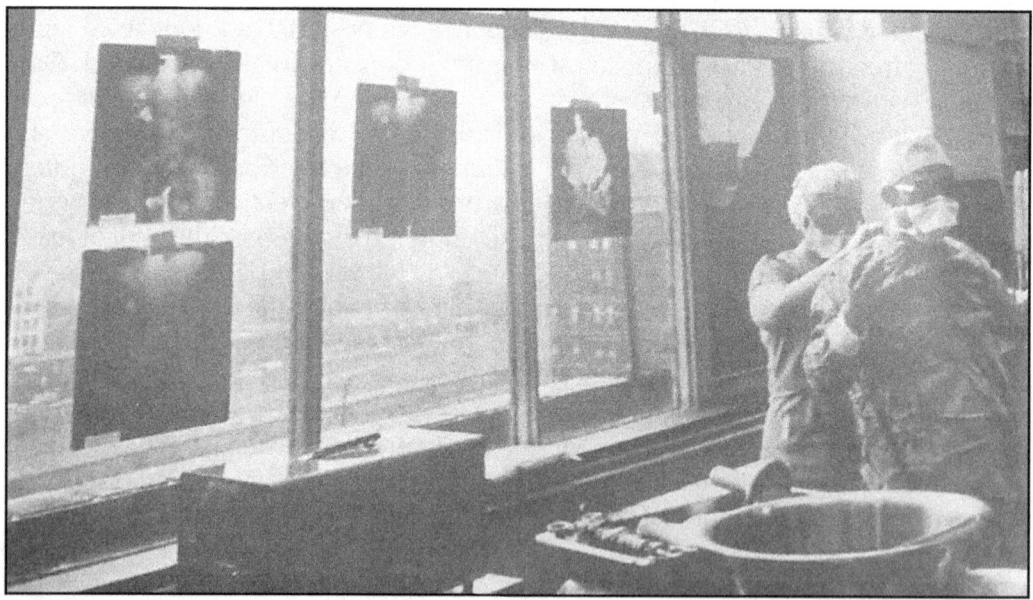

*Figure 2–2  Operating room with a large window. The window was often used as an X-ray box.*

served as the official fly swatter, especially at night. A poignant remembrance of these windows described by an intern during the 1950s makes one recall similar experiences in the past:

*We had a wonderful time at County. We, who were there, especially during the winter, can never forget the sounds; those wondrous, weird, melodious sounds made by the windows in surgery. It was like the haunting melody of an Aeolian harp unlike the sound of any other building, anywhere.*[1]

On opposite ends of the operating room floor were the female locker, toilet, and coffee break area and the corresponding male locker, toilet, and bath. There were six elevators installed in the main building, five of which accessed the operating suites, one on each end of the building and three others for bringing patients up to the OR. The elevators opened directly to the main operating room corridor, which in turn opened directly to the different operating suites. The eighth floor of the children's hospital, which housed the children's operating rooms, was connected to the main operating room corridor in the eighth floor of the main building by a covered bridge, allowing patients to be wheeled in either direction. When OR staffing was limited at night or weekends, older pediatric patients requiring an operation were taken to the main operating room for surgery. All operations performed on neonates and infants were performed in the children's operating room.

The narrow corridor of the main operating room, which opened directly to the elevators, was made part of the operating complex that could be accessed only with proper OR attire. Every so often, house staff bringing patients to the OR in an emergency would simply wheel the patient to the OR corridor to be received by appropriate personnel. Elective cases were taken to the operating room utilizing the east-end elevators and sent directly to a preoperative receiving area.

The operating room at the time was managed with an iron hand by the OR supervisor, and, for the most part, she tried her best to get elective cases done so that very few cases were still going on after the morning shift and very few cases were cancelled. The morning staffing appeared to be adequate, although the afternoon and night shifts were always understaffed. Major cases going beyond 3:00 p.m. were staffed by the morning-shift nurses who volunteered—after much encouragement—to stay until completion of the operation on overtime pay. Staffing for the afternoon shift was only sufficient to open two operating rooms; one team was always on standby for obstetrical (OB) emergencies. The other shift was available for other emergency cases, which were prioritized primarily in consultation between the nursing staff and the night surgeon. Occasionally, when several emergency cases needed to be done simultaneously, volunteer OR nurses were requested to return to staff another operating suite. This resulted in some delays in operating stable trauma patients with stab wounds of the abdomen—at times they were not operated upon until the day following admission—so much so that a template for a clinical study on the nonoperative treatment of selective penetrating injuries of the abdomen was initiated. A protocol was developed and guidelines were then followed. Clinically stable patients with no obvious peritonitis who remained stable for several hours were observed and simply underwent additional X-ray studies to determine hollow viscus injury. Eventually, peritoneal lavage and analysis of the lavage fluid were used to determine the need for operative intervention in those patients who were clinically stable and had no clinical evidence of hollow viscus injury.

Outpatient clinics were established for postoperative visits and for evaluation of new patients referred from other clinics or from the emergency room of the hospital. Despite adequate documentation, the lack of attending supervision and designation of specific clinical responsibility made long-term follow-ups difficult due to the frequent change in resident assignments. This was further compounded with the patient's failure to follow instructions and lack of compliance for regular follow-up visits. Even when a breast clinic was organized and directed by Dr. Louis Rivers, a volunteer senior attending surgeon, some patients who had breast biopsy were lost to follow-up, only to return weeks or months later to realize that additional surgery and treatment was necessary for a lesion that was malignant.

Patients with surgical problems usually presented themselves to the hospital or to the clinics with long-standing problems that had been ignored due to lack of access to medical care. Malignancies were frequently far advanced and no longer amenable to surgical extirpation. Patients suffering from peptic ulcer disease were admitted through the emergency room because of perforation, bleeding, or obstruction at which point operative intervention was the only recourse of treatment. It seemed that, aside from inguinal hernia, gallbladder disease, and trauma, the most common operation performed during this period was a subtotal gastric resection (80%) with a Bilroth II reconstruction. Later, total vagotomy was likewise added to the procedure, except that instead of an 80% resection, antrectomy was done.

The care of pediatric patients, especially neonates, was likewise deficient due to the absence of surgeons who limited and dedicated their practice to pediatric surgery. At the time, general surgeons were confident that they were capable of performing all surgical procedures in the pediatric age group.

**The Late 1960s and 1970s**

Major renovations took place during the late 1960s and 1970s to comply with regulatory bodies such as the JCAHO, IDPA, and Residency Review Committees of the Accreditation Council on Graduate Medical Education (ACGME). Air conditioning was installed—initially, individual window air conditioners, later replaced by central air conditioning in 1967. The seven main operating suites were separated from the adjacent smaller suites by a scrub sink, and separate access was provided to each of the operating rooms. The problem of the elevators directly opening into the OR corridor, which was considered a part of the sterile operating environment, was never resolved and continued to be a source of constant citation by inspectors of various accrediting bodies, especially those from the State Health Department.

Toward the mid-1970s, the number of general surgery male and female wards drastically dropped to half the number previously occupied, with an average daily ward census of 25–30 patients, less than half of what it had been. This change in inpatient census can be attributed to a number of factors:
1. reduction in the length of postoperative stay for routine surgical procedures;
2. outpatient preoperative workup of nonemergent surgical cases prior to admission for definitive elective surgery;
3. advent of same-day surgery where patients undergoing elective surgery for common problems such as cholecystectomy, herniorrhaphy, and the like, were discharged within 24 to 48 hours of surgery with appropriate postoperative follow-up; and
4. a shift in the admission pattern of patients with specific surgical problems such as cancer or colorectal disease to the newly organized subspecialties of surgical oncology and colon-rectal surgery, respectively, rather than to general surgery as practiced in the past.

Additionally, the rapid acceptance and use of the gradually evolving technology of minimally invasive surgery further influenced a shorter postoperative hospital stay for patients. This change in surgical practice actually increased the volume of operations performed in the department. Consequently, patients who were now admitted to the various services, including the surgical intensive care unit, had a higher acuity of illness requiring a more intensive service by physicians and nurses. Furthermore, the introduction of newer diagnostic tools required the services of proficient and better trained health care providers.

## The Era of All Voluntary Staffs

### Attending Surgeons

In 1877–1878, an agreement was made among the Chicago Medical College (now Northwestern University Medical School), Rush Medical College, and members of the medical profession not engaged in teaching on the one side and the Board of County Commissioners on the other. The attending staff was organized by the nomination of one-third of the staff by each of the two colleges and one-third by the outside profession, then elected by the Board of County Commissioners. The plan proved satisfactory, and some of the best physicians were appointed, including Edmund Andrews, Moses Gunn, Charles T. Parkes, Christian Fenger, D.A.K. Steele, Ralph Isham, Edward W. Lee, John H. Hollister, William Quine, Lester Curtis, Norman Bridge, Joseph P. Ross, and Isaac N. Danforth, all of whom were representatives of the best in Chicago.[1] The close relationship of two leading colleges set an example for the other local medical schools of stature, such as Loyola and the College of Physicians and Surgeons (now University of Illinois), and Chicago Medical School that followed at a later date. Over the course of the next 30 years, the formula worked reasonably well until political maneuvering of appointments became a concern. In the 1880s, the county commissioners added homeopathic and eclectic physicians to the staff of the hospital. The real impetus for a change in the appointment formula came in the early 1900s with the realization that members of the County Board, who had the ultimate responsibility for appointment of the medical and house staff, were actually selling positions to even the most qualified applicants. Christian Fenger, an internationally known pathologist, was forced to come up with $1,000 to ensure appointment to the voluntary staff at County as a Rush appointee in the late 1870s. This activity became so rampant that under the administration of Edward Brundage, the president of the hospital, instituted civil service examinations for both attending staff and house staff, which had to be retaken every six years.

This is not to say that all physicians were pleased with the system. The story was circulated that Dr. Albert Ochsner, Chief of Surgery at Augustana Hospital and at the College of Physicians and Surgeons (later the University of Illinois College of Medicine), who had recently authored a textbook of surgery, referenced each of his answers to a page in his book and then wrote his resignation from the County staff on the last page of the examination.[4] He did, however, continue to be a formidable figure in Chicago surgery until his death in 1925.

From the time Christian Fenger was at County, first as a pathologist and later as a surgeon, he established himself as a great teacher. Whether or not it was his teaching of pathology, bacteriology, or surgery that established Fenger as the consummate medical educator of his times is immaterial. What is important and impressive is the group of people he trained in all these areas. He nurtured John B. Murphy and Nicholas Senn, two of the leading surgeons in Chicago, and his academic influence extended to pathologists and internists as well.

When one looks at the history of early surgical education in Chicago, it is interesting to note that these giants did not necessarily spend their entire careers at one medical school. As a matter of fact, the opposite is really the norm, especially with respect to the big three schools that continue to serve to the present day. For example, J. B. Murphy is thought of as a Northwestern (Chicago Medical College) surgeon, but he started as Lecturer in Surgery at Rush, followed by Professor of Surgery at the College of Physicians and Surgeons (University of Illinois), and only then went to Northwestern University.

He moved to Rush to co-chair with Arthur Dean Bevan but ended up again at Northwestern as the Chair of the Department of Surgery until his death. Christian Fenger began academically at Northwestern University, gravitated to the College of Physicians and Surgeons, and returned to Northwestern University. He ended his career at Rush Medical College. What remained constant among these professionals was their affiliation with County. The same could be said of other pre-eminent Chicago surgeons: Moses Gunn, Edward Lee, Ralph Isham, and Edmund Andrews, who practiced at Rush or Mercy but kept their teaching appointments at County. Nowadays, we would call this type of faculty arrangement a geographic full-time appointment, which indicates that the surgeon actually makes his living operating at a hospital other than where he teaches. This was indeed the case with the surgeons who taught at the large charity hospitals throughout the United States. The surgeons at County fit this mold, and it would have deep implications for the doctors in training as time went on.

After Senn and Murphy, two other influential surgeons joined County in the early 1900s. In 1914, at the age of 28, Karl Meyer (Figure 2–3) was appointed attending surgeon and superintendent of CCH. Raymond McNealy was appointed attending surgeon in 1917 and in 1931 was named president of the medical staff, a position he held until retirement.[5] Soon, the Meyer-McNealy Surgical Service became one the greatest surgical services in the country. All interns remember McNealy's deft drawings and teachings. McNealy came to the operating table with all the dignity of a king or a general leading his troops into battle. He admonished interns to stand up straight and keep both elbows by the body. Those who knew them say that Meyer was a better surgeon but McNealy was the better teacher. Meyer served as chair and director of the surgical program from 1940 to 1958. He trained numerous surgeons who practiced in many small towns across the country. Surgical training under Meyer followed the Midwestern School of Surgery for the training of clinical surgeons.[6]

Despite the fact that the patient population was dominated by African Americans, there were few Afro-American surgeons at CCH. The first Afro-American surgeon was Dr. Austin Maurice Curtis. He was born in Riley, North Carolina, on January 15, 1868. He graduated from Northwestern University Medical School and did his internship at Provident Hospital (now Cook County/Provident Hospital) in 1892. He joined the staff as attending surgeon at Cook County Hospital in January 1896. Another well-known Afro-American surgeon was Dale Williams, also a graduate of Northwestern University. Dr. Williams was the first surgeon in Chicago to operate on the heart.

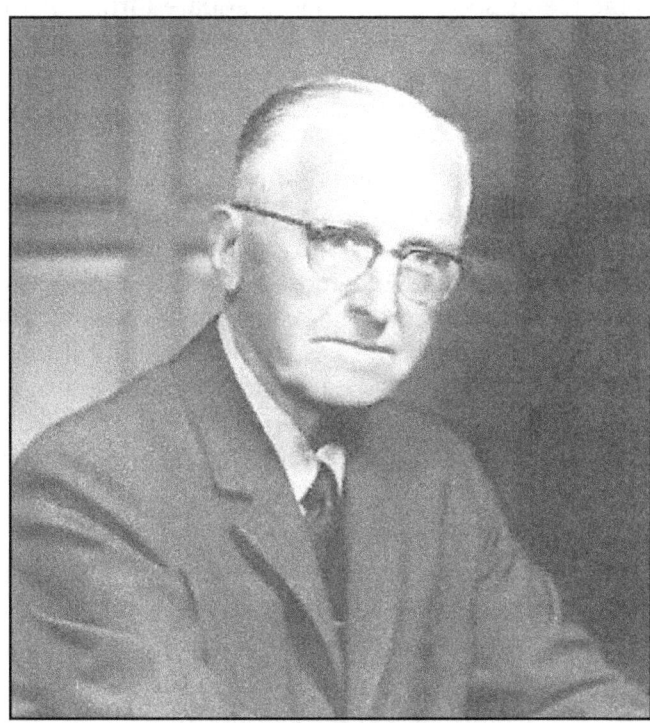

*Figure 2–3 Karl A. Meyer*

Cook County Hospital started as an intern hospital and gradually became a resident's hospital in the late 1930s when residency was offered for training. The program started with three years of training and later expanded to four. The program has been ACGME-approved since 1939. Prior to having full-time surgeons on staff, teaching or supervision of an operative procedure relied on the voluntary staff (attending or associate) and residents. Some attendings were very good, and some were not. Similarly, some residents were good teachers and some were not. As a result, learning was somewhat unguided and unstructured. The saying of "see one, do one and teach one" became a tradition of trial and error, and it only perpetuated mistakes. Many procedures were done by residents without prior knowledge of or even having assisted in the procedure. While there were rich case materials from which one could learn, there was also more opportunity to make avoidable mistakes. Surgery is essentially a craft, and there is no substitute for learning the craft from one with good surgical skills, sound judgment, and experience. As time went by, it was apparent that teaching by voluntary staff was not meeting the standard of surgical training set by the governing bodies.

## Internship

The internship is the focal point of the transition of medical student to physician. It probably evolved from the concept of apprenticeship first described in 1773 at the Pennsylvania Hospital, Philadelphia.[7] In the United States, Cook County Hospital was the first hospital to establish an internship (1866).[1] In the early days, internship was optional, and it was perfectly fine for one to enter practice as soon as one had graduated from medical school. Yet internship was appreciated as a most valuable experience for it gave the opportunity of putting theory into practice. Therefore, the best students wanted to take an internship before entering practice. As Bill Beck, one of the prominent Chicago surgeons, said, "The best of the best, the crèmè de la crèmè, desired an internship in an institution which provided ample and varied clinical material, hands-on experience, and good, but also forbearing supervision."[4]

The internship at Cook County Hospital was one of the most popular in the country. To be selected, one had to pass a highly competitive examination, usually held in April. The examination was an oral quiz by attending staff, and students worked for months to prepare. The internship was 12 months and later, in 1867, extended to 18 months with one intern accepted every six months.

The 18-month internship at County was structured with the first six months as junior assistant, the second six months as senior assistant, and the third six months as the house physician and surgeon. The responsibilities for these three positions from 1866 to 1937 were as follows:[3]

*First six months: Junior Assistant (three months each in surgery and medicine)*
- *Accompanied the head of the medical staff on rounds*
- *Wrote histories*
- *Wrote prescriptions*
- *Compounded prescriptions*

- Wrote out requisitions for supplies
- Conducted primitive laboratory examinations

**Second six months: Senior Assistant (five periods of five weeks each—examining room, obstetrics and children, contagious hospital, nervous disease, pathology)**

- Surgical dresser
- First assistant of surgical operations
- Conducted post-mortem examinations
- Assisted the eye and ear surgeon
- Kept record of his work

**Third six months: House Physician and Surgeon (three months surgery, three months medicine)**

- Supreme command in the wards, both medical and surgical
- Assumed all responsibilities outside of those assumed by the head of staff
- Assumed all emergency and obstetrical cases
- Made rounds morning and evening
- Supervised the writing of histories and prescriptions
- Ordered the discipline of the wards
- Expelled patients if necessary
- Supervised preparation of monthly reports for the medical board

In the days prior to beepers or even phones, emergencies were much more difficult matters to manage. Noted expert Dr. Frank Billings is quoted as saying that the house physicians had the responsibility of reporting the circumstances of the emergency to the attending in charge.

While there appears to be defined assignments of duty for interns at different levels, the work increased constantly. Nothing has changed about the scutt (noneducational) work that interns have to perform, which includes blood tests, starting all IVs in the ward, urine analysis, and, worse yet, personal transportation of patients for X-ray examination in emergency cases.

The large volume of cases, poor physical facilities, and inefficiency often frustrated the interns. In writing about Cook County Hospital, Dr. Freeark vividly described his frustration when he was an intern at the hospital.[8] "One of the less publicized unofficial duties of the intern and junior resident was to secure donated blood from the family of patients. Each service maintained a balance credit with the blood bank to ensure there was blood available for elective surgery. A negative balance would result in cancellation of elective surgery, a cardinal sin for every surgical resident. In order to maintain a positive balance, interns and residents made blood rounds on Saturday or Sunday when families were around. When the balance was low, even hernia or hemorrhoid surgery would bear a price of two units of blood. Blood donated by the family was credited to the service, or alternatively, the family could purchase the blood at a price of $10 per unit. One could say about the blood bank at CCH, 'it is a big bank, with a little bank inside'."

The house physician and surgeon were under the authority of the head of the staff, and the warden had no jurisdiction over the doctors in training. This slightly elongated rotating internship was designed to provide the maximum exposure to the conditions that a busy general practitioner, both in the city and downstate, was likely to experience.

Nils T. Quales (Figure 2–4) of Rush Medical College, having triumphed in a competitive examination for the position, began his career as the first intern at CCH on January 12, 1866. At this time, there was only one patient in the hospital, a German girl with a palmar abscess.[1] Three months later, James M. Hutchinson began his service as an intern.

Dr. Quales was born in 1831 and obtained an education in veterinary medicine in Copenhagen. He immigrated to the United States and reached Chicago in mid-1859. He obtained a medical degree from Rush Medical College in 1866. He completed a 12-month internship and subsequently served as city physician. He also was active in the Chicago Medical Society.

On March 1, 1871, Dr. Quales became Surgeon and Chief of the U.S. Marine Hospital. He played a major role in the founding of Lutheran Hospital and the Norwegian Old People's Home. He held membership in the Chicago Medical Society, the Illinois State Medical Society, and the American Medical Association. On account of his service to the Norwegian people in the city of Chicago, Dr. Quales received the order of St. Olaf from King Haakon VII of Norway in April 1910.

Dr. S. Root, who began in April 1867 and graduated in October 1868, was the first intern to serve 18 months.[1]

The first woman intern at Cook County Hospital was Mary Elizabeth Bates

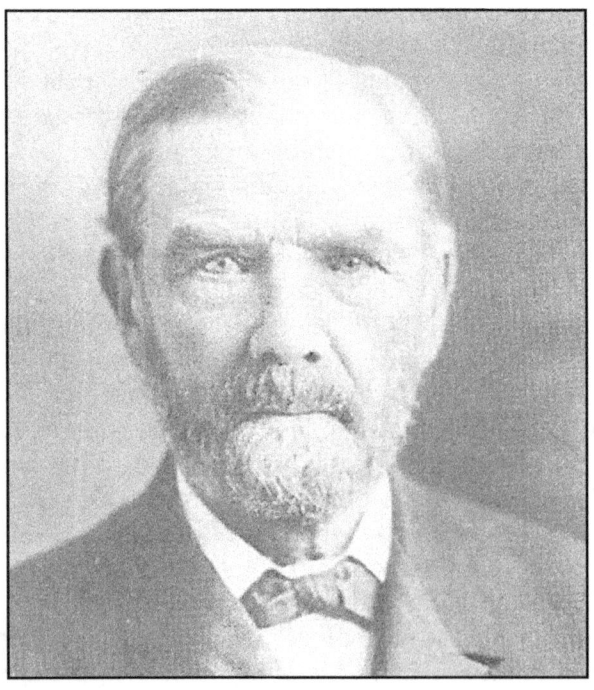

*Figure 2–4 Nils T. Quales*

(Figure 2–5). As described in the Cook County Award Dinner program, Dr. Bates was a graduate of the Women's Medical College and together with Frank Billings, was appointed as an intern in 1881, one of the first two finishers of the competitive examination. She worked closely with Dr. Fenger in the morgue and took part in 14 amputations. Later, she described her 19 months at Cook County Hospital as follows:

*The first six months were hell; the second six months were purgatory.*
*The third six months were heaven; when it came time for me to leave,*
*I wept bitter tears.*

Dr. Bates and Dr. Billings were instrumental in petitioning the hospital committee and the County Board to provide physicians with new stethoscopes and pocket cases of instruments.

Dr. Bates later taught at the Women's Medical College, her alma mater, and built a private practice. Due to poor health, she was forced to leave the city and spend the rest of her life in Denver, Colorado. In Colorado, she promoted the passage of several state laws to improve the condition of women and children, which were later taken as models by other states. She also succeeded in having a law passed to require physical examination of school children and the treatment of any uncovered medical conditions.

In 1905, the Cook County Board of Commissioners mandated that future appointees to the attending staff and interns must pass the civil service examination.

During the 20 years after 1900, the internship became a defined entity. The AMA established its Council on Medical Education (CME) in 1904, which one year later recommended an "ideal standard" for medical education: a one-year internship in a hospital after completion of medical school.[7] Pennsylvania

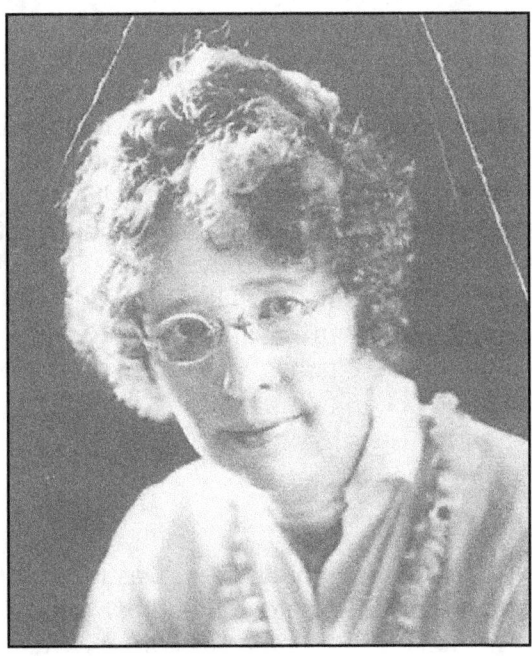

*Figure 2–5 Mary Elizabeth Bates*

became the first state to require that every candidate for medical licensure must have served one year as an intern in an approved hospital. The CME completed its first survey and published a list of "Approved Training Hospitals." Cook County Hospital was among them.[9] The internship program was accredited officially by the AMA in 1914.[10] By the time the report was published in 1914, it was estimated that 75 percent of graduates were completing an internship. The 1910 Flexner report indirectly affected the internship.[11] Many schools that did not meet the standards set forth in the report were forced to close. In 1905, there were 160 medical schools, but by 1922, there were only 81. In 1919, the Council of Medical Education and Hospitals (now renamed ACGME) published standards for internship entitled "The Essentials of an Approved Internship."[7,12]

After World War II, one of the major revolutions in internship was the introduction of a National Internship Matching Program conceived by the Association for American Medical Colleges.[7] It was introduced in the 1951–52 school year. The matching program served the needs of both senior students and hospitals. In 1960, internship continued to evolve, and many hospitals no longer offered a rotating internship but instead a straight internship to a given specialty. The requirement for a rotating internship was terminated in the 1960s.

In 1970, further change of the structure of internship occurred. The AMA approved the incorporation of the accreditation of the first graduate medical education year (internship) into the resident review process. The AMA announced that after July 1975,

> *No internship program shall be approved which is not integrated with residency training to form a unified program of graduate medical education. The term PGY 1 has effectively replaced the internship.*[7]

From the beginning of 1866 to the early 1900s, internship was the most sought-after position at CCH. The list of surgeons who did their internship at CCH reads like a "Who's Who" in American surgery, including Nicholas Senn, John B. Murphy, L.L. McArthur, Albert Halstead, Samuel Plummer, Rosewell Park, Raymond McNealy, Kellogg Speed, William Morgan, Frederick Besley, Dean Lewis, Vernon David, Sumner Koch, and many others. Many surgery department chairmen at various medical schools did their internships at CCH. These include Dallas Phemister at University of Chicago, Edmund Andrews, Jr., Weller van Hook, Allen Kanavel, Harry Richter, Loyal Davis at Northwestern University,[13] and Arthur Dean Bevan at Rush Medical College. The list goes on and on, and virtually every famed surgeon in Chicago at one time or another received training at CCH.

**Residency**

In the beginning, there was no training program for surgeons, and learning surgery was by watching surgery (amphitheatre teaching) or via an internship. Assistanceship, popular in Europe, was not accepted here in the United States until the 1900s. In 1913, the Council of Medical Education of AMA became more involved in postgraduate training of surgeons. They recommended two years training plus one year of internship. There was, however, no distinction between well-trained and inadequately trained surgeons. In 1926, the AMA-approved Residency Program in Surgery listed approximately 15 institutions throughout the country, which included Cook County Hospital, the only approved program in Chicago at that time.

In the early years, training of surgeons relied heavily on the leader of the surgical department, and two schools of training emerged: the William Halsted School of Hopkins[14] and the Midwestern School of Surgery by Christian Fenger.[6] The Halsted school was designed to train academic surgeons or professors with strong interest in research whereas the Midwestern school focused on training clinical practicing surgeons. Both schools were needed for training surgeons in the United States. The Halsted school was introduced in 1889 and was a transformational progressive and science-based, but steeply pyramidal, program, adapted from the German model.[14] A single individual might emerge as a fully trained potential professor of surgery after prolonged intensive apprenticeship. The superior surgeon, if produced, led many centers to follow suit.

Regardless of what school was used for training, there was a growing concern and need for establishing a professional standard to define surgeons. The American Medical Association, spurred by the efforts of Arthur Dean Bevan of Rush, supported improvement in medical education proposed in the Flexner report in 1910 but resisted setting specialty standards in deference to the constituency of practitioners who wished to continue to perform surgery without restriction.[15] In 1919, the American College of Surgeons (ACS) first defined requirements for Fellowship of the College as follows:

1. One year internship, usually rotating
2. Two years assistance under a preceptor
3. Visiting surgical clinics
4. Submission of a list of 50 consecutive cases.[16]

After 1920, graduation from an approved medical school was added. Evarts Graham, Professor of Surgery at Washington University, was critical of the lax standards of the ACS. At the 1935 meeting of the American Surgical Association, President Edward Archibald appointed a committee to investigate the "elevation for surgical standards."[15] Graham chaired the committee and decided a more representative national body should be invested with the authority to organize a qualifying board of surgery. Under the leadership of Graham, the American Board of Surgery (ABS), a non-profit organization, was founded in 1937 for the purpose of certifying surgeons who met a defined standard of education, training, and knowledge.[15] The Board's training requirement for examination evolved gradually. In 1950, a Resident Review Committee (RRC) for surgery was formed under the auspices of the Council of Medical Education, ABS, and ACS. The RRC inspects training programs for approved surgical training that complies with the guidelines of the training curriculum.[10] At present, ABS is one of the 24-member boards of the American Board of Medical Specialties.

After the establishment of the American Board of Surgery, a second transformation occurred in surgical residency: the "rectangular" program of residency formulated by Edward Delos Churchill of Massachusetts General Hospital, Harvard Medical School.[16] The rectangular residency provided complete training to a small number of candidates, emphasizing peer group education in a school of surgery not dominated by a single individual. The steep pyramid system was eliminated. Soon after its introduction, many surgical training programs elected to follow the rectangular system. The "pattern" of the Churchill residency has stood the test of time extraordinarily well.[15] It has served as a model for modification of surgical education throughout the United States.

Commencing in the 1930s, there were residents training at CCH. The first residents were in ophthalmology and ENT, and then in pediatrics. The surgical residency was not started until the late 1930s, and as time went on, the hospital became less and less an intern's hospital and instead a resident's hospital. In 1939, the ACGME approved the residency in General Surgery at County. Residencies in the other surgical specialties followed soon after.

The first surgical resident was John W. Howser (Figure 2–6), a graduate of Northwestern University Medical School in 1937. From January to June of 1937 he served an internship at the old Wesley Hospital on 26th Street. He then served a regular 18-month internship at Cook County Hospital from January 1937 to June 1938.

At the completion of his internship, Dr. Howser asked Dr. Karl Meyer for an appointment as surgical resident. Dr. Meyer told him the hospital was awaiting

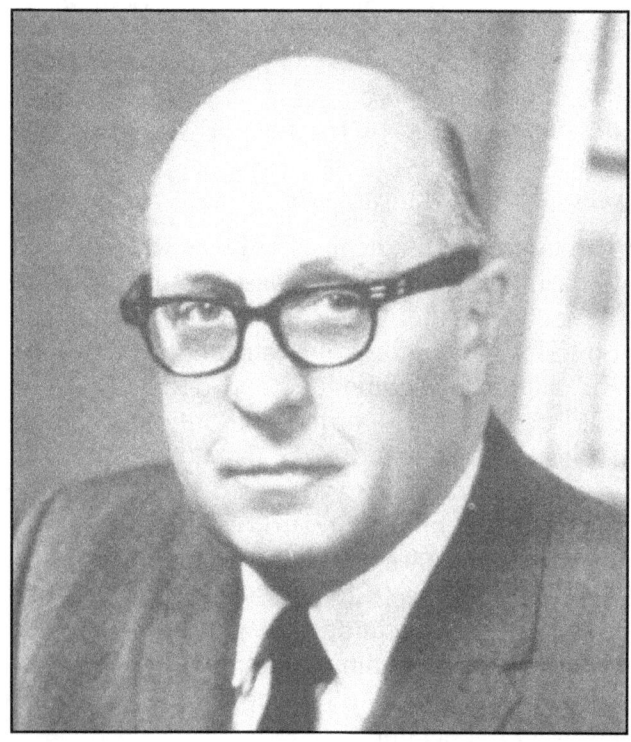

*Figure 2–6 John W. Howser*

approval of such a residency and suggested he take a temporary appointment elsewhere. Howser then started a residency at Grady Hospital in Atlanta in July 1938 where he remained until he was invited back to County by Dr. Meyer to be the first surgical resident, a position he served from January 1939 to December 1942.

After certification by the American Board of Surgery in 1942, he was given an appointment at CCH as the associate of Dr. Arkyll Vaughn, as well as an attending appointment at Oak Park and West Suburban Hospitals. He was made a full attending surgeon at County after passing the civil service examination in 1950 and was night surgeon (Wednesday and Saturday) from 1951–1954. He was truly a man on whom legends were made: first as the intern who swallowed his cigarette when Dr. Meyer got on the elevator with him, and second as the attending who took a good friend's son who was thinking of a career in surgery to the OR to help on a cholecystectomy. He gave the young man a stick sponge and a large clamp to hold "so that they will be there when I need them." While the student watched the procedure with riveted attention and expectation for use of his tools, Dr. Howser finally asked for them back when the last skin suture had been placed. With residents of this nature, it is no surprise that as time passed, County became known as a resident's hospital.

Dr. Howser's academic appointments include Associate in Surgery at Northwestern University Medical School, and Associate Professor of Surgery at Loyola and Rush Medical Schools. He was a trustee of Cook County Graduate School of Medicine.

The first female surgical resident was Vera Markovin. She graduated with a B.A. from Syracuse University in 1939 and an MD from Rush Medical College (University of Chicago) in 1942. She did an internship and residency in general surgery from 1942 to 1946 at CCH and a chief residency in surgery at the American Hospital of Chicago in 1946–1947. She became Diplomate of the American Board of Surgery in 1949. She practiced general surgery at various hospitals in the Chicago area from 1947 to 1965. Later, she became interested in emergency medicine and was active in the professional organizations of emergency medicine. She co-founded the emergency medicine residency at the University of Illinois College of Medicine. In 1983, she moved to Michigan where she continued her work in emergency medicine where she became an Associate Professor of Emergency Medicine at Michigan State University.

From 1940 to 1958, Karl Meyer was the Chair of Surgery and program director of the surgical training program. In this period, all training was under the supervision of voluntary attending staff. Each of the attending staff was assigned one or more attending associates nominated through the dean's office of the school with which the attending surgeon was affiliated as an undergraduate teacher. Five medical schools had service for student and resident teaching at CCH: Northwestern University Medical School, University of Illinois, Rush Medical College, Loyola University, and Chicago Medical School. The Cook County Residency Program was an independent, rectangular training program with residents rotating from these medical school services for training. As stated previously, there were shortcomings with supervision solely by voluntary staff.

In order to comply with training standards set by governing bodies, a full-time Director of Surgical Education position was created: Dr. Robert J. Freeark was chosen to fill the position, and a new era of surgical education was begun.

**Surgical Amphitheatre Teaching**

Teaching surgical procedures in an amphitheatre was a common practice in the early days of surgical education. The practice evolved from anatomy or pathology teaching. Throughout the 19th century, amphitheatres were commonplace in metropolitan medical centers. In the United States, the oldest surgical theatre was built in 1804 at Pennsylvania Hospital at Philadelphia.[17] It was designed to function as lecture hall and operating room, with a gallery on the operating level as well as the mezzanine. Visiting surgeons or trainees were all in street clothes without a cap or a mask. On the east coast, the clinics of Hayes Agnew and Samuel Gross were well known.[15]

In Chicago, the first surgical amphitheatre was built in 1870 at the Cook County Hospital. Rush also had a theatre at the top of the building with oil paintings of Gunn and Ross, and sloping seats. All leading surgeons such as Nicholas Senn and Christian Fenger had their own operating clinics (Figure 2–7). Fenger conducted his clinic at the Davis Hall next to the Northwestern Medical School on Dearborn Street. While an attending surgeon at County, John B. Murphy conducted a surgical clinic on Friday mornings at County Hospital. The clinic was attended by students from all medical colleges (Figure 2–8). The clinic started

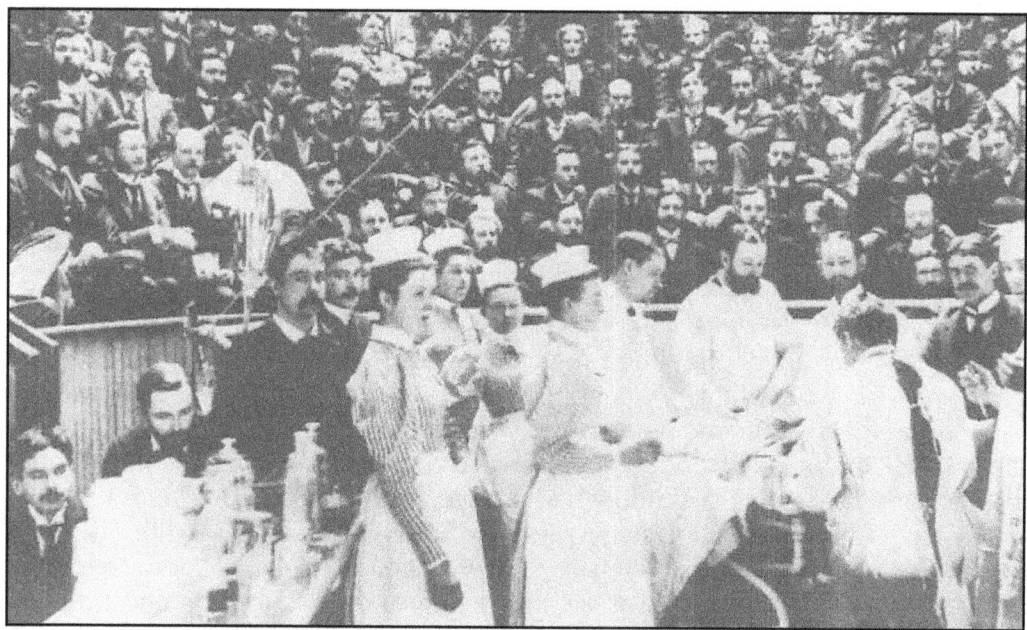

*Figure 2–7  Operating clinic conducted by Christian Fenger in 1886*

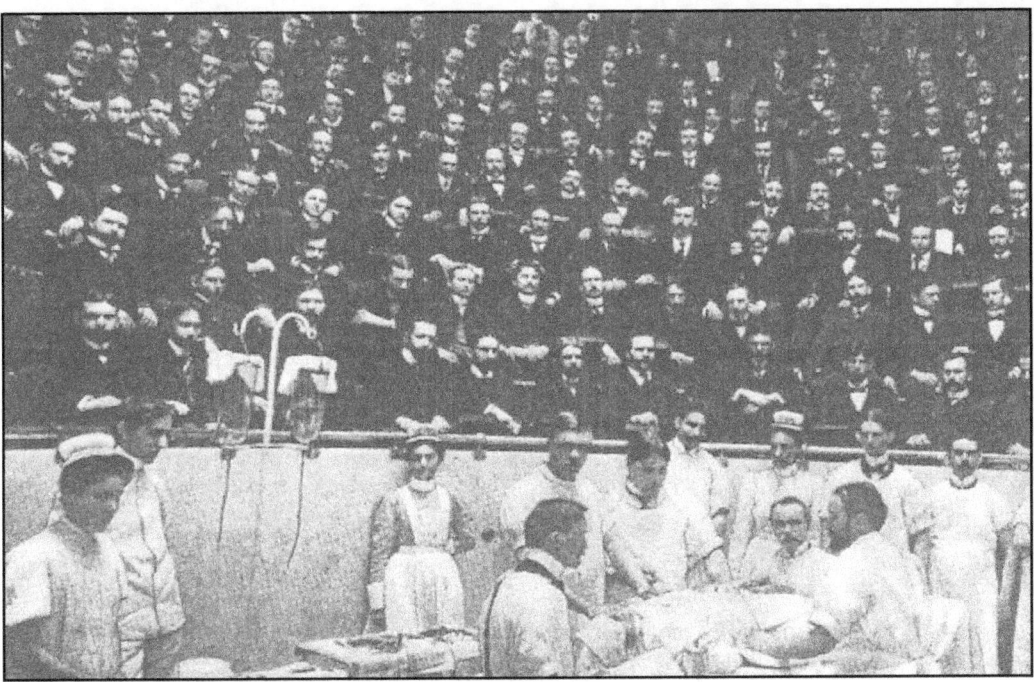

*Figure 2–8 Operating Clinic sponsored by John B. Murphy on Friday mornings at CCH*

with an intern or resident making a presentation of the clinical history of the patient, followed by sharp questions from Dr. Murphy. This was followed by the operation and the discussion of highlights of the procedure. Later, John B. Murphy went on to conduct the famous surgical clinic at Mercy Hospital with publication of a monograph. The monograph, called *Surgical Clinics of John B. Murphy* was so popular that when Murphy died, the W. B. Saunders Co. kept the format of quarterly publication and renamed it *Surgical Clinics of North America*. Many well-known surgeons were invited as guest editors to develop the volume on the subject of their choice. Today, the *Surgical Clinics of North America* remains popular reading for many surgeons.[18]

The amphitheatre at the new County Hospital was located on the seventh floor and was used by many surgeons. Of these surgeons, the Saturday clinics conducted by Meyer in the morning and by McNealy in the afternoon were legendary. For Meyer, a favorite operation was the gastric resection, which he always performed with ease. For McNealy, visiting surgeons always remembered his explanation of the procedure by drawing on the blackboard simultaneously with both hands. Both these surgeons were master surgeons and many surgeons from downstate came to watch them operate.

In 1923, concern about the increased infection rate caused a gradual decline in the use of amphitheatre teaching. The amphitheatre, however, was still in occasional use for the wet clinic of Illinois State Surgical Society meetings or for Cook County Graduate School of Medicine. Gowns, caps, and masks were used by visitors to minimize infection. The practice of amphitheatre teaching finally ended in the late 1950s but remains a historical part of surgical education in America.

**The Night Surgeon**

The night surgeon position was a unique part of surgical heritage at Cook County Hospital. It was designed to develop the skill of the attending surgeon and also for trainees to develop independent surgical judgment. Early on, the man who contributed most to the legend of the night surgeon was a 1903 graduate of Rush Medical College who interned at St. Elizabeth Hospital and then at Cook County Hospital, finishing in March 1907. Dr. Roger Throop Vaughan (Figure 2–9), who was in private practice at St. Luke's Hospital with offices at the fashionable 30 N. Michigan address, was initially a faculty member at the College of Physicians and Surgeons (University of Illinois) in 1910. With the exception of two months on active duty with the U.S. Army in late 1918, Dr. R.T. Vaughan spent the time from 1917 to 1950 as the attending surgeon for night emergencies and assistant warden of the County Hospital.[4] The other assistant warden for medical affairs was Dr. Karl Meyer, who was appointed in 1918. The night surgeon was usually an assigned attending surgeon, responsible for all emergencies after 5:00 p.m. Dr. Vaughan was regularly scheduled as night surgeon on Thursday; however, for the 33 years that he served as the night warden, he spent

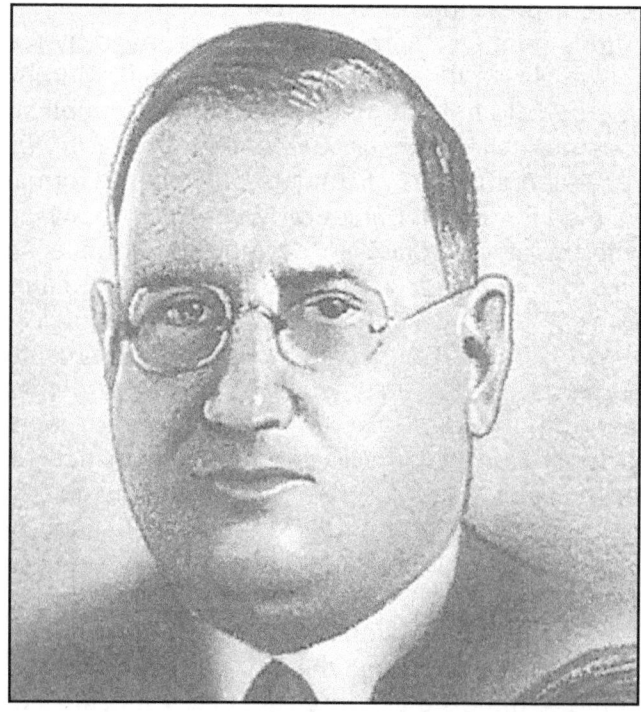

*Figure 2–9  Roger T. Vaughan*

every weekday night at CCH and went home to his farm in Homewood for the weekends. He worked the night shift from about 8:00 p.m. until 5:00 or 6:00 a.m. Not only did he provide clinical instruction and care during this time, but he contributed extensively to the surgical literature on a wide variety of topics from osteomyelitis of the sternum to retrograde amnesia following skull fracture. When X-ray was first introduced, he quickly adapted this new technology in the diagnosis of acute abdomen. He did experimental work by injecting air in cadavers and found only 10cc of air was needed to produce free air under the diaphragm by X-ray. He was an expert on the management of mechanical small bowel obstruction secondary to adhesions. He also was active in moving the hospital forward in areas other than patient care and teaching, such as in the areas of hospital budget, development of physical therapy, improvement in laboratory testing, and improving the general cleanliness of the hospital.[18]

A word should be said about the manner in which emergency surgery was approached in the world according to R.T. Vaughan. According to Dr. William Beck, a noted Chicago surgeon of the early 20th century who was a long-time attending and member of the night surgeon coverage team, the process for admitting surgical emergencies was in rotation just like nonemergencies, but with a note from the admitting intern to have the intern on call see the patient immediately or as soon as possible.[4] This note imitated the performance of a "Vaughan history and physical," which required an extensive notation of each and every symptom, all food and drink ingested, and what was excreted from the first onset of symptoms to the present time. The physical examination was equally complete, and together, the information would cover 10–12 pages. From this information, a differential diagnosis was developed and pertinent laboratory examination attached, although these really did not interest Dr. R.T. Vaughan very much. Armed with this information, the responsible intern, often in company with his fellow intern, would make the trip up the stairs to the second floor of the main hospital to the administrative area of the large lobby, where there were three desks fronting the area set off by a counter. The middle desk was reserved for Dr. R.T. Vaughan while those on either side, though usually empty at night, belonged to Dr. Meyer and the hospital warden. Other surrounding desks were also empty at night but the chairs filled with interns to discuss the cases that were being presented, with questions for all from Dr. R.T. Vaughan. At the end of the discussion, Vaughan would arrive at a diagnosis, sign a form, and send it with the intern and the patient to the night surgeon for surgery. These diagnoses usually were made without Dr. R.T. Vaughan examining the patient, but according to eyewitness observers, the diagnoses were correct most of the time. If, however, it was necessary to examine the patient, the patient—bed and all—would be wheeled to the second floor lobby and Dr. R.T. Vaughan would perform the examination. Only rarely did he ask the patient any questions.

This, then, was the process, but Dr. William Requarth, a resident in the 1940s, attending surgeon, night surgeon, and author of the well-written and often-read classic on the diagnosis and management of the acute abdomen, leaves us with a graphic representation of what the intern would find when he arrived in front of that big desk at the top of the stairs in the second floor lobby:

> *(a man) ... of slight posture with thin, unkempt hair, wearing a visor, with often a cigar perched alongside a single protruding upper tooth. Behind this rather unimpressive appearance was a man of wide interest and much knowledge outside of medicine, for example he had a keen interest in Spanish literature and was fluent in the Spanish language. He did not appear to be the man of independent means that he was, a person who was able to live his life as he desires—one whom I would call a brilliant eccentric.*

As one might suspect, Dr. Vaughan worked until the very end. Late in the first week of November 1950, he suffered a coronary event, went into nonresponsive congestive heart failure, and was dead within a week, leaving behind the legacy of the night surgeon as the master curer of all things surgical that presented after the sun had set.

In the early years, appointment to the night surgeon list was not a given for attendings as the following vignette from Dr. William Beck, a noted Chicago surgeon of the day, demonstrates:

> *Dr. Beck found himself at County one Sunday morning seeing one of the patients, when an intern asked Beck to see a patient with a perforated ulcer. Beck realized the need for immediate surgery, so Beck joined him on the trip to the second floor office of the warden. Dr. Meyer was the only person there. Beck explained the situation and Meyer said softly, "I am the Sunday surgeon." I (Beck continues) wanted to sink through the floor. My embarrassment must have showed for he graciously said, "Why don't you take the patient up and operate on him, then come down and tell me about it." I did so. Later he said, "You know, I've been tied down here every Sunday and holiday. You could do me a favor by becoming the Sunday and holiday surgeon." So Dr. Beck, after petitioning both Drs. Meyer and Vaughan on several occasions, finally got the position on the night service through dogged persistence.[4]*

The last use of an attending as night surgeon was probably in the late 1940s. Dr. John Keeley was the night surgeon from 1941 to 1949. When the surgical residency became extended to four years, the chief surgical resident became the night surgeon. He or she had independent surgical privileges and served as supreme commander of surgical affairs of the hospital. The night surgeon tradition, through the years, spawned the tales of which legends and reputations were made. The prestige of being an appointed surgeon at County carried the aura of something special. In the late 1950s, a medical student was told facetiously by a senior ward medical resident that the "night surgeon speaks only to God."[19] Somehow, the tradition of surgeon on emergency call and warden remained even into the early 1960s. The on-call schedule of 1964 shows that the assistant night surgeon doubled up as night warden (Figure 2–10) and in most instances, his duty was to sign death certificates.

The night surgeon was one of four chief residents, usually in the fifth year of training. He or she headed an operating team consisting of a fourth-year resident (senior) as an assistant surgeon, a runner, a third-year resident, and the intern of the respective service (Figure 2–10). The night surgeon usually stayed in the operating room with the senior surgeon to make final decisions for cases that needed surgery. The runner oversaw the interns in preparation of patients for the operating room. He also ran among wards for surgical consultations. The system worked well and was the backbone for delivery of care for emergency cases. In the 1940s and 1950s, most routine emergency cases such as bowel obstruction, gunshot wounds, and appendectomy were handled by the fourth- or fifth-year surgical residents with approval from the attending surgeons. For some problems such as bleeding ulcers, an attending surgeon, usually Peter Rosi, came in and performed an emergency gastric resection. For some pediatric problems such as

SURGICAL RESIDENTS - May 1964

| | | Night Surgeon | Assistant Surgeon | Jr. Resident | Warden's Office |
|---|---|---|---|---|---|
| | 1 | Mogan | Bransfield | Go, C. | Ruffalo |
| Sat. | 2 | Reyes | Corley | Pletsch | Adamski |
| Sun. | 3 | Carey | Hagstrom | Adamski | Corley |
| | 4 | Cunningham | Mittelpunkt | Neal | Bransfield |
| | 5 | Mladick | Vanecko | Wenzel | Mittelpunkt |
| | 6 | Sanders | Ruffalo | Boyles | Pletsch |
| | 7 | Mogan | Bransfield | Bass | King |
| | 8 | Reyes | Corley | Drake | Vanecko |
| Sat. | 9 | Carey | Hagstrom | Adamski | Boyles |
| Sun. | 10 | Cunningham | Mittelpunkt | Okada | Drake |
| | 11 | Mladick | Vanecko | Kennedy | Fitzgerald |
| | 12 | Dippel | King | Boyles | Bass |
| | 13 | Mogan | Bransfield | Yao | Chang |
| | 14 | Reyes | Corley | Somerville | Okada |
| | 15 | Carey | Hagstrom | Adamski | Kennedy |
| Sat. | 16 | Cunningham | Mittelpunkt | Bernstein | Hagstrom |
| Sun. | 17 | Mladick | Vanecko | Go, C. | Ruffalo |
| | 18 | Dippel | King | Boyles | Adamski |
| | 19 | Sanders | Ruffalo | Pletsch | Corley |
| | 20 | Reyes | Corley | Neal | Bransfield |
| | 21 | Carey | Hagstrom | Adamski | Mittelpunkt |
| | 22 | Cunningham | Mittelpunkt | Wenzel | Pletsch |
| Sat. | 23 | Mladick | Vanecko | Bass | King |
| Sun. | 24 | Dippel | King | Boyles | Vanecko |
| | 25 | Sanders | Ruffalo | Drake | Boyles |
| | 26 | Mogan | Bransfield | Okada | Drake |
| | 27 | Carey | Hagstrom | Adamski | Fitzgerald |
| | 28 | Cunningham | Mittelpunkt | Kennedy | Bass |
| | 29 | Mladick | Vanecko | Yao | Chang |
| Sat. | 30 | Dippel | King | Boyles | Okada |
| Sun. | 31 | Sanders | Ruffalo | Somerville | Hagstrom |

Warden's Office - Weekends and Holidays - 8 a.m. to 4 p.m.

| | | |
|---|---|---|
| Sat. | 2 | Carey |
| Sun. | 3 | Cunningham |
| Sat. | 9 | Dippel |
| Sun. | 10 | Mogan |
| Sat. | 16 | Reyes |
| Sun. | 17 | Sanders |
| Sat. | 23 | Carey |
| Sun. | 24 | Mladick |
| Sat. | 30 | Cunningham |
| Sun. | 31 | Dippel |

*Figure 2–10 Residents' call schedule in 1964*

duodenal atresia or imperforate anus, Drs. Fell or Keeley came in to do the operation. In those days, the Fire Department did not have ambulances, and patients were brought to County Hospital by the police in "squadrols." These were small police wagons with rear doors that could hold two stretchers. One benefit of this system was that doctors working in the emergency rooms got to know many of the police by name. As a result, the police, who were usually superstitious by nature, would seldom give a "County Doc" a traffic ticket.

At the time of the example schedule (1964), the attending surgeon supporting the chief surgical resident as a night surgeon was Dr. William Norcross. Norcross worked after 5:00 p.m. every day and was always available for the night surgeon asking for diagnostic help or assistance in the operating room. The presence of Norcross was always nonintrusive, but when need was apparent, he would always be there for the night surgeon. This arrangement allowed the trainee to mature and to develop sound surgical judgment, an experience unique to the Cook County training program. Bill Norcross graduated from Northwestern University Medical School in 1959 and did his internship and residency in surgery at CCH, where he stayed on as attending surgeon for emergencies. During the day, he served as chief surgeon at the Cermak Memorial Hospital (serving the House of Corrections/Cook County Jail). He was there when Richard Speck, the notorious murderer of eight student nurses, was captured and sent to the hospital at the county jail for examination and detention. The hospital at the county jail was also a place for approved "moonlighting" night calls for surgical residents who needed extra cash. Norcross was hardworking, intelligent, and totally dedicated to the training of surgeons at CCH to deal with emergencies. He was, indeed, an unsung hero in the history of the Department of Surgery at CCH.

## The Cook County Graduate School of Medicine

The Cook County Graduate School of Medicine was the first institution to embark on continuing education, which many academic centers now offer to practicing surgeons. By the early 1930s, Dr. Meyer had become convinced that a formalized mechanism to provide postgraduate medical education for the practicing surgeons was in order. The concept built upon the postgraduate clinics held with the cooperation of the Chicago Medical Society, which ran in two-week sessions during the summer of 1926 and drew approximately 500 practicing physicians for the grueling 9:00 a.m. to 4:00 p.m. daily curriculum. On October 1, 1932, under the direction of Dr. Meyer, the staff of Cook County Hospital organized and incorporated the Cook County Graduate School of Medicine. The building was located at 427 South Honore Street. Later, because of the widening of Congress Street, the graduate school was moved to a new building located on the southeast corner of Flournoy and Wood Streets opposite the Cook County Children's Hospital (Figure 2–11). This organization was very closely associated with Northwestern University faculty. Raymond McNealy from Northwestern was a constant contributor with his operative clinic. McNealy also served as trustee and professor of surgery as well as secretary-treasurer at the graduate school. Any person on the hospital staff, attending or associate, could be on the faculty of the graduate school if he or she had the ability to attract students.

According to Meyer, the concept of a postgraduate school at County was conceived by John B. Murphy. Indeed, Murphy had philanthropic support to establish such a school but failed due to lack of support from a few of the staff.[18]

The school specialized in giving short courses. An animal laboratory was also available for students to practice certain techniques under supervision. The Chicago Medical Society (CMS) was an ad hoc partner in these early courses as it publicized the offerings and tuition costs regularly in its journal, *Chicago Medicine*. This was especially helpful in a day when nearly all practicing physicians in the city were members of CMS. At the height of the graduate school activity, there were some 60–70 courses offered per year by surgeons and non-surgeons. For surgical experience, the school featured classroom and wet clinics with Dr. McNealy performing either a thyroidectomy or cholecystectomy on Saturday morning, and Dr. Meyer performing a gastric resection in the afternoon. It was noted by several residents of the 1950s that Dr. Meyer preferred patients with gastric ulcer since there was more for the visiting physicians to feel and see when the specimen was passed around the audience than when the operation was performed for duodenal ulcer. In the 1970s and 1980s, one of the sought-after courses was the general surgery review course for the American Board of Surgery examination. The course was spearheaded by Robert J. Baker, faculty

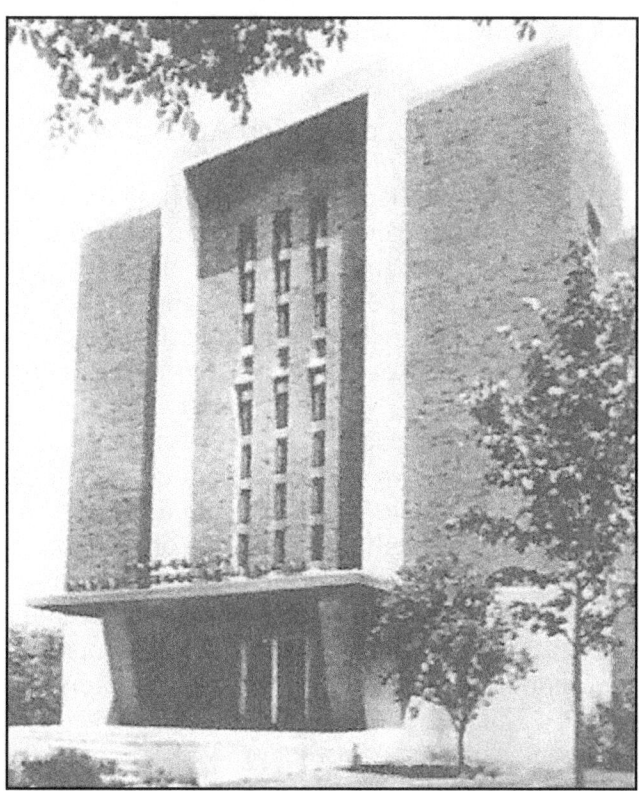

*Figure 2–11 Cook County Graduate School, 707 South Wood Street*

member and also professor of surgery at the University of Illinois College of Medicine. The course made use of the best platform lecturers of the combined medical school faculties of the city and attracted an estimated 1,000 attendees each for just the surgery and internal medicine board review courses. In a report by Meyer, some 20,000 physicians from all over the world had registered and taken special courses over a 17-year period.[13]

The wet clinic died out after Meyer stepped down as the chair in the early 1960s, though some courses in learning new techniques (primarily vascular surgery) continued to be held in the Graduate School Building at 900 S. Wood Street for many years.

In the 1980s, with the increase of continuing medical education courses both within professional organizations such as the American College of Surgeons and the American College of Internal Medicine and by a variety of entrepreneurial enterprises, the Graduate School began to experience financial difficulties, and the administration, which included Dr. S. Waldstein as the executive director and Dr. Robert Baker as the dean, decided to sell the building on Wood Street to the newly resurgent Rush Medical College. They moved the school now known as the National Center for Advanced Medical Education to the neighborhood of Northwestern Medical School's campus east of Michigan Avenue, the "Magnificent Mile." In the mid-1990s the school was sold to the Kaplan network, and after about 2006, CCH stopped being involved in presenting these medical courses, according to Dr. Robert Wilson, Professor of Surgery at Wayne State College of Medicine, who coordinated the last course. Cook County Graduate School of Medicine finally faded silently into the history of the surgical education of CCH.

## The Era of Full-time Salaried Attending Staff

The appointment of Dr. Robert J. Freeark (Figure 2–12) as Chair of the Department of Surgery at Cook County Hospital in 1963 ushered in a new era of surgical education and clinical care that reflected a new trend at all major medical centers in this country. Dr. Freeark was the first full-time salaried attending and he painstakingly built a staff of full-time salaried attending surgeons in a variety of surgical subspecialties. He laid out a vision and set out a goal to revitalize the resources of the hospital in order to promote quality health care and establish a superior postgraduate training program in surgery and the surgical specialties that would equal any of the academic medical centers of the era. The foundation was crafted and laid out so that trainees not only benefited from the wealth of experience obtained from the care of patients, but also that the patients themselves received the same type of care previously accorded only to those able to afford the services of a private physician and the facilities of a private institution. Generations of surgical specialists were produced during this period to share their educational experiences to benefit their respective patients throughout the country. This evolutionary process represented the golden age of surgical practice and education at this institution.

## The Freeark Era—1958–1968
### Interim Chairs: Robert J. Baker, 1969; Frank Folk, 1970–1972

Dr. Robert J. Freeark, a graduate of Northwestern University Medical School, was in the Cook County Hospital Intern Class of 1952. He completed his residency in general surgery at CCH in 1958 and soon after was appointed the first full-time salaried attending surgeon at the institution, an associate of Dr. Karl Meyer and director of surgical education. This appointment heralded the era of education by full-time salaried surgical staff. In 1963, he was appointed as chair of the Department of Surgery and immediately embarked on an ambitious goal of developing a full-time system with salaried attending surgeons in the department, a drastic deviation from the organizational structure of the past. Toward the end of the decade, Dr. Freeark established a strong and dedicated full-time faculty comparable to that of any medical school or medical center in the country. A culture of accountability by a full-time attending staff in patient care, resident education and supervision, and research had been accomplished through his vision, tenacity, and uncanny ability to interact with surgeons with different backgrounds, training, and personalities, ignoring the personal agendas and big egos of some of them, provided they were fully committed to their responsibilities. He recruited Dr. Robert Baker (Figure 2–13), a former co-resident, who was enticed to return from his private practice in California, and together, they established the first trauma and burn unit in the country. Dr. Freeark also recruited Frank Folk (Figure 2–14), who was in private practice in the western suburbs of Chicago following his two years in the service in the division of general surgery. Eventually, both in succession (Dr. Baker in 1968 and Dr. Folk from

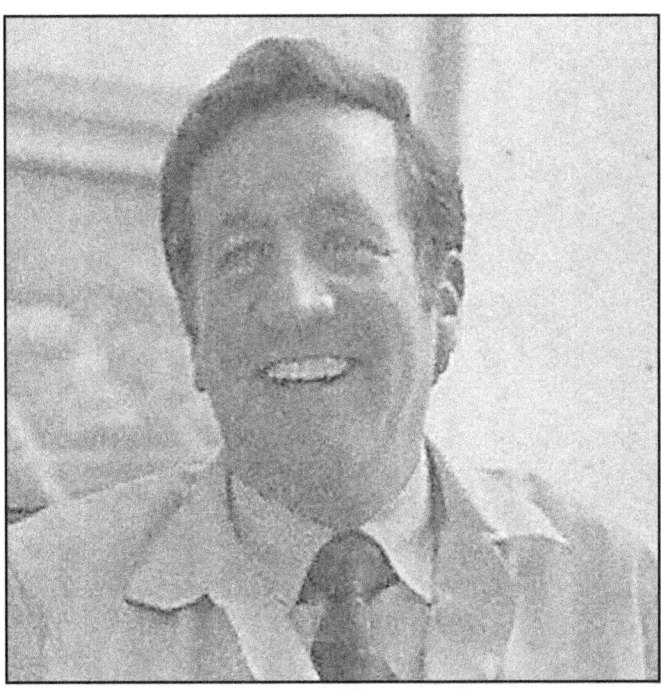

*Figure 2–12*
*Robert J. Freeark*

1969 to 1972), took over as chief of surgery upon the promotion of Dr. Freeark to the position of medical superintendent of the hospital. Dr. Folk subsequently took over full oversight of the breast service and contributed innovations in the care of these patients. Together with Dr. Freeark, Drs. Baker and Folk served as full-time mentors of the surgical residents, and supervised their clinical work in addition to their active participation in the educational programs. Dr. Baker also assumed the position of director of the blood bank until his departure in 1968. Dr. William Norcross, who completed his surgical residency in 1959, stayed in the hospital at night and supervised emergency night surgery. Dr. John G. Raffensperger was made chief of pediatric surgery and acting chair of thoracic surgery, replacing Dr. Milton Weinberg who decided to devote his time to private practice at Presbyterian Hospital. Dr. Constantine Tatooles subsequently took over the chairmanship of the Division of Thoracic Surgery. Dr. William Shoemaker (Figure 2–15) from the Harvard Medical System, a true academic surgeon, was recruited in general surgery and critical care. He was given the responsibility of directing surgical research at Hektoen Institute and also at the shock trauma unit. He organized a group of elite nurses on the trauma unit who were able to do many procedures previously performed by physicians (an early version of nurse practitioners). Dr. Joseph Carey, then a junior resident assigned to the trauma unit, organized a basic science research seminar for the surgical residents at Hektoen, which evolved into the Saturday grand round conference for the residents. Other recruitments included: Dr. Anthony Raimondi in neurosurgery; Dr. David Long for thoracic surgery; Dr. Jack Kerth in otolaryngology; and Dr. John Boswick on the burn and hand service, later joined by Dr. Nelson Stone, Dr. Jack Stevens, Dr. Theodore Hartman, and Dr. Richard "Crash" Corley.

The increased supervision provided by the full-time attending staff early on

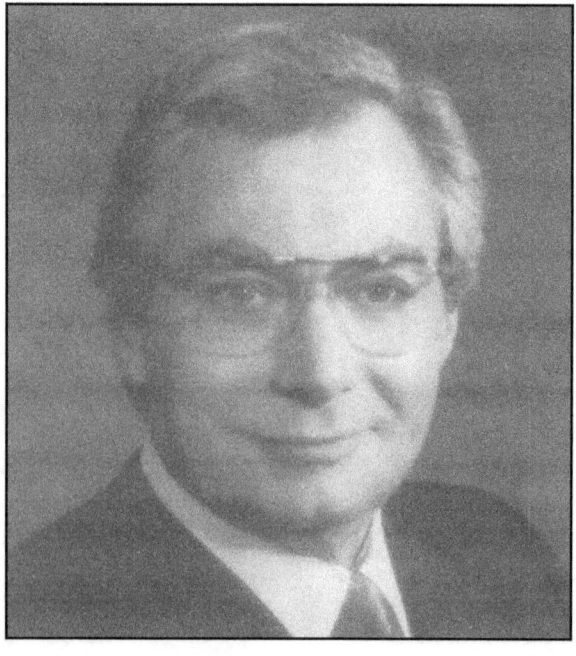

*Figure 2–13 Robert J. Baker*

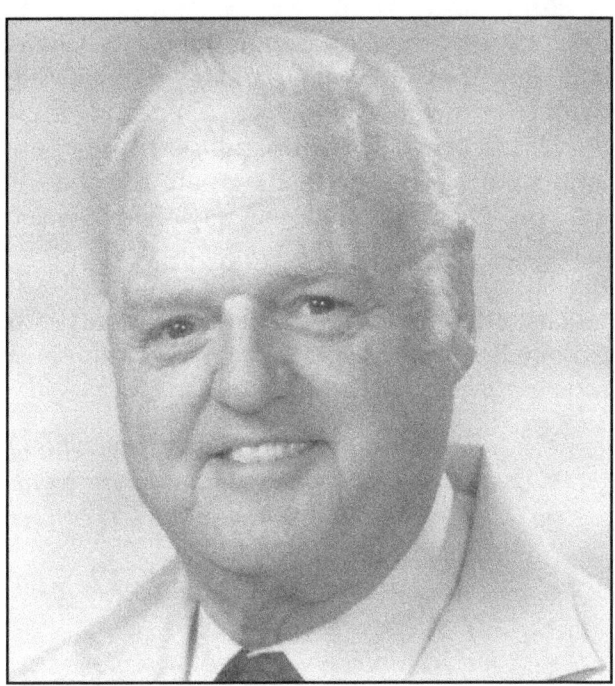

*Figure 2–14 Frank Folk*

was resented by the surgical residents, especially those in their last year of training. It became apparent as the years went by that the full-time system allowed a better supervision of patient care activities. More structured conferences were organized, research activities were encouraged, and clinical work of the house staff was better supervised and scrutinized.

In the late 1960s, Freeark made two moves to improve residents' training. First was the Lahey Clinic rotation. Two senior residents were selected for a two-month rotation with world-famous surgeons Drs. Kenneth Warren, Bentley

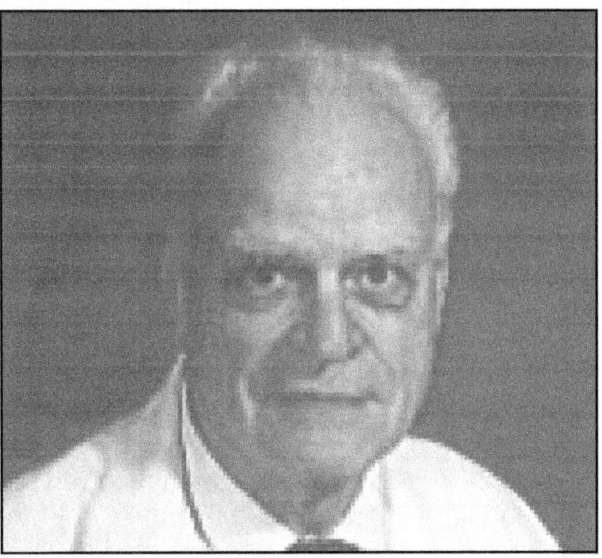

*Figure 2–15 William Shoemaker*

Colcock, and John Braasch at the Lahey Clinic. This proved to be an invaluable experience, especially in pancreatic-biliary surgery. The second was the recruitment of renowned surgeons in Chicago like George Block and Don Ferguson of the University of Chicago, and Otto Trippel and John J. Bergan of Northwestern to join the volunteer attending staff. These were leading surgeons in Chicago and their presence at County one day a week was most welcomed by residents.

Dr. Freeark eventually assumed the position of medical superintendent of the hospital on September 20, 1968, replacing the legendary Dr. Karl Meyer, much to the dismay of the latter's supporters in the medical staff and the Cook County Board, who had full control of the hospital. Ensuing raging political turmoil embroiled the hospital due to:

- *a lack of physician input in policymaking for the hospital*
- *a patronage system with an inefficient workforce*
- *inability to hire new employees or fire nonperforming political appointees*
- *lack of funding for critical patient care activities*
- *chronic shortage of nurses*
- *lack of ancillary services to relieve nonphysician functions from the house staff*
- *patient overcrowding*
- *lack of state-of-the-art laboratory facilities*

Dr. Freeark eventually resigned as medical superintendent of the hospital during early 1970 and was replaced by the then associate director, Dr. Clyde Philips, a well-trained and highly respected African-American general surgeon. Dr. Robert J. Freeark eventually became professor and chair of the Department of Surgery at Loyola Stritch School of Medicine and went on to establish a premiere academic surgical department at that institution. He also was instrumental in the establishment of a hospital and medical center for Loyola University in Maywood, Illinois, a suburb of Chicago.

After Dr. Freeark departed from CCH in 1969, Robert Baker took over as interim chair for the year of 1969. He was succeeded by Frank Folk who served as chair of surgery from 1970 to 1972. Both tried to manage the department in very difficult times.

The turmoil that engulfed the hospital (a continuum of a chronic problem since the hospital's establishment in 1866) did not abate until the late 1970s with recurring threats to close the hospital; house staff sit-ins and strikes; and frequent conflicts between the attending physicians, hospital administration, and the Cook County Board, especially over budget matters. In July of 1969, the State Legislature established the Health and Hospitals Governing Commission of Cook County, charged with planning and coordinating health care and overseeing the management of the County Hospital, the School of Nursing, and the Oak Forest Hospital. In 1973, the Commission received the added responsibility of operating the Cermak Memorial Hospital at the Cook County Jail. on November 23, 1970, Dr. James G. Haughton was appointed as the executive director of the Hospital

Commission. At the very beginning, conflicts occurred between the Hospital Commission, the attending physicians, and the house staff represented by the House staff Association, and led to the firing and resignation of competent and highly regarded physicians and the jailing of House staff Association leaders for contempt of court. Eventually, the Health and Hospitals Governing Commission was dissolved on November 30, 1979, by the Governor of the State with return of hospital control to the Cook County Board and eventual resignation of the executive director.

All of the old problems were never truly corrected, and crisis after crisis subsequently surfaced, including ongoing citations by JCAHo, old physical plant (it was considered substandard by the American College of Surgeons as far back as 1935), unjustified firing of an AIDS-infected physician, overcrowded and decrepit outpatient clinic, long waiting lines of patients to fill prescriptions (sometimes as long as eight hours), and many other problems resulting in rapid turnover of hospital directors. Repeated re-accreditation inspections made by JCAHo and IDPH were a constant source of dismay for the medical staff, Many of whom were frequently made scapegoat for institutional deficiencies that were beyond their control and responsibility.

## The Moss Era—1972–1977
### Interim Chair: Dr. Robert Moody, 1977

Dr. Gerald Moss, who completed his surgical training at Massachusetts General Hospital in Boston, a researcher and an expert in shock, was an assistant professor of surgery at the University of Illinois College of Medicine at Chicago and Chief of Surgery at the Westside VA Hospital in Chicago when he was recruited by Dr. John Beal, Chair of the Department of Surgery at Northwestern, and Dr. Lloyd M. Nyhus, Chair of the Department of Surgery at the University of Illinois, to the chairmanship of the Department of Surgery at Cook County Hospital. Moss assumed the position on August 13, 1972. At that time, due to the ongoing turmoil in the hospital, the previous attraction for a County internship diminished among graduates of American medical schools, especially those schools based in Chicago. In 1970, there were only 50 applicants through the National Intern Matching Program from American medical schools for the 140 intern positions, the rest filled with graduates of foreign medical schools, many of whom were from Cuba, Mexico, the Philippines, Thailand, India, and Hong Kong. Later, there was an influx of physicians from the Middle East, especially Iran.

At the time of Dr. Moss' appointment, the freestanding residency program in general surgery was on probation. He recruited outstanding graduates of the program, including Dr. John Saletta (Figure 2–16) who was then in private practice, as chair of the Division of General Surgery, and Dr. Hugh Firor, who replaced Dr. John Raffensperger as chair of the Division of Pediatric Surgery. He also retained outstanding surgical residents who completed their training at County, including Drs. Herand Abcarian in colon and rectal surgery, Ernestine Hambrick in general surgery, Leo Lim in vascular surgery, and Miguel Teresi and Avram Kraft in general surgery. With changes in the residency program, full accreditation was obtained. To relieve the house staff from nonphysician functions, Dr. Moss and Dr. Saletta developed a 15-month nurse practitioner program in the department. This program performed much of the nonphysician activities previously provided by the house staff. It was of great importance to the department and for patient care activities because at the time, the Residency Review Committee (RRC) in surgery reduced the number of surgical resident trainees, not only at County but throughout the United States with more stringent rules regarding supervision, scheduled educational activities, and scholarly activities with specific timelines for these activities. Dr. Avram Kraft was given the responsibility of directing the established nurse practitioner program. Trained nurses were assigned to the various surgical specialties with responsibilities that included attendance at all patient rounds, dressing changes, evaluation of wounds, initial evaluation of patient admissions in the hospital and in outpatient clinics, insertion of NG tubes and IV fluids including central lines, and assisting the physicians with the various functions needed to provide better care to the patients. In effect, the program supplanted some of the ward nursing functions but on a more comprehensive and focused patient care activity in the surgical services. Thirty-five nurses took this program, and nearly half of them were still in the Department of Surgery 15 years later.[2]

Dr. Moss appointed Dr. Robert Moody as chair of the Division of Neurosurgery in 1974. At this time, the freestanding residency program in neurosurgery lost its accreditation and became affiliated with the University of Illinois program. Other appointments included: Dr. Takayoshi Matsuda, a former County

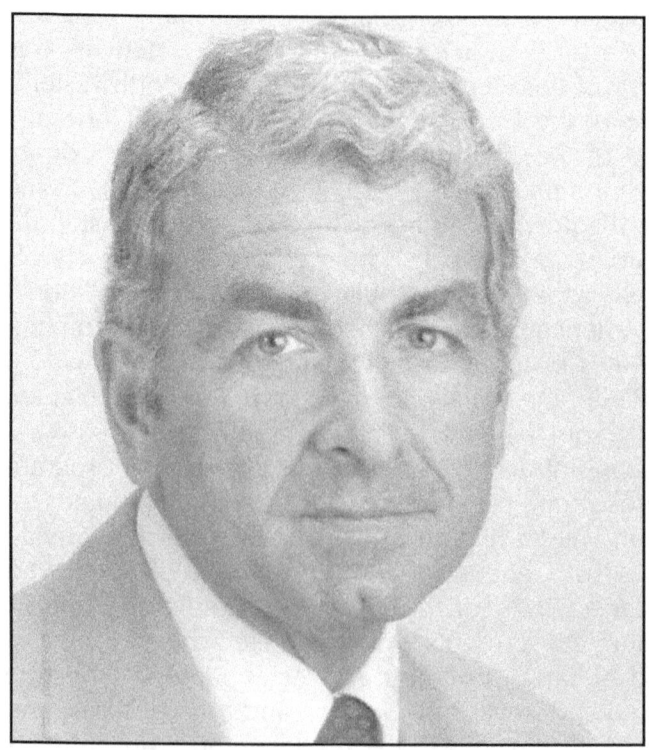

*Figure 2–16 John Saletta*

intern and surgical resident who returned from Japan to take over as Chair of the Division of Burn Surgery; Dr. Arsen Pankovich as Chair of Orthopedic Surgery; Dr. Sidney Blair as Chair of the Hand Service; Dr. Conrad Tasche, also a County intern, surgical resident, and plastic surgery resident as the Chair of the Division of Plastic Surgery; and Dr. Hernan M. Reyes as the combined Chair of the Division of Pediatric Surgery at County and Chief of the Section of Pediatric Surgery at the University of Illinois College of Medicine and Hospital in 1976. He was recruited jointly by Drs. Moss of CCH and Lloyd Nyhus of University of Illinois.

During this era, the surgical residency program was fully accredited, the faculty was greatly enhanced in all the surgical specialties, a nurse practitioner program was established and functional, and a much closer academic relationship with the University of Illinois was developed.

By 1976, 70 percent of the house staff were graduates of American medical schools. This was due in part to restrictions made by the government on foreign medical graduates entering this country for postgraduate education, an increased awareness of health care issues among the poor with a corresponding social consciousness among graduates of medical schools in this country, and an improved house staff work environment at County.

Dr. Moss resigned in 1977 to assume the chairmanship of the Department of Surgery at Michael Reese Hospital and Medical Center, where he continued his research in shock and blood volume replacement with nonblood products. He would later return to the University of Illinois College of Medicine and University Hospital as chair of the Department of Surgery, and following the upheavals that took place at that institution, he was subsequently appointed dean of the College of Medicine at the Chicago campus and executive dean of the University of Illinois College of Medicine systems.

## The Jonasson Era—1978–1986
### Interim Chair: Dr. Herand Abcarian, 1986

Dr. Olga Jonasson (Figure 2–17), a talented and skillful academic surgeon, was both a general surgeon and a renal transplant surgeon. She graduated from the University of Illinois College of Medicine at Chicago and obtained her surgical residency at the University of Illinois under Dr. Warren Cole. She completed her fellowship training in transplant surgery, and at the time of her recruitment and subsequent appointment as chair of the Department of Surgery at County, served as professor of surgery and chief of the section of transplant surgery at the University of Illinois College of Medicine and the University of Illinois Hospital.

There were ongoing conflicts between the House staff Association (approved by arbitration since 1974 as a bargaining unit representing the entire house staff) and the executive director of the Health and Hospital Governing Commission regarding salary structure and patient care issues, which led to a number of unsettling house staff strikes, several of their leaders going to jail for contempt of court charges, and firing of highly regarded attending physicians, including the then Chair of the Department of Medicine, Dr. Quentin Young. Despite these conflicts, the Department of Surgery, as well as the other clinical departments, continued on with their mission of providing quality health care to the poor and excellent education to the house staff. The volume and variety of clinical problems were of a magnitude that made the training programs attractive to applicants from medical schools in this country and abroad.

One of the very first things that took place during Dr. Jonasson's tenure was the full integration of the general surgery residency program with that of the University of Illinois residency program in general surgery. The freestanding General Surgery Residency Program at County had graduated hundreds of general surgeons and other surgical specialists throughout the country, some of whom gained prominence in their respective fields in clinical practice, academics, hospital administration, and research; it was eliminated. While there was a lot of resentment from the medical staff, especially the House staff Association, with the changes, the integration eventually proved to be the right decision in order to improve the quality of the educational program. Conjoined appointments of attending physicians from the various surgical divisions and sections of CCH and the University of Illinois were made, and postgraduate training affiliations took place.

In general surgery, Dr. Philip Donahue, an associate professor of surgery and attending surgeon at the West Side VA Hospital, was appointed chair of the Division of General Surgery and professor of surgery at the University of Illinois. Drs. Katherine Liu, a graduate of the University of Chicago residency program, and Subash Patel were recruited as junior attending surgeons; Dr. Samuel Appavu became the chair of the Division of Surgical Critical Care; and Dr. Robert J. Lowe, a trainee of Dr. Freeark, remained as chief of the trauma unit. Following his death from cancer in 1982, Dr. Lowe was succeeded by Dr. John Barrett. Dr. William Powell, chair of the Division of Otolaryngology, had residents rotating to the

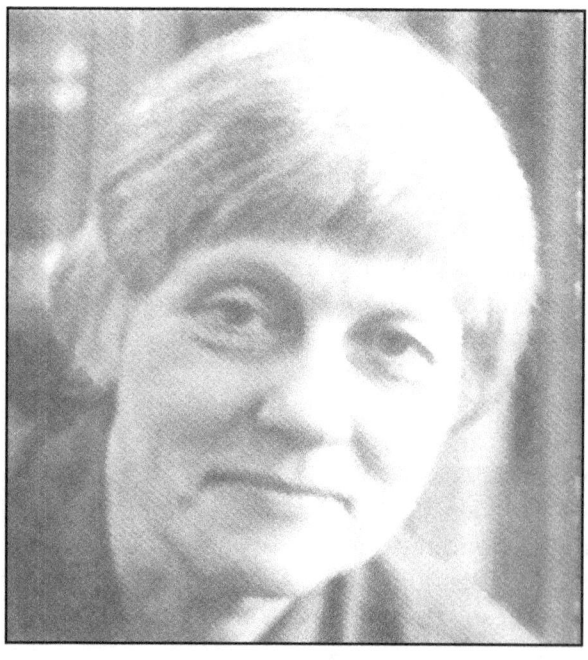

*Figure 2–17  Olga Jonasson*

service as an affiliated institution from the University of Illinois and Northwestern University programs. Dr. Alan Axelrod, chief of ophthalmology, along with his staff, maintained a freestanding residency in ophthalmology. Dr. James Stone, who succeeded Dr. Robert Moody as acting chair of the Division of Neurosurgery, received a faculty appointment at the University of Illinois and had residents rotating from the University of Illinois program.

Dr. Robert Hall, who succeeded Dr. Arsen Pankovich as acting chair of the Division of orthopedic Surgery, maintained an extremely busy service (probably the busiest and most productive in the Department of Surgery); he had two orthopedic services staffed separately by rotating residents from the University of Illinois and Northwestern University orthopedic programs. Most members of the attending staff were part-time salaried physicians. It was impossible to recruit full-time staff in the Division of Orthopedic Surgery because of the low salary offered at County.

The Division of Surgical Oncology was a unified service with the University of Illinois. Dr. Tapas Das Gupta, the professor and chief of the Division of Surgical Oncology at the University of Illinois simultaneously occupied the chair of the division at County. Members of the staff at the University of Illinois were all part-time salaried attending staff at County. This service, together with the Division of Pediatric Surgery, had a unified and integrated attending staff with parallel services at the University and the County. This relationship was actually the best example of an ideal symbiotic system of patient care and education in a county hospital and a university hospital. The Division of Oral Surgery and Dentistry, with its freestanding residency program in general dentistry and oral surgery, was headed by Dr. John Sisto. While thoracic surgery was performed at County, patients who were candidates for cardiac surgery were transferred to the University of Illinois for care. Dr. Takayoshi Matsuda remained as chair of the Division of Burn. The hand service was effectively integrated with the Division of Orthopedic Surgery, although some cases were done in the plastic surgery service. An acting chair was in charge of the Division of Plastic Surgery upon the appointment of Dr. Conrad Tasche as Director of Medical Education and Coordinator of the Internship program. A sex-change operation that was being performed at that time was discontinued upon pressure from the hospital administration. The Division of Urology, chaired by Dr. Patrick Guinan, received residents from the University of Illinois program in addition to a surgical intern assigned to the service.

A sense of relative calm settled in during the decade of the 1980s, although chronic problems associated with an old and outdated facility continued to plague delivery of services at the hospital. Numerous deficiencies were cited regarding cleanliness in the wards and other patient care facilities, lack of nurses, overcrowding, and long waiting lines in the outpatient clinics, pharmacy, and emergency room.

In 1986, Dr. Jonasson resigned as chair of the department and accepted a position as Zollinger Professor and chairperson of the Department of Surgery at Ohio State University and Surgeon-in-Chief of the University Hospital. Dr. Herand Abcarian, Chair of the Division of Colon and Rectal Surgery, served as the acting chair of the department until November of 1986. He subsequently went on to become the professor and chair of the Department of Surgery at the University of Illinois College of Medicine and the University Hospital upon the retirement of Dr. Lloyd Nyhus.

## The Reyes Era—1986–1998

Following a national search that lasted more than six months, Dr. Hernan M. Reyes, who was then the chair of the Division of Pediatric Surgery, was recommended by the search committee for appointment as chair of the Department of Surgery. He received this appointment from the hospital director in December 1986 on an acting basis and full appointment as the permanent chair by the Cook County Board on January 6, 1987.

Under the leadership of Reyes, the department was reorganized as follows.

### Organization

An overall organizational structure was reviewed. Permanent chairs of the various divisions were appointed and sections within the divisions were created where needed to improve patient care activities.

Initially, there were 13 surgical divisions:
- *Burn: Dr. Takayoshi Matsuda remained as chair of the Division of Burn.*
- *Cardiothoracic: A series of part-time chairs of the Division of Cardiothoracic Surgery were appointed following the departure of Dr. Constantine Tatooles: Drs. Robert Gasior, Vincent Kucich, and Cyrus Serry. Dr. William Warren was appointed section chief of Thoracic Surgery*
- *General Surgery: Dr. Philip Donahue was recruited as full-time chair of the Division of General Surgery.*
- *Neurosurgery: Dr. James Stone headed Neurosurgery.*
- *Ophthalmology: Dr. Alan Axelrod headed Ophthalmology.*
- *ENT & Head/Neck Surgery: Dr. William Powell headed ENT*
- *Orthopedic Surgery: Dr. Robert Hall headed Orthopedic Surgery.*
- *Oral Surgery/Dentistry: Dr. John Sisto headed Oral Surgery/Dentistry.*
- *Pediatric Surgery: Dr. Reyes retained his position as chair of the Division of Pediatric Surgery.*
- *Plastic and Reconstructive Surgery: Dr. Mimis Cohen, who was then chair of Plastic Surgery at the University of Illinois, was recruited as chair at County in a dual role.*
- *Surgical Oncology: Dr. Tapas Das Gupta remained as chair of Surgical Oncology and also as Section Chief of Oncology at the University of Illinois.*
- *Trauma: Dr. John Barrett was chief of Trauma.*
- *Urology: Dr. Paul Ray headed Urology.*

The new surgical divisions immediately created were:
- *Colon/Rectal Surgery: with Dr. Charles Orsay as chair.*
- *Surgical Critical Care: with Dr. Samuel Appavu.*
- *Theoretical Surgery: Dr. Harry Richter was appointed chair of*

*Theoretical Surgery, the division given the responsibility of monitoring and enhancing research activities in the department, which were conducted at the Hektoen Institute of Medical Research. Dr. Robert Walter, who had a PhD in microbiology, was made supervisor in the division.*

In 1994, the Divisions of Trauma and Burn were made into the Department of Trauma Surgery. This was agreed to because of the inordinate amount of resources needed to maintain a Level I Adult Trauma Center, which was draining the resources allocated for the Department to the disadvantage of the other surgical divisions. Subsequently, the Divisions of Breast Oncology and Vascular Surgery were created with Drs. Elizabeth Marcus and Richard Keene as chairs, respectively. In the year 1995, there were 16 administrative divisions in the Department of Surgery with their respective sections. This organizational structure remained until the end of the 20th century.

**Attending Staff**

The most obvious reason for failure to recruit well-trained and motivated full-time attending staff was the low salary at County, which was not competitive with the academic and private sectors. This dilemma was similarly experienced in the retention of faculty who after a few years would move elsewhere, either in academia or in private practice for economic reasons. Difficulty in recruitment greatly affected surgical education of residents. This problem was especially critical in all of the surgical subspecialties where a physician who recently completed fellowship training in a subspecialty would receive a salary much higher than a senior surgeon at County. A solution to this problem was partially implemented by a conjoint faculty recruitment with the University of Illinois in which an attending physician received part-time salary from both institutions that when combined, was nearly equal to that offered in the job market. There are obvious disadvantages to this arrangement in that the physician is committed to each institution on a part-time basis and eventually, the service provided in one of the participating institutions could be less than the other for a variety of reasons. The arrangement did not foster loyalty and individual performance in clinical work or education of students and house staff, and scholarly productivity was fragmented and far from focused.

In order to improve the situation, the department chair worked with the hospital administration to upgrade attending surgeon salaries to the 50th percentile of the AAMC in the Midwest. With attrition from part-time attending surgeons and converting part-time positions to full-time positions, the upgrade in salaries was shown to be budget-neutral. This plan was subsequently approved by the Cook County Board, and when fully implemented, the total number of salaried attending staff in the department was 73 (35 full-time, 38 part-time) as compared to a previous staffing of 81 attending surgeons (38 full-time and 43 part-time). The new salary scale became more attractive and allowed recruitment of full-time faculty so that new programs (a distinct breast service, implementation of an upgraded tumor registry in compliance with the requirements of the ACS Cancer Committee, a full-time peripheral vascular service, resumption of the cardiac surgery program at County, availability of consultants to sister institutions such as Provident Hospital and Oak Forest Hospital, development of newer technology such as the evolving advances in minimally invasive surgery, and more time allotted for teaching, supervision of patient care activities, and research) could be implemented. Additionally, an in-house attending surgeon on call was initiated primarily for coverage of emergency general surgery cases and to act as an administrator for the Department of Surgery to resolve problems that might occur during the night, weekends, and on holidays for which the department chair or a specific division chair was not available. The reduction in the number of attending physicians did not, in fact, decrease the clinical productivity but had the opposite effect as repeatedly shown based on annual reports.

**Clinical Activity**

The clinical work in the department consisted of both outpatient and inpatient activity. Outpatient clinics were established in all the surgical divisions. For the most part, each service within the division conducted a minimum of two half-day clinics each week. All residents assigned to the service were expected to participate in all outpatient clinic activity. Patients were referred to the clinic from outside sources as well as from the emergency room of the hospital or other specialties in the institution. Additionally, postoperative patients were followed up on a regular basis in these clinics. All clinics were supervised by the attending physician assigned to the specific service. The increase in clinical activity was observed despite the reduction in the number of attending physicians: 81 (1994) versus 73 (1996) and a corresponding decrease in the total number of surgical residents from 108 (1995) to 99 (1996) to 85 (1998). The decrease in the total residents was a result of cutbacks required from new regulations promulgated by the various residency review committees of the ACGME, as well as the result of a study made on the department regarding the work load of general surgery residents and its impact on their education.[4]

There were sentinel improvements during this era. First, the cardiac surgery program was re-instituted in 1991. Prior to this date, an agreement was made that patients requiring open-heart surgery were to be transferred to the University of Illinois for the procedure. Unfortunately, the patients from County were frequently delayed in receiving needed operative intervention, oftentimes cancelled with preferential treatment given to patients at the University. It reached the point where the CCH Department of Medicine threatened to transfer their patients requiring operative intervention to institutions other than the University of Illinois. Unfortunately, the threat was hollow, because other institutions rarely accepted patients being transferred from County. This dilemma prompted the chair of the Department of Surgery to re-institute the cardiac surgery program. While sporadic cases were being done at County under the leadership of Dr. Robert Gasior, who started the program, a more consistent schedule was accomplished when Dr. Vincent Kucich was recruited on a full-time basis, and agreed to come to County despite the low salary that the department could offer. The first 100 cases done by Dr. Kucich, which included complex coronary bypass procedures with valve replacement, had no mortality whatsoever. Despite these efforts, close scrutiny was implemented to the program with thorough review of each case, and any mortality or morbidity that followed. Unfortunately, Dr. Kucich decided to join a group in the southwest suburbs of Chicago in private practice and the program was taken over by the attending staff from the Rush Department of Cardiovascular Surgery.

In an attempt to improve the care of patients with breast cancer, the department chair recruited Dr. Elizabeth Marcus, a graduate of Rosewell Park Cancer Center surgical oncology program, to be the full-time director of the breast surgery service. The mandate was to make sure that a patient with a breast lesion who was seen in the clinic would undergo mammography and/or needle aspiration biopsy, and would be advised the same day as to whether additional surgery or other treatment was needed. It was an ambitious program, but it was one way of making sure patients were not lost to follow-up, especially those patients whose initial biopsy revealed a cancerous lesion. The program was developed to prevent occurrences as in the past when a patient would return several months after an initial biopsy only to find a more extensive disease.

As part of an ongoing process to improve patient care, an outdated cancer registry was replaced with an electronically automated record system utilizing current programs recommended by the Cancer Committee of the American College of Surgeons. Dr. John Greager—who subsequently succeeded Dr. Das Gupta as chair of the Surgical Oncology Division, in conjunction with Dr. Emily Pang, chair of Medical Oncology—installed and implemented this new program. While there was discord and lack of acceptance from the older members of the tumor registry staff, it was obvious that a modernized system was needed for better patient care.

The advent of laparoscopic surgery changed the way surgeons were trained. In the early 1990s, with medical centers throughout the country establishing their own minimally invasive programs, the department chair established a learning (skill) laboratory and operating room at the Hektoen Institute of Medical Research for both the resident and attending staff. Dr. Philip Donahue, chair of the Division of General Surgery, took the leadership in recruiting Dr. Miguel Teresi to oversee the program and make sure that all members of the attending staff in general surgery attended courses and received hands-on experience in the laboratory prior to implementing the procedure in clinical practice at the institution. Equipment was procured and laparoscopic surgery was initiated, starting with cholecystectomy, hernia repair, and appendectomy, later expanding to advanced laparoscopic procedures. The operating room in the laboratory at Hektoen was maintained for instruction of residents and attending surgeons.

A summary of the individual divisions' clinical achievements towards the beginning of 1997 showed the following:

- *The Division of Breast Oncology, which was created in August 1996, changed the clinic functions from a resident-run to an attending-driven model, thereby ensuring proper continuity of care and improving the overall quality of care provided to the patients.*
- *A multidisciplinary clinic was started in conjunction with the staff of the medical oncology service to develop a unified rational approach to the treatment of patients with locally advanced breast*

cancer. Drs. Elizabeth Marcus, division chair, and Kambiz Dowlat, a part-time member of the attending staff from Rush, led the changes in this division.

- The Division of Colon and Rectal Surgery, led by Dr. Charles Orsay, fully realized a functioning computerized video-endoscopic unit with close to 2,000 gastrointestinal endoscopic procedures performed. The division was the only unit that actively placed esophageal stents for malignant lesions of the esophagus to facilitate oral intake. Additionally, the staff closely worked with the HRD (HIV-related disease) clinic to provide leading edge treatment and computerized registry for patients with ano-rectal disease infected with HIV. The stoma registry of the division was claimed to be the most comprehensive and the largest in the world.
- The Division of General Surgery, under the leadership of Dr. Philip Donahue, continued to excel in its laparoscopic program. The practice at County of laparoscopic surgery included routine cases (cholecystectomy and appendectomy) as well as advanced laparoscopic procedures such as adrenalectomy, splenectomy, hiatus hernia repair, achalasia, and vagotomy. Over 80 percent of the patients with cholelithiasis had laparoscopic procedures.
- In the field of endocrine surgery, led by Dr. Subash Patel, the volume and complexity of the case load increased substantially.
- In the Division of Surgical Critical Care headed by Dr. Samuel Appavu, the observed patient survival rate was 90 percent despite an increasing acuity of the patients' illness. Several improvements in care included the elimination of manually injected cardiac output technology to eliminate the risk of nosocomial bacterial infections, inclusion of hypercapnia ventilation with their ventilation application techniques, improved blood gas measurements at bedside, and introduction of a technique for continuous blood gas monitoring.
- On the research side, the staff was involved in evaluating the pathophysiology and risk factors of perioperative myocardial infarction from inpatient and outpatient surgery.
- The Division of Surgical Oncology under Dr. John Greager pioneered an aggressive multimodal, neo-adjuvant treatment approach for esophageal and head and neck cancer patients, and initiated new efforts to further improve survival utilizing new agents such as Gemzar.

Since the establishment of Level I pediatric trauma centers in Chicago, the trauma center at the Children's Hospital of CCH experienced a steady increase in the number of patients admitted to the service. Through the initiative of Dr. John

R. Hall, section chief of pediatric trauma, which was supported by the department chair and division chiefs of neurosurgery and orthopedic surgery, unified treatment protocols were established for major traumatic conditions, leading to an improved survival of severely injured children. Furthermore, this dynamic protocol allowed changes to practices that did not work and usage of those that did without the random changes initiated by the physician on duty that day, especially illustrated in severely injured children suffering from head injuries, major orthopedic injuries, and blunt and penetrating injuries of the head and neck, torso, and abdomen. At the time, the observed mortality rate at the Pediatric Trauma Center at County was less than the expected mortality rate as reported by the National Pediatric Trauma Registry when comparing various pediatric trauma centers in the country. Furthermore, the Pediatric Trauma Center at County had one of the top three outcomes in head injury in children in North America, and was the sole unit where the outcome of infants with severe head trauma was as good as that of older children as reported by the National Pediatric Trauma Registry. The division was an early advocate for the nonoperative treatment of solid organ injuries secondary to blunt trauma of the abdomen, evaluation of blunt injuries of the abdomen by a double contrast CT scan instead of an invasive peritoneal lavage, selective operative treatment of penetrating Zone II neck injuries, and the nonoperative treatment of small vessel injuries of the lower extremities from gunshot wounds.

**Education**

As it has always been in the past, third-year medical students from Rush Medical College, University of Illinois College of Medicine at Chicago, and Chicago Medical School obtain part of their surgical clerkship at Cook County Hospital. In the biennium covering the years 1995–1996, 208 third-year medical students from the above medical schools rotated through the various surgical specialties but primarily in general surgery at County. There were 85 residents in the various surgical specialties assigned to three freestanding residency programs (Ophthalmology, General Dentistry, and Oral Surgery), three integrated programs (General Surgery, Plastic and Reconstructive Surgery, and Colon-Rectal Surgery), five affiliated (Cardiothoracic, Neurosurgery, Plastic and Reconstructive, Otolaryngology, and Orthopedics) ACGME/ADA approved residency and fellowship programs, and one unapproved fellowship program in surgical critical care. Thirty-six surgical residents were assigned to the general surgery services including surgical oncology, pediatric surgery, and vascular surgery at County through the Rush integrated program. Although affiliated programs remained with the University of Illinois, Northwestern, and Loyola University Medical Schools, the primary integrated and affiliated programs were with the Rush Medical College and Rush Medical Center. The 26 percent downsizing of the resident staff was justified by a departmental study as alluded to above, in which a typical resident worked 3,990 hours annually or 81 hours per week exclusive of a three-week vacation but inclusive of eight hours of didactic lectures and conferences per week. This approximated that described in another study[4] as ideal work hours for an ideal general surgery workload. This carefully crafted program was geared toward education without consideration of service needs in an urban public hospital. It was made possible by proper coordination of clinical activities, eliminating overlapping services, on-site attending physician supervision and active participation with resident clinical activities, and appropriate utilization of nonphysician extenders for ancillary, noneducational functions. This program allows a humane resident workload without compromising patient care.

A long-standing identity problem has existed with regards to the educational programs at Cook County Hospital. Prior to 1960, almost all voluntary attending physicians were from Rush Medical School. There had been numerous recommendations in the past to divide clinical services and turn the control of the educational programs to two or three of the Chicago area medical schools. The recommendation was either ignored or simply not implemented, resulting in multiple institutional affiliations based on the department chair's or the division chair's established relationships and preferences while maintaining freestanding residency programs. The system lent itself to a morass of agreements, especially with respect to resident salary reimbursement to the affiliated institutions, often leaving the County at a financial disadvantage.

In 1993, the hospital administration and the executive medical staff discussed the relevance of the various postgraduate training programs and the multiple medical school affiliations that currently existed. While there were deeply rooted relationships between clinical departments or divisions with specific medical school programs, it was obvious to everyone that the ideal partnership was a single institutional academic affiliation. It was believed that this relationship would allow better integration of services and sharing of resources, enable the County patient to utilize the University's tertiary care services such as transplant and cardiac surgery, and increase research collaboration and productivity, all of which would ultimately enhance patient care at County. Despite the advantages of a single-institution academic affiliation, it was also obvious that certain clinical services such as neurosurgery and orthopedic surgery, where the number of residents trained in a single program were limited, could not be fulfilled by a single program at County.

One of the considerations relevant to the educational program of the Department of Surgery was the need for an integrated program that would allow exposure of a surgical resident to the volume and variety of patients seen in a public hospital, as well as the type of patients seen in a private medical center. At the same time, it was believed that part-time salaried attending physicians who maintained a private practice in a major private medical center in close proximity to County were a better arrangement as compared to those currently on the staff whose practices were quite a distance from County. With the consent and approval of the executive medical staff, the hospital director sent a letter to all the Chicago area medical schools requesting a dialogue for a single academic affiliation with County. To the medical staff's surprise, Rush University Medical Center, which was located a block away from Cook County Hospital, was the sole institution that offered to affiliate and/or integrate all their postgraduate education programs with Cook County Hospital. After repeated discussions and meetings between the hospital administration and the leaders of the medical staff at both institutions, a master affiliation agreement was signed and approved by the Cook County Board as well as the trustees of Rush University Medical Center (at the time it was named Rush-Presbyterian-St. Luke's Medical Center) in 1994.

Prior to implementing such an agreement, the department chair at County wrote a letter to the chair of general surgery at Rush and the chair of surgery at the University of Illinois, suggesting a discussion on having a unified general surgery residency program at the Westside VA Medical Center consisting of an integrated program between the University of Illinois, Rush, and Cook County Hospital. While the chair at Rush was in favor of exploring the possibility of joining the individual programs, the concept was not considered at all by the other parties.

Since the various surgical specialties at Rush were separate departments whereas they were divisions at Cook County Hospital. It was agreed that the chairman of surgery at County would co-ordinate all integrations or affiliations with Rush, thereby requiring that he be involved in all the discussions between the division heads of a specialty at County and the corresponding chair at Rush. The integrated general surgery program was gradually phased in, starting with the first-year residents during the first year of the integration and a gradual phasing out of the University of Illinois residents. This arrangement was implemented without any adverse impact to individual residents from both the Rush and the University of Illinois programs. Implementation of the integration with Rush and disaffiliation with the University of Illinois was approved fully by the Residency Review Committee for Surgery of the ACGME. Dr. Reyes, who previously served as associate program director of the general surgery residency at the University of Illinois, resigned that position and assumed a similar position with the Rush program. Furthermore, because of his involvement with the other surgical specialty affiliations, he was appointed assistant dean at Rush Medical College.

By 1998, the following residency programs were integrated with Rush University Medical Center: general surgery, neurosurgery, cardiothoracic surgery, vascular surgery, and orthopedic surgery. Affiliated programs were maintained with the University of Illinois in colon-rectal surgery, plastic surgery, orthopedic surgery, and ENT/head and neck surgery; with Northwestern University in orthopedic surgery and ENT/head and neck surgery; and with Loyola University in neurosurgery.

Affiliations with multiple institutions in orthopedic surgery, neurosurgery, and ENT/head and neck surgery were inevitable because of the small number of trainees from each program and the larger number of residents needed at County. The plastic surgery program at the University of Illinois only graduated one resident per year, and the division chair at County was also the section chief at the University of Illinois. The colon-rectal surgery program likewise graduated one fellow per year, and there did not appear to be any advantage to changing the existing affiliation. The Division of Urology opted not to have any residents and decided to be an attending-run service with a junior general surgery resident assigned to the service. Three programs remained freestanding because of the large size of the program at County: oral surgery, general dentistry, and ophthalmology.

The result of this affiliation was having a number of general surgery attending physicians admitted to the staff at Rush University Medical Center, thereby enabling them to have a limited private practice. Conjoined recruitment of attending surgeons in cardiac surgery, general surgery, pediatric surgery, and surgical oncology was facilitated with a base salary funding from County. The opportunity to enhance the individual's income with a private practice at Rush made the appointment to County an attractive option to a young, talented, and potentially productive surgical specialist.

Dr. Reyes strongly recommended that County, being a public hospital, should ensure that medical students at the third- and fourth-year level from all the Chicago area medical schools be allowed rotations to Cook County Hospital to be exposed to the care of the poor and uninsured patients in a public hospital setting. The following members of the attending staff in the department were assigned responsibilities to supervise medical student rotations from schools that requested such a rotation: Drs. Subash Patel and John Greager for Rush, Drs. Harry Richter and Samuel Appavu for the University of Illinois, and Drs. Janet L. Meller and Katherine Liu for Chicago Medical School.

In 1998, Dr. Reyes opted for the early retirement that was offered all County employees. He stayed on for six months beyond the deadline set for the early retirement period at the behest of the hospital administration and the Cook County Board. Toward the end of his tenure in office, construction started on the new Cook County Hospital building, implementing all the recommendations of the Department of Surgery with regard to the physical structure and configuration of the surgical wards, operating rooms, surgical and neurosurgical intensive care units, and specialty surgical outpatient clinics. Upon Dr. Reyes' retirement on August 30, 2008, Dr. Philip Donahue, then chair of the Division of General Surgery, was appointed interim department chair. He served until the County Board appointed a new chair recommended by the search committee and the hospital administration.

## The New Cook County Hospital/John H. Stroger Jr. Hospital—2000–

In 2002, a new replacement hospital was completed with significant cost overruns, and all medical services were transferred to this facility. There was no open surgical ward in the new facility. The hospital was renamed John H. Stroger Jr. Hospital in memory of Cook County President John H. Stroger Jr. With the name change, the illustrious Cook County Hospital ended its 136 years of service as a center for medical education and a hospital for all, regardless of race, wealth, or creed. A new health care delivery system had just begun.

# References

1. *History of Medicine and Physicians and Surgeons of Chicago*. Chicago: The Biographical Publishing Corporation; 1922.
2. *Chicago Med J*. 1866;23.
3. Raffensperger JG, Ed. *The old Lady on Harrison: Cook County Hospital, 1833–1995*. New York: Peter Lang Publishing Group; 1997.
4. Beck C, Beck WC, Moody R. Clinical Activity at Cook County Hospital: Reminiscences of Three Eras. *Proc Inst Med Chgo* (Part I-1987;40:50-51; (Part II-1987;40:133-140; Part III :1988;41:14-15.
5. McNealy RW. The Influence of Cook County Hospital on Medical Education in the United States. *Q Bull N U Med Sch* 1957;31:169–173.
6. Dragstedt LR. Christian Fenger and the Midwestern School of Surgery. *Guthrie Clin Bull* 1963;33:13–24.
7. Wentz DK, Ford CV. Brief History of the Internship. *JAMA* 1984;252:3390–3394.
8. Freeark RJ. In Lewis S, *Hospital: An oral History of Cook County Hospital*. New York: The New Press; 1995; 109.
9. History of Accreditation of Medical Education Programs. *JAMA*. 1983;250: 1502–1508.
10. Britt LD. Graduate Medical Education and Residency Review Committee: History and Challenges. *Am Surg*. 2007;73:136–139.
11. Flexner A. *Medical Education in the United States and Canada: A Report to the Carnegie Foundation for the Advancement of Teaching. Bulletin 4*. Boston: Merrymount Press;1910.
12. Hart D. Historical Aspects of Surgical Residency Programs. *N C Med J* 1964;25:43–48.
13. Meyer KA. Historical Background of Cook County Hospital. *Q Bull NU Med Sch*. 1949;23:271–275.
14. Halsted WS. The Training of the Surgeon. *Johns Hopkins Hosp Bull*. 1904;15:267–275.
15. Rutkow IM. *American Surgery: An Illustrated History*. Philadelphia: Lippincott-Raven; 1998.
16. Grillo JC. Edward D. Churchill and the "Rectangular" Surgical Residency. *Surgery*. 2004:136:947–952.
17. Wangensteen oH, Wangensteen SD. The Surgical Amphitheatre. In Wangensteen oH, Wangensteen SD. *The Rise of Surgery: From Empire Craft to Scientific Discipline*. Minneapolis: University of Minnesota Press; 1978:453–473.
18. Meyer KA, Hyman S. *John B. Murphy: An Inquiry into his Life and Scientific Achievements*. J. B. Murphy Memorial Lecture, Chicago Medical Society, Chicago, September 16, 1959.
19. Printen K. Personal communication.

# Section II

*Contribution of Chicago Area Medical Schools to Surgery at CCH*

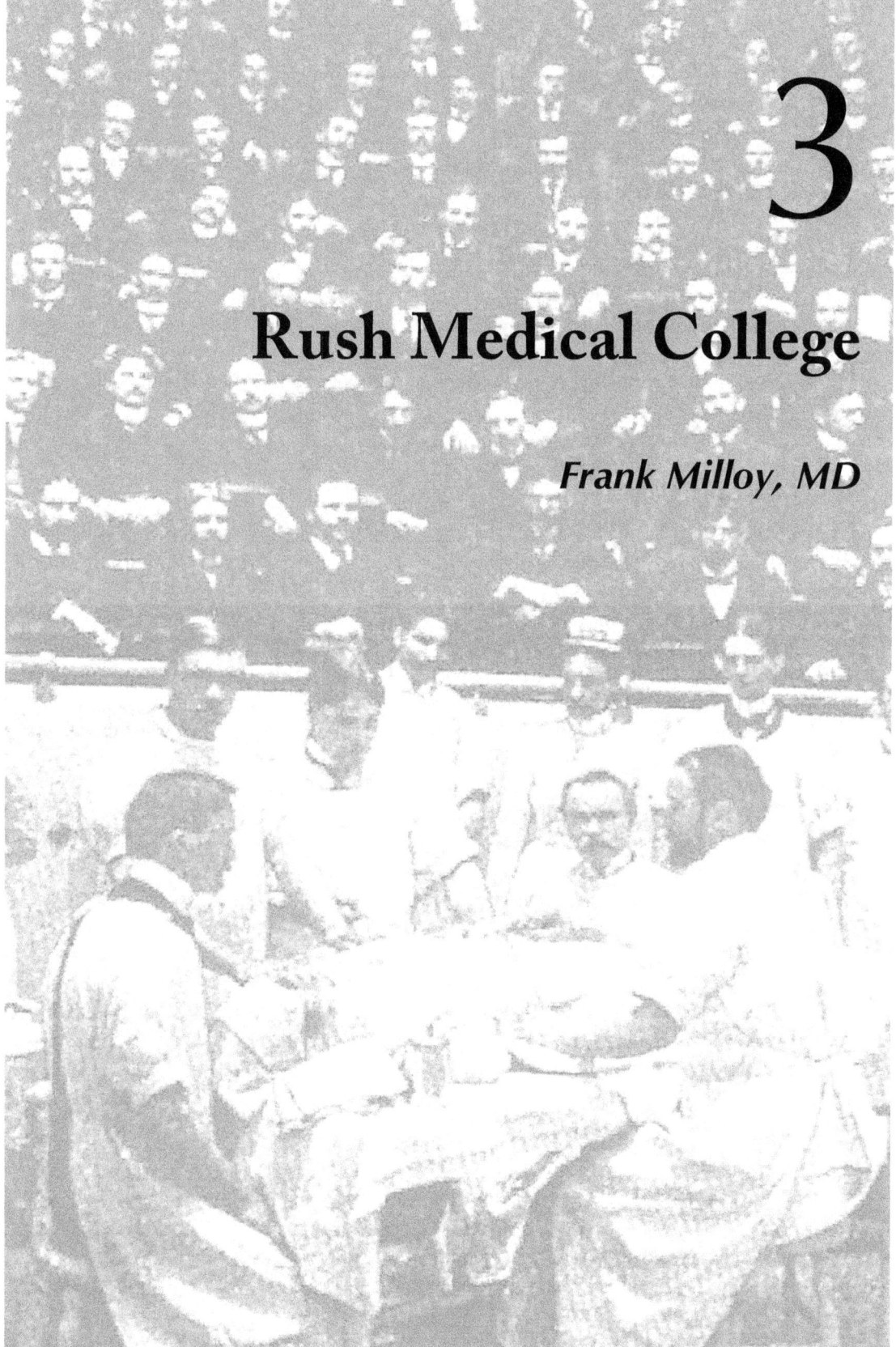

# 3
# Rush Medical College

*Frank Milloy, MD*

- Rush Medical College
- Daniel Brainard
- Moses Gunn
- Charles Parkes
- Edwin Powell
- Christian Fenger
- Nicolas Senn
- John B. Murphy
- Arthur Dean Bevan
- Rush and University of Chicago
- Rush Faculty at Cook County Hospital
- Presbyterian/St. Luke's Merger
- Reopening of Rush Medical College and Renewing Old Acquaintances with CCH
- References

## Rush Medical College

Rush Medical College, the first medical school in Chicago, was founded by Dr. Daniel Brainard. This new college, like its city, gained its charter in the first week of March 1837. The school was named after Benjamin Rush, MD, physician, statesman, and a signer of the Declaration of Independence. During the first century of operation, more than 10,000 physicians received their training at Rush Medical College; a "Rush Doctor" was a highly prized commodity in the American West of the 19th century. Rush physicians were of driving force at County Hospital, and many of Chicago's leading physicians (Nathan Smith Davis, William Quinne, James Herrick, Frank Billings, George Amerman, Joseph Ross) were faculty members. After the Chicago fire of 1871, Rush built a medical school at 761 West Harrison Street, close by Cook County Hospital (Figure 3–1).

Rush Medical College was affiliated with the University of Chicago from 1898 until 1942. With the onset of World War II, Rush suspended its educational program and moved its faculty to the University of Illinois. In 1969, the Charter of the Medical College was reactivated when it became part of Presbyterian-St. Luke's Medical Center, which changed its name to Rush University Medical Center. In 1971, Rush Medical College reopened with a class of 66 first-year students. In 1994, Rush renewed its academic affiliation with Cook County Hospital, and the Department of Surgery at County is now part of the Rush University Medical Center program.

## Daniel Brainard

Daniel Brainard was born May 15, 1812, in the town of Western, Oneida County, New York. At age 16, he decided on a career in medicine. He was apprenticed first to Dr. R. S. Sykes, his family's physician, for a year, and then for two years to Dr. Harold H. Pope of nearby Rome, New York. After these three years of preceptorship, he entered Fairfield Medical College, also known as the College

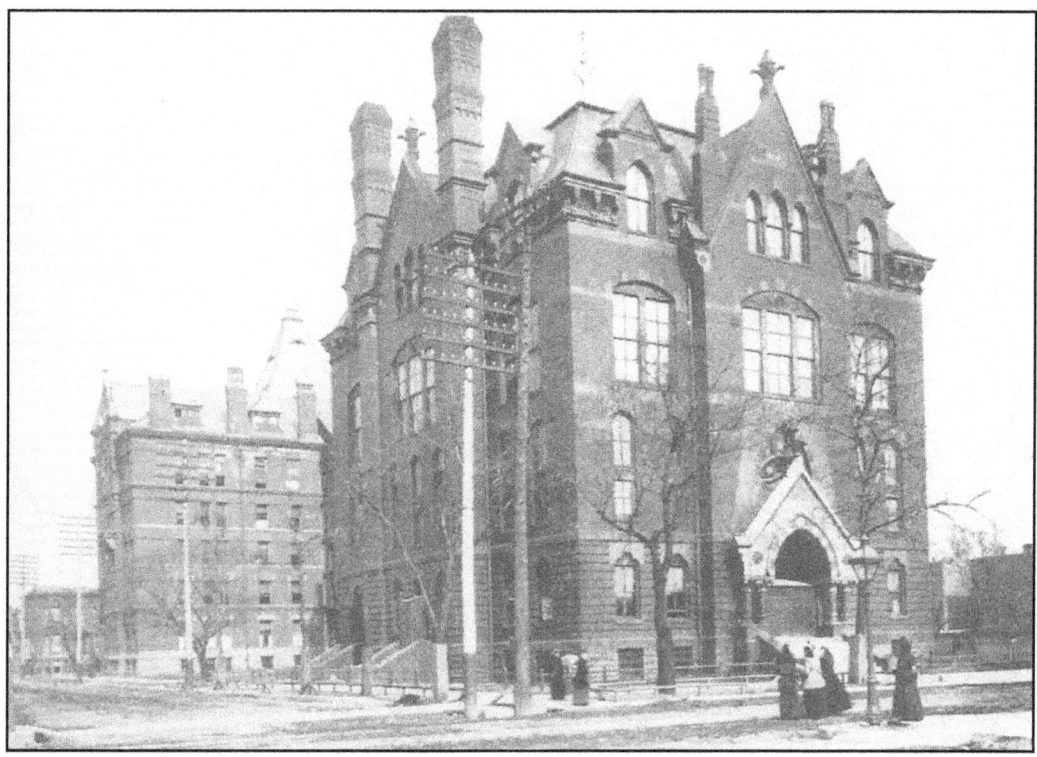

*Figure 3–1 Rush Medical College, 761 West Harrison Street*

of Physicians and Surgeons of the Western District of the State of New York. The school had been founded in the small town of Fairfield in 1809 and numbered 205 students when Daniel arrived in the autumn of 1831.[1]

In 1832, after a year at Fairfield, Brainard entered Jefferson Medical School in Philadelphia (Figure 3–2). In those days, Philadelphia was the largest city in the United States and had two medical colleges. The University of Pennsylvania College, America's first medical school, was founded in 1765 at America's first hospital, founded in 1752. Jefferson was founded in 1825, and like other medical schools, it had a four-month series of lectures from November 1 to March 1, the time of year when farming activity was at a minimum. For graduation as an MD, a student was required to attend the same series of lectures twice, in two consecutive years.[1-2]

After graduation from Jefferson, Brainard returned to his home town where Dr. Sykes had offered him an association. However, Daniel preferred to leave New York State and go west. He took a boat to Detroit where he bought a pony and followed the trail to Chicago.

In the autumn of 1835, a bedraggled Dr. Daniel Brainard rode up to the Chicago office of John Dean Caton, a lawyer and friend he had known during his time in Rome, New York. His sole possessions were the contents of his saddlebags and the Indian pony, which he soon sold for needed cash. John Caton offered him a table in his office where he could sit to see patients and where he

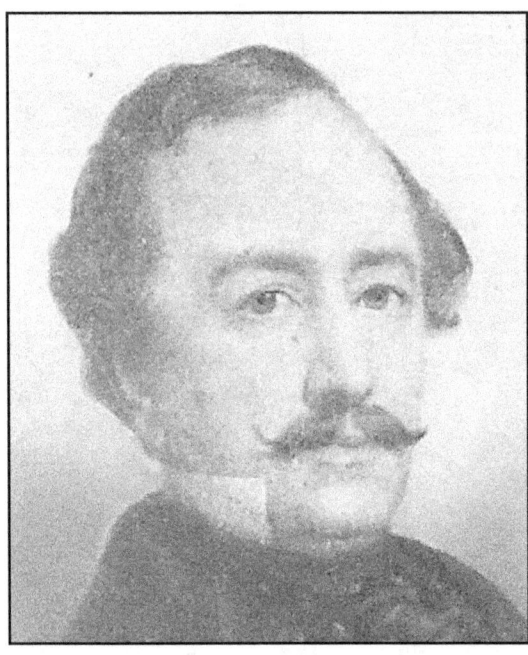

*Figure 3-2 Daniel Brainard*

slept, using his knapsack as a pillow.

In January 1837, Dr. Brainard saw a patient who was no longer able to work on the Illinois-Michigan Canal because of a painful swelling in his thigh, the site of a previous femoral fracture. Brainard performed a high amputation and femoral disarticulation of what was evidently a sarcoma of the femur. The patient died on the 48th postoperative day, and an autopsy revealed widespread tumor. The case was reported in the August 1838 issue of the *American Journal of the Medical Sciences*. The surgical ability and knowledge of anatomy exhibited by Brainard in this case established him as the leading surgeon in Chicago. Later, he was the first in the city to use ether for a finger amputation at Tippecanoe Hall Dispensary on January 12, 1847,[2] shortly after ether was first used in Boston.

In the late autumn of 1836, Brainard and his good friend Dr. Josiah Goodhue, who assisted Brainard at the above hip disarticulation , had drawn up an Act of Incorporation for "Rush Medical College" and submitted it to the Illinois State Legislature. Goodhue, a native of Vermont and a Yale Medical School graduate, was described as a man of tremendous charm and boundless energy. He had come to Chicago in 1832 and by 1837 had the largest practice in the city. The charter, granted to Rush Medical College on March 2, 1837, by the Illinois Legislature in Vandalia (then the capital of the state, which had been admitted to the Union in 1819) was the first institution of any type to be charted by the Illinois State Legislature.[2] The College had been named after Benjamin Rush (1745–1813) who was George Washington's physician and the only physician to sign the Declaration of Independence. Brainard had hoped that the Rush family might give financial aid to the school. The Rush family proved to be grateful but not helpful. Tragically, Dr. Goodhue died young, in 1847, when he fell into an open well after making a nighttime house call.

Much of the information on this period is taken from the excellent biography of Daniel Brainard written by Dr. Janet Kinney of Chicago. I knew her well when we shared an office in the 1960s. She was a fine physician and a fascinating historian.

On March 4, 1837, two days after it had chartered Rush Medical College, the Illinois State Legislature chartered the City of Chicago, which then had a population of 3,300. It had been chartered a village of 350 inhabitants only four years before. The rapid growth of Chicago from a village to a city was ascribed by some to the large amount of funds made available to Illinois by the federal government for construction of the Illinois-Michigan Canal. Unfortunately, in April of 1837, a financial panic and depression hit Chicago. This economic problem was caused in part, some believed, by the closure of the First Bank of the United States by President Andrew Jackson, and its effects were experienced throughout the country. Work stopped on construction of the Illinois-Michigan Canal, and the opening of Rush Medical College were delayed.

In the autumn of 1839, Brainard went to Paris for postgraduate studies. In France he heard lectures at Hotel Dieu by Philippe Roux and Alfred Velpeau in the hospital where Dupuytren and Larrey had operated and where the great internist Laennec had practiced. After two years of hard study in Paris, Brainard returned to Chicago in 1841 where the city was recovering from the economic depression and where work had resumed on the Illinois-Michigan Canal. He reopened his office and resumed practice. However, in the fall of 1841, he accepted an offer to teach anatomy for a year at the then-opening Saint Louis Medical College.

When Brainard returned from St. Louis, he brought with him James V.Z. Blaney to teach at Rush Medical School. In Chicago, Brainard found that two medical schools had opened in the area in 1842, one in St. Charles, Illinois, and another in La Porte, Indiana. And the Illinois College Medical School was about to open in Jacksonville, Illinois in 1843. As a result, Brainard hurriedly rented two small rooms south of the river at Lake and Clarke Streets, and Rush Medical College opened on December 4, 1843, with 22 students seated on two wooden benches. This first term of Rush Medical College was completed in 16 weeks in the spring of 1844.

At the same time, Brainard and Blaney founded the *Illinois Medical and Surgical Journal*, which had its inaugural edition in April of 1844. This was the first medical journal in the states of Illinois, Indiana, and Wisconsin. In the summer of 1844, a permanent home for Rush College was built north of the Chicago River at the corner of Grand and Dearborn Streets. The building, built of brick with a basement and two stories, measured 60 x 30 feet and cost $3,500.[1-2] Later, in 1855, a companion building was added. The original building at Grand and Dearborn is now the headquarters of the Chicago Medical Society.

By 1847, the Chicago population had grown to 7,500, and it became obvious that a hospital was needed, not only for the growing city but to provide clinical experience for the medical students at Rush. One effort was made to convert Tippecanoe Hall to a hospital: it was described as a rickety old warehouse at Kinzie and North State Street.[1] Cook County officials agreed to furnish supplies for this purpose, and Bowman[2] considers this the first Cook County Hospital.

Drs. Brainard, Blaney, and Herrick of Rush Medical College served on the first medical staff of the institution. This undertaking did not last long, however, and another effort was made in 1847 when Brainard rented rooms for 12 beds in the Lake House Hotel on the north bank of the river near the present location of the *Chicago Tribune* building. It so happened that Brainard had befriended a group of Mercy nuns who had come to Chicago to found a school, and he convinced four of them to volunteer to care for the patients at Lake House. By August of 1853, the nuns built their own hospital at Wabash and Van Buren Streets, and this became Chicago's first private hospital.[3] The medical staff consisted of Rush faculty physicians, and medical education was an important part of its mission.

A previous agreement had been reached that while the county was responsible for the chronic sick and elderly, the city would handle communicable diseases, such as the frequent epidemics of typhoid, typhus, cholera, and smallpox. The first city hospital for this purpose was a temporary structure built in 1843 that burned down two years later.[4] A cholera epidemic in 1854 prompted the city to build a more substantial structure at 18th and Arnold (LaSalle) Streets. This location on the edge of town was chosen to avoid exposure of the population to the communicable diseases. The city physician, Brockholst McVickar, convinced the city to build a more substantial three-story building with a basement in the same location at a cost of $75,000. It was completed in 1857. The city appointed a medical staff that included several homeopathic "physicians." The "regular" doctors considered the homeopathics to be "quacks" and refused to serve on the staff with them. The building then stood empty for two years until two physicians (Joseph Ross, an internist, and George Amerman, a surgeon) offered to run it as a private hospital with an agreement to care for the city's charity patients for a "unified fee of $3.00 per week." This arrangement lasted for three years until the American Civil War. Then, on October 29, 1862, the Army took over the hospital and operated it until November 12, 1865. After the war, Dr. Amerman got himself elected to the Cook County Board of Supervisors. He persuaded his fellow supervisors to buy the building and operate it as a charitable county hospital.[4] It opened as such on January 10, 1866, and this, in the opinion of some, was the true beginning of the present day County (Stroger) Hospital. The first two interns, N.T. Quales (a native of Norway) and Jim Hutchinson were appointed in February 1866. The building was later enlarged to 220 beds, and when the original Rush College burned in the fire of 1871, Rush used the clinical amphitheatre at County Hospital temporarily for classes four days after the fire. In 1876, County Hospital moved to its new location on the southwest corner of Wood and Harrison Streets.[5] Rush then built its new building kitty-corner from County on the northeast corner of the same intersection (Figure 3–1). The new Rush building also reopened in 1876.

The death on October 10, 1866, at age 54 of the great Daniel Brainard marked 1866 as a watershed year in the history of medicine in Chicago. Brainard had awakened the morning of his death in apparent good health. After breakfast at 9 a.m., he had a spell of diarrhea. His condition deteriorated rapidly, and by 9:15 p.m., he was dead of cholera. This was a common course in the dread disease, which was epidemic at that time in Chicago.

In retrospect, the tall, austere Brainard had been a giant of accomplishment in his 30-year career in Chicago. Best known for the establishment and promotion of Rush Medical College, he had continued to improve Rush's faculty by appointing leading Chicago physicians as well as attracting prominent physicians from other medical centers. Austin Flint had come from New York to teach for three years before returning to East Bloomfield, New York to become a leading cardiologist, and the remarkable Nathan Smith Davis had continued in Chicago after his career began in the East.

In the 23 years from 1843 to 1866, Rush Medical College had grown to an enrollment of 374 students, and as a result of the high-quality faculty developed by Brainard, was on course to become one of the leading medical schools west of the Alleghenies.

In addition to medical education, Brainard, along with James Blaney, had founded the first medical journal in the Chicago area. By the time of his death, he had published 60 scientific articles on a wide variety of subjects, most of which appeared in the aforementioned journal.[1] It is rumored that Brainard was once considered for appointment to the Medical College of Pennsylvania faculty. In addition, he was responsible for the transient Tippecanoe Hall and hospital and may well have encouraged Amerman (who he had placed on the Rush faculty in 1860) to become Cook County supervisor in his successful effort to establish the first version of Cook County Hospital with its legendary internship. Brainard's encouragement of the Mercy nuns to volunteer for patient care in the Lake House Hotel laid the foundation for the first private hospital in Chicago. In short, Brainard had been the leader of the practice of medicine in Chicago for 30 years.

Looking forward, the new half-century from 1866 to 1916 would be dominated by a quintet of leading Chicago surgeons: Moses Gunn, Charles Parkes, Christian Fenger, Nicholas Senn, and John B. Murphy.

## Moses Gunn

Moses Gunn, who replaced Brainard in 1866, was born on April 20, 1822 in East Bloomfield, New York.[8] As a youngster of Scottish descent, he asked his mother why she named him "Moses." He was told he was named for his grandfather, a courtly old gentleman, who his parents hoped he would emulate. His reply was he could emulate his grandfather without being named after him.

Gunn attended East Bloomfield Academy, followed by preceptorship under Dr. Carr in Canandaigua, New York. Then in October 1849 he entered Geneva Medical College. After completing his medical education in 1850, he was appointed to the faculty of newly opened University of Michigan Medical College in Ann Arbor.

His wife described him as tall and stately with brown wavy hair and a blonde goatee (Figure 3–3). He was nearsighted and required glasses. With the onset of the Civil War, he entered the Army on September 1, 1861. His wife states he served in "the 5th Army of the Potomac" until July, 1862, when he received a medical discharge. Among several articles mentioned in Jane August Gunn's memoire[6] was one on hip and shoulder dislocations: *Luxation of the*

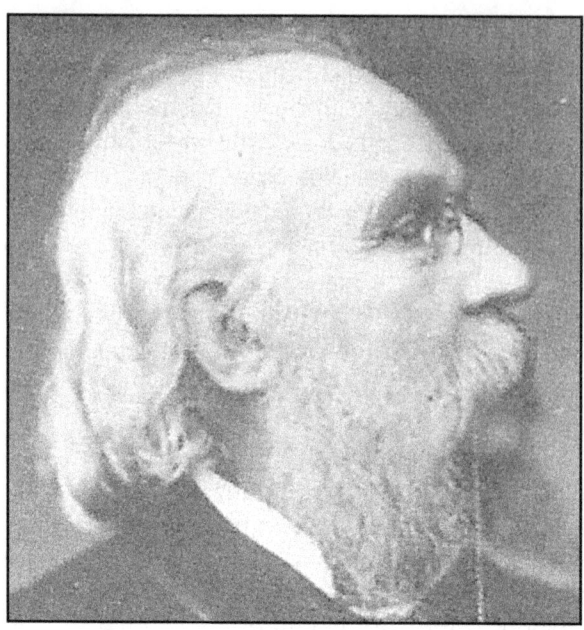

*Figure 3-3 Moses Gunn*

*Hip and Shoulder Jointts and the Agents Which Oppose Their Reduction* (1859). Another article was on *Union of Nerves,* which was his presidential address to the American Surgical Association of which he was a founding member.[7] In that address, Gunn mentioned his duties at Cook County Hospital where he had been an attending surgeon. James Herrick[8] describes Gunn as less than scholarly, but earnest and understandable.

Unfortunately, a manuscript Gunn wrote entitled "A Compendium on Surgery" was destroyed in the Great Chicago Fire of 1871. Had it been published, it might have improved Gunn's reputation as a scholar. Bowman[2] states that having begun his work in the early days of anesthesia, Gunn was used to operating rapidly. Gunn withheld belief in the germ theory and is credited with the observation that a surgeon must have the heart of a lion and the eye of an eagle. Although he was able to attend a meeting in San Francisco early in 1887, he developed cancer and died on November 4, 1887.

## Charles Parkes

Gunn was succeeded in late 1887 by Charles Parkes (Figure 3–4) who was described as "having a majestic, magnetic personality, and had he lived, would have been one of America's outstanding surgeons."[8] Parkes died tragically of pneumonia four years later in 1891. He was the first Rush surgeon to scrub his hands and forearms vigorously before operating and to sterilize instruments in carbolic acid. Charles Parkes was the first western surgeon to carry on experimental research in gunshot wounds of the small intestine.[9] In 1884, he wrote monographs entitled *Gunshot Wounds of the Small Intestine,* which were influencial in establishing new lines of clinical treatment for gunshot injuries. For several years before his premature death, Parkes began to write for a textbook in general and

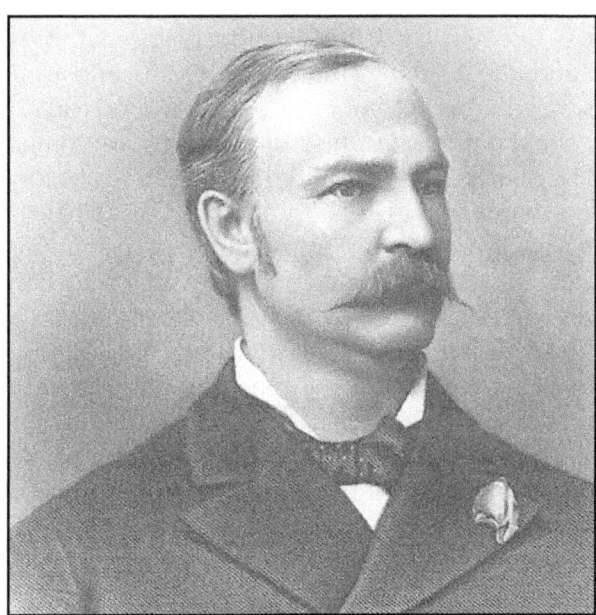

*Figure 3-4 Charles Parkes*

abdominal surgery. His wife had the unfinished manuscript published as *Clinical Lectures in Abdominal Surgery and Other Subjects* (1896) with Albert Ochsner serving as editor.[9]

## Edwin Powell

The antiseptic surgical technique was introduced at County Hospital by Dr. Edwin Powell in 1878. He had observed Lister in England.[9] Powell was a pioneer in abdominal surgery and an active proponent of animal experiments. He was attending surgeon at Presbyterian Hospital and also at Cook County Hospital.[10]

## Christian Fenger

One of the legendary Chicago surgeons of the era was Christian Fenger from Denmark. He studied medicine at the University of Copenhagen in the winter of 1860-61 and interned at the Royal Fredrick Hospital in Copenhagen. Fenger served in the 1865 War against Germany[11] and later studied under Bilroth and Rokitansky, after which he became a pathologist in the Copenhagen City Hospital. When he did not get a desired professorship in 1875, he left Denmark and went to Egypt. There, he served under the Khedive for three years before coming to Chicago in 1877. Although he was an accomplished pathologist, he still had to pay the requisite $1,000 to a county commissioner to obtain the job of pathologist at Cook County Hospital.[12] For 15 years (1878 to 1893), the autopsy room at County was the Mecca of learning for the medical students, interns, and the doctors of Chicago. Fenger's achievement was to demonstrate the association between pathology and surgery. He introduced surgical pathology as the basis for surgical treatment.[2] From 1880 to 1884, he served as Curator of Rush Medical

College Museum. In addition to his pathological duties, he substituted for vacationing County Hospital surgeons and in 1880 secured for himself a regular surgical appointment that he continued for 12 years. Although Fenger was an excellent pathologist, his abilities left something to be desired in surgical technique. His operations were lengthy, sometimes as long as six hours, and he occasionally operated with an open anatomy text at hand. His incisions were reminiscent in length to those seen in the autopsy room. He also had a high mortality rate.

In 1893, he became Professor of Surgery at Northwestern Medical School and Attending Surgeon at Mercy Hospital. In 1899, he returned to Rush and Presbyterian hospital as Professor of Surgery, Rush Medical College-University of Chicago. He died three years later on March 7, 1902, at age 62. Fenger is credited as the mentor for two great Chicago surgeons, Nicolas Senn and John B. Murphy.

## Nicolas Senn

Nicholas Senn (Figure 3–5) was born on October 31, 1844 in northeast Switzerland near Lichtenstein. His parents were farmers who migrated to Ashford, Wisconsin, in 1852 when Nicholas was eight years old. He graduated from Fond du Lac High School in 1864. In 1865, he entered the Chicago Medical College (now Northwestern University) and graduated with honors in 1868. In 1868-1869, he interned at Cook County Hospital. Senn then practiced medicine for five years in Ashford. He moved to Milwaukee, Wisconsin, in 1874. There he purchased a building at Juno Avenue and North 3rd Street with a drugstore on the first floor. His office was on the second floor, and his laboratory was in the basement. After settling in Milwaukee, Senn met Dr. Christian Fenger. They became close friends, and Senn visited Chicago often. In 1877, he entered the University of Munich where he studied under Professor Van Nussbaum.

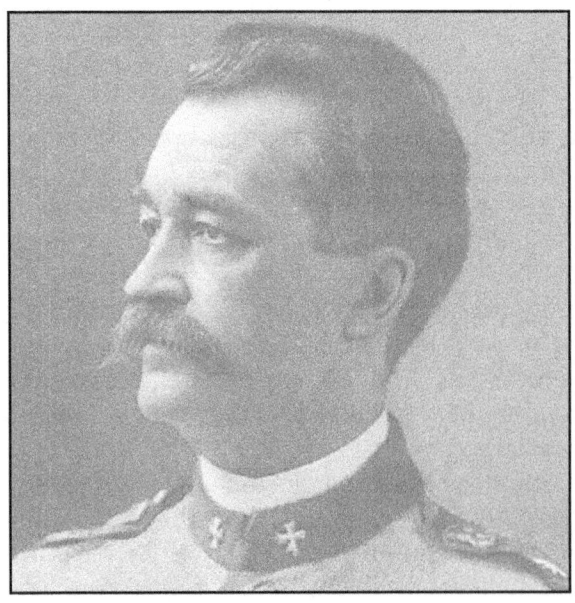

*Figure 3-5 Nicholas Senn*

Upon his return to America, Senn was elected Professor of Principles and Practice of Surgery in the College of Physicians and Surgeons of Chicago in 1884, and in 1888 he became Professor of Principles of Surgery and Surgical Pathology at Rush. For several years, he commuted between Chicago and Milwaukee twice a week, lecturing in Chicago and maintaining his practice of surgery and scientific work in Milwaukee. In 1891, after the death of Parkes, Senn became the fourth chairman of the Surgery Department at Rush. Senn's tie to Cook County Hospital is through Fenger who was his friend and advisor, and these two men—with John B. Murphy—formed the celebrated triumvirate of scientific genius at the western front of American Surgery.

Senn wrote several books including *Experimental Surgery* (1899), *Intestinal Surgery* (1889), *Principles of Surgery* (1890), *The Pathology and Surgical Treatment of Tumors* (1895), and *Practical Surgery for General Practitioners* (1902). Among Senn's most important papers were one on surgery of the pancreas (1899), one on the use of rectal insufflations to test for colonic perforation (1888), and a historical review of intestinal sutures and anastomosis (1893). Senn was President of the American Surgical Association in 1893 and the American Medical Association in 1897. He traveled extensively and gained an international reputation. He served in the U.S. Military during the Spanish-American War (this fact thanks to Dr. Alexander Doolas who has studied Senn's life).[13] Senn did much to improve military surgery and founded the Association of Military Surgeons of the United States in 1891. In his later years, he traveled the world extensively and documented his journeys in a series of books entitles *Around the World via Siberia* (1902), *Tahiti, the Island Paradise* (1906), and others.[14] Senn was also a bibliophile and collected one of the best private medical and surgical libraries in the United States, which was given to the Newberry Library and later transferred to John Crerar Library, both in Chicago.[14] He died on June 2, 1908.

## John B. Murphy

The fourth surgeon of this remarkable era and arguably its most prestigious, was John Benjamin Murphy. He was born on December 21, 1857, in a log cabin in Appleton, Wisconsin, to parents who had migrated from Ireland.[15] He graduated from high school in 1876, taught school for two terms, and then spent a year preceptorship with Appleton physician Dr. H.W. Reilly. A year later at the age of 19, he entered Rush Medical College where tuition was $65 a year. Rush had been suggested by Dr. Reilly because it neighbored Cook County Hospital.

Among his attending at County, Murphy admired Dr. Gunn and later Dr. Edward Lee. Lee encouraged Murphy to attend lectures by Dr. Fenger, both at the hospital and at Dr. Fenger's home. The doctors of Chicago learned a great deal from Fenger because of his ability to relate autopsy as well as microscopic tissue findings to surgical therapy. Murphy, in later years, would acknowledge his debt to Fenger for the instruction early in his career, and considered himself a protégé of Fenger.

After completing his internship in 1881, Murphy went into practice with Dr. Lee in offices at Harrison and Halsted Streets. After a year of Family Practice, at the suggestion of Dr. Fenger, Murphy spent 18 months in Vienna, Berlin, and Heidelberg. Murphy then returned to Chicago in 1884, and at age 26 resumed his private practice with Dr. Lee who referred him to Dr. Nicholas Senn. Senn appointed Murphy Instructor of Surgery at Rush Medical College, and at the same time, Lee also got Murphy appointed to the surgical staff of Cook County Hospital. For 18 years, Murphy was an Attending Surgeon at Cook County Hospital and conducted a clinic at the amphitheatre on Friday mornings attended by students from all medical colleges.

In 1892 after several years at Rush, Murphy was appointed Clinical Professor of Surgery at the College of Physicians and Surgeons of Chicago ( the precursor of University of Illinois Medical School). In 1900, at the invitation of Christian Fenger, he joined Northwestern University Medical School as Professor of Clinical Surgery and moved his practice to Mercy Hospital. Before this time, he had by mutual agreement separated from Dr. Lee and moved his office to the Loop, limiting his practice to surgery. By then, Rush Medical College had become affiliated with the University of Chicago, and William Rainey Harper, President of the U of C, requested that Murphy be made Chairman of the Department of Surgery at Rush. Loyal Davis,[13] in his biography of Murphy (P. 208), vividly describes the scene when Harper and Billings visited Murphy in his home to offer him the position. In 1905, Murphy returned to Rush and Presbyterian Hospital as Co-Chairman of Surgery with Arthur Bevan. After three years, Murphy left Rush to become Chairman of the Department of Surgery at Northwestern Medical School where he served until the end of his career.

As the years passed, Murphy was increasingly troubled by angina pectoris, to the point that eating gave him severe attacks. He went to Mackinac Island in the summer of 1916 where he died suddenly on August 11 with L.L. McArthur, his junior intern at Cook County Hospital, at his side.[15]

## Arthur Dean Bevan

Arthur Dean Bevan (Figure 3–6) was on the surgical staff of Chicago Presbyterian Hospital from 1892 on and continued as Chief of Surgery at Rush until 1934. A remarkable personality, Bevan served during World War I as director of general surgery in the surgical division of the Surgeon General's Office. Bevan also held many important positions throughout organized surgery. He was chairman of the AMA committee that produced the Abraham Flexner report on medical education in 1910. In that report of 54 medical schools in Illinois, only six gained approval.[2] Bevan was a member of the first Board of Governors of the American College of Surgeons. He was elected President of the American Surgical Association in 1932. As a surgeon, Bevan developed several operative procedures, and his name was long associated with an operation for cryptochidism. He also developed the "hockey-stick" incision for cholescystectomy and performed the first operation in which ethylene oxide was used as an anesthetic.[16]

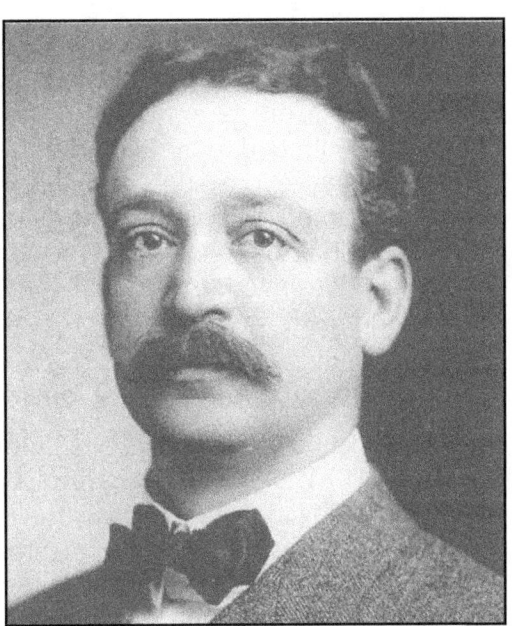

*Figure 3-6 Arthur Dean Bevan*

## Rush and University of Chicago

The Presbyterian Hospital opened with 45 patient beds in September 1884 on land adjacent to Rush Medical School. By 1889, the hospital had been enlarged to over 300 beds, and by 1897, Rush was the largest medical school in the United States with 847 students and a faculty of 80. From 1887 to 1894, 66 of 147 Cook County interns were Rush graduates.

In June of 1898, an affiliation between Rush Medical College and the University of Chicago became final. Some considered this "a marriage made in heaven:" Chicago's outstanding medical school joining the glamorous new University of Chicago, which was supported by America's wealthiest benefactor, John D. Rockefeller. However, a tectonic fault marred this union. The Rush Presbyterian County Hospital attitude was focused on the pragmatic art of healing, as practiced by Chicago's leading clinicians. Rockefeller, on the other hand, wanted to replicate Baltimore's Johns Hopkins Medical School. He visualized full-time salaried scientists looking through their microscopes seeking disease causes, with a sideline interest in actual patient care. There was no place in that concept for Cook County Hospital. The mismatch in these two institutions would only widen until their divorce in 1943. So much for the marriage made in heaven.

It is of interest that in the first decade of the century, all three of Chicago's leading surgeons—Senn, Fenger, and Murphy—were operating at Presbyterian Hospital, and all three had close County Hospital connections. James B. Herrick in his autobiography[8] devotes a chapter to his observations of, and experiences with, these three surgeons. In this same period, three of America's leading internists—Frank Billings, Herrick (coronary disease), and Bertram Sippy (peptic ulcer)—were also present at Rush Presbyterian.

On July 1, 1929, the young Dean of Yale Law School, Robert Maynard Hutchins, became President of the University of Chicago. He earlier proclaimed Rush Medical College a "jewel in the crown of the University." However, the University continued to build medical facilities on the south side of Chicago, and in spite of great efforts such as a suggestion that Rush-Presbyterian move to the south side campus, all attempts at reconciliation failed, and in June of 1940, the union of Rush and the University of Chicago was dissolved. As reported below, the staff at Presbyterian Hospital then joined the faculty of the University of Illinois, and Rush Medical College closed.

## Rush Faculty at Cook County Hospital

Rush doctors had always been close to County since their original building burned in 1871, and they waited to see where County built before erecting the new Rush Medical College across the street.

The surgeons of Presbyterian Hospital maintained their close association with Cook County Hospital. Dr. R. Kennedy Gilchrist—associate of Dr. Veron David, Dr. Egbert Fell (an associate of Dr. Edward Miller), and Dr. Francis Strauss—were all attending surgeons at County. Dr Miller interned at County in 1914 after graduation from Rush.[9] After studies in Europe, he joined the staff of Presbyterian Hospital in 1915. He served in the Army in both World Wars and was Chief of Surgery at Rush and Presbyterian Hospital from 1939 to 1954 and Attending Surgeon at Cook County Hospital from 1935 to 1954. He published 66 papers. Dr. Miller was a very polite and soft spoken gentleman, and was known as "Silent Ed."

When World War II started for the United States on December 7, 1941, several surgeons at Presbyterian Hospital served in the Presbyterian Hospital Unit, which saw duty in New Guinea, the Philippines, and the southwest Pacific. Dr. Fell played an important role in taking care of patients with cardiovascular disease, especially children. Dr. Francis Strauss and Dr. Frank Theis were also on the staff from Presbyterian Hospital and Rush Professors. Other Rush surgeons included Fred de Peyster (Figure 3–7), William Shorey, William Diffenbaugh, John Reynolds, and E. Lee Strohl (Figure 3–8). All were leading surgeons in Chicago.

## Presbyterian/St. Luke's Merger

In 1954, James A. Campbell, a cardiologist who performed the first cardiac catheterization in Chicago, became Chairman of Medicine at Presbyterian Hospital.[17] He was a strong-minded activist with many social contacts among trustees of both Presbyterian and St. Luke's Hospitals as a result of his residence in Lake Forest, Illinois. On February 10, 1956, the trustees voted to merge the hospitals and move the staff of St. Luke's on Michigan Avenue to Presbyterian Hospital. The merger was completed on June 26, 1959.[2] Dr. Edward Beattie became Chairman of Surgery and of the section of Cardio-Thoracic Surgery of Presbyterian/St. Luke's (PSL). He also served as president of the newly merged Presbyterian-St. Luke's Medical Center. But on July 1, 1965, he left for New York

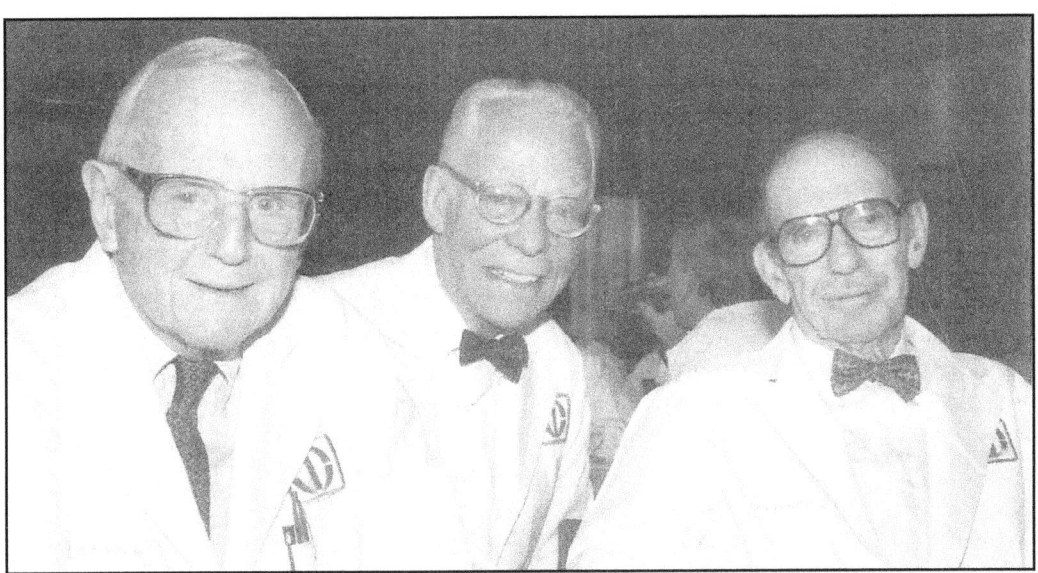

*Figure 3-7 Fred de Peyster (center) with colleagues*

to become Chairman of Surgery at Memorial Cancer Hospital. He was succeeded by Ormand Julian, a leading cardiovascular surgeon in Chicago. In 1971, Harry Southwick became the Chairman, and Rush reopened its medical school. He was succeeded in 1985 by Dr. Steven Economou.

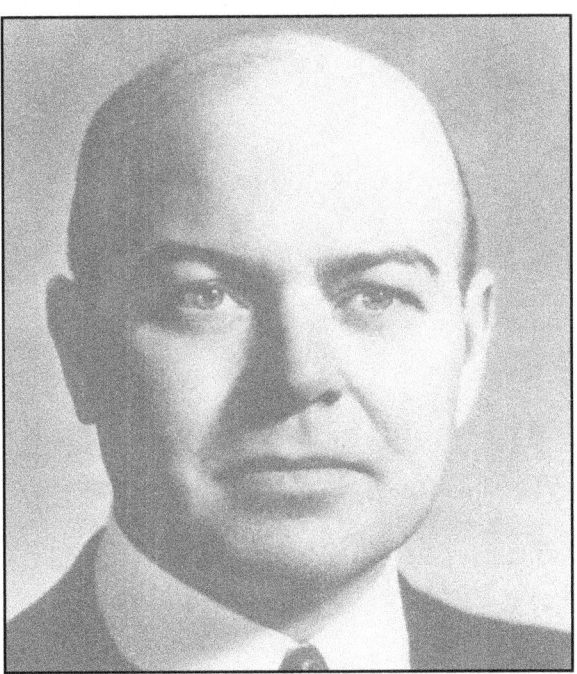

*Figure 3-8 E. Lee Strohl*

## Reopening of Rush Medical College and Renewing Old Acquaintances with CCH

On September 27, 1971, Rush Medical College reopened with 66 first-year students and 33 third-year students after a 30-year period of closure.[2] This was accomplished through the efforts of Dr. James Campbell[17] who had previously been a medical school dean for a brief period in New York State. The Charter of Rush Medical College was reactivated in 1969 when it became part of Rush/Presbyterian/St. Luke's Medical Center, which changed its name to Rush University Medical Center to reflect the important role that education and research played in its patient care.

When Dr. Richard Prinz became Chairman of Surgery at Rush in 1993, the opportunity to develop an academic relationship with Cook County Hospital arose. Dr. Hernan Reyes (Chief of Surgery at County) and Dr. Prinz sought the support of colleagues to develop the Rush University Presbyterian-St. Luke's Hospital/Cook County Hospital Integrated Surgical Residency Training Program. This academic affiliation took advantage of the geographic proximity of the two institutions and rekindled the historical bonds that had linked both centers since Daniel Brainard founded the Medical College and Cook County Hospital in the mid-19th century.

On July 1, 1994, Cook County Hospital staffs renewed their academic affiliation with Rush Medical College. The affiliation called for the Rush Medical students to complete surgical rotation at County Hospital, and the surgical training program was merged with the Rush program. Academic faculty positions were offered to attending staffs at Cook County Hospital. Thus the close and mutually beneficial relationship between Rush and Cook County Hospital, begun in 1866, was resumed and has progressed into the 21st century.

# References

1. Kinney, J. *The Saga of a Surgeon: The Life of Daniel Brainard MD* Southern Illinois University School of Medicine: Springfield IL: 1987.
2. Bowman, J. Good Medicine. *The First 150 Years of Rush-Presbyterian-St. Luke's Medical Center*. Chicago Review Press; Chicago: 1987.
3. Clough, Sr. J RSM. *The History of Mercy Hospital*. Mercy Hospital and Medical Center: Chicago: 1979.
4. Bonner TN. *Medicine in Chicago 1850-1950, 2nd Ed*. University of Illinois Press: Chicago: 1991.
5. Johnson C B. *Growth of Cook County Vol. 1*. Board of Commissioners of Cook County: Chicago: 1960.
6. Gunn JA. *Memorial Sketches of Doctor Moses Gunn*, W. Kenner: Chicago; 1889.
7. Gunn, M. *The Union of Nerves of Different Function, Considered in its Pathological and Surgical Relations*. Address of the President, Transactions of the American Surgical Association, Vol. 4 P1, 1886.
8. Herrick J.B. *Memories of Eight Years*. University of Chicago Press: Chicago: 1949
9. Rutkow I. Charles Parkes in *American Surgery- An Illustrated History*. Philadelphia: Lippincott-Raven Publishers: 1998: 206.
10. Raffensberger J. *The Old Lady on Harrison Street, Cook County Hospital, 1833-1895*. Peter Lang: New York; 1997.
11. Hirsch EF. *Christian Fenger, MD 1840-1902*. Dartnell Press: Chicago; 1972.
12. Arey L. *Northwestern University Medical School 1859-1979*. Northwestern University Medical School: Chicago; 1979.
13. Doolas A. Notes for a Talk on Nicholas Senn.
14. Rutkow I. Nicolas Senn. In: *American Surgery-An Illustrated History*. Philadelphia: Lippincott & Raven Publishers; 1998:275-276.
15. Davis LE. *J. B. Murphy, the Stormy Petrel of Surgery*. GP Putnum Sons: New York; 1938:208.
16. Rutkow I. Arthur Bevan. In: *American Surgery-An Illustrated History*. Philadelphia: Lippincott & Raven Publisher, 1998: 310-312.
17. Flanagan MJ. *To the Glory of God and the Service of Man. The life of James A. Campbell MD* FHC Press: Winnetka, Illinois; 2005.

# Northwestern University

*James S.T. Yao, MD*
*Robert M. Vanecko, MD*

- *Evolution of Northwestern University Medical School*
- *CCH and its Academic Affiliation with Northwestern University*
- *The Internship*
- *Attending Staff*
- *The Fenger-Murphy Era*
- *The Meyer-McNealy Era*
- *The Freeark Era*
- *References*

From the beginning, Cook County Hospital was a center for medical education and has been called an institution of learning. Raymond McNealy, the famed Chicago surgeon, declared that Cook County Hospital has had a tremendous influence on medical education in the United States.[1] All medical schools in Chicago at one time or another had an affiliation with Cook County Hospital, and Northwestern University is no exception. This chapter attempts to trace the affiliation between Northwestern and Cook County Hospital from the beginning until it ended in the 1970s. Since Northwestern University Medical School developed at the same time as Cook County Hospital, a brief review of the evolution of the medical school is needed to understand the intricate relationship with Cook County Hospital.

## Evolution of Northwestern University Medical School

The first medical school in Chicago was Rush Medical College, founded by Dr. Daniel Brainard. The school was chartered in 1837, 12 days before the city of Chicago. The charter was the first granted to an institution of learning. The school opened with 22 students on December 4, 1843. The name "Rush" was in honor of Dr. Benjamin Rush, the only physician to sign the Declaration of Independence. In 1855, Hahnemann Medical College, a homeopathic college, came into existence. In 1854, due to a difference of opinion on the improvement of medical education by introducing a new curriculum, several members of Rush Medical College (Drs. Nathan S. Davis, Homer A. Johnson, Edmund Andrews, William H. Byford, and John H. Hollister) quit and joined Lind University to establish a Medical Department in Chicago. Classes at the Medical Department of Lind University began on October 9, 1859. In the spring of 1863, the Lind University trustees changed the University's name to Lake Forest University. The Medical Department then reorganized and adopted a new name: Chicago Medical College. In the summer of 1869, an agreement on a union of Chicago Medical College and Northwestern University was reached. Chicago Medical College thus became the precursor of Northwestern University Medical School. During this period, females had difficulty gaining admission to medical school, which led to the establishment of Woman's Medical College in 1870. In 1875, Woman's Medical College became Northwestern University Woman's Medical

School. In 1891, Northwestern University took a giant step merging the NU Woman's Medical School and Chicago Medical College into Northwestern University Medical School (NUMS).[2] The late Ruben Feinberg, who died in 2002, was instrumental in directing gifts from the Joseph and Bessie Feinberg Foundation to Northwestern University Medical School, which resulted in the school's renaming to Northwestern University, Feinberg School of Medicine.

At the beginning of the 20th century, there were 14 medical schools in Chicago, many of which were night schools, correspondence schools, and homeopathic, osteopathic, or chiropractic schools.[3] In 1908, the Carnegie Foundation for the Advancement of Teaching commissioned Abraham Flexner, an external reviewer, to study medical education in U.S. and Canadian medical schools.[4] The 1910 Flexner Report predicted that only Rush, Northwestern, and the College of Physicians and Surgeons would survive. The Flexner report set the standard of medical education, and it inspired the alignment of medical schools with universities. As a result, many nonregular, homeopathic schools disappeared from the scene of medical education.

At present, there are six recognized medical schools in Chicago: Feinberg School of Medicine, Northwestern University; University of Illinois College of Medicine; Rush University Medical College; Stritch School of Medicine, Loyola University; Pritzker School of Medicine, University of Chicago; and Chicago Medical School, Rosalind Franklin University. From the beginning of Cook County Hospital to 1978, these schools provided volunteer staff coverage for surgical services at the Hospital. In addition to general surgery, faculty members of Northwestern University Medical School also provided attending staff for orthopedic surgery, otolaryngology, head and neck surgery, and plastic surgery. In 1978, the Cook County surgical residency program merged with University of Illinois, and in 1994, the affiliation changed to Rush Medical College. The academic affiliation of the Department of Surgery of Cook County Hospital with Rush Medical College had come full circle, from the beginning in 1837 to the renewal in 1994.

## Cook County Hospital and its Academic Affiliation with Northwestern University

All medical schools need a hospital to teach their students, and all hospitals would like to have academic staff to care for their patients. This symbiotic relation remains the engine to advance the field of surgery. Since the medical school or university had never maintained a general hospital of its own, interactions between the hospital and the school on education or patient care depended either on a friendly agreement or on more binding contracts of affiliation. Both arrangements had their own risks, and it appeared good faith and strong commitment to academic and clinical excellence substitute for absolute control. Affiliation must work both ways, and Northwestern University Medical School began its affiliation with Cook County hospital dating back to when the hospital began to take care of patients.

## The Internship

Internship, the first step taken by medical graduates to enter the real world of medicine, was first started at Cook County Hospital in 1866. It preceded the internship at Johns Hopkins Hospital when their hospital opened in 1899.[5] In the early part of the history of CCH, neither the intern nor attending surgeons was paid, but they gained valuable experience in treating a wide variety of disease. To gain internship at CCH was a highly competitive undertaking, and candidates had to pass a tough oral examination. Candidates often prepared for months. The internship was 12 months in the beginning and later extended to 18 months. The first six months were spent as junior house physicians on medicine and surgery, the second on the various specialties such as obstetrics, and the third six months as senior physicians. Thus, the senior became what we would now call a resident physician, capable of both teaching the junior and accepting responsibility for certain patient care. The amount of care left to him was the responsibility of the attending staff.

The first intern at CCH was Dr. N.T. Quales. He started on January 12, 1866, and three months later was joined by Dr. James M. Hutchinson.[6] Figure 4–1 shows the Directory of interns in the beginning years at CCH. Dr. D. S. Root, who began in April 1867 and graduated in October 1868, was the first to serve 18 months. In 1914, the internship at CCH received official accreditation by the American Medical Association. The number of interns gradually increased, and in the 1960s, there were 120 interns at CCH.

In the early years, graduates from Chicago Medical College (now Northwestern) sought internship at CCH, and the majority did well in competitive examination. In the year of Samuel Plummer's examination (1886), seven of eight were NU graduates, and in the year of Albert Halstead's examination (1891), again seven of eight were NU graduates.[2] Both Drs. Plummer and Halstead eventually held the post of Professor of Surgery at Northwestern. Many famed surgeons from Northwestern in-

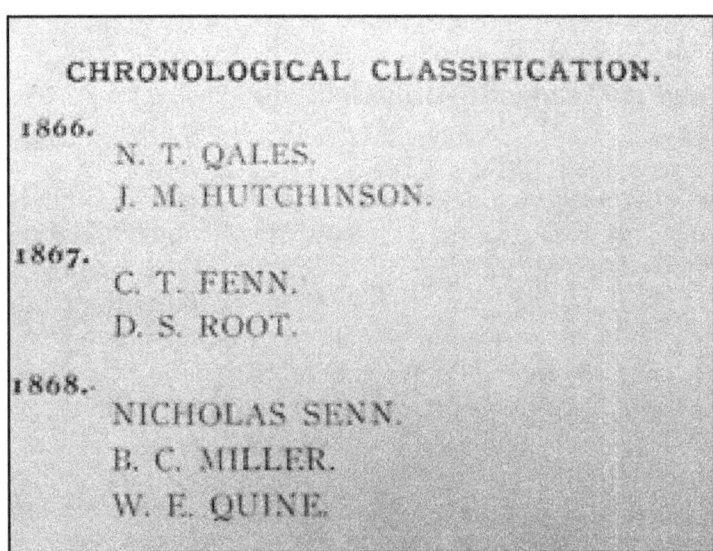

Figure 4–1
N.T. Quales, first intern at CCH. He was joined by Hutchinson three months later.

terned at CCH, including Drs. John B. Murphy, Walter Van Hook, Albert Halstead, William E. Morgan, Frederick Besley, Harry Richter, Samuel Plummer, Allen Kanavel, Raymond McNealy, Loyal Davis, Karl Meyer, Jacob Buchbinder, Sumner Koch, Michael Mason, John Bell, William Stromberg, and others, a historic all-star cast of Chicago surgeons. Modern-day Northwestern Surgical faculty who did internships at CCH include Drs. Robert Freeark, John Raffensperger, Paul Nora, Robert Vanecko, and James S. T. Yao.

## Attending Staff

The first hospital in Chicago was Mercy Hospital, founded by the order of Sisters of Mercy in 1850. In the beginning, Cook County paid Mercy Hospital to care for patients. After the first county hospital, known as Almshouse, was built by the Board of Commissioners, Rush physicians were the staff members. In the early development of Cook County Hospital, Rush Medical College dominated the presence at Cook County Hospital. In 1876, when a new hospital was built on the block between Harrison and Wood Streets, an agreement was reached between Rush Medical College and Chicago Medical College (now Northwestern University) that one-third of the staff would be from Rush Medical College, one-third from Chicago Medical College, and one-third from outside physicians appointed by County Commissioners. This plan worked well and many of the best surgeons in Chicago were on the staff (Figure 4–2). Among the members of the staff at this time were such well-known surgeons as Drs. Edmund Andrews (NU), Moses Gunn (Rush), Charles Parkes (Rush), and Christian Fenger (NU). In 1881, a newly elected Board decided not to follow this plan. Instead, homeopathic physicians and surgeons were given one-fifth of the patients, and political interference with medical activities brought further unrest. In 1882, in protest against the dismissal by the board of Dr. Edward Lee for his experiment with skin grafting using the skins of chicken and lambs, the whole staff of the hospital resigned. The Board of County Commissioners, with no great concern over the loss of academic prestige of the hospital, continued to appoint staff without regard for professional qualification. They doubled the size of the attending staff, and in addition to the homeopathic physicians, allowed eclectic physicians to control one-fifth of the hospital. This period, ending in 1905, was, on the whole, the darkest in the history of the hospital.[7]

In 1905, the County Board implemented the civil service examination for appointment and tenure of interns and attending staff. Competitive examination was required for the appointment of attending physicians, surgeons, and specialists who served for a period of six years. The interns, too, were appointed on the basis of competitive examination to serve for 18 months. The medical schools were now again represented through the attending physicians of the respective schools who passed the examination. Despite these safeguards, there remained irregularities in grading of the examinations and the results were not entirely on the merits of the scientific response.[8]

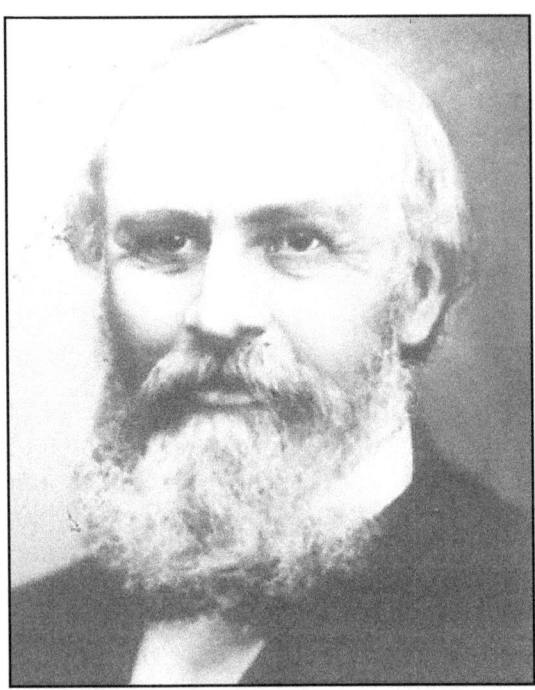
*Figure 4–2 Edmund Andrews*

Northwestern University's contributions to Cook County Hospital started with Dr. Edmund Andrews, one of the 12 Founders of the Northwestern University Medical School. From the start of the new school, Dr. Andrews held an academic appointment to the Chair of the Principle and Practice of Surgery and Clinical Surgery at Northwestern University. At the outbreak of the Civil War, Dr. Andrews enlisted as a surgeon in the Illinois regiment. In 1866, he made a trip to visit Lister to learn about the carbolic spray as an antiseptic technique in the operating ward. Returning to Chicago, he tested the technique first in Mercy Hospital, and in 1870, he popularized antiseptic surgery at CCH.[3] In fact, one of the jobs of Dr. J. B. Murphy while he was an intern was to spray carbolic acid in the operating room while the attending surgeon was operating.[9] Dr. Andrews was also a pioneer in neurosurgery and was the first to develop a urethroscope. Dr. Andrews contributed largely and soundly to the medical literature; his treatise, *Rectal and Anal Surgery*, went on for several editions. He was also the first to test gas-oxygen anesthesia and to report the results. He wrote many papers on injuries incurred in war. He was also a geologist, naturalist, and a founder of the Chicago Academy of Science.

## The Fenger-Murphy Era

Despite the turmoil during the period from 1882 to 1905, Dr. Christian Fenger joined the staff at Cook County Hospital in 1877 as a pathologist, and in 1879, Dr. John B. Murphy passed the competitive examination and became an intern at CCH (Figure 4–3). Both Drs. Fenger and Murphy soon rose to be major figures in Chicago surgery. Both men were appointed Chairman and Professor of Surgery at Northwestern University Medical School, with Dr. Fenger serving as the first Chairman of the Medical School from 1896 to 1899 and Dr. Murphy as the third Chairman from 1908 to 1916. Dr. Christian Fenger was born and educated as a pathologist in Denmark and immigrated to America. When he was invited to conduct a few autopsies, his superb knowledge of pathology from Virchow and the scientific demonstration of pathology made such a strong impression on Dr. Isaac N. Danforth, founder of Wesley Hospital who then held the appointment of chief pathologist, that Danforth resigned in order to open the position to Fenger. As was protocol at that time, Dr. Fenger had to borrow $1,000 from friends to buy the appointment.[2] There was also a rumor that Dr. Fenger raised the money by selling an Egyptian mummy.[10] Others also received appointment through political influence. Dr. David Graham of Woman's Medical College later confessed his appointment was obtained "through the political influence of a friend." The appointment of Dr. James Herrick was secured through a friend sitting on the County Board. The only price Dr. Herrick had to pay for his appointment "was an annual note of thanks, with a box of cigars to my sponsor."[3,8]

Dr. Fenger was well-suited for the position of pathologist, and soon the autopsy room at County Hospital became a Mecca for students, interns, and medical professionals of Chicago. Performing surgery at the County Hospital as a replacement for vacationing staff members, Fenger secured a regular surgical appointment in 1880 and served on the staff for 12 years. In 1893, he became Professor of Surgery at Northwestern. His contributions in surgery include the practice of antiseptic surgery: he was the first to use rubber gloves in the operating

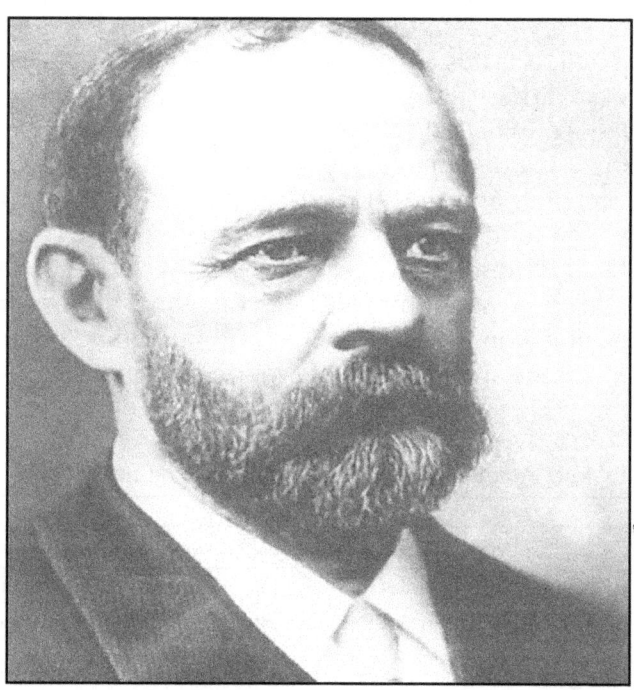

*Figure 4–3 Christian Fenger*

room. He was also the first to change street clothes and shoes for clean cotton clothing in the hospital. Dr. Fenger was known to be the first to remove a gallstone from the common bile duct and to perform a vaginal hysterectomy. He was a prolific writer and contributed to the literature of surgery, special pathology, and diagnosis, and his writings were translated into many languages. Dr. Fenger has been hailed as the "Osler of the Middle West" and compared to Theodor Billroth, Claude Welch, Howard Kelly, and William Halsted of East Coast surgeons.[2,10,11] Table I shows the academic appointments of Dr. Fenger.

Dr. Christian Fenger was probably the most influential figure of his time and a pioneer in antiseptic surgery. For years, he conducted teaching sessions for interns at CCH on every Thursday evening at his house. The teaching often lasted until midnight. It was through his influence that many young physicians visited European clinics and returned to America to become leaders in surgery. His influence extended not only to the younger generation of surgeons such as Drs. Nicolas Senn, John B. Murphy, William J. Mayo, and Lewis L. McArthur, but also to physicians such as Drs. Frank Billings, James Herrick, and William Faveill and pathologists such as Drs. Ludwig Hektoen, Edwin LeCount, and Gideon Wells. His influence was unequaled by any other individual of the period in Chicago. The era he presided over has been termed by Dragstedt, in a broad sense, the Midwestern School of Surgery, or, in a narrow sense, the CCH-Chicago School of Surgery.[10] In 1899, Weller Van Hook assumed the Chair after the death of Dr. Fenger. He was also an attending surgeon at CCH.

In 1879, after graduating from Rush Medical College, Dr. John B. Murphy (Figure 4–4) prepared for the competitive examination to become an intern at County Hospital. At that time, only students of Rush and Chicago Medical College were eligible for a coveted place on the staff of the large charity hospital. Service as an intern was not required of a graduate before he or she could practice as it is today, and those who did not take the examination regarded those who did as fellows who "want to stay in school all their lives." But each year, the examination was an important event and was attended by a large audience that included practically the entire senior class of both schools. The examination was oral, and the spectators often offered free and sometimes wrong advice to the candidates as they were examined. The result, of course, was a good show. Dr. J. B. Murphy stood firm and calm during the examination, and the result was that Professor Moses Gunn, following the examination, congratulated him on having won first place.[9] The hospital had no equipment except a large amount of medicine and an adequate supply of bandages. The windows of the hospital were

**Table I. Academic Appointments of Christian Fenger**

| Year | Title and Institution |
|---|---|
| 1882–85 | Professor of Pathology, Northwestern University |
| 1884 | Professor of Surgery, College of Physicians and Surgeons |
| 1893 | Professor of Surgery, Chicago Medical College (NU) |
| 1899 | Professor of Surgery, Rush Medical College |

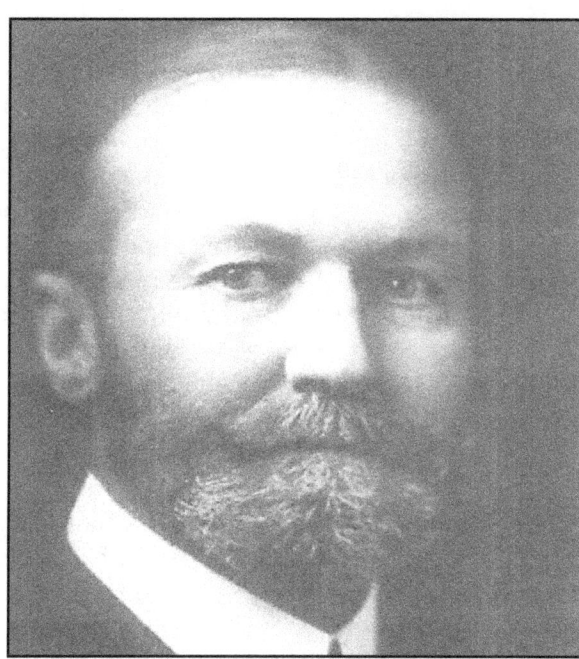

*Figure 4–4 John B. Murphy*

kept open just like in the 1960s. At that time, the CCH capacity was 450 patients. There were six interns in surgery on two services. Dr. Murphy was on Dr. Edward Lee's service, and he later joined Dr. Lee in private practice.

Dr. Murphy became attending surgeon in 1880. During his career, Dr. Murphy changed his academic appointments on several occasions. He was first with Rush and later joined the Northwestern faculty (Table II) but at all times he was on staff at CCH. Dr. Murphy performed several landmark operations at CCH. On March 2, 1889, while making rounds at the Cook County Hospital, he recognized and operated on an early case of appendicitis or "perityphlitis," as he called it then. The patient had symptoms for only eight hours. At operation, he found a typical red appendix with pus in it but without perforation.[12] He claimed that his operation antedated Charles McBurney's operation only by 20 days. In 1892, he performed the first successful Murphy button for intestinal anastomosis in a woman[9] and became the first surgeon to reconstruct an injured femoral artery and vein due to a gunshot wound in October 1896.[13]

**Table II. Academic Appointments of John B. Murphy**

| Year | Title and Institution |
|---|---|
| 1884 | Lecturer in Surgery, Rush Medical College |
| 1892 | Professor of Surgery, College of Physicians and Surgeons |
| 1895 | Professor of Clinical Surgery, Postgraduate Medical School |
| 1900 | Professor of Clinical Surgery, Northwestern University |
| 1906 | Professor of Surgery, Rush Medical College |
| 1908 | Professor of Principles and Practice of Surgery and Clinical Surgery and Chairman of Surgery, Northwestern University |

Dr. Murphy had an interest in vascular surgery and was first to perform many operations, including arterial anastomosis in human,[13] removal of cervical ribs causing aneurysm formation of a subclavian artery,[14] and iliac-femoral embolectomy.[15] He also was a pioneer surgeon in thoracic surgery, in particular the treatment of tuberculosis. In later years, he became a leader in bone and joint surgery, making numerous contributions in the literature.[16,17]

In 1895, Dr. Murphy was appointed Chief of Surgery at Mercy Hospital. At Mercy, he conducted a surgical clinic several times a week with 400 to 500 attendants. The Surgical Clinic of John B. Murphy was so popular that it made "Murphy" and "Mercy" interchangeable. He published all operative cases with discussion in a quarterly publication, *The Clinics of John B. Murphy, MD, at Mercy Hospital, Chicago*. (After his death, W. B. Saunders Co. continued the series and changed its name to *Surgical Clinics of North America*.) In 1900, Murphy was appointed Professor of Surgery at Northwestern, and he continued to maintain a busy practice at Mercy Hospital. He became Chairman of Surgery at Northwestern in 1908 and served three years. Dr. J. B. Murphy received many honors and awards in the United States and abroad; he has been ranked with Galen, Hippocrates, William Harvey, and Joseph Lister. Murphy was also an early advocate for a Cook County Graduate School of Medicine for postgraduate education.[12]

Dr. Murphy was a flamboyant surgeon. He was not well liked by his colleagues for his publicity-hound attitude. Some thought he only presented good results of his surgery. He married rich and enjoyed his high-society life. In Chicago, he made his name known from taking care of wounded policemen and others in the Haymarket riots. He is also known for stealing President Theodore Roosevelt as a patient from other surgeons.[9] Although he eventually was admitted to the American Surgical Association and Chicago Medical Society, his first try for membership to these two societies was rejected outright. In the book *Stormy Petrel*, Dr. Loyal Davis wrote:

> *There was good and bad in this man—and in abundance on both sides—but there were other things too. There was great brilliance and downright stupidity; there was charm and the power to irritate; ambitions, with all of ambition's ugliness as well as its beauty....*[9]

After Dr. Murphy, Chicago surgery entered a more quiescent period. Following Drs. Fenger and Murphy, the Chairman of the Department of Surgery at Northwestern continued to serve as Attending Surgeon or Consultant at CCH. In 1883, Dr. E. Wyllys Andrews (Figure 4–5) served as Surgeon-in-Chief at Cook County Hospital. Dr. Andrews was the son of Dr. Edmund Andrews, founder of Northwestern University Medical School. Dr. Andrews became Professor of Surgery at Northwestern in 1888 and was the fourth Chairman of the Department of Surgery from 1916 to 1919. A true son of Northwestern, he was known for his contribution in hernia surgery and the use of a glass tube for subdural drainage of hydrocephalus. He also had interest in thoracic surgery and served as President of the American Thoracic Surgical Society.[18]

Two African-American surgeons, both graduates of Chicago Medical

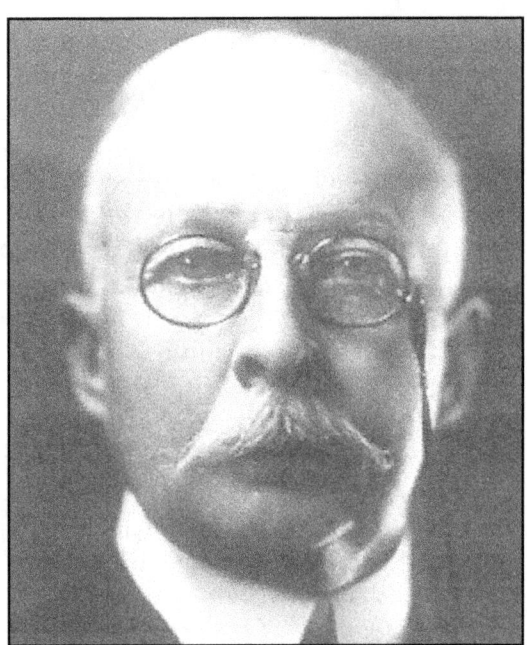

*Figure 4–5 E. Wyllys Andrews*

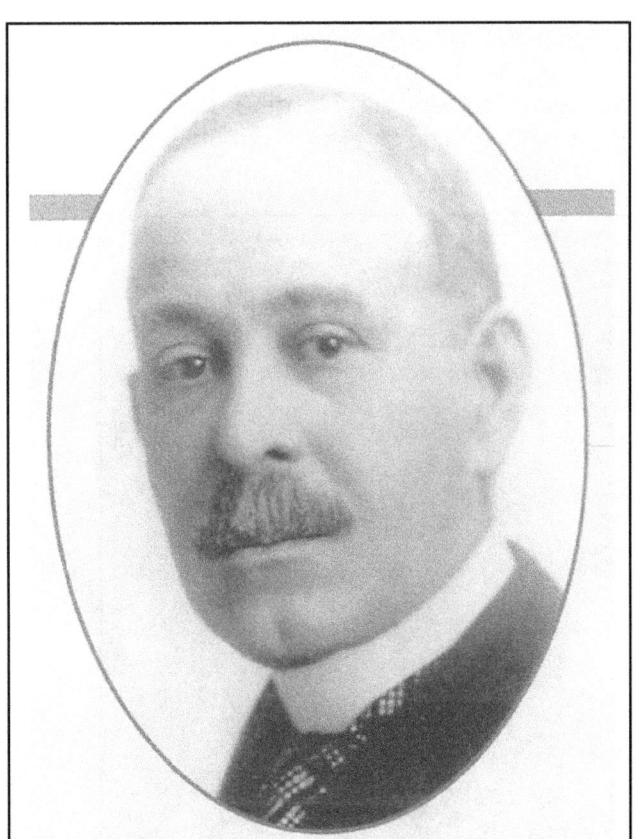

*Figure 4–6 Daniel H. Williams*

College, made black history in Chicago. In 1896, Dr. Austin Maurice Curtis became the first African-American physician to receive a regular staff appointment at a white Chicago hospital (Cook County Hospital) when the County Commissioners agreed to open a staff position for one African-American doctor.[18] He was considered among the most prominent African-American surgeons of his era. In 1883, Dr. Daniel Hale Williams (Figure 4–6) performed a groundbreaking operation. At Provident Hospital, he repaired the torn pericardium of a young black patient who sustained a knife wound of the heart. This was the second repair of a wound to the pericardium on record. Provident Hospital is now a part of the Cook County health care system. Dr. Williams was instructor in anatomy at Northwestern University and served as attending surgeon at Cook County Hospital from 1900 to 1906. In 1913, he became a charter member and the only African-American in the American College of Surgeons.[18]

Dr. Allen Kanavel (Figure 4–7), the fifth Chairman of the Department of Surgery at Northwestern, began his surgical career first as an assistant in the clinic at Northwestern. He gradually rose to be Professor of Surgery in 1919 and served as Chairman of the Department from 1919 to 1929. He published a book entitled *Infections of the Hand*, which became a classic in hand surgery. Under his direction, Dr. Sumner Koch and his partners Drs. Harvey Allen, Michael Mason, John Bell, and William Stromberg, established a Hand Surgery Service at Cook County Hospital. The Hand Surgery Service was one of the very first in the country and became known as the Chicago School of Hand Surgery.[19] All these surgeons were interned at County and all were in private-practice hand surgery at Passavant Memorial Hospital. They also had extensive interests in patients with burn injuries. The first burn unit at Cook County Hospital, the Sumner Koch Burn Unit, again made valuable contributions to patients with burn injuries. The Burn

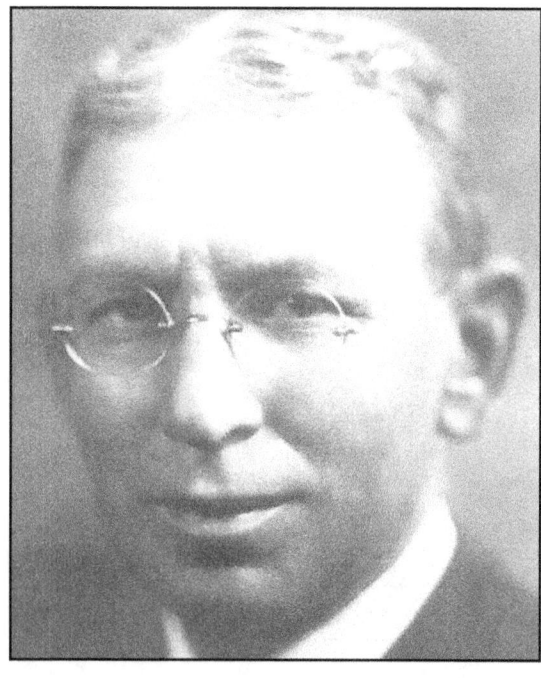

*Figure 4–7 Allen B. Kanavel*

Unit became the center of learning and training of all students and residents of Chicago-area medical schools. The Hand and Burn Units represented a notable contribution of Northwestern University to Cook County Hospital. Dr. Kanavel was also known for his expertise in abdominal surgery and neurosurgery. He was elected President of the American College of Surgeons in 1931.

Dr. Harry Richter (Figure 4–8), the sixth Chairman of Surgery at Northwestern, completed his internship at CCH in 1894 and served as Attending Surgeon afterward. He was named Professor of Surgery at Northwestern in 1920 and became Chairman of Surgery from 1929 to 1932. Dr. Richter is known for thyroid surgery and had a special interest in pediatric surgery. He was also known for using a vacuum cleaner motor to make a respirator to save a patient with polio.

In addition to the many contributions by the chairmen of surgery, there were also professors of surgery of Northwestern who served as attending surgeons at CCH. Dr. Albert Halstead, a graduate of Northwestern, joined CCH as attending surgeon 1891 and served until 1914. He joined the academic faculty at Northwestern in 1898 and was Professor of Surgery from 1907 to 1914. Dr. Halstead was interested in vascular surgery and published articles on arteriovenous anastomosis for gangrene of extremities, arterioplasty for aneurysm, and together with Dr. Roger Vaughan, presented to the American Surgical Association on aortic aneurysm. Other professors of surgery who served at CCH included Drs. William Schroeder (1903–15), Frederick Besley (1915–44), Jacob Buchbinder, and Herbert Potts. Dr. Schroeder was Chief of Surgery at Wesley Hospital. Dr. Besley was known for his contribution in industrial injuries and was elected President of the American College of Surgeons. Buchbinder became attending surgeon at CCH in 1925. Dr. Potts was a dentist first and then attended Northwestern University Medical School. He organized oral surgery at CCH and became the chief oral surgeon at CCH for 14 years.

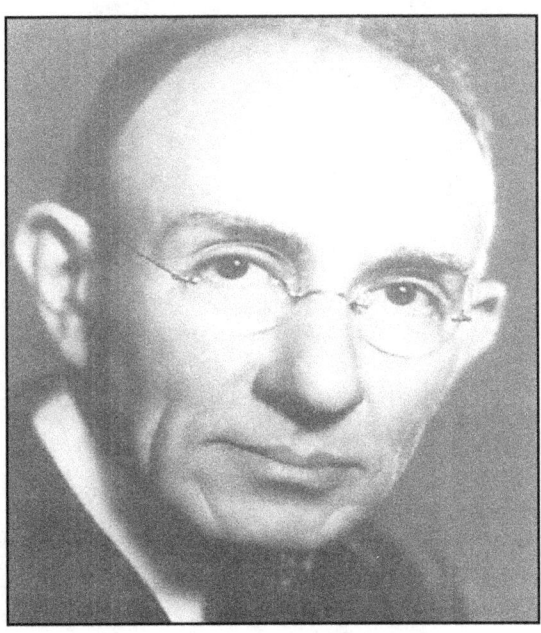

*Figure 4–8 Harry Richter*

## The Meyer-McNealy Era

In 1912, the new Cook County Hospital opened its doors and soon became the center for medical education. The Northwestern University Medical School continued its affiliation with Cook County Hospital. Two leading surgeons, Drs.

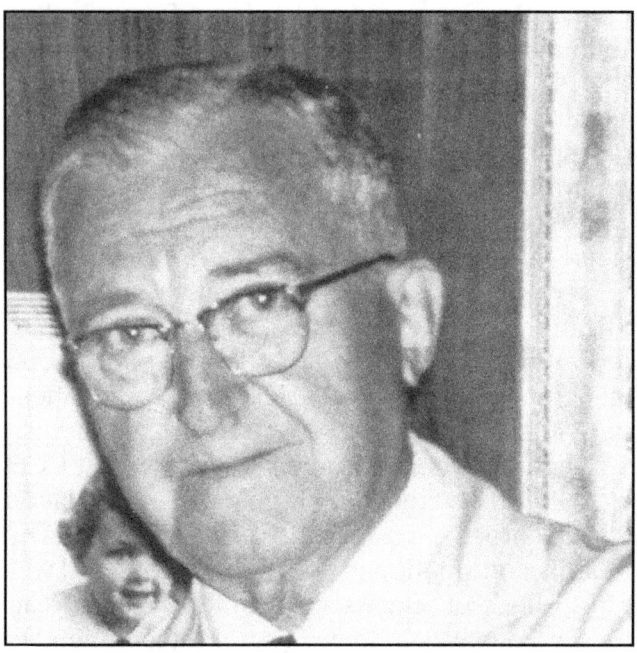

*Figure 4–9 Karl Albert Meyer*

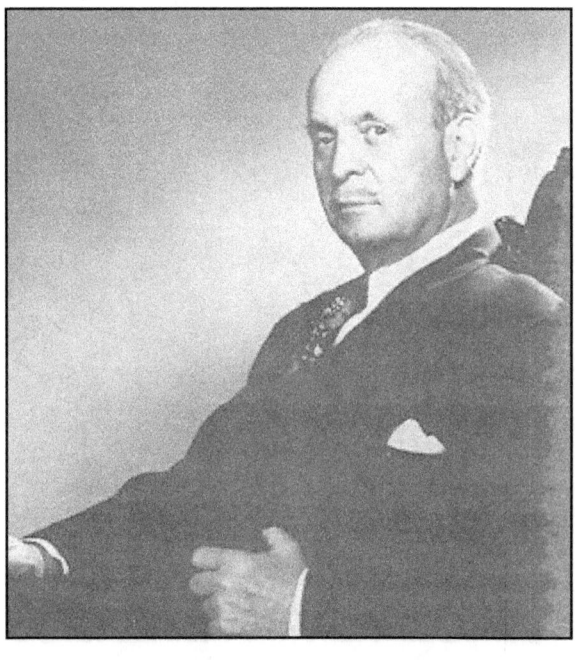

*Figure 4–10 Raymond McNealy*

Karl A. Meyer (Figure 4–9) and Raymond W. McNealy (Figure 4–10) emerged to continue the tradition of Drs. Christian Fenger and John B. Murphy as great teachers of surgery. Both took their internship at County, Dr. Meyer in 1908 and Dr. McNealy in 1910. Dr. McNealy became Attending Surgeon at County in 1917 and Dr. Meyer in 1918. Dr. Meyer was also appointed as superintendent of the hospital at the age of 28 and was universally known as Mr. County Hospital. When the new Wesley Hospital was built, Dr. McNealy took time off from his practice and served as superintendent of Wesley Hospital. In addition to attending to patient cares at CCH, both had busy private practices. Dr. McNealy was also Chief of Surgery at Wesley Hospital and became Associate Professor of Surgery at Northwestern in 1926, a position he held until he retired. Dr. Meyer was appointed Professor of Surgery at Northwestern from 1945 to 1952. Both men were superb technical surgeons. Karl Meyer also practiced at Columbus Hospital and was the busiest surgeon in Chicago at that time. He reportedly performed more than 100,000 operations, often as many as 10 a day.[20]

The Meyer-McNealy era at Cook County Hospital was legendary. Dr. McNealy served as Attending Surgeon from 1918 to 1958. He was a skillful surgeon, ambidexterous, and operated with decisive moves. He often explained his procedure by drawing on the blackboard simultaneously with both hands. His Saturday afternoon clinic at CCH was one of the highlights of teaching for many visiting surgeons. Dr. McNealy was elected President of the Medical Staff at CCH in 1931. He also served as Trustee and Professor, Cook County Graduate School of Medicine after its establishment in 1932. His surgical interest included hernia, abdominal surgery, and blood vessel surgery. At Wesley, he maintained a busy surgical practice and was the master surgeon at that hospital.

No one has contributed more to Cook County Hospital than Dr. Karl Meyer. Under the leadership of Meyer, the attending staff made regular rounds and either actually carried out the surgical procedures or supervised them. Each member of the staff was permitted an associate, who he personally could appoint. In most instances, however, the associates were recommended by the deans or department heads of the medical school with which the attending staff was affiliated.[9] As a surgeon, Dr. Meyer performed more operations than anyone on the staff. He had special interest in gastric surgery, and for years, Ward 56 was specifically for the care of patients with GI bleeding. All patients with GI bleeding were admitted to Ward 56 under Dr. Meyer's service. Dr. Meyer also played a role in the introduction of partial gastroenterostomy in patients with vagotomy to prevent gastric stasis. He, together with Dr. Peter Rosi, had a special interest in Crohn's disease. Dr. Meyer was the first in Chicago to repair a tracheal-esophageal fistula in a baby.[21] Every Saturday morning, he conducted a surgical clinic at the amphitheatre of CCH and quite often performed a gastric resection for visitors to observe. As superintendent, he led and oversaw the development of CCH. Under his direction, 21 buildings were added to the campus of CCH. In 1928, expansion of CCH to include a children's hospital, the morgue, and Men's Hospital took place, and Cook County Hospital became the largest public hospital in the United States with a 3,000-bed capacity. In 1932, Dr. Meyer started the Cook County Graduate School of Medicine for post-graduate education.[22] The Board Review Course conducted by staff of the Graduate School was sought after by many preparing for the Board examination. Most of the staff at Cook County Graduate School were Northwestern faculty, and many gave short courses.

Dr. Meyer did not live at home with his wife. He lived in the rooftop apartment on the fifth floor of County Hospital with his aunt, Mrs. Grant. His automobile, a black stretch limousine, license plate #106, was always parked at the front door of the hospital. Every evening, Mrs. Grant or Leo, Dr. Meyer's chauffeur, would go through the recovery room on their way to walk her dogs. Dr. Vincent Collins, who ran the unit, was very upset but didn't have any power to stop it. Every Wednesday, Dr. Meyer held a staff meeting at his apartment, and a nice lunch was served by the head nurse of the operating room. Definitely, Dr. Meyer was from the old school and a well-known disciplinarian for interns and residents. He demanded absolute quiet in the operating room. No one spoke but Dr. Meyer. He would ask a question, and the expected response from the residents was "Yes, Sir", "No, Sir", or "I don't know." He hated smokers, and his passion for anti-cigarette smoking was legendary.

While Meyer and McNealy dominated the surgical scene at County, there were many equally distinguished and skillful surgeons on the Northwestern Surgical Service. All these surgeons had busy private practice and volunteered their service to County Hospital. Table III shows the names of Northwestern attending staff serving at County Hospital since its inception. They often were paired to ensure coverage at all times. Of these surgeons, Dr. Peter Rosi (Figure 4–11) deserves special mention. Dr. Rosi came to this country at the age of five.

**Table III. Northwestern Surgical Faculty Who Served at Cook County Hospital**

| | |
|---|---|
| Edmund Andrews | Manuel E. Lichenstein |
| Christian Fenger | Ted Lescher |
| Weller Van Hook | Samuel Fogelson |
| John B. Murphy | Durand Smith |
| E. Wyllys Andrews | William McMillan |
| Dale Williams | Michael Govostis |
| Albert Halstead | Harold Method |
| William E. Schroeder | Stephen E. Reid |
| Frederick A. Besley | John Bell |
| Herbert Potts | Robert J. Freeark |
| Harry Richter | William Stromberg |
| Allen Kanavel | James Hines |
| Jacob Buchbinder | Harold Laufman |
| Karl Meyer | Marion C. Anderson |
| Raymond McNealy | John J. Bergan |
| Sumner L. Koch | John G. Raffensperger |
| Jerome Head | John Boswick |
| Peter Rosi | Clyde Philips |
| Orion Stuteveille | Otto Trippel |
| Harvey Allen | Michael Mason |

He attended University of Chicago and Rush Medical School. He interned at St. Luke's Hospital and completed the surgical residency at CCH. He stayed on as attending surgeon for 30 years afterward and was elected to chief of staff. Dr. Rosi joined Dr. Meyer in private practice and earned a reputation as a surgeon's surgeon. He was well-known for gastrointestinal surgery, and his contribution to colon cancer surgery was classic. Although small in statue, Dr. Rosi had extraordinary stamina and often operated the whole day at Wesley and then spent time with the night surgeon at County Hospital. At Columbus Hospital, many residents rotating from CCH would recall the midnight rounds with Rosi to see patients. He joined the academic faculty at Northwestern in 1948 and was appointed Professor of Surgery in 1965.

Dr. Rosi was well-liked by his residents. At his retirement, a group of residents from CCH held a private dinner for him in his favorite restaurant, The Italian Village (Figure 4–12).

Surgical residency training in the United States started in 1924. In 1926, Cook County Hospital was among the 15 AMA-approved residencies in general surgery throughout the country and the only approved program in Chicago. In the beginning, there was no system designed for the training of surgeons. It was not until 1937, with the charter of the American Board of Surgery, that a systematic approach to surgical training was initiated. In 1939, AMA's Council on Medical Education approved the freestanding residency in general surgery at CCH; it was approved again by the Conference Committee on Graduate Training in Surgery for surgery in 1950.[22] The surgical residency program at County was a unique independent program with academic affiliation with four medical schools: Northwestern, University of Illinois-Rush, Loyola, and Chicago Medical School. Each of these schools maintained a service at a designated ward with medical students from these schools rotating to the ward for bedside teaching. The surgical residency started as a three-year program in 1939 and expanded to four years in 1950. Surgical residents of the County program rotated to these four medical school services at one time or another, depending on their level of training. Each school had two designated wards; Wards 61 and 56 (Meyer-Rosi-McNealy) were assigned to the Northwestern Service. Loyal Davis, Chair of the Department of Surgery at Northwestern, provided academic affiliation and attending surgeons to staff the service. Attending surgeons from Passavant and Wesley were selected, and each spent one day a week at CCH. Dr. Davis did his internship at County in 1919 and was on the staff as a neurosurgeon for a brief period after passing the civil service examination. After discovering that every general surgeon wanted to demonstrate that he could operate on neurological patients as well as he could, Dr. Davis resigned.[23] His star pupil, Dr. Thomas Starzl, the world-renowned transplant surgeon, was attending surgeon in Ward 56 in 1959.

In the 1950s, when homograft was introduced as an arterial graft for aortic aneurysm, Dr. Ormand Julian established an artery bank at University of Illinois. Later, the artery bank was transferred to Cook County Hospital with support from all the medical schools in Chicago. Dr. Harold Laufman of Northwestern played a vital role in the Chicago Artery Bank and a subsequent development of the artery bank at Passavant Hospital.

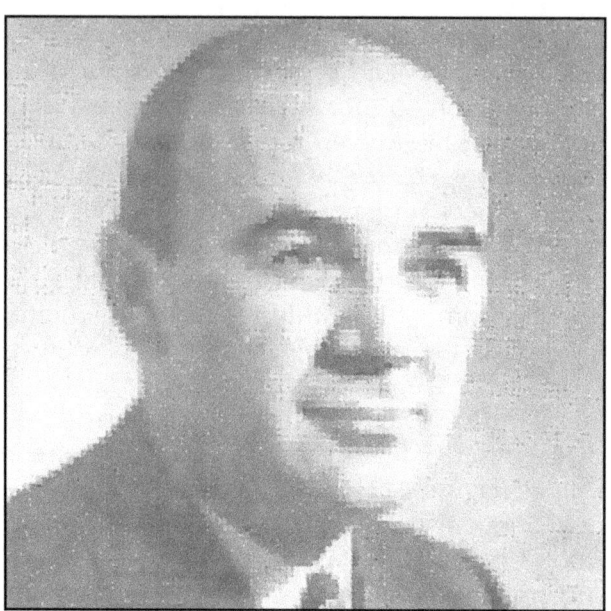

*Figure 4–11 Peter Rosi*

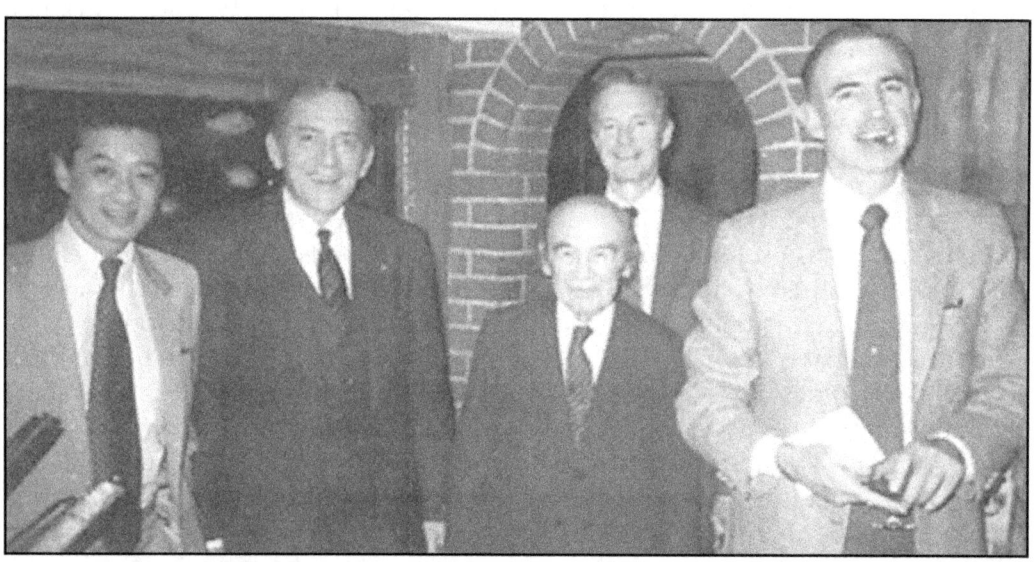

*Figure 4–12 Peter Rosi with former residents at Italian Village Restaurant*

In 1959, Dr. Meyer resigned from the position of Chairman of Surgery, and Dr. Manuel Lichenstein served as Interim Chair. In his letter of resignation, Meyer wrote,

*I have held high the torch of healing and hope, I feel the time has come to pass the responsibility onto younger hands.*

The Cook County Board of Commissioners passed a Resolution containing the following paragraph:

*Truly, greatness and goodness have been with us in the person of Dr. Meyer all of these many years, and our Cook County Hospital may indeed be regarded as a living symbol in his honor of man's humanity to man. All of mankind is indebted to Dr. Karl A. Meyer and we in Cook County are especially fortunate that he belongs to us.*

Dr. Lichtenstein was a graduate of Rush Medical College and received an MS degree from Northwestern. He was appointed attending surgeon at CCH in 1932 and a professor of surgery at Northwestern in 1965. A master surgeon and a great teacher, Dr. Lichenstein was well-liked by surgical residents.

## The Freeark Era

The Freeark Era began in the 1960s. Dr. Robert Freeark grew up in the South Shore of Chicago, attended University of Chicago Laboratory School, and then University of Illinois as an undergraduate. After a stint in the U.S. Marine Corps during World War II, he attended Northwestern University Medical School and graduated in 1952. He completed his surgical residency at Cook County Hospital and was appointed Director of Surgical Education in 1959. In 1960, he was named Chairman of the Department of Surgery and served until 1968 when he was appointed to the office of Hospital Superintendent, a post he kept until his resignation in 1970.

The appointment of Dr. Freeark heralded a change in surgical staffing at Cook County Hospital. At the same time, Dr. Robert J. Baker of University of Illinois was also appointed as Vice-Chairman of the Department of Surgery. From there on, Drs. Freeark and Baker were linked together as the modern-day surgeon-educators at Cook County Hospital. This was the first time that County had full-time salaried surgeons on the staff. In times past, appointment to attending staff was highly competitive. In more recent years, there appeared to be less interest by practicing surgeons to take the qualifying examination because of the demands of their practices. An attending position thus became a burden to all but the most dedicated academic surgeons. The change to a salaried staff was also necessary in order to provide closer supervision of residents, and to improve student teaching and educational conference. The full-time staff then gradually increased and supplemented the teaching by volunteer staff. Teaching for Northwestern medical students was more organized, and senior residents who were on the Northwestern Service began to receive academic appointment as Instructor in Surgery from Northwestern University. Drs. Robert Bass and James S.T. Yao were the first two County surgical residents appointed to the NU Medical Faculty. Dr. Freeark was appointed as Associate Professor of Surgery at NU in 1965 and became a Professor of Surgery in 1967. During his tenure, he elevated the training standards of the program. Teaching rounds, surgical grand rounds,

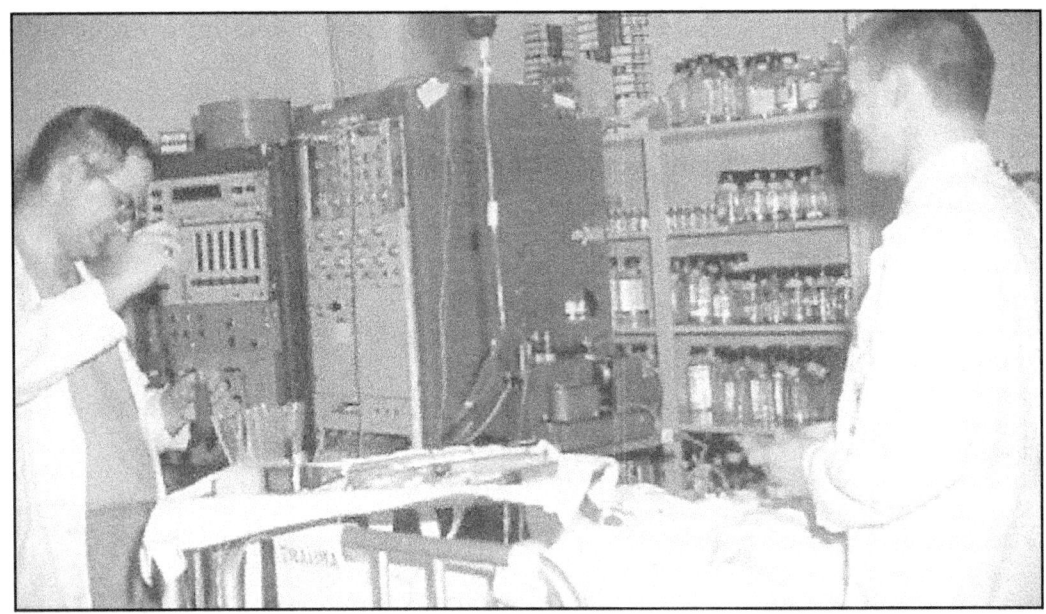

*Figure 4–13 Shock study team: K. Printen and D. Monson*

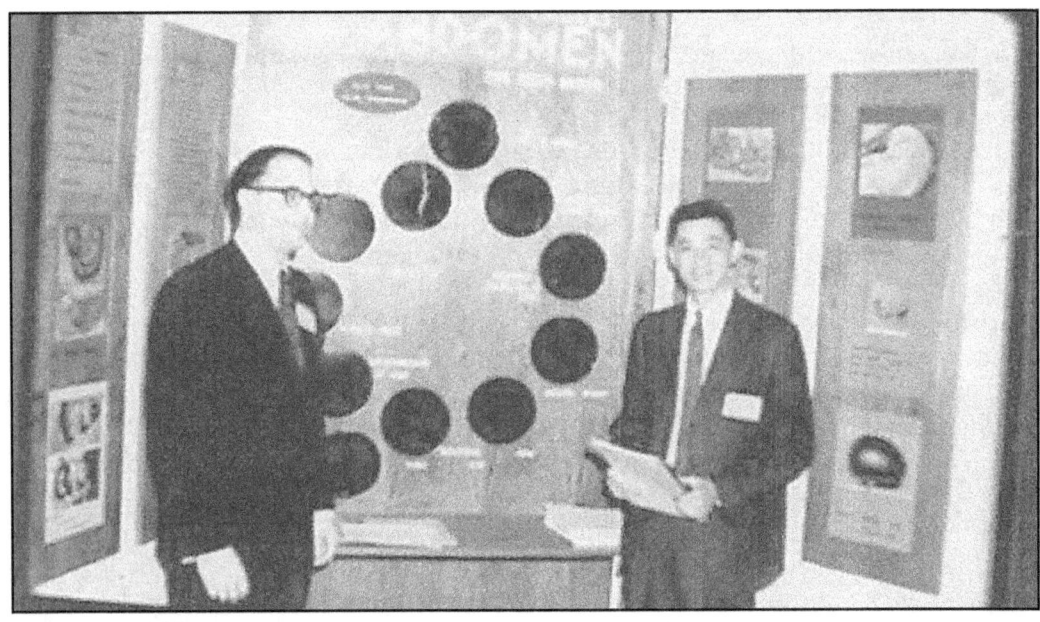

*Figure 4–14 Scientific exhibit by Vanecko and Yao*

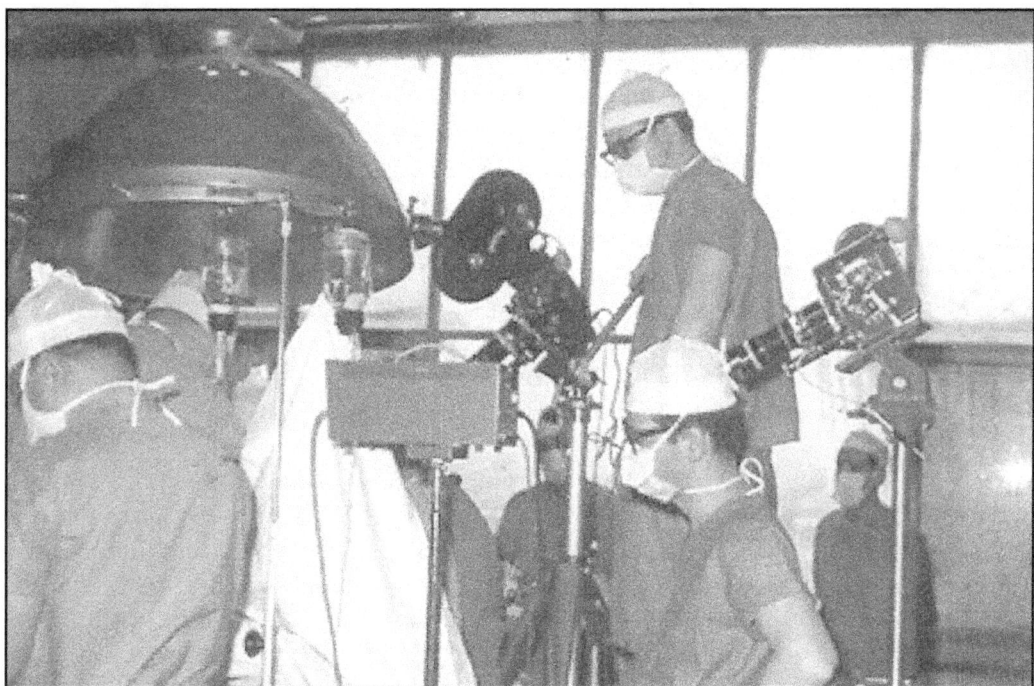

*Figure 4–15 Movie-making by Bob Vanecko*

journal club, and mortality and morbidity conferences were much improved. Residents were encouraged to publish and to make presentations at national or regional meetings, and to participate in surgical research. In 1964, Dr. William Shoemaker, a renowned researcher in shock was added to the staff to expand research at the Hektoen Institute of CCH. The shock study under his direction exposed many surgical residents to surgical research. Bedside measurement of cardiac dynamics carried out by residents became a common sight in the Trauma Unit (Figure 4–13).

Many residents also participated in animal research at the Hektoen Institute. One of the residents most inspired by Dr. Shoemaker to pursue research was Dr. Joseph Carey. With Dr. Carey's leadership, the shock study made great strides in surgical research and won the group of residents the first surgical research prize ever awarded to residents at CCH by the Chicago Surgical Society. Other academic activities under Freeark's leadership included exhibits and movies that were shown in surgical meetings. Figure 4–14 shows the exhibits built by Robert Vanecko and James Yao presented at the American Medical Association convention. Color photographs displayed in the exhibits were shot by Dr. Yao. Many movies that were shown in the Cine Clinic of the American College of Surgeons convention were produced by Dr. Vanecko (Figure 4–15).

Dr. Freeark was also instrumental to the establishment of the Trauma Unit, the first in the country. He also established the Hand and Burn Unit named for Dr. Sumner Koch. The Burn Unit became the prime location for training of burn care for many surgical residents from all six medical schools in Chicago. Finally, Dr. Freeark initiated the recruitment of specialty surgeons: Drs. John Raffensperger for Pediatric Surgery, John Boswick for Hand Surgery and Burn, William Shoemaker for Surgical Research, Milton Weinberg for Cardiothoracic Surgery, Anthony Raimondi for Neurosurgery, Irving Bush for Urology, Nelson Stone for Plastic Surgery, and David Long for Thoracic Surgery. Dr. William Norcross was fully in charge of emergency surgery performed at night, which eventually developed into a surgical subspecialty, Trauma Surgery. In the late 1960s, under Dr. Freeark's direction, many surgeons from Northwestern and University of Chicago faculty were recruited to provide volunteer service to CCH. This new generation of famed surgeons included Drs. Marion C. Anderson, John J. Bergan, and Otto Trippel of Northwestern; and George Block and Thomas Ferguson of University of Chicago.

Unfortunately, the Freeark era was plagued with political turmoil involving the control of administering the hospital (i.e., the Cook County Board versus a Health and Hospital Governing Commission). Because of the political and acrimonious nature of the conflict, Dr. Freeark resigned as Hospital Superintendent and went on to become Professor and Chairman of the Department of Surgery at Loyola University Medical School where he built an outstanding academic center in Chicago. From the day he resigned from the hospital, Dr. Freeark never again set foot in the hospital.[24]

In 1972, Dr. Gerald Moss from University of Illinois was appointed to the Chairman of Surgery at County Hospital. After the resignation of Dr. Freeark, Northwestern University also suspended their service at CCH. In 1978, under Dr. Olga Jonasson, then Chairman of the Department of Surgery at CCH, the freestanding CCH training program integrated with the University of Illinois Surgical Program. With that integration, Cook County Surgical Residency Program, long an independent program with academic affiliation with several medical schools in Chicago, officially ended. It also ended the long affiliation of Northwestern University with Cook County Hospital. Northwestern faculty members, particularly those who served at CCH since the beginning (Table III) always can look back with pride and honor at this unique affiliation of nearly one hundred years of volunteer service to patients at Cook County Hospital. There will never be another service like this by Northwestern University. Undoubtedly, it is a milestone in postgraduate education in America.

# References

1. McNealy RW. The influence of Cook County Hospital on medical education in the United States. *Q Bull NU Med Sch*. 1957; 31: 164-173.
2. Arey LB. *Northwestern University Medical School, 1859-1979*. Evanston IL: Northwestern University: 1979.
3. Bonner TN. The expansion of medical education in the twentieth century. In: Bonner TN. *Medicine in Chicago, 1850-1950: A chapter in the social and scientific development of a city*. Madison WI: The American History Research Center, Inc.: 1957.
4. Flexner A. *Medical education in United States and Canada*. New York: The Carnegie Foundation for the Advancement of Teaching: 1910.
5. Wentz DK, Ford CV. A brief history of the internship. *JAMA*. 1984: 252:3390-3394.
6. Chicago Medical Society. *History of medicine and surgery and physicians and surgeons of Chicago*. Chicago: The Biographical Publishing Corporation: 1922.
7. Meyer KA. Historical background of Cook County Hospital. *Q Bull NU Med School* 1949: 23:271-275.
8. Beck C, Beck WC, Moody R. Clinical activities at Cook County Hospital. *Proc Inst Med Chgo*. 1987: 40:50-51.
9. Davis L. *J.B. Murphy, Stormy Petrel of Surgery*. New York: GP Putnam's Sons: 1938.
10. Dragstedt LR. Christian Fenger and the Midwestern School of Surgery. The fifth annual Guthrie Memorial Lecture. *Guthrie Clin Bull*. 1963: 33:12-24.
11. Hirsch EF. *Christian Fenger: A physician who inspired his associates to greater goals*. The Dartnell Press: Chicago: 1972.
12. Meyer KA. *John B. Murphy Memorial Lecture. Three great Chicago surgical pioneers: N Senn, JB Murphy, C Fenger*. 24th Annual Congress of International College of Surgeons: September 16, 1959.
13. Murphy JB. Resection of arteries and veins injured in continuity--end-to-end suture. Experimental and clinical research. New York: The Publisher's Printing Company;1897 (Reprint from *Medical Record* 1897: 51:73).
14. Murphy JB. A case of cervical rib with symptoms resembling subclavian aneurism. *Ann Surg*. 1905: 41:399-406.
15. Murphy JB. Removal of an embolus from the common iliac artery, with re-establishment of circulation to the femoral. *JAMA*. 1909: 12:1661-1663.
16. Davis L. *Surgeon Extraordinary, the Life of J.B. Murphy*. George G. Harrap & Co. LTD: London: 1938
17. Schmitz RL, Oh T. Bibliography of John B. Murphy, MD, FACS. *Proc Inst Med Chgo*. 1969: 42:24-27.
18. Rutkow IM. *American surgery: An illustrated history*. Philadelphia: Lippincott-Raven Publishers: 1998.
19. Nagle DJ. The Chicago School of Hand Surgery. *J Hand Surg*. 2003;28: 724-728.
20. Founder Dr. Karl Meyer dies in Chicago. *Int Surgery* 1972: 57:176.
21. Raffensperger J. Personal communication: 2007.
22. Reyes HM. Introducing the Department of Surgery at Cook County Hospital. *Curr Surgery* 1997: 54:280-282.
23. Davis L. *A Surgeon's Odyssey*. Garden City NY: Doubleday & Co.: 1973:251
24. Freeark R. Dr. Robert Freeark. In: Lewis S. Hospital: *An Oral History of Cook CountyHospital*. New York: The New Press; 1994:109.

# 5

# University of Illinois

*Phillip E. Donohue, MD*
*Kenneth Printen, MD*

- *Introduction*
- *Bayard Holmes*
- *Albert Ochsner and Carl Beck*
- *Warren Cole*
- *Rush-University of Chicago-University of Illinois*
- *Lloyd Nyhus*
- *Gerald Moss*
- *Olga Jonasson*
- *Hernan Reyes*
- *References*

## Introduction

When the Flexner Report was published in 1910, only three of the plethora of homeopathic, regular, osteopathic, and other types of full-time and part-time (night school) medical schools in the state of Illinois were judged by Flexner himself to be in good enough standing for full certification.[1] While two of these, Rush and Northwestern, come as no surprise to anyone familiar with the early history of Chicago medicine (since both schools had their academic roots in the educational system begun by Dr. Brainard and his associates based at Mercy Hospital in the 1870s), the third is generally less well-known.

## Bayard Holmes

The third of Flexner's most qualified Illinois schools, like the other two, was located in Chicago. The College of Physicians and Surgeons had been organized in 1881 as a strictly proprietary enterprise. As a prerequisite for the privilege of teaching at the institution, potential faculty members were required to purchase stock in the school. The price list ranged from $500 for an instructor to $2,000 for a full professor. In its early existence, the school and its board were both run by Dr. William Quinne, one of the most accomplished internists in the city. In the early 1890s, he had the good sense to hire Dr. Bayard Holmes (Figure 5–1), a former Cook County intern, as the college secretary. Holmes, who had an interest in bacteriology, collaborated with Fenger in early studies relating to the prevention and treatment of surgical sepsis. He actually set up the first microbiology laboratory in Cook County Hospital in a bathroom between two of the wards.[2] Besides his expertise in applied microbiology, Holmes proved to be a prodigious educational innovator who by 1895, much in advance of Flexner's curriculum recommendations, modified the undergraduate medical curriculum to one that survives largely unchanged to this day. To bolster the teaching staff of the College of Physicians and Surgeons in support of this new curriculum, Holmes hired Albert Ohlmacher, Ludvig Hektoen, Weller van Hook, John B. Murphy, and Henry Byford, all men with ties to Cook County Hospital, to teach endocrinology,

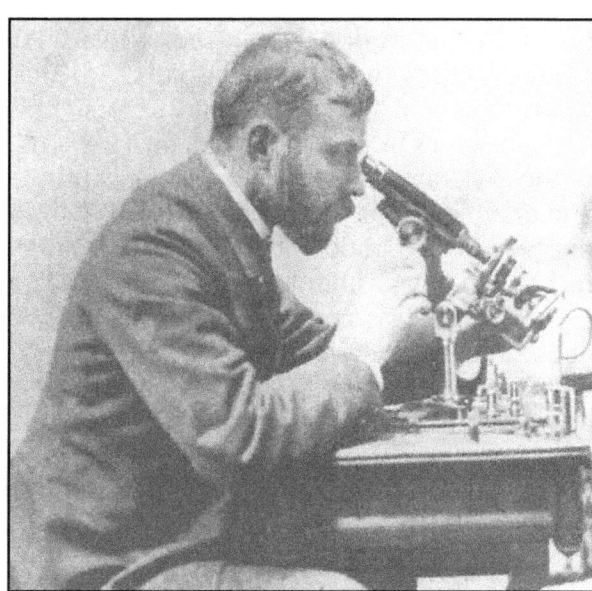

*Figure 5–1  Bayard T. Holmes*

pathology, surgical pathology, surgery, and obstetrics and gynecology, respectively. He himself taught bacteriology. This combination of a new curriculum and a new widely respected faculty helped triple the school's enrollment between 1895 and 1900. In addition, Holmes negotiated a loose informal affiliation with the University of Illinois in 1897. This ensured that the College of Physicians and Surgeons, which was already using Cook County Hospital for clinical teaching, would continue to have a strong academic base nearby.

The affiliation agreement with CCH remained in effect until 1913, when in the face of the Flexner Report and the pressure that it created for predictable uniformity of undergraduate medical curricula and university control of the educational system at large, the physician stockholders decided it was in their best interest to sell the College of Physicians and Surgeons to the University of Illinois. However, with all-too-familiar apathy and indecision, the state legislature could not reach a decision on the purchase. In order to be free of what might turn out to be a costly white elephant, the board donated the medical school to the University.

## Albert Ochsner and Carl Beck

The new University Medical College maintained the long-standing surgical relationship with CCH under the direction of its first chairman, Dr. Albert Ochsner (Figure 5–2), who besides being professor and chairman at the medical school and a long-time County attending, was also a busy surgeon in the community as Chief of Surgery at the Augustana Hospital in the fashionable Near North Side's Gold Coast. He also operated at the not-so-fashionable St. Mary's Hospital in the Polish ethnic neighborhood immediately to the west of the Gold Coast. Dr. Ochsner was one of the giants of early Chicago surgery. Along with J.B. Murphy and Franklin Martin, Ochsner was a founder of the American College of Surgeons, of which he was president in 1923–24 and an editorial board member of *Surgery, Gynecology, and Obstetrics* from its beginning in 1905 until his death. He was also a president of the American Surgical Association and published his own book on the care and treatment of acute appendicitis in 1902.[3] Unlike Murphy and McBurney, he believed in the nonoperative management of the patient with spreading peritonitis, recommending gastric decompression and Fowler's position.

Ochsner was not the only world-class surgeon at the College of Physicians and Surgeons in the early years of the 20th century. Dr. Carl Beck (Figure 5–3), who graduated from medical school in Prague and had studied subsequently in pathology with Virchow and on the Billroth surgical service in Vienna, was on a first-name basis with many of the leading surgical figures in Europe. There is no telling what he might have accomplished in the European surgical circles of his day were it not for several bouts of hemoptysis that necessitated several tours in the sea air as a ship's physician. This got him into contact with fresh clean air, the recommended and only treatment for pulmonary tuberculosis in those days. The trips also put him into contact with Harry Newman, who along with Franklin Martin and Frank Billings founded the Post Graduate Medical School of Chicago. Newman was so impressed with the knowledgeable ship's physician that he offered him a professorship at the school. Beck accepted and began a career that saw him rise to co-founder of the American College of Surgeons and the Chicago Surgical Society. Because of his international connections, which he maintained and fostered, he was a leader in the exchange of ideas in surgical innovation between the United States and Europe. These affiliations are evident in his smoothing the path for Dr. Alexis Carrel's sojourn at the University of Chicago

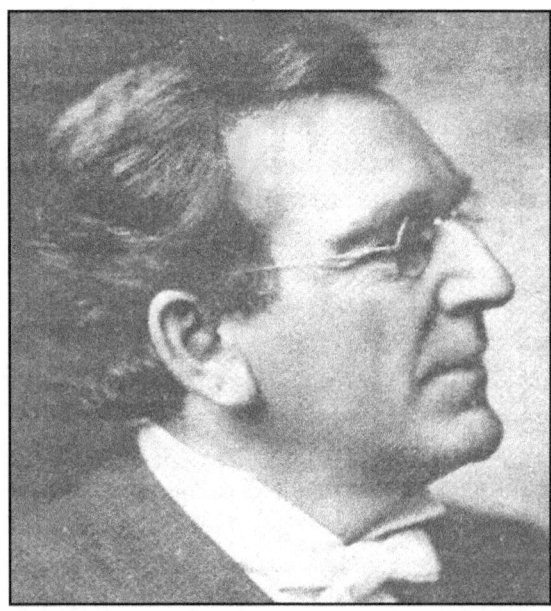

*Figure 5–2*
*Albert J. Ochsner (1858–1925)*

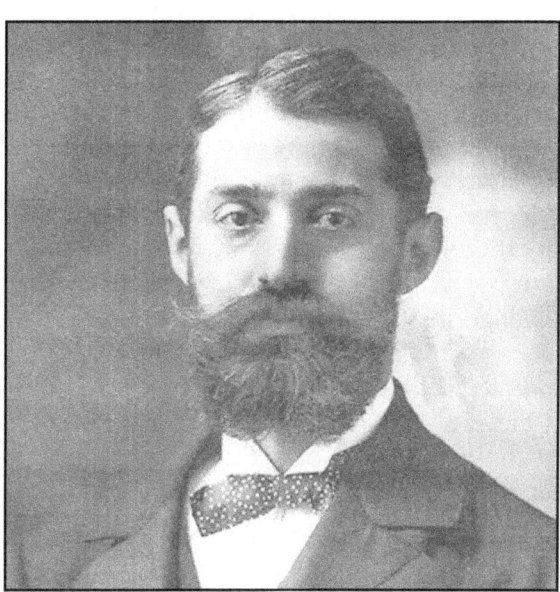

*Figure 5–3  Carl Beck (1864–1952)*

from 1904 to 1906 when the two collaborated to develop a surgical approach to esophageal replacement. While Dr. Carrel departed Chicago for the Rockefeller Institute in late 1906, Dr. Beck continued his international activities, traveling to Europe in 1920 with Dr. Ochsner to supervise distribution of American food and aid to European refugees. In addition, he encouraged his friend Albert Einstein to consider relocating to the United States. Dr. Beck accepted a professorship in surgical pathology at the College of Physicians and Surgeons in 1898, which he retained until his resignation from active practice in 1928. He was also a surgical attending at County from 1898 until 1917.[3]

The Beck name remained in evidence at CCH and the University of Illinois through the efforts of two of Dr. Beck's brothers, Emil and Joseph. Both were educated at the College of Physicians and Surgeons, and both were initially general surgeons. Emil developed an interest in radiology, especially stereo-roentgenography and is best known for his work as a radiologist. Joseph became a founder of the American Board of Otolaryngology and professor at the University of Illinois from 1902 to 1932, as well as an attending at CCH during the same period.

While Drs. Ochsner, Beck, and their associates held academic rank at various of the Chicago-based medical colleges, their teaching at County and other hospitals was largely volunteer and thus uncompensated, a situation very surprising to physicians brought up in the European tradition. The income of these teachers depended on their private practices of surgery at a community hospital of their choice, or as in the case of the Beck brothers, a proprietary hospital of their own. This led to some strange situations. For example, Dr. Arthur Dean Bevan, Professor of Surgery at Rush and attending at the Presbyterian Hospital, served as the surgical consultant at the Lake Forest Hospital. The hospital was located a mile north of "Half-Day Road," which was how long it took a horse and carriage to travel the distance. It was a long way to go to make daily post-op rounds.

## Warren Cole

For the University of Illinois, this situation began to change with the 1936 appointment of Dr. Warren H. Cole as Professor and Chairman of the Department of Surgery, with the status of full-time faculty member. In brief, this meant that his income was totally the province of the University. As more full-time faculty were recruited, there was less and less incentive for the University's instructors to become involved in the uncompensated care system of Cook County Hospital. This change in status was not helped by the fact that the two most imposing surgical personalities at the Westside Medical Center—Dr. Cole, the world-renowned academician, past president of the American College of Surgeons and the American Cancer Society, and noted medical researcher, and Dr. Karl Meyer, master surgical technician, Professor of Surgery at Northwestern, member of the Board of Trustees at the University of Illinois, medical superintendent of Cook County Hospital, and powerful Democratic political figure—just plain didn't like each other very much. It was rumored that Dr. Cole used his influence at the American College of Surgeons (ACS) to keep Dr. Meyer and Dr. Max Thorek, a U of I nontenured Professor of Surgery, who operated twice a week at County and was on the faculty of the Cook County Graduate School of Medicine from 1934 to 1960, out of the American College of Surgeons. All this in spite of the fact that Thorek was widely acknowledged as at least a local expert in breast and plastic surgery.[4] It was also rumored that Meyer and Thorek were largely responsible for the formation of the rival International College of Surgeons, also headquartered in Chicago.

## Rush-University of Chicago-University of Illinois

A fortuitous upheaval in medical school-private hospital alignments occurred at this time that allowed the University of Illinois to maintain its affiliation with County without sacrificing adherence to the full-time faculty model. In 1937, the administrations of the Rush Medical School and the University of Chicago reached agreement that some time in the near future, but certainly within five years, they would cease their collaboration. The University would maintain its own medical college, teaching both the clinical and preclinical segments of the curriculum.

This transition actually took place in 1941 and left a large number of the Presbyterian Hospital surgical staff without an academic home. The University of Illinois affiliated with Presbyterian Hospital for the teaching of medical students and residents under a volunteer "geographic" basis. It turned out to be a win-win situation for all concerned, and the County House staff and U of I students assigned to the wards were the beneficiaries of the talents of a host of surgical attending, such as Fred dePyster, E. Lee Strohl, Frank Theis, and the always gentlemanly and ever-patient Dr. Willis Diffenbaugh. A bit later in time came the originators of the cardiac surgery service, Drs. Egbert Fell and Milton Weinberg, followed by the Julian cardiovascular group, which limited its activity in the County Surgical Program largely to consultative and conference participation.

As in the days of the Flexner Report some 50 years earlier, the late 1950s and early 1960s brought with them calls for standardization of teaching programs and tightening of attending supervision at both the resident and student levels. Dr. Robert Freeark was hired as the first full-time chief of surgery at County in 1958, and one year later Dr. Robert J. Baker became the second full-timer in the Department of Surgery, although he had to be hired as the Chief of the Blood Bank because there was only one full-time salary budgeted in the Department of Surgery: Dr. Freeark's. Dr. Baker, who completed his internship and residency in the same class at County as Freeark, previously served as an Army physician in the Far East, and after a period of time in private practice in southern California returned to do a year of research with Dr. Donald Kozoll, an associate of Dr. Meyer's, at County. Dr. Baker subsequently became Chief of Surgery in 1968–69 after which he left to become a full-time professor at the University of Illinois. A gifted surgeon and operating room teacher, Dr. Baker was the consummate platform lecturer with a quick wit and a bottomless fund of medical knowledge, especially in his favorite areas of pathophysiology and treatment of shock and fluid and electrolyte disturbances. His knack for "grilling" all available target students and residents on ward rounds and the conferences in the ward lecture rooms was legendary but never fatal.

## Lloyd Nyhus

In 1967, Dr. Lloyd Nyhus (Figure 5–4), a surgeon's surgeon with a strong academic background, succeeded Dr. Cole as Chairman at the University of Illinois. Unlike Dr. Cole, Dr. Nyhus had an immediate influence on County and encouraged his faculty to become involved in the teaching program on the north side of Polk Street. Dr. Robert Condon arrived with Nyhus from the University of Washington. While Dr. Condon spent most of his time at the University, he was an attending surgeon at County from 1968 until 1970, when he left to become

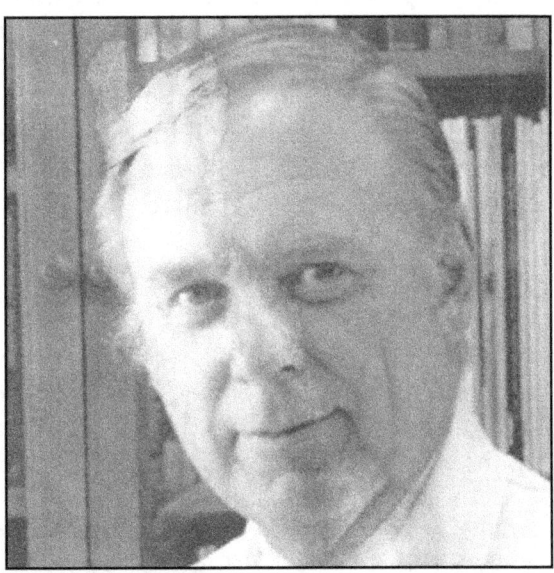

*Figure 5–4 Lloyd Nyhus*

chief at the University of Iowa and later the Medical College of Wisconsin at Milwaukee. Encounters with Dr. Condon on rounds were always lively, sometimes traumatic, but always informative. His previous experience as an officer in the U.S. Marine Corps was generally evident in his approach to teaching rounds. Dr. Nyhus also was active in recruiting Dr. Gerald Moss as the chief of surgery at County in 1970, after the resignations of both Dr. Baker as head of surgery and Dr. Freeark as medical director of Cook County Hospital.

## Gerald Moss

Dr. Moss, a graduate of the Ohio State residency program, was a Vietnam era veteran who had served with the Naval Area Medical Research Unit. At County he continued his work on shock and resuscitation of the injured patient, including important work on the pathogenesis of shock lung. He had an abiding interest in trauma and hemorrhagic shock and was a good fit with the hospital that only four years previously had formed the first comprehensive Trauma Unit in the United States. He and his team made important strides in working with solubilized hemoglobin (Polyheme), which was later tested extensively in the critical care arena as a substitute for blood in acute hemorrhagic shock, especially in situations where banked blood was not available. Dr. Moss encouraged a variety of research and educational activities among the residents and students assigned to County. Among the most notable on the clinical research side was the innovation in antibiotic bowel prep devised at County under the inspiration of Dr. Sherwood Gorbach, head of the Division of Infectious Diseases. This Neomycin-Erythromycin combination, later known as the Condon-Nichols prep (after Dr. Robert Condon and his resident Dr. Ronald Nichols), rapidly became the gold standard in bowel surgery since it was the first combination to address eradication of the huge numbers of anaerobic flora in the gut. On the educational side, Moss combined the weekly County surgical conference, which had been started by the house staff in the mid 1960s, with the U of I College surgical conference. This lively, comprehensive, and wide-ranging give-and-take session lasted until the early part of the 21st century when it fell victim to the constraints of the 80-hour work week for residents. In 1977, Dr. Moss left County to become chief of surgery at the University of Illinois-affiliated Michael Reese Hospital. In 1990, he returned to the Westside Medical Center as the chief of surgery and later dean of the U of I College of Medicine.

## Olga Jonasson

In 1977, Dr. Olga Jonasson, the first woman to head a major surgical department in the United States, became the department head at County. Like Drs. Baker and Moss before her, her academic appointment was at the University of Illinois. She had been a protégé of Dr. Cole and initiated the renal transplant services at the U of I College. She and Dr. Nyhus recognized the importance of a major academic partner of the County Department of Surgery and proposed a combined residency in 1980. Dr. Jonasson was the prime mover in the integration of the County and University of Illinois surgical residencies, which produced a monolith that for several years contained more than 100 residents and finished 12 chief residents per year. Under her aegis, the most cherished teaching conferences were those that were held in her home on nearby Jackson Boulevard. In addition to her activities as chief of surgery at County, Dr. Jonasson was in charge of the National Institutes of Health (NIH) Fellowships at the University of Illinois Hospital. In that capacity she was able to provide learning experiences for residents in the medical center at both County and University of Illinois Chicago. As luck would have it, one of the residents who she helped to get one of these fellowships, for esophageal surgery in 1975, did the seminal work in establishing the floppy Nissen fundoplication as "a standard method of performance worldwide." That same resident, Dr. Phil Donohue, after a successful career at the University of Illinois and County, became the chief of general surgery at the Stroger Hospital, the successor to County in all but name.

Dr. Jonasson left County in the late 1980s to become the chair of surgery at the Ohio State College of Medicine and subsequently headed the Department of Education at the American College of Surgeons.

## Hernan Reyes

Dr. Hernan Reyes, a noted pediatric surgeon, followed Dr. Jonasson as chair at County and as professor of surgery at Illinois as well. He salso erved as the chief of pediatric surgery and was active in the management of pediatric trauma. It fell to Dr. Reyes to oversee the transition of the County surgical services from the purview of the University of Illinois to Rush College of Medicine in 2001 when the latter assumed the mantle of academic sponsorship. While there is still the opportunity for residents and students from the U of I to rotate through various County services, there is no question that the major input of the University was accomplished before the 2001 transition. However, we would be remiss if we did not include at this juncture the mention of some U of I individuals and programs that were in evidence in times past or may have assimilated in the new institutional education structure.

In the period of the 1950s to the 1980s the University of Illinois wards at County had the benefit of a number of attending with University of Illinois affiliations. One of those remembered by a number of residents was Dr. Sidney Black, who combined his knowledge of surgery with an advanced degree in anatomy, which he taught to the underclassmen at the University of Illinois College. No herniorrhaphy or cholecystectomy on Dr. Black's service could pass without a full-scale anatomy lesson complete with quiz and a real life practical exam. He was as diligent in ward rounds as he was in OR attendance and could usually be counted on to make his opinions known at the Monday afternoon surgical pathology conferences.

The Colon and Rectal Surgery Unit was established by Dr. Hernand Abcarian, a graduate of the County Surgery Residency in the mid-1970s after he completed a fellowship in Colon and Rectal Surgery at St. Mark's Hospital in

London. At the time, it was the first such teaching service in Chicago. As one of the earliest surgeons in Chicago to utilize flexible fiberoptic endoscopy to diagnose colon disease, Dr. Abcarian was a leader in the endoscopic field as it progressed into the age of new optics and better tools. In 1981, he and two foregut surgeon-endoscopists from the University of Illinois, Drs. Tom Bombeck and Phil Donohue, were among the founding members of the Society of American Gastro Endoscopic Surgeons (SAGES). Dr. Abcarian went on to become chief of surgery at the U of I, and after his retirement from that position, returned to become fellowship director of the colon and rectal training program at County.

The creation of Surgical Critical Care as a separate surgical specialty occurred around 1980 as the specialized support for postoperative patients including ventilators and cardiac support became more widespread. County Hospital surgeons, however, had a long history of interest in postoperative care. Dr. Karl Meyer believed in frequent checks on postoperative patients and knew that there was no substitute for personal surveillance of the patient after surgery. For years house officers in medicine and surgery practiced the art of "evening rounds," which included a bedside visit to every patient on the service, figuratively tucking the patients into bed for the evening. It was a custom most appreciated by the patients and a way to avoid a lot of 0200 calls for things that could have been avoided. Eventually, much of this activity took place, at least for the critically ill surgical patients, in the Surgical Intensive Care Unit. Dr. Samuel Appavu, who finished the County Program under Dr. Moss in 1975, was the first director of the County Hospital Surgical Intensive Care Unit. In 2001, he received ACGME accreditation for a Surgical Critical Care Fellowship at Cook County Hospital. Although Dr. Appavu has left to assume the chairmanship of surgery at the University of Illinois Medical School at Rockford, the unit and the program continue to provide support and care for some of the sickest patients in the hospital.

## References

1. Flexner A. *Medical Education in the United States and Canada: A Report to the Carnegie Foundation for the Advancement of Teaching*, Bulletin No. 4. New York City; The Carnegie Foundation for the Advancement of Teaching: 1910.
2. Bonner TN. The birth of Modern Medical Science 1850-1900. In: *Medicine in Chicago 1850-1950*. Madison: The American History Research Center: 1957:37
3. Rutkow I M. Albert Ochsner. In: *American Surgery: An Ilustrated History*. Philadelphia:Lippincott-Raven: 1998:286.
4. Thorek M. *A Surgeon's World: The Autobiography of Max Thorek*. Philadelphia, New York; J B Lippencott Co: 1943.

# Loyola University

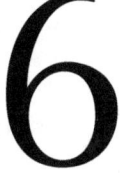

*Harold Haley, MD*
*Frank Folk, MD*
*Kenneth Printen, MD*

- *Stritch School of Medicine*
- *Surgical Department Chairs and CCH*
- *Loyola Surgical Faculty at CCH*
- *Dr. Harold Haley—First Full-time Faculty at CCH*
- *Mercy-Loyola Faculty at CCH*
- *References*

## Stritch School of Medicine

Loyola University was founded in 1870 as St. Ignatius College. It is the largest Jesuit Catholic University in the United States. The School of Medicine originated in 1909, when an affiliation was formed with the Illinois Medical College that became the Medical Department of Loyola University. This affiliation preceded the publication of the AMA's Flexner Report in 1910 that recommended standardization of undergraduate medical education and the closure, or at least the consolidation, of proprietary and notoriously weak medical schools. Nowhere was this dictum more important than in Illinois, where it had long been recognized that the majority of the medical schools fell below any acceptable standard of education, both in faculty and curriculum. In Chicago, the report led to the formation of the University of Illinois College of Medicine in addition to Loyola and the Chicago Medical School as independent entities.

In 1910, the Bennett and Reliance Medical Colleges merged to form the Bennett Medical College, which became affiliated with Loyola University. With the combination of these three medical schools, at this juncture the medical department had grown large enough to form a separate college within the university, which was formally designated as the Loyola University Medical School. The school continued to expand, and in 1917 it purchased the Chicago College of Medicine and Surgery complete with its buildings (Figure 6–1), which were located at 706 South Lincoln Street (later Wolcott Street), immediately to the east of the main County Hospital building and directly opposite the exit road from the County emergency room. The location was extremely convenient for the new school since it could continue to make use of the County teaching arrangements that its recently amalgamated medical colleges had previously established. In addition, Loyola developed a very productive affiliation with Mercy Hospital beginning in 1919 that provided many years of excellent clinical training for the medical students and seasoned surgical clinicians for the Loyola wards at County. As in the present day, funding for a private medical school was always a tenuous situation, but with the financial assistance of Samuel Cardinal Stritch)—who felt very strongly that Chicago should have a Catholic medical school)—Loyola was able to manage without its own university hospital, making extensive use of both County and Mercy for clinical education.

In recognition of the Cardinal's support, the school was renamed Stritch School of Medicine in 1948.

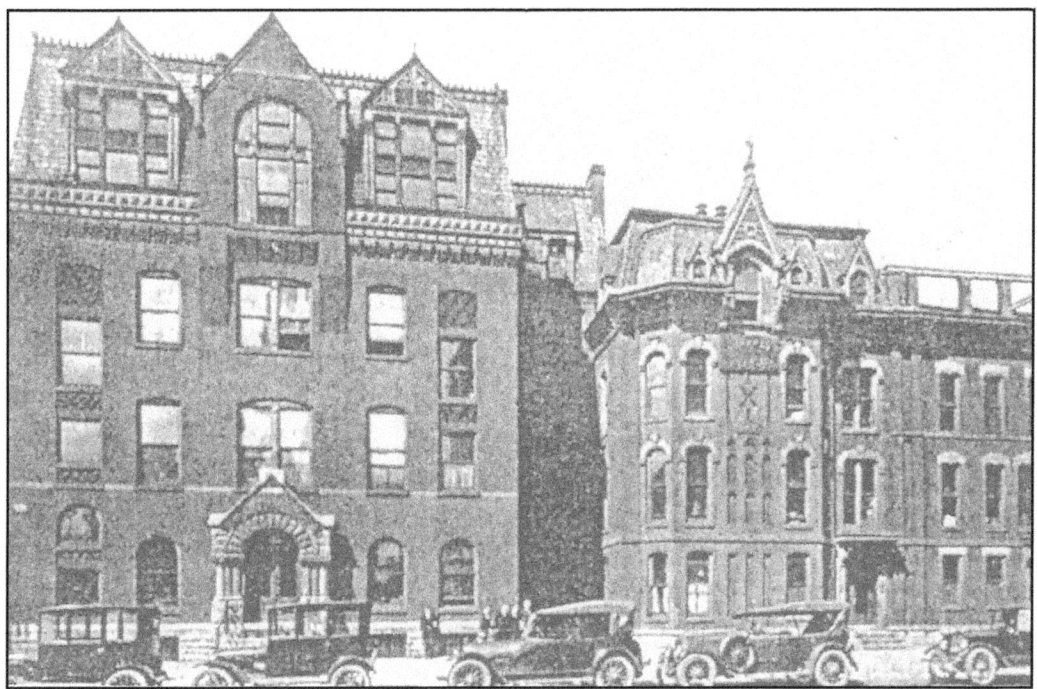

*Figure 6–1 Strich School of Medicine, Loyola University, 706 South Lincoln Street*

## Surgical Department Chairs and CCH

The importance of Cook County Hospital to the new medical school is evident from the fact that the earliest chairmen, Dr. John D. Robertson, 1909–1916 (Figure 6–2), and Dr. Lawrence Ryan, 1917–20, were already attendings at County when the Loyola Medical School was organized, and both kept their appointments even after they stopped being department chairs of the school. The second chairman was Dr. Hugh Mackechnie, 1916–1917 (Figure 6–3). While there is no ready reference as to his status at County, the proximity of the school to the hospital plus the affiliation agreement for student teaching, lead one to believe that he was at least a consultant, given his status in the surgical community at the time.

These earliest of the Loyola surgical chiefs were all interesting figures. Dr. Robertson advertised himself as a surgeon and practicioner of public health. In fact, he was the Chicago Commissioner of Health from 1915 to 1922. In addition to his work as a physician, he did quite well as a real estate broker and seems to have been involved in the sale of the Wolcott Street property to several medical schools in the early 1900s. While both Drs. Mackechnie and Ryan were prominent Chicago surgeons with practices at South Shore, Illinois Masonic, and St Anthony's Hospitals, Dr. Robertson's resume does not even show that he had a private office. The same notable absence is observed in memberships in organizations. Both Drs. Mackechnie and Ryan list a number of medical organizational memberships including the Chicago Pathological Society, the B&O Railroad Surgeons Society,

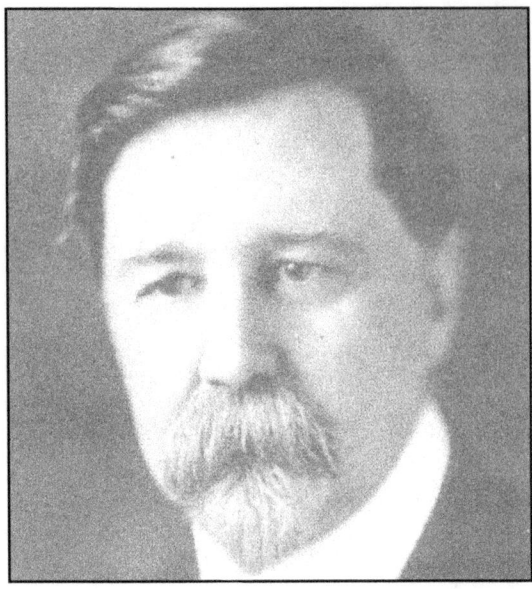

*Figure 6–2 John Dill Robertson*

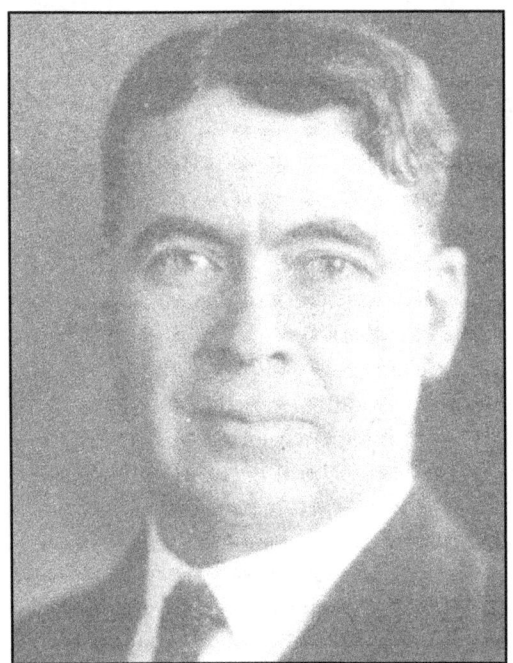

*Figure 6–3 Hugh Neil Mackechnie*

and in Dr. Ryan's case, the Chicago Surgical Society, which was quite a prestigious honor then as now. Robertson tended more toward public health and Masonic organizations. His publications were mostly pamphlets on public health topics, while his successors wrote on jejeunal diverticula and hernias in children in recognized surgical journals.[1]

There is no question that, at least administratively, the department of surgery was the province of the Moorhead family from 1920 to 1940. Dr. Edward L. Moorhead served as the chief of general surgery from 1920 to 1928. His son, Dr. Louis D. Moorhead, was the dean of the medical school from 1920 to 1928 and the chairman of surgery from 1928 to 1940. The Moorheads were primarily in private practice and did most of their work at Mercy Hospital. They were close to the Catholic archdiocesan hierarchy, with Dr. Louis serving as the personal physician to both Cardinal Mundelein and Cardinal Stritch. As a member of the Papal household in service to the Pope, Dr. L.D. Moorhead was sealed with the College of Cardinals in the Vatican when Pope Pius XII was elected in 1939.[2]

## Loyola Surgical Faculty at Cook County Hospital

Despite the fact that the majority of the Loyola faculty was centered in private practice at Mercy, St. Joseph's, and Loretto Hospitals in the city, there was an increasing presence of Loyola attending and associate physicians on the surgical staff of County. Whether this was because of an increasing number of County-trained individuals on the staff of the medical school or for other reasons is uncertain, but the influence of County on the surgical faculty is clear. The subsequent chairmen—Dr. Harry Oberhelmen, 1940–1960 (Figure 6–4), Dr. John Keeley, 1960–1968 (Figure 6–5), Dr. Paul Fox, 1968–1970 (Figure 6–6), and Dr. Robert Freeark, 1970–1995—were or had been very active members of the County surgical teaching staff. Oberhelmen, Keeley, and Fox were all attending pediatric surgeons on Ward 46, mostly in the days before this branch of surgery was recognized as an independent specialty. Both Drs. Keeley and Oberhelmen were accomplished pediatric thoracic surgeons, and especially Dr. Keeley who was an attending night surgeon from 1941 to 1949, who regularly came in to help

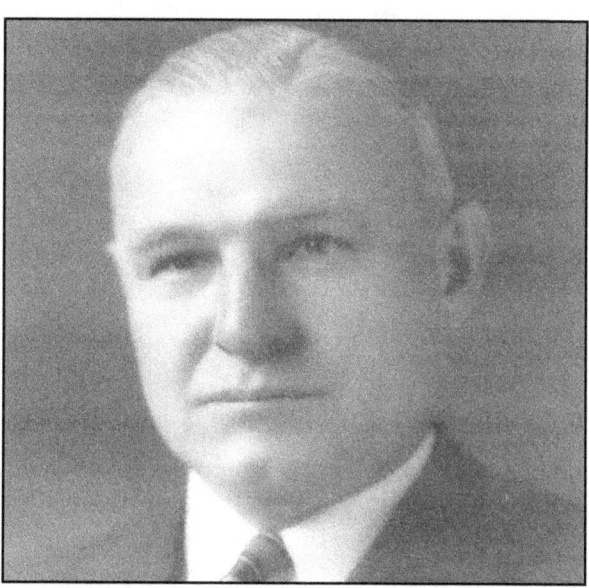

*Figure 6–4*
*Harry Oberhelman (1940-1960)*

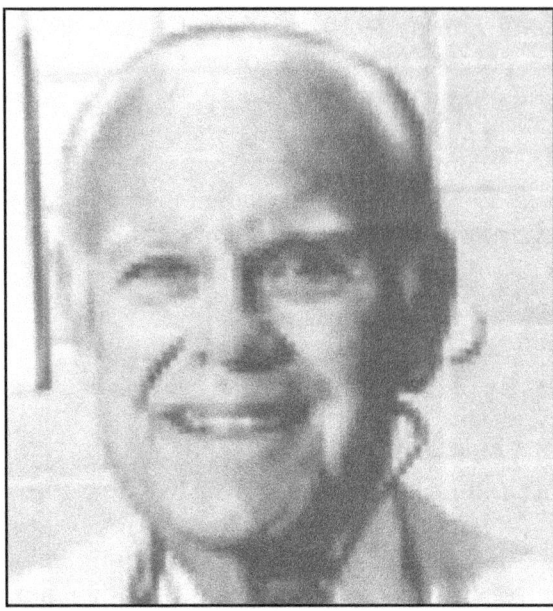

*Figure 6–5*
*John Keeley (1960–1968)*

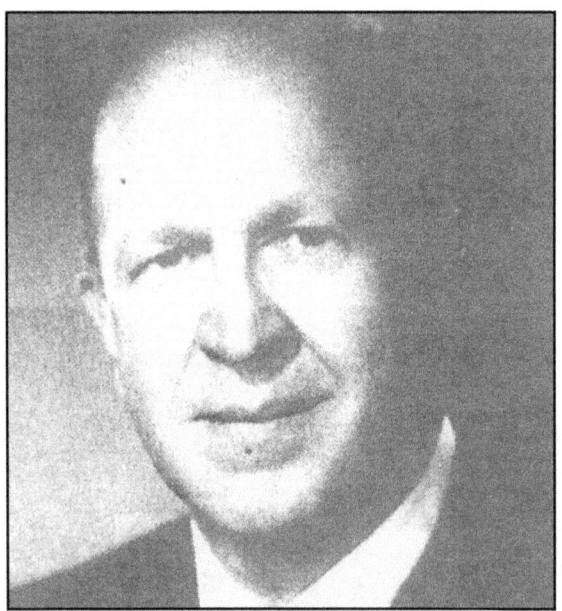

*Figure 6–6 Paul Fox (1968–1970)*

on complicated emergency cases such as pediatric tracheo-esophageal fistulae.[3] Dr. Fox, who had worked with Dr. Willis Potts at Children's Memorial Hospital in Chicago in the early days of pediatric cardiac and vascular surgery, had a long history of attending service on Ward 46 and could always be counted on to provide sage advice on patient care, usually from the bedside, not the telephone.

## Dr. Harold Haley—First Full-time Faculty at CCH

The volunteer faculty with Loyola academic appointments exerted quite an influence on the teaching program of both students and residents in County's department of surgery. As a matter of fact, by the late 1950s, Loyola-associated surgeons were assigned to so many services that students couldn't be assigned to all of them all the time. However, as Dr. Harold Haley (Figure 6–7), the first and only full-time salaried Loyola surgeon at County during that time, recounts:

> Cook County was a place where the medical schools could help serve the general public. It also provided a mechanism for interaction and cooperation between various clinical departments and among the different schools. Interrelationships among the schools occurred in both teaching and research. Ward lectures were open to anyone who showed up regardless of academic affiliation. On any given ward there were usually four separate services, often with attendings from different schools. When making rounds most attending would include any students on site without regard to what medical school they came from. This comaraderie and collegiality among the physicians, residents, and students was one of the great things about Cook County Hospital Surgery. Being an attending was meaningful for both the volunteers and the full-time staff.

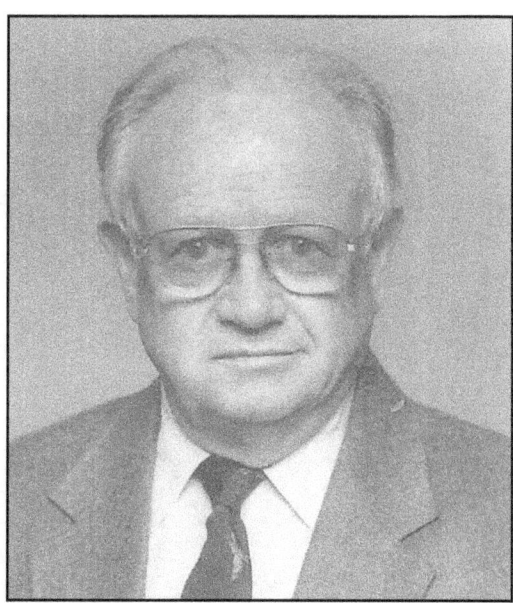

*Figure 6–7  Harold Haley*

## Mercy-Loyola Faculty at CCH

Initially, the majority of the Loyola graduates were surgeons who had their practice based at Mercy, which was Loyola's major private hospital affiliate. But as time passed and more County graduates remained in the city and suburbs to practice following completion of their training, the spectrum of practice loci widened considerably.

Of the Mercy faculty, Dr. Arkell Vaughan was always recognizable by his string ties, Stetson hat, and cigar, which from time to time was known to shed an ash on healing wounds during rounds, an event followed by the reassurance, "That's OK. It'll make the wound heal faster." And it most often did. Dr. John B. O'Donohue, who will be mentioned in more detail in Chapter 24: Historical Vignettes, was a surgeon of the old school who was imposing in manner and delighted in carrying off the popular version of the successful physician in practice. Dr. Robert Schmitz (Figure 6–8) came from a family of physicians . He was a tall, patrician figure who trained at the Mayo Clinic and brought with him an air of gentleness and respect for the patients, residents, and students. He was as precise in manner as he was in surgical technique, with a wit as sharp as his scalpel. He was likely the first attending on rounds to have called a third-year student "Doctor," meaning it as a compliment. A great admirer of John B. Murphy, he edited a book on the surgical contributions of J.B. Murphy.[4]

The volunteer Loyola attending with County ties who staffed the many surgical services included Dr. John Howser, the first County surgical resident and the intern who actually did swallow his cigarette when Dr. Meyer stepped into his elevator. Dr. Everett Nicholas was a long-term attending from the western suburbs who enjoyed a long relationship with County. Drs. John Condon and Ed Sinaiko were two of the only attendings to practice on both the pediatric and adult surgical services. Dr Morris Friedell, the long-time owner of the Jackson Park Hospital,

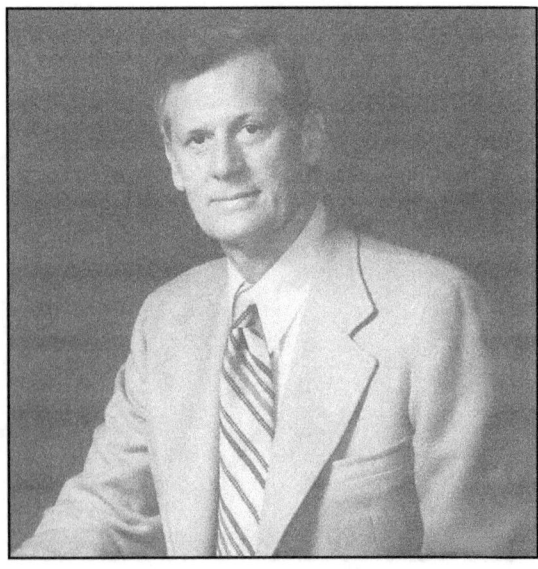

*Figure 6–8  Robert Schmitz*

was the thyroid expert of his day, and residents lined up to get cases for him on his Monday afternoon OR time. Drs. James Kane Sr., Warren Clohissey, and Henri Conti all served long terms as associates to a host of older attendings. Almost all of the residents experienced two rotations on the Breast Clinic begun by Dr. Louis River just before WWII. Dr. River was a Loyola faculty member, as were his associates on the service, Drs. Joseph Silverstein, John Tope, and Frank Folk.

The connection between Loyola and County diminished after 1970 when Loyola was finally able to build its own medical center complete with a teaching hospital in the suburb of Maywood, some distance from the West Side Medical Center. However, the roots of the surgical service at the new location showed evidence of the shadows of County with the recruitment of Dr. Freeark as the first Chairman of Surgery at the new Loyola Medical Center; Dr. Frank Folk, a former County Chairman of Surgery and long-time attending on the Breast Service; John Bartizal and Frank Banich, products of the County training program; and later Jim Kennedy (Figure 6–9), also a former County surgical resident, hired as professor of surgical anatomy.

There are a host of other Loyola faculty who contributed to surgical education at County, especially in the days before the construction of the logo for University Medical Center (LUMC) in Maywood. While we have mentioned some of them and others will appear in Chapter 24, we could not cite them all here but know that all of them fit the model described by Dr. Haley:

> *Attending and associate surgeons had many positive characteristics. They were unpaid volunteers who enjoyed giving their time, knowledge, and skills in service to the County patients. They valued their teaching time and the opportunity to see patients with a wide gamut of diseases. Interrelationships with colleagues were important and there was prestige associated with appointment as a County Attending.*

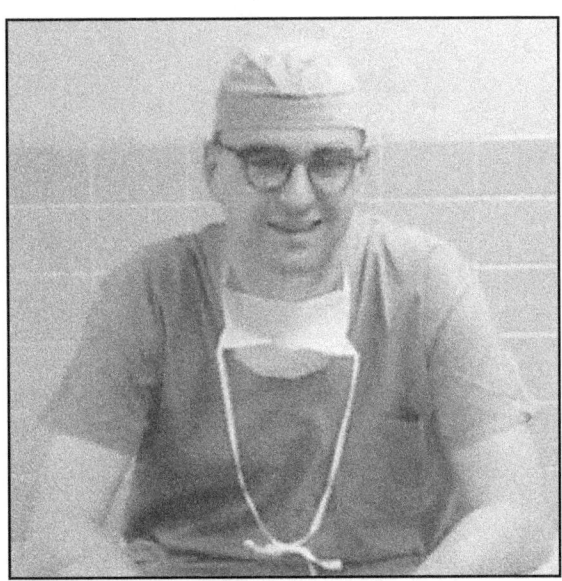

*Figure 6–9 Jim Kennedy*

## References

1. Chicago Medical Society. *History of Medicine and Physicians and Surgeons of Chicago.* Chicago: The Biographical Publishing Corporation: 1922.
2. Loyola University Health Systems. *Department of Surgery: News and Events.* January, 2009.
3. John Raffensperger: Personal Communication.
4. Schmitz Robert L and Oh, Timothy T. *The Remarkable Surgical Practice of John Benjamin Murphy.* Champaign, Illinois: University Of Illinois Press: 1993.

# 7

# Chicago Medical School

*Michael J. Zdon, MD*

- *History of Chicago Medical School'*
- *CMS and its affiliation with Cook County Hospital*
- *AMA Accreditation*
- *CMS and Jewish Business Community*
- *CMS and its Affliliated Hospitals*
- *University Health Sceincies*
- *CMS and Downey VA in North Chicago*

The Chicago Medical School (CMS) has enjoyed a fruitful relationship with Cook County Hospital since the first formal agreement was entered between the two institutions in 1924. Of all the medical schools in Chicago, Chicago Medical School is probably the least understood, but it has a rich history and a relationship with Cook County that continues through to the present day. In the following pages, I will briefly recount the somewhat stormy history of the school and its relationship to both Cook County Hospital and the many physicians who have been associated with County and Chicago Medical School.

## History of Chicago Medical School

In January 1912, two physicians—Drs. Norbert Odeon Bourke and Frederick Leusman—along with Frederick Landwer, a local minister, formed a medical school called the Chicago Hospital-College of Medicine. The school was located in a building that originally housed the Hering Medical College (a homeopathic teaching institution) in the 3800 block of South Rhodes Avenue. It was located about two blocks east of what is now Martin Luther King Drive and two blocks north of Pershing Road, in the middle of what became the Ida B. Wells housing project. It was chartered in the state of Illinois as a nonprofit educational corporation and was recognized by the Illinois Department of Registration and Education as an accredited medical school. The four-story building housed laboratories, classrooms, a library, and a 300-seat amphitheatre. In addition, there was an adjacent clinic building and free dispensary. Within two years, the school erected its own hospital—the Fort Dearborn Hospital—directly behind the Rhodes Avenue building (Figure 7–1).

In 1917, the Chicago Hospital-College of Medicine absorbed the Jenner Medical College that had been in existence in Chicago since 1893, and in 1919, the school was renamed the Chicago Medical School. Originally, the institution was proprietary in that the owners of the school served as its Board of Directors, Board of Administrators, and faculty, an arrangement that unfortunately resulted in later difficulties.

Although most people nowadays associate the school as an institution with strong Jewish ties, this ethnic affiliation did not occur until the 1940s. Indeed, the school had always prided itself on the fact that admission was based on academic qualifications and not sex, race, religion, or national origin. The early cur-

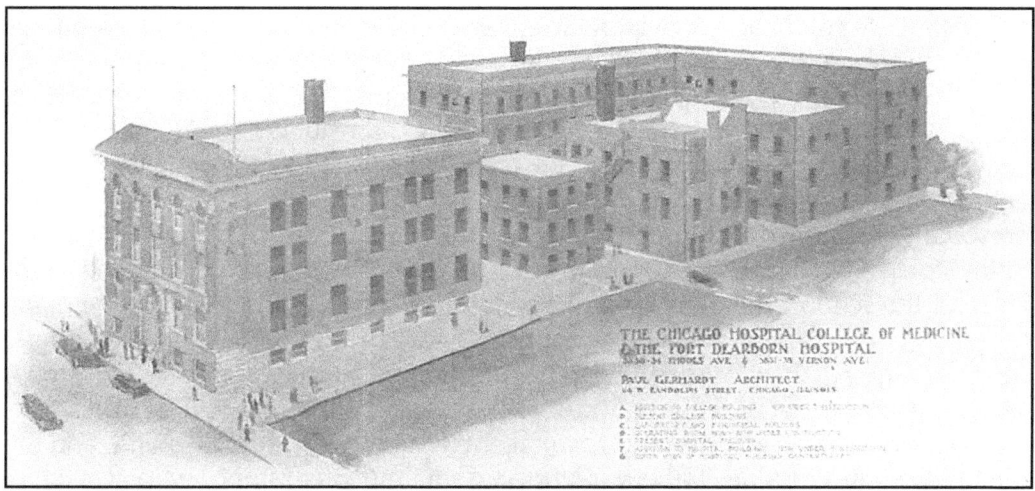

*Figure 7-1   Chicago Hospital College of Medicine and the Fort Dearborn Hospital on South Rhodes Avenue*

riculum was a relatively standard four years with one notable exception: Classes were scheduled in the late afternoons and evenings. The founders' intention in this regard was to have a school where "employed men and women who wished to become physicians could study medicine at night." Although somewhat unorthodox, this was at the height of the Progressivism movement in which social activists from a variety of professions demanded that greater attention be paid to the lower and middle classes of society, and this deviation from the norm was generally considered an enlightened view that allowed working students to attend classes in their off-duty hours in some social quarters. Unfortunately for the school, the medical community at large was not so enlightened.

The 1910 report on Medical Education in the United States by Abraham Flexner recommended the reduction of medical colleges throughout the United States and improvement in the standards of existing schools. The report was enthusiastically endorsed by the AMA. At the time of the Flexner Report, the AMA had instituted a policy of grading medical schools A, B, or C corresponding to acceptable, doubtful, and unacceptable, and set up the Council on Medical Education to inspect and rate schools. At the time, the major recommendation of the Council was for independent medical colleges to either affiliate with major universities and acquire substantial financial endowments or close their doors.

These recommendations had a major impact. Between 1906 and 1929, the number of medical colleges in the United States decreased from 161 to 79. The number in Illinois dropped from 14 to five, and four had major university affiliations. These were the Rush Medical College of the University of Chicago, The College of Physicians and Surgeons of the University of Illinois, Bennett Medical College of Loyola University, and Northwestern Medical School. Only CMS remained independent. If left up to the AMA, there would have been no CMS at that time, but since the Illinois Department of Registration and Education recognized the school, its graduates were allowed to take state exams and practice in Illinois (and Massachusetts).

That the school did survive is a testament to the will of one of its founders, Dr. N. Odeon Bourke (Figure 7–2). Bourke was considered a highly qualified surgeon in Chicago. He was born in Paris, France, and received his medical education at the University of Paris and University of Tennessee. His aggressive personality and unconventional views on nighttime classes did not endear him to the conservative medical community of the city. This wound up creating problems for the school. The early faculty of the school numbered 92, including many prominent surgeons in the city. Among these was Rudolph Menn, who briefly served as the Chair of Surgery in 1918 and trained at the University of Vienna. Menn was Professor of Surgery at the former Jenner Medical College and an attending surgeon at Cook County Hospital, German (now Grant) Hospital, and the Illinois Central Hospital. Others included Benjamin Breakstone, who was chief surgeon at the West End Hospital, a former attending at County and professor of general and genito-urinary surgery at the Bennett-Loyola medical school, as well as at Rush. He was the author of a textbook on ambulatory surgery and a series of papers on the value and abuses of medical charity. George C. Hall (president and chief surgeon of the Provident Hospital) and John McKeller were additional members of the early surgical staff.

The school experienced financial difficulties in the early 1920s, and in the fall of 1923 a crisis occurred when the state withdrew the school's accreditation. It seems that the main reason for this withdrawal was the presence of Dr. Bourke. If the school found a suitable replacement for Dr. Bourke, the state would consider restoring its accreditation. Much to the amazement of everyone, Dr. Bourke agreed to resign, and on the recommendation of the State Board, Dr. A. Augustus

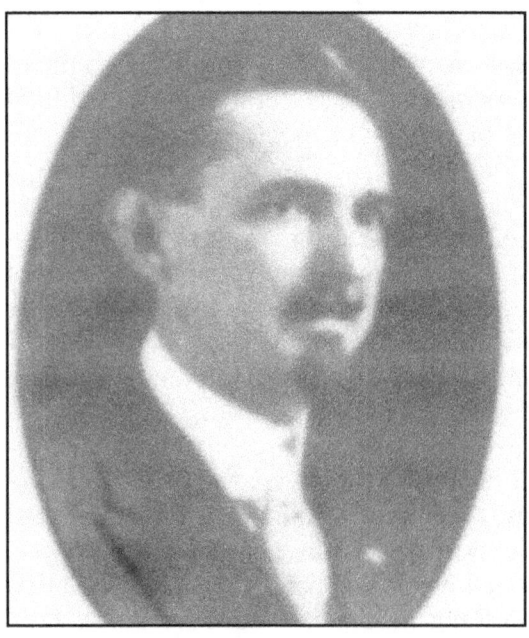

*Figure 7-2 N. Odeon Bourke*
*Founder of Chicago Medical School*

O'Neill was approached and agreed to become the school's administrator, a fortuitous choice for the school.

Although he was 64 at the time, O'Neill was a highly respected figure in Chicago medicine. Trained at Kansas Medical College, Jefferson Medical College in Philadelphia, and the New York Polyclinic, O'Neill came to Chicago where he developed a large surgical practice. He was a fellow of the American College, and among his accomplishments were President and Surgeon in Chief of the Columbia Hospital, President of the Chicago Medical Society (1916–1917), Chairman of the Illinois Influenza Commission, Regional Director of the American Red Cross appointed by Woodrow Wilson, and President of the Chicago Physicians Club. Dr. O'Neill in turn recruited many prominent physicians to the faculty, including Bayard Holmes, a nationally noted heart specialist who some 20 years previous had modernized the undergraduate medical curriculum at the College of Physicians and Surgeons (now the University of Illinois) well in advance of the Flexner Report; Frank Maple from Rush Medical College to chair Obstetrics; and Dorrin Rudnick, a prominent pathologist at Cook County Hospital. This period also saw the recruitment of several strong deans, among them A. Newman Dorland, author of *Dorland's American Medical Illustrated Dictionary*. In addition, the school finally transitioned to a day curriculum, and in 1927 the night extension was formally dropped. With all these changes in place, the school easily won reaccreditation by the state in 1925.

## Chicago Medical School and its Affiliation with Cook County Hospital

The departure of Dr. Bourke also terminated the relationship with the Fort Dearborn Hospital and thus began affiliations with multiple institutions to provide clinical training, which continues to this day. In 1924, the school reached a formal agreement with Cook County Hospital where clinics and classes were arranged for CMS students on Tuesday and Saturday afternoons and all day and evening on Thursdays. Among the County staff who provided instruction but were not formal faculty were Karl Meyer, David Strauss, Alex Goldsmith, and Clarence McMullen. Karl Meyer, in particular, remained a strong friend and supporter of CMS throughout his life.

By the late 1920s, the school was beginning to outgrow the facilities on Rhodes Avenue. In addition, in 1927 the City of Chicago decided to condemn the building in order to create the park that still exists in that location. The combination forced the school to seek new accommodations.

In 1930, the school located a vacant building next to the Loyola Medical School on Wolcott (then Lincoln) Avenue (Figure 7–3). Previously, the building housed the Francis Willard Temperance Hospital and was literally across the street from the County Hospital, proving ideal for both the faculty and students. This new home of Chicago Medical School consisted of five stories with two substantial amphitheaters and adequate space for offices, classrooms, laboratories, a library, and a large museum.

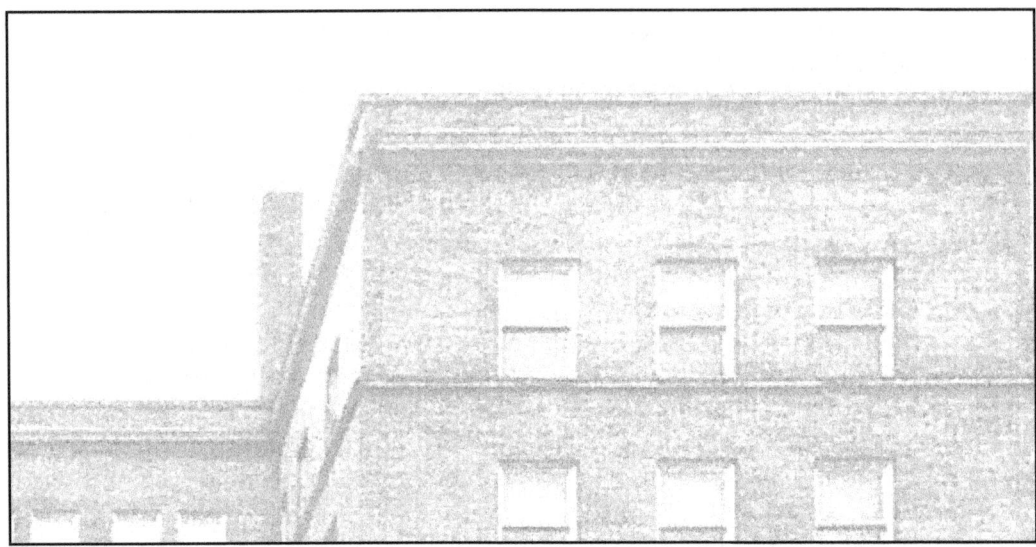

*Figure 7-3  Chicago Medical School Building, 710 S. Wolcott Street*

## AMA Accreditation

Despite the advancements made in the 1920s with regard to organization, administration, faculty, and new facilities, national accreditation through the AMA was not forthcoming primarily due to the lack of university affiliation. In 1930, the state once again threatened to withdraw accreditation. Although Dr. O'Neill was much more respected than his predecessor Dr. Bourke, his advanced age at the time, as well as the fact that the school was still organized as a proprietary entity with Dr. O'Neill wielding complete power, prompted the state to demand that new leadership with a reformed organizational structure and a more secure endowment be put in place. After some discussion with a faculty committee, Dr. O'Neill agreed to step down. In addition, the president of the school forfeited his absolute veto power, and the status of hospital affiliations underwent review and reorganization, as required both by the AMA and the state. Most of these responsibilities fell to Dr. Abel Larrain who was appointed acting dean.

In addition to abolition of the president's veto power, a new constitution and a completely reorganized board was formed with increased membership (to 25), including staff members of the affiliated hospitals and several physicians from Cook County, faculty, alumni, and various respected business leaders. The new constitution was approved in 1932. The first president of the board was Dr. Henry Mundt, an opthamologist and graduate of the University of Illinois Medical School with ties to the AMA and the State Board of Education. For vice president, the highly regarded surgeon Leslie MacDiarmid was elected. Dr. MacDiarmid also served as chair of surgery from 1931–38.

The third and most impressive prong of reform was faculty reorganization. This resulted in the recruitment of an impressive list of basic scientists to join the school. Among these was an anatomist, John J. Sheinin. The addition of Dr. Sheinin proved to be probably the most important addition in the history of the school.

On the clinical side, Larrain decided the school would try to develop a closer relationship with Cook County Hospital. However, this seemed a difficult proposition as nearly all of County's attending staff already was associated with other medical schools. The new administration came with what for the time was a radical idea: They would offer salaries to clinical faculty. CMS appears to be the first medical school in Chicago to offer to pay physicians in private practice to teach medical students. With the commitment to provide compensation for physician-teachers, a number of eminent clinicians at Cook County Hospital accepted faculty appointments at CMS. These included Maxwell Phillip Borovsky as chair of pediatrics, Egon Walter Fischmann in gynecology, and in surgery, Drs. John Ross Harger, Leslie MacDiarmid, and Cassius Rogers. Other surgeons of note to join the school were the noted proctologist Charles Drueck and general surgeons Wade Harker, Paul Papsdorf, and Edwin Sloan.

With this major transformation complete, the expectation of everyone was that accreditation would easily occur as the school was now positioned on the same level or one better than the other existing schools. Unfortunately, because of continuing administrative difficulties with the AMA accrediting body, another reorganization of the school was required. On December 5, 1935, John Sheinin (Figure 7–4), the chair of anatomy, reluctantly agreed to take the position of dean, a decision that turned out to be the most fortuitous in the school's history.

Sheinin's first action was to propose revisions to the constitution including elimination of faculty members on the board as well as the establishment of two executive officers—a president to act as the school's executive officer, and a chairman of the board to preside over the board's activity. The first chair of the revised board was surgeon Leslie MacDiarmid who resigned from the faculty to assume office. Following his faculty resignation, Edward A. Christofferson (Figure 7–5 ) assumed the role of chair of surgery and held that position from 1938–1954.

Sheinin next turned his attention to strengthening the clinical association with Cook County Hospital and appointed several new faculty members from County, including the noted allergist Samuel Taub, Arthur Conely in orthopedic surgery, Peter Gaberman in physical diagnosis, and Edward Christofferson in surgery.

The school was visited by the AMA again in 1942. In its report the AMA acknowledged the impressive progress but once again denied recognition. Herman Weiskotton, the new head of the AMA Council on Medical Education, suggested that the school put its impressive new board to work on raising funds to ensure solvency.

## CMS and the Jewish Business Community

It was suggested to Dean Sheinin that one potential source of philanthropy might be wealthy Jewish businessmen who in the past had recognized the need and service of medical education. Dean Sheinin was introduced to Rabbi Solomon Goldman, one of the most respected spiritual leaders in the Jewish community

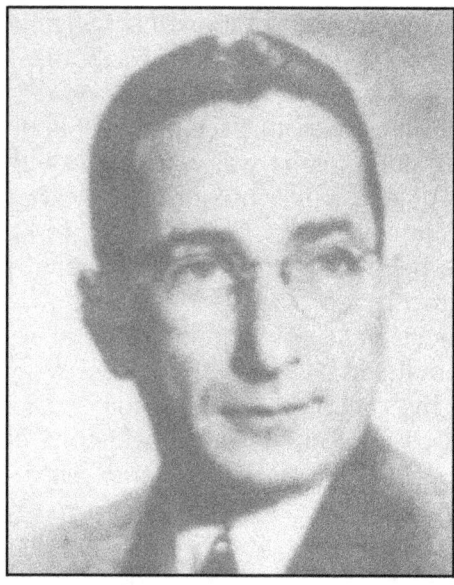

*Figure 7-4 John Sheinin*

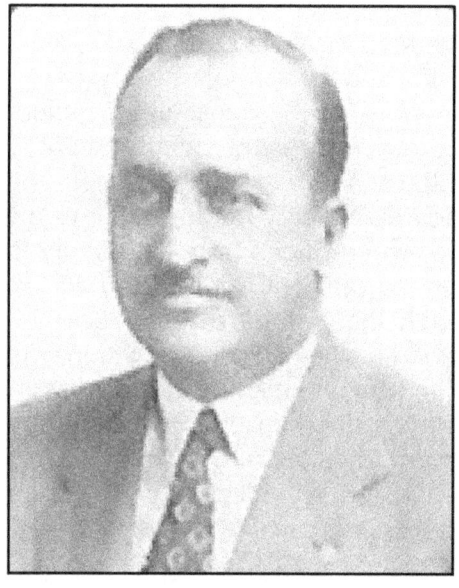

*Figure 7-5 Edward A. Christofferson*

who became convinced that CMS must be allowed to continue. This was the beginning of Chicago Medical School's long affiliation with the Jewish business community. It is of note that at about the same time Loyola University College of Medicine was having the same type of discussion with Samuel Cardinal Stritch, the archbishop of Chicago, who felt much the same about the Catholic medical school as Rabbi Goldman felt about the Chicago Medical School.

One of the people to answer the call for contributions to sustain CMS was Lester Selig, president of the General American Transportation Corporation. For the next 20 years, his main interest was CMS. He joined the board of directors and within a short period of time was elected chairman and launched a nationwide fund-raising effort.

In June of 1946, Selig called a group of his business friends together for a meeting at the Tavern Club in Chicago. After a presentation by John Evans and John Sheinin, the group was persuaded to establish a Guarantee Fund that would ensure an annual subsidy of $200,000 for five years for the school if it were looked on favorably by the AMA.

It was with much anticipation that the AMA site visit of 1947 took place. One month following the three-day inspection, the school was notified that the first two years had been approved and had received an "A" rating. There were some concerns regarding the clinical program, but the school was informed that if these could be resolved, the entire curriculum would be given "A" accreditation. The board immediately convened to consider its options. Affiliation with Mt. Sinai Hospital was finally considered the best course of action. It was close to the school, had 290 beds, 45,000 outpatient visits, and was considered to be one of Chicago's better medical institutions. Despite the new affiliation with Mt. Sinai, the relationship with Cook County continued and improved. On October 18, 1948, the AMA returned, and on November 9 the school received the official word that it had received full accreditation. It is worth noting that out of some 80 unapproved medical schools in the United States, all of which at one time or another were ordered closed, CMS was the only one to receive accreditation.

The next several years were marked by increases in both basic science and clinical faculty. Prior to accreditation, the number of faculty was 109. By 1949 there were 233 faculty members, and by 1958 the number had increased to 472. Dr. Leo Zimmerman (Figure 7-6), a well-known County attending, took over the chair of surgery in 1955, a position he held until 1961.

The years of the early 1950s were busy ones for the school, with many firsts. The administration recognized the importance of research endeavors and decided that all faculty should be allowed 50 percent of their time to pursue research. In the surgery department, several members of the faculty were among the first to successfully transplant a heart into a dog. Dr. David Movitz pioneered the use of angiography and was one of the first to perform a resection of abdominal aortic aneurysm and replacement. Along with Dr. James S.T. Yao, he evaluated the use of catheter arteriography. He also investigated the usefulness of splenosis in myocardial revascularization in the days before direct coronary bypass was possible. Most of this work was done in the labs of either the Hektoen Institute or the Old Post-Graduate School. For most who worked in and around surgery at County at that time (the late1950s to the 1970s), Dr. Movitz was best known as the co-ordinator and chief instructor for the third-year CMS students on rotation in the County complex. His counterpart from the other "orphan" medical school (Loyola) was Dr. Harold Haley. Both men were dedicated teachers of junior medical students and junior residents and a willing pair of hands for any senior resident who asked for their help. Both men were totally dedicated to their young charges and always tried to teach them the human side of what being a doctor was all about. Although their names and presences may have slipped by

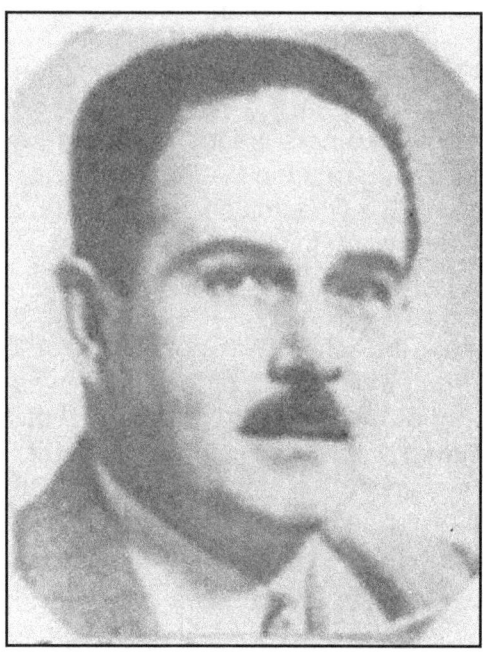
*Figure 7-6 Leo Zimmerman*

unnoticed, they were unforgettable to any of those privileged to work with them.

The school hired Dr. Vera Morkovon, a former County resident and the first female diplomate of the American Board of Surgery in Illinois, as a faculty member. The school also hired Dr. Roscoe Giles as an assistant professor of surgery. He was one of the first four African-American members of the American College of Surgeons and was president of the National Medical Society. In addition, he was a 50-year member of the Illinois State Medical Society, which was at that time quite rare for a physician of color. An acknowledged leader in Chicago medicine, Dr. Giles was selected by the Jesuit Centennial in 1957 as one of the "One Hundred Outstanding Citizens of Chicago," an award presented to him by Samuel Cardinal Stritch in December of that year. In 1962, Richard De Wall took over as chair of surgery, a position he held until 1971.

## CMS and its Affliliated Hospitals

The affiliation with Mt. Sinai and Cook County Hospitals remained strong throughout the 1950s and 60s. For a brief time, the school also had affiliations with Michael Reese and the West Side VA. As a part of the County affiliation in the mid-1960s, CMS helped to provide the basis for a return to basic research into surgical physiology and more scientific approaches to the treatment of critically ill surgical patients by helping to recruit Dr. William Shoemaker to head the division of surgical research at County and to serve as a professor of surgery at Chicago Medical School. While the "Shoe's" exploits in the fields of critical care and basic physiology are detailed elsewhere in this book, suffice it to say that he and his staff provided all the encouragement and much of the scientific background for a number of interested residents and students who presented a lot of questions with mostly rudimentary ideas of how to arrive at the answers. With the proper guidance, some of these questions were actually answered, and from about that time, graduates of the surgical program began—at least in small numbers—to seek and actually obtain postgraduate and faculty positions at academic medical institutions.

## University Health Sciences

In 1967, a new era in the school's history began with the establishment of the University of Health Sciences. The medical school became one of the first schools in the country to develop interlocking education programs for physicians and related health professionals. In addition to the medical school, the University encompassed a School of Graduate and Postdoctoral studies awarding M.S. and/or PhD degrees in anatomy, biochemistry, clinical psychology, medical physics, microbiology, pathology, pharmacology, and physiology. A School of Related Health Sciences provided more choices with B.A. and M.S. degrees in medical technology, physical therapy, and nursing (in conjunction with Barat College).

## CMS and Downey VA in North Chicago

In 1971, Thomas Baffes took over the chair of surgery, and in 1973, the school was approached by the Downey VA in North Chicago, a primarily long-term psychiatric facility with 550 medical/surgical beds, to relocate to its campus and run the medical facilities in North Chicago. In addition, the school could affiliate with the Great Lakes Naval Hospital, a significant-sized acute care facility at the time with 563 beds, as well as with other interested local hospitals (Figure 7–7). After discussions with the state director of Comprehensive Health Planning, the deans of the Chicago area medical schools and the Liaison Committee on Medical Education (LCME), a move was agreed upon. In July 1974 the clinical faculty moved into Building 50 on the North Chicago campus. The move also coincided with a very acrimonious split between the school and Mt. Sinai that would take many years to begin to mend. The school recruited new clinical chairs with the split from Mt. Sinai, and in 1974 William Schumer, a CMS alumnus, assumed the chair that he held until his death in 2000. With the move to the North Chicago campus several new faculty were recruited to the Department of Surgery. These included David Rollins, Dale Buchbinder, and Deborah Lange in vascular surgery; and Krishnan Sriram, John Clark, Michael Zdon, and Stephen Wise in general surgery.

The size of the entering class in 1980 was 160 compared to the 1967 class of 74, and the faculty numbered some 560. Although the VA endeavor progressed well, the number of veterans served in North Chicago began the same decline that all VA's in the northern midwest began to experience in the decade of the 1980s. In addition, the acute care facilities at the Naval Hospital experienced similar decreases in size. In 1982, the school opened the Robert R. McCormick Clinic in the new building, which consisted of both primary care specialties and

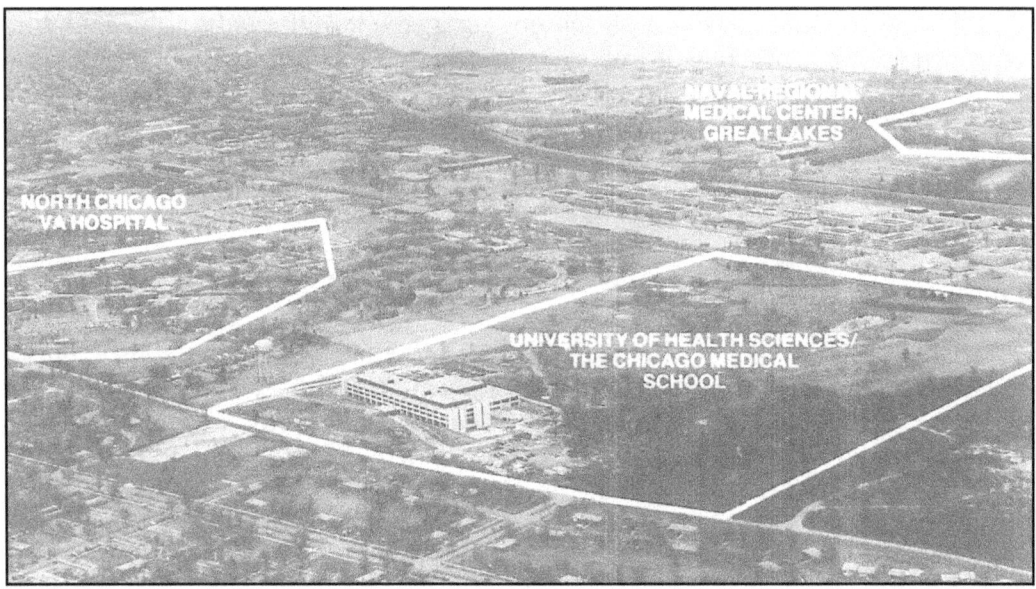

*Figure 7-7   North Chicago Campus: Chicago Medical School, North Chicago VA, and Great Lakes Naval Hospital*

surgical specialties. School physicians obtained hospital privileges, primarily at Highland Park Hospital, where patients seen in the clinic could be hospitalized when requiring inpatient services.

With decreasing patient resources on the north campus, the late 1980s saw reconciliation with Mt. Sinai and the return to using the facility for both student and resident training. The rotation of medical students to Cook County Hospital continued uninterrupted during this period.

In 1988, Bill Schumer negotiated to combine the then-independent surgery residency at Mt. Sinai with the CMS program in North Chicago, and a single CMS residency program with a north and south campus was established. In addition, Dr. Schumer was named chair of surgery at Mt. Sinai Hospital.

Following the death of Dr. Schumer in 2000, Michael J. Zdon, MD, assumed the position of acting chair until the recruitment of Joseph LoCicero, MD, by Mt. Sinai and the medical school. Following a period of 18 months, Dr. LoCicero accepted the chair at the University of Alabama. After another period of acting chair by Dr. Zdon, Thomas Vargish, MD, was recruited as the chief of surgery at Mt. Sinai Hospital and interim chair of the Department of Surgery at Chicago Medical School, positions which he currently holds.

In 2001, a major addition occurred when the Dr. William M. Scholl School of Podiatry joined the University and decided to relocate from their site in Chicago to the North Chicago campus.

Following the death of Herman Finch in 1998, the board of directors underwent a major reorganization. The newly reorganized board under the chairmanship of Marshall Falk, who had previously been dean of the school from 1974 to 1991, felt a major change in leadership was needed. Following a national search in December 2002, Dr. K. Michael Welch, a neurologist and the head of the Research Institute at the University of Kansas Medical Center in Kansas City, was chosen as the university's new president. With the new president came a major reorganization of the university's administration. Part of the changes included major strategic planning initiatives to redefine the goals and vision of the university in the 21st century. One result of this initiative was the decision to rename the university in an effort to have a name that identified with the school's new vision. The university faculty participated actively in the process, and a decision was made to rename the university after Rosiland Franklin, a young Jewish physical chemist who had worked with Nobel Prize-winners Watson and Crick on the structure of DNA at the University of London in the early 1950s. Unfortunately, she died of ovarian cancer in 1958, four years before the prize was awarded for her work.

In October 2002, a new 140,000 square foot health sciences building was added to the campus, which allowed the relocation of the Podiatry School and united the university, giving students a reasonably priced place to reside on campus grounds.

Clinical affiliations continue to evolve. Recently, the VA and Navy have combined their facilities into a single entity utilizing the facilities of the VA to treat both veterans as well as Navy trainees, retired naval personnel, and their dependents, including children. While maintaining a strong relationship with Mt. Sinai and Cook County Hospitals, recent years have seen increasing affiliation with the Advocate Medical System and Lutheran General Hospital in particular. In addition, recent changes in leadership and acquisition of Condell Medical Center in Libertyville by the Advocate Health System has generated increasing medical school involvement in Lake County.

The University currently is comprised of four colleges: Chicago Medical School with 750 Students; the College of Health Professions with 481; the Scholl College of Podiatric Medicine with 322; and the School of Graduate and Post Graduate Studies with 126. The University has over 14,000 living alumni, with more than 6,500 from the medical school alone. As recently as 10 years ago it was estimated that one of every 10 physicians in the Chicago area was a graduate of CMS. All owe a debt of gratitude to Cook County Hospital and its hospital staff for providing uninterrupted quality training for the past 84 years.

# Section III

*Prominent Surgical Services at Cook County Hospital*

# 8
# Trauma Unit

*David R. Boyd, MDCM, FACS*
*Kimberly Kay Ormsby Nagy, MD, FACS*
*Kenneth J. Printen, MD*
*James S.T. Yao, MD*

- Introduction
- America First Trauma Center
  - Reflections of Robert J. Freeark, MD
    - Educational Impact
    - Trauma System
  - Reflections of Robert J. Baker, MD
    - Trauma Care Prior to 1966
    - Addressing the Problem
    - Staffing the Trauma Unit
    - The Model Trauma Unit
    - The Trauma Team
    - The Triage System
  - Reflections of the First Trauma Director of Nursing
    - Norma Shoemaker, RN
- Trauma Nursing: Contributions of Teresa H. Romano
- Department of Trauma
- Trauma Unit Research Programs
  - Biomedical Investigations
  - Trauma Registry
  - Clinical Investigations
  - Patient Management
  - Diagnostics
  - Complication and Sequelae
  - Repair and Prosthetics
  - Laboratory Studies
  - Protocols and Practice Guidlines
  - Multicenter Studies
  - Public Health Impact
  - The County Way and Protocols
- The University of Maryland Hospital
- Leadership Surgeons: The Second Generation
  - David Boyd
  - Robert Lowe
  - Max Ramenofsky
  - John Fildes
  - John Barrett
  - Kimberly Ormsky Nagy
- Continuing History of the World-Famous Trauma Unit (WFTU ) 1982-2008
  - Department Overview
  - Training and Education
  - Physical Change in the Trauma Unit
  - The Famous and the Infamous

*Outreach Efforts*
*Research Endeavors*
*Where We are today*
*Trauma Care as Public Health Policy*
*Summary*
- *References*

## Introduction

The increasing number and severity of illnesses in critically injured patients admitted to Cook County Hospital in the 1960s led to the establishment of the Trauma Unit (TU). It was a practical response to a constellation of pressing problems caused by the growing complexity of patients' clinical problems and the expanding professional training requirements. These increasing demands made it more difficult to provide optimal trauma care and surgical training within the existing system, which had remained largely unchanged since the hospital was first opened a century earlier. The Cook County Hospital Trauma Unit (CCHTU), established in March 1966, was, as a concept, an extension of surgical knowledge and practices gained from previous military and mass-casualty experiences. But for a large inner-city public hospital, it was an experiment in team-building and development of newly minted job tasks without parallel at any level of the health care delivery spectrum.

The key organizing principle was to establish the trauma victim as the centerpiece of the clinical focus. The plan called for a readily available general surgical team with essential consultant and support personnel and adequate logistic assets, concentrated in a designated area within the larger general hospital. The always-available trauma team and dependable resources were prime reasons for initial and continuing success.

The CCHTU was an early and progressive success story. After 1971, it became the conceptual model and professional nucleus and training center for organizing hospital trauma care, along with the regionalization of trauma care in Chicago and the state of Illinois. The CCHTU pioneered new techniques in resuscitation and initial trauma management, injury evaluation, diagnostic protocols, surgical treatment, operative techniques, critical care innovations, and standards of care. In short, it became the generator of new concepts for the organization of Trauma and Emergency Medical Services (EMS) systems and essential professional training requirements on a nationwide basis.

The 1996 National Academy of Science-National Research Council's (NAS-NRC) report, "Accidental Death and Disability, the Neglected Disease of Modern Society," outlined a set of deficiencies in our nation's trauma care and EMS response capability.[1] The CCHTU concept and operations overcame these stated deficiencies and influenced national recognition of and response to the "trauma problem." The Cook County Hospital Trauma Unit became a major professional performance, public education, and political policy change agent. Under the influence and guidance of a series of outstanding surgeons and directors, the CCHTU was instrumental in developing a wide spectrum of clinical, biomedical systems, and epidemiologic research. The computerized Trauma Registry originated there. CCHTU surgeons have been well respected leaders in trauma centers, national care-standards organizations, research and professional policy committees as well as governmental trauma care and EMS systems-related activities.

The CCHTU was the original idea of Drs. Robert J. Freeark and Robert J. Baker. Heretofore, patients, after a rapid triage in the emergency room screening area, were transported in rotation to the respective admitting general surgical and specialty services throughout the hospital. In those days, the trauma patient probably received the best surgical care available in Chicago. These critical patients, however, produced a recurring challenge and onerous demand on the limited medical and nursing staff available on the various admitting services. Trauma patients were typically admitted during busy periods at night when the more-senior residents were actively involved in operations on previously admitted patients. Many times, this left the less experienced staff—interns and untrained nurses with limited resources—to perform resuscitation, stabilization, evaluation, and diagnosis without the benefit of effective supervision or consultative guidance. Trauma patients could, and did, deteriorate because of unanticipated or unsuspected problems. Further, many patients with serious multiple or occult injuries went directly to subspecialty wards that were unprepared for and inexperienced with these critical cases.

This mismatch of critical patient needs to expert care and available resources was immediately corrected by the trauma unit approach. On the CCHTU, an always-available experienced surgeon and nurse trauma team provided evaluation, stabilization, consistent diagnosis, educated operative interventions, and aftercare. In the new setting, the critically injured patient became the central focus of the surgical and nursing staffs' attention.

The stark differences in improved consistency, quality and efficiency of trauma care, the much enhanced educational experience, and the research potential were immediately recognized. The new approach had the approval of the hospital's Senior Medical Officer, Dr. Karl Meyer, and in turn led to a growing recognition by certifying agencies (Residency Review Committee, American Board of Surgery, and Medicare) of the value of improved full-time staffing and supervision in the various surgical disciplines. There was a parallel wide-ranging impact of enhanced focus and development of emergency radiology, anesthesiology, and laboratory support.

## America's First Trauma Center
### Reflections of Robert J. Freeark[2]

Cook County Hospital was, for most of its existence, the only hospital serving the indigent sick for the entire County of Cook, which includes the City of

Chicago and adjacent suburbs, a population of more than seven million people. Prior to 1966, all trauma patients were seen by interns in an emergency department that averaged over 1,000 patients per day with minimal triage and often prolonged delays before being seen.

Patients requiring admission were assigned to a service and ward based on the emergency department intern's assessment of their principal problems or needs. Patients with multiple injuries, including fractures, were assigned to one of the three fracture wards (two male, one female) staffed by general and orthopedic interns and residents. Similarly, head injuries went to neurosurgery, hematuria to urology, stab wounds of the neck to ENT, and so on. During evenings and holidays, each of the special units was staffed by an intern who could request consultation from a resident if he recognized the need. Full-time staffing was uncommon, and in the surgical specialties, voluntary attending staff visited only on certain days, primarily to cover elective operative procedures.

Cases with missed injuries, delayed consultation or treatment, or inadequate or inappropriate follow-up were common and rarely brought to the attention of those responsible for either patient care or house staff education. The over-900 surgical beds were largely run by house officers who, though in theory worked under the supervision of a largely volunteer attending staff, had remarkable freedom to act in its own best interests. It is a real tribute to these house officers that patient care in the face of limited facilities and staffing was generally superior to that available to indigent patients in private hospitals in the city.

The County Hospital Trauma Unit established in 1966 was the first comprehensive trauma center in the United States. Important components included:

1. A designated ward of the main hospital was established exclusively for adult trauma patients. This unit consisted of an admitting area for stretchers, resuscitation area, and ward beds including intensive care and research laboratory beds.
2. The staff was comprised of full-time general surgeons, nurses, and surgical house staff who had no other patient care responsibilities.
3. All major trauma patients were admitted directly to the unit, bypassing traditional emergency department evaluation or treatment.
4. Patients requiring operative intervention were taken to surgery by the trauma team with appropriate surgical specialists called in for consultation.
5. Following operation and post-anesthesia recovery, trauma patients returned to the trauma unit for necessary care ranging from intensive to rehabilitation.
6. All patients discharged from the hospital unit were followed by the surgical staff in an outpatient clinic.
7. Patients requiring primarily surgical specialty care (e.g., orthopedic, neurosurgery, burn) were transferred to those hospital units either preoperatively or for post-operative care, depending on the overall seriousness of the patient's general condition.

### Educational Impact

Improved supervision and education of the house staff in all the surgical disciplines were immediate consequences of the oversight and controls imposed by the unit. Since each of the full-time attending surgeons was a part-time director of surgical clerkships for one of the four medical schools using County and was assigned junior and senior students at the Cook County Hospital, the unit exposed literally hundreds of medical students to trauma care. Led by the surgical trauma unit nurse, the time-honored restrictions on nurse responsibilities began to buckle as trauma center nurses were trained to catheterize patients, start IVs, perform cut-downs, suture lacerations, and assume responsibilities that previously were performed or exercised only by doctors.

### Trauma System

Part of the motivation for planning the trauma center was the flawed Chicago area-wide system for care of the injured. While a senior orthopedic surgeon (Dr. Sam Banks) had spent years training Chicago Fire Department first responders, the majority of trauma patients were brought to Cook County Hospital in police vans manned by officers who had received no formal instruction in the care of the injured. Even worse, a city ordinance called for taking all emergencies to "the nearest hospital." Often, the nearest hospital was inadequately staffed for, or not interested in, trauma care, particularly for an indigent patient, and would have to arrange transport to Cook County Hospital, again relying on the police squadrol (vans) to transport the patient, often causing hours of delay for appropriate resuscitation and injury assessment. One day after losing a young patient to exsanguination from a major liver injury following this delay in treatment, Dr. Baker wrote a letter to the editor of the City News Service decrying "the nearest hospital" concept, using this patient as a glaring example. It must have been a slow news day because the letter was published in all of the Chicago newspapers, and the trauma center staff became the focus of a number of reporters who demanded to know what should be done to improve the system. This publicized the importance of having designated hospitals throughout the Chicago area that were both capable of, and committed to, trauma care.

## Reflections of Robert J. Baker

Dr. Baker was the Associate Director, Division of Surgery, Cook County Hospital, from October 1959 to September 1968; founder of the trauma unit in 1966; chief of the trauma unit, Cook County Hospital, from 1966 to 1969; and Chief of Surgery, Cook County Hospital, from 1968 to 1969.

### Trauma Care Prior to 1966

Cook County Hospital was a 3,400-bed hospital. Essentially, it provided care to the indigent, which was supported and funded by the County of Cook, including Chicago and adjacent suburbs, and to a much lesser extent, by the State of Illinois. Then as now, the Cook County Board of Commissioners was the governing body, responsible for funding, setting policy and implementing programs at the hospital. The board appointed the medical superintendent, who was effectively both the chief executive officer and medical chief of staff. Dr. Karl Meyer was appointed in 1912, and he continued to serve in this capacity until well into the 1970s.

The attending staff of the hospital, responsible for all patient care on their services, was appointed following a competitive written examination. Dr. Robert Freeark was the first full-time salaried surgeon, appointed as director of surgical education in 1958, after he completed his surgical residency at Cook County Hospital. I was recruited as associate director of surgical education, also a full-time position, in 1959.

The emergency room, the primary site of entry to the hospital for the sick and injured patients, was a first-floor facility that occupied the center of that level of the main hospital building facing on Harrison Street, just west of the Chicago Loop. Staffing was by both interns and residents assigned to the Emergency Department, largely medical and surgical house staff.

Most of the surgical services were located in this building, as were the operating rooms, radiologic facilities, and inpatient surgical beds. These wards, 45- to 60-bed units, were geographically separated from one another and had nursing stations (one per ward), as well as a house staff lab where blood counts, urinalyses, and microscopic study of specimens could be done, almost invariably by the interns. Surgical specialties, including fractures (a separate service from orthopedics), urology, neurosurgery, otolaryngology/plastic surgery, and thoracic surgery were housed on similar wards with different attending staffs but similar house staffs. A few specialties had advanced trainees (fellows), but most of the care was provided by rotating interns (undesignated) and general surgery residents.

Children up to the age of 14 were seen, treated, and admitted through a separate pediatric emergency room in the Children's Hospital building, separated from the main hospital building by several hundred yards and staffed by rotating interns and pediatric residents with support on-call by the pediatric attending staff. Consultation for surgical problems, including trauma, was provided by on-call interns and residents from the Department of Surgery. The Children's Hospital had its own operating rooms, in which all surgical patients in the Children's Hospital were operated. Roughly 20 percent of the patients in the Children's Hospital were adults, on cardiac surgery and cardiology, orthopedic surgery, or Dr. Karl Meyer's adult surgical service on Ward 56. The operating room staffs of the main operating room and the Children's Hospital operating rooms were treated as entirely separate units, with different supervisors and nursing staffs. Burn patients were admitted to general surgical services, irrespective of the severity of their burns, and trauma patients were admitted at random to the admitting surgical service.

There was no intensive care unit prior to the mid-1960s. This changed only when Dr. Vincent Collins was recruited from Bellevue Hospital in New York City to chair the revamped Department of Anesthesiology. The anesthesia service was previously headed and staffed by a group of nurse anesthetists with an anesthesiologist occasionally recruited to work with the nurse anesthetists. Anesthesia provided by doctors was generally used for the longer cases and to teach the obstetrical and general surgical residents assigned to anesthesia for one month rotations. With Dr. Collins' arrival, and with the tacit approval of Dr. Meyer, anesthesia services were immediately modified. The nurse anesthetists no longer controlled the service, which had now become a department.

Most of the nurse anesthetists welcomed this restructuring, and Dr. Collins responded by immediately starting an educational program for them that upgraded their knowledge and level of performance. The advent of an anesthesiology residency marked the first semblance of an academic program in that specialty at the Cook County Hospital.

All trauma patients entered the patient care system through one of the two emergency rooms, mostly through the main emergency room in the main hospital, but children under 14 years of age were brought to the Children's Hospital emergency room. The surgical house staff on call would rush down to the emergency room and more or less direct the resuscitation effort, stop bleeding, and try to assess the patient. Portable X-rays were often used but seldom proved particularly useful. Attending surgeons were rarely involved in trauma evaluation or even operative treatment. The senior surgical residents at that time were, in essence, the surgeon in charge, although not the admitting surgeon who was always an attending surgeon. Surgical residents at all levels spent a great deal of time and effort, often at a run, going from place to place to provide and/or oversee care provided by more junior house staff, even interns. Medical students from the Universities of Illinois, Northwestern, Loyola, and Chicago Medical School were variably present and often were vital components of patient care.

**Addressing the Problem**

The major issue that confronted Dr. Freeark and myself was how to more efficiently manage the care of critically ill trauma patients in large numbers. This was complicated by the different locations to which these patients might be sent after admission and the various attending surgeons whose management of these patients was highly variable and occasionally even questionable. The surgical resident staff always initiated patient care for trauma, as well as all other acute surgical problems. In some instances, the senior resident made certain that the attending surgeon agreed with the treatment plan, and then instituted appropriate management. The problem of variability of trauma care by different surgeons, some without adequate trauma experience, was not unique to Cook County Hospital and was substantially worse in community hospitals.

Cook County Hospital received the vast majority of penetrating trauma cases in the Chicago area. It was not unusual for a busy Friday or Saturday night to yield 15 to as many as 30 emergency surgical admissions, many critically injured and requiring operative treatment. Coupled with the usual array of nontraumatic surgical emergencies, the surgical residents on call often had patients lined up on carts in the operating room corridors awaiting treatment and operated almost nonstop until they got to the end of the line. This might be 24 hours or more after the injured patient was received and initially evaluated. While the chief surgical resident served as the de facto night surgeon until the early 1950s, when Drs. Roger Vaughan and later William Norcross during the 1960s and 1970s served as the in-house on-call staff night surgeon. While it seems Dr. Vaughan was largely involved in establishing correct diagnoses and making sure that appropriate preoperative testing was amalgamated into the surgical decision-making process, Dr. Norcross would often show up in the operating room unannounced just to ask what was happening. If the progression was not to his liking, he was not above scrubbing in to improve the situation as he saw it. Both men were incredible sources of clinical knowledge, and in their appropriate circumstances, dispensed very useful information to resolve the problems at hand.

Another issue of concern was the quality and quantity of the nursing service available to care for the injured. The hospital wards were sparsely staffed, and routine nursing functions often had to be provided, if at all, by interns and other junior house staff. A large surgical intensive care unit was in the planning and construction stages, but it was of concern that critically injured patients required more by way of continuous nursing care than they were receiving.

A third concern was that this large number of trauma patients did not provide the staff the opportunity to develop new information and publish research about diagnoses and care of the injured that should have accrued from such a large volume of patients. Clinical papers were written in much larger volume than previously, but prospective studies of diagnostic and monitoring techniques, as well as clinical outcomes, were relatively rare, primarily because all of the medical staff were involved with patient care issues on patients spread around the various surgical services in the hospital. Also, as in many other urban public hospitals, medical-record management was not a high priority in a huge institution with limited resources. Once a record left the ward or service, it would likely never be seen again, except by accident.

At an International Society of Surgery meeting in Europe, Dr. Freeark and I met Professor Jorg Bohler, an Austrian trauma surgeon of international recognition whose basic interest and training was in general and orthopedic surgery. His major clinical interest was in the trauma management system in Austria. All road-accident victims were taken to one of six trauma hospitals, arranged at strategic intervals along major freeways. These hospitals had been planned and built immediately following the end of World War II. Surgeons were facile in managing all facets of vehicular accidents, including head injury, torso trauma, fractures and dislocations, and extensive soft tissue injury. Most importantly, all accident patients, regardless of patient or family wishes, were taken to the closest of these highly efficient, well-staffed, and equipped hospitals where the surgeons were devoted to trauma care in all of its aspects.

Dr. Freeark and I subsequently met Professor Bohler's son, also a renowned Austrian trauma surgeon, who invited Freeark to come to Austria and see how their system functioned. He did, and after due deliberation, we decided to open the Chicago version of the trauma hospital, the Cook County Hospital Trauma Unit. All trauma patients would be sent to this unit on admission, except for relatively trivial and nonlife-threatening injuries that could still be cared for on a surgical ward. The unit was to be located on the third floor of the main hospital building with a dedicated medical and nursing staff, as well as dedicated attending surgeons and residents. In addition, the plan was that it would have 12 beds, eight intensive trauma care and four study beds, for ongoing scientific exploration of critically injured trauma and shock patients. The geography of the unit was, unfortunately, determined by the available space, which had to be allocated by Dr. Meyer. The hospital had built a house staff residence for residents and interns. And the staff dining room, previously on the third floor of the main building, had been moved to the new building, freeing up a modest amount of space for the proposed trauma unit. With the help of Dr. Collins and several influential surgical attendings, Dr. Meyer agreed on the space allocation, and the project was implemented in 1964.

### Staffing the Trauma Unit

Having the seriously and critically injured patients in one place with intensive attending, house staff and nursing service was the primary aim. The assignments were simultaneously two senior residents (fourth or fifth year), three or four junior residents (second or third year), and several attending surgeons, including both Freeark and myself as senior staff. Senior residents had a total of four to six months on the trauma service, and juniors had four months. Dr. Freeark was the first director, and I succeeded to that role in 1967. Dr. William Shoemaker became the third full-time attending on the service when he was recruited to be the director of surgical research for surgery, focusing primarily on the trauma/shock patient. Dr. Shoemaker recruited a number of talented residents, both from County and outside academic programs, to spend varying periods of time in his laboratory and conduct meaningful research on the trauma unit.

Nurse staffing was addressed when Norma Shoemaker R.N. Dr. Shoemaker's wife, volunteered to head the dedicated nursing service in the trauma unit. Norma recruited a group of spectacularly talented nurses, held extensive training and educational seminars for them, and was the power that drove the nursing engine. She had superior relations with everyone, was remarkably knowledgeable, and was always willing to share her experience with attendings (who sometimes needed it), residents (who almost always needed it), and medical students. She ultimately was succeeded by Teri Romano, who refined and improved the trauma nursing service even further. Nurses throughout the hospital correctly believed that the educational opportunity for nurses on the trauma unit made it a highly desirable assignment, and there were always nurses who wanted to become part of the trauma nursing team.

### The Model Trauma Unit

The trauma unit initially consisted of 18 beds (this varies with reports and bed configurations). It provided centralization of available hospital resources for comprehensive resuscitation, initial evaluation, and peri-operative care of seriously injured patients. The capital outlay for establishing this unit was minimal. Existing available equipment, resources, and personnel were mobilized from the various surgical wards.

The CCHTU was initially organized into the following four sections:

1. A four-bed receiving and triage area available for resuscitation and evaluation. All trauma victims with potentially serious injuries were taken directly to this area, thereby separating them from the larger mass of emergency room patients. A variety of procedures could be

and were performed here, including pericardiocentesis, thoracentesis, and emergency thoracotomy under extraordinary life-threatening circumstances.
2. A 13-bed intensive care unit adjoined the resuscitation area. Two beds were located close to the nursing station and a resident's call room for the very critical or respirator-dependent patients. Three types of patients were admitted to this intensive care unit: (a) patients who required further observation to determine if operative treatment was needed, (b) patients with major multi-system injuries requiring several consultants, and (c) patients with major chest and abdominal injuries requiring operative treatment.
3. A single-bed area provided intensive physiologic monitoring and investigations.
4. A laboratory where routine and special determinations could be obtained. An X-ray unit was maintained here as well (Figure 8–1).

**The Trauma Team**

The most important component of a trauma center is a well-trained, well-functioning trauma team. This team is directed by a trauma surgeon and includes other surgeons, anesthesiologists, emergency physicians, other consulting specialists and intensivists, trauma nurses, respiratory therapists, laboratory and radiology technicians, and other ancillary support personnel. The trauma team functions were as outlined below:[3]
1. Immediate identification of the injured patient and provision for transport to the trauma care area.

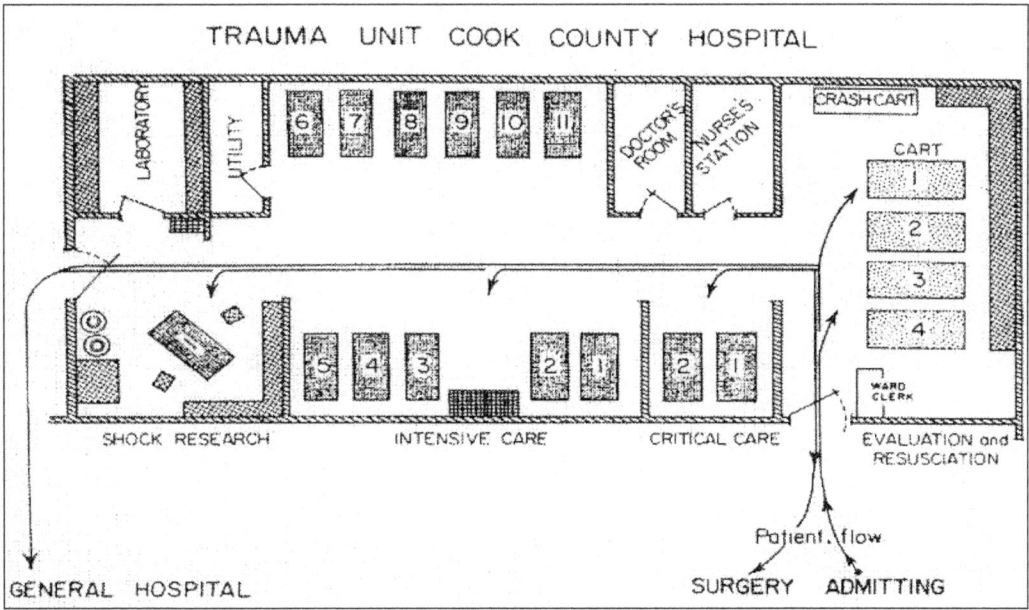

*Figure 8–1 Floor plan of the trauma unit at CCH*

2. Triage of all hospitalized trauma victims in a single location by a team of experienced surgeons.
3. Resuscitation and comprehensive initial evaluation in a fully staffed and equipped area of the trauma unit.
4. Utilization of a team approach to in-dividual patient care with the general surgeon functioning as the team co-ordinator.
5. Upgrading the level of training of the trauma team coordinator to that of a senior experienced surgeon.
6. Establishment of an integral intensive care area dedicated to the needs of the critically injured patient.
7. Specially trained nurses and other health professionals developed to staff the unit, with continuing education courses for these personnel.
8. Consolidation of all related hospital resources for the injured patient in this central location.
9. Necessary supporting laboratory services available in the unit.
10. Establishment of a priority system in the hospital's X-ray Department and blood bank, in which trauma patients are given appropriately high priority at any time of the day or night.

Leadership of the TU later evolved to a recognized medical director, a surgeon with trauma care background and a commitment to optimal trauma care. The director had overall responsibility for developing protocols, training, supervision, and management of the TU. Consultant surgeons were assigned to the TU from neurosurgery, vascular, orthopedics, and plastic surgery, with other specialties on an as needed basis

### The Triage System

The large numbers of trauma cases brought to CCH were immediately triaged directly to the TU. There they were the responsibility of the second-year general surgery resident who had completed his or her first two-month rotation on thoraco-cardiovascular service before he or she could be assigned to the trauma unit. The TU provided comprehensive resuscitation, initial evaluation, and full stabilization of all critically injured patients. Backup was always available from advanced residents rotating on service or in-house. After the patient was stabilized, additional diagnostic procedures and operations were undertaken. Those with a single system injury were transferred to specific on-call surgical services (e.g., vascular, chest, orthopedics, and neurosurgery). Most of these transfers were initially managed on the unit with continuing assistance of the TU team.

Patients with critical and undetermined abdominal injuries were managed by the TU team. Patients with combined injuries with suspect thoracic or vascular injuries were co-managed as appropriate. Postoperative care for these and other complicated cases was provided in the TU intensive care unit. Initially, patients were discharged from the TU to a general surgery ward in rotation. A step-down ward and a follow-up clinic were established later.

The organizational principles underlying the development of the Cook County Hospital trauma unit described here were extended to the trauma centers through the Illinois Statewide Trauma System. This was the operational goal of the program and an expectation of practicing surgeons previously trained at the CCHTU.

## Reflections of the First Trauma Unit Director of Nursing, Norma Shoemaker R.N.

In 1964, Chicago, like many large urban areas, was overwhelmed with trauma patients. It was the decade of the hippies and new drugs that let users think they could fly without benefit of wings. It was the time when we were stunned and frightened by the murders of John F. Kennedy, Martin Luther King, Jr., and Robert Kennedy. It was also a time when Chicago gangs went to war for control of their territories, and a time for hospitals to look at the problem of care delivery and provide a comprehensive, workable solution. Cook County was a huge hospital licensed for more than 3,000 beds. There were multistory buildings devoted to just one category of patients, such as a psychiatric building, a medical building for men, and another for women. There was a large burn unit, pediatric facilities, and, of course, a very busy emergency service that was in gridlock. In late 1964, I was contacted by Drs. Robert Baker and Robert Freeark for discussions about starting a trauma unit at Cook County Hospital. There was a severe problem in providing timely care to all Chicago's emergency patients; but as the busiest ER service in the city, the problem was especially apparent for trauma patients at CCH.

The question is, of course, why Norma Shoemaker? The answer was I was there and had experience. In 1953, I had graduated from a three-year nursing program at Hahnaman Hospital in Philadelphia in the days when trauma patients came into the ER via paddy wagons, and student nurses staffed the hospital.

In my discussions with Drs. Baker and Freeark, I shared my convictions concerning the factors that would be essential for a trauma unit to function optimally. I felt that the administration would have to provide the funds for equipment and personnel and then leave the unit to function autonomously insofar as it was possible. I envisioned an atmosphere of camaraderie where the doctors weren't captains of the ship but rather rowers in the same boat with the nurses, technicians, and other medical staff. The medical and nursing directors absolutely had to share a common vision. Drs. Baker and Freeark wanted a top-notch trauma service that would provide teaching opportunities for their surgical residents and a clinical research program that could produce work that would be published in the finest peer-reviewed journals. After we had discussed our concepts and goals, we agreed that we could do it. We would set up a trauma service that handled all of the trauma patients presenting at CCH. The patients would by-pass the ER and go directly to the trauma unit. Any bumps in the road would be solved by our wonderful communication system. There were bumps, but the system worked because we did communicate, and the hospital administrator in charge of our program was most helpful.

Following our discussions, the two doctors took me to see the physical space allotted to the trauma unit. Our hopes and dreams agreed upon, I found myself on the elevator to the third floor. The door to the right of the elevator was opened, and there sat a large empty room with another room behind it. And if we didn't mind going outside, we could use a third room, complete with fireplace, as a staff room. I didn't know whether to laugh or cry. This abandoned storage area, this ugly duckling, was to be our trauma unit, our swan.

I spent the next six months as an employee at CCH assigned to the nursing director's office. During that time, I actually gave nursing care in the ER and on the wards, attended nursing department meetings, and generally learned how things worked. The nursing director became a friend and believer.

The results of my time floating were the creation of policies that had a huge effect on the success of the unit. One example was the idea that the trauma unit nurses were never to be floated to other floors. By the same token, we would never have nurses floated in. I had three reasons for wanting this policy:

1. Of all the morale killers, floating nurses is at the top of the list.
2. The trauma unit nurses were highly experienced. At the end of two years of operation, all but one of the original nurses were still working in place. Two years on the CCH trauma unit could not be duplicated by the same experience on a general ward. Therefore, there was no guarantee that the nurses floated in could provide the type of care required in a unit that could have five seriously wounded patients at the same time.
3. What was good for the goose had to be good for the gander. You don't take our nurses; we won't take yours. It just wouldn't be fair. And I wanted the general floor nurses to know we respected them.

Another benefit of these six months was a chance to get to know the non-nursing staff on the surgical units. This made it possible to recruit ancillary staff that was experienced and wanted to be part of this new venture. All transfers were by choice, not conscription. The upshot was that we had the best clerks and assistants in the hospital. We became "the" place to work. While I am on the subject of staffing, let me point out some realities. I was told I had an unlimited line for registered nurses. Of course I did! The availability of nurses was limited beyond belief. For a nurse to walk onto a trauma unit and function well, she (and it was always a she) had to have had experience in an ER or on a surgical floor. In the early 1960s, not many nurses had ever seen an ICU. So they came, one at a time, usually by word of mouth. They stayed and perfected their skills, then taught the less experienced nurses as they joined us. Remember, the doctors had to learn the way of a trauma unit also, so doctors and nurses learned together and built mutual respect and interdependence. The unit clerk at CCH was crucial, especially with the admission load that the trauma unit had. He or she had a tremendous responsibility and could positively impact patient flow and public relations.

A trauma unit does not function without ancillary personnel. Hiring technicians and non-nursing personnel was really easy. I would just call "downtown" and give them the job description of the person I needed, and "they" would send me a new hire. If the person was acceptable, she stayed. If not, I called "downtown" again, and they would send another applicant. I was never quite sure how "downtown" worked, but it had something to do with ward bosses. Even our "downtown" people became team members: none of the "them vs. us" attitude that is so destructive to morale. Laboratory technicians, orderlies, and nursing assistants were all valued, and the rest of us went out of our way to make it so.

Drs. Freeark and Baker hand-picked the first residents for the unit. Without mentioning names, let's just say that we realized we had to have doctors who were open-minded, willing to work in a team setting they had not encountered before, and become a cheering squad to inoculate the rest of the surgical staff. Consequently, the first few months were critical for setting the culture that would lead to success.

The unit itself had to go from a storage room to a limited space that could do all that needed doing. The admitting area was much too small. On a busy Friday night, you could hardly get between the stretchers. The nurses' station was an oversize closet, and the doctors' on-call room had a cot and a desk. It was decided in the very beginning that we would have two holding beds for critical patients and 16 beds for short-stay patients. We also had a study room with a stat lab. Many were the confabs we had about design and function. It became obvious that there had to be many tradeoffs. When the remodeling was finished and the stocking began, we found that in spite of limitations, it would work. And work it did. Many a month we cared for more than 600 patients with unbelievably good morbidity and mortality statistics.

Why did our patients do so well? People always ask how, including a trip from the ambulance bay on the first floor to an elevator for a ride to the third floor, we beat the clock. And that, of course, is the answer. The four or five minutes extra to get to the unit was more than made up for by the speed with which care was carried out on the unit. Nursing staff covered the holding and research patients as well as the admitting room. Nurses took patients in the order in which they arrived and when needed, the nurses in the "back" would help in the admitting area. At least one resident was on the unit at all times, and additional physician coverage was as close as the telephone. There was always physician back-up available. Lab tests were done without leaving the unit. The OR was always ready. We had a well-oiled machine, and the patients were the winners.

As time went by, we started to host physicians from other hospitals and countries. We had caught the interest of the press. High-profile patients raised our reputation, and the visitors increased. CCH had its own Chicago Police Department precinct station on the premises, so we had a lot of interaction with the police. Many patients arrived with their own assigned officer. No night was more memorable than when a nurse, cleansing the arm of a bleeding patient, identified the tattoo "born to raise hell." That patient was mass murderer Richard Speck. He had killed eight nurses in their quarters at a suburban hospital and then disappeared for a week. Every staff member had a detective assigned to them, supposedly to prevent the nurses from doing him harm. Ironically, the one nurse that survived by hiding under a bed was a classmate of a nurse on duty in the trauma unit when Speck was admitted.

During the gang wars, we had as many as eight patients with serious gunshot wounds admitted on one eight-hour shift. The stories make TV seem calm. But what the stories did was raise the public consciousness about trauma and the difference an organized delivery system can make. Prior to the trauma unit opening, patients would wait hours in the ER only to lose their place in line to a trauma patient. Trauma patients cared for in the ER had to be triaged and the appropriate doctor notified. Without a team and system, optimal care could not be delivered. It was no wonder we could lower the mortality and morbidity statistics so dramatically. We had both a system and a team, and an intangible spirit that made all of the difference.

It is usually easier to start something new than it is to sustain the enthusiasm for the long term. We used several strategies to keep the team spirit. First, we fostered mutual respect between the medical and nursing staffs. There was no going to Drs. Freeark or Baker to complain about the residents. If the nurses couldn't work out the problem, we would have a discussion with the senior resident who could usually resolve the situation. And we had lots of fun. Any excuse for a party! And we spent a lot of time at the Greek's, the local watering hole.

One rule that I was very strict about was that every nurse had to have one long weekend a month. Since weekends were our busiest time, those four days in a row could be in the middle of the week, but it did give the staff a day to wind down and three days to recover. I believe that one simple rule increased the time the nurses could work in trauma. Trauma is very demanding, both emotionally and physically. From the nursing perspective, trauma is different from ICU. With rare exceptions, once the patient was stable or in surgery, we didn't know what the outcome was; therefore, we didn't have the emotional satisfaction of knowing we had done a good job. And, of course, the pace is much faster in a busy trauma unit. During critical times, there simply is not time to take a break. Meals are eaten on the fly. Since families are not as apt to be involved at the time of admission, the patient is not really known to the staff. Histories are sketchy. With many patients only surmises can be made. Unfortunately, a very large percentage of our patients were under the influence of alcohol or drugs, which presented a challenge in itself. Consequently, communication with the patient was minimal compared to the intense communication among staff members. And as a result of the staff communication level, the interdependence, and respect of trauma unit members is unique. In some part, that interdependence resulted in low work-lost statistics and an unusual retention rate for all levels of staff. The trauma unit experience is best described as the *Mash Mentality*, reflecting the esprit de corps reflected in that popular TV series.

## Trauma Nursing: Contributions of Teresa H. Romano

Teresa H. Romano, a young and enterprising TU staff nurse, developed a trauma nurse specialist core curriculum for the knowledge and training requirements of graduate R.N.s to actively participate as qualified trauma nurses on the CCHTU.[4] She was later recruited by Dr. Boyd in 1971 for the statewide trauma program as trauma nursing director, and she became the nation's first trauma R.N. coordinator. Romano established her nurse specialist educational and training program for emergency and ICU nurses in the developing trauma centers across the state. This was a four-week intensive course, basically a mini-internship for new trauma nurses, which included both didactic and clinical experience. This original Illinois Trauma Nurse Specialist (TNS) Training Program was replicated in many trauma centers across the country and is still ongoing in Illinois. The core concepts evolved into nationally recognized trauma and emergency medical clinical nurse training programs (Figure 8-2). Romano also established the trauma nurse coordinator (TNC) position, a most important concept and position. This new professional role soon became recognized as essential for all hospital trauma centers and the public health department Trauma/EMS Lead Agency. Now it is called the trauma program manager (TPM) with the critical role and responsibility of organizing, coordinating, and improving trauma care to national standards.[5]

## Department of Trauma

In 1994, Dr. Barrett and colleagues established the Trauma Department (TD) as a way to ensure a more coordinated approach to the care of the trauma patient. It was developed around the concept that trauma is a disease and needs to be handled in a comprehensive and coordinated fashion. The TD is interdisciplinary with interests in injury prevention, pre- and in-hospital initial resuscitation, stabilization, operative intervention, intensive care, rehabilitation, trauma research, and education.

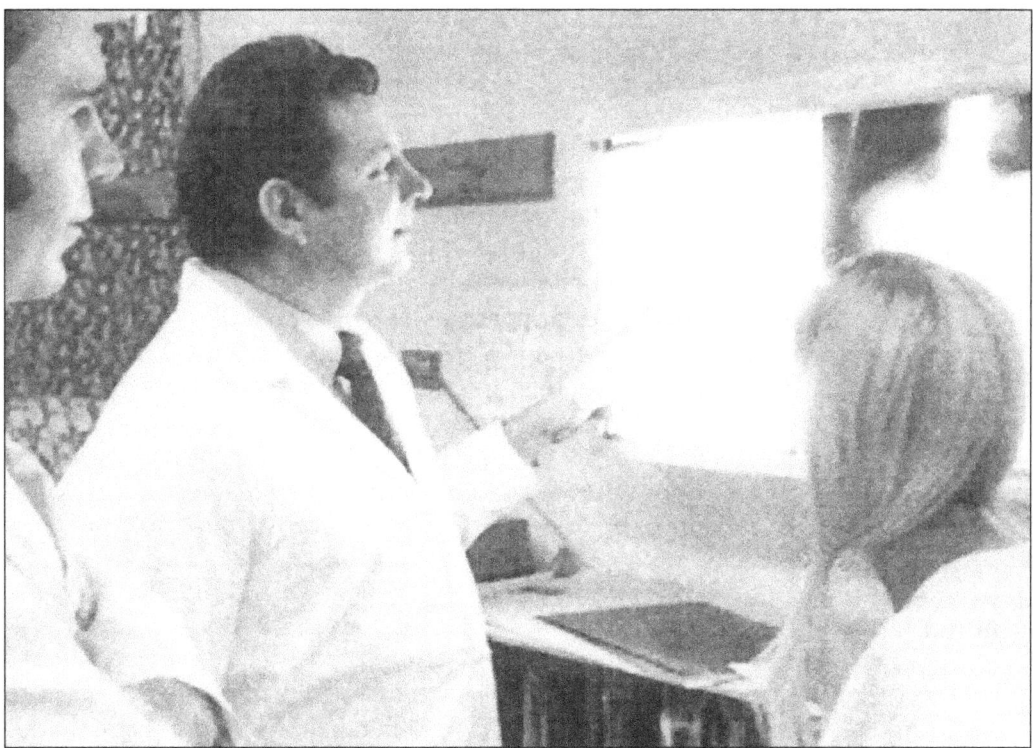

*Figure 8–2 David Boyd, Robert Lowe, and Terry Romano*

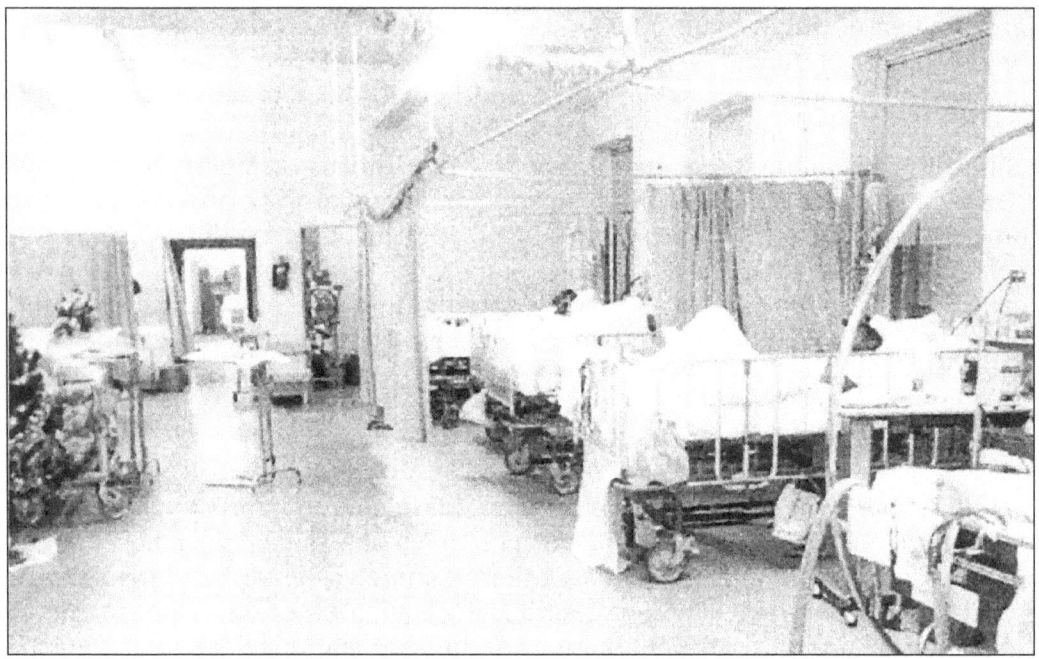

*Figure 8–3  Original trauma unit of the third floor of the old hospital*

Continuing on this theme of coordinated comprehensive care, the same trauma nursing team works in both the resuscitation area and the intensive care unit. The TD professional staff consists of full-time attending surgeons, emergency physicians, burn and rehabilitation attending, clinical trauma fellows, nurse epidemiologists, a trauma resources coordinator, a nurse researcher, and data trauma registrar. All phases of trauma care are represented among the medical staff disciplines, specialty training, and research activities.

Admission records of the initial years of the trauma unit are not available. Boyd[5] reported the total number of admissions in 1969 as 6,863. From this report, a sample showed that 68.3 percent were the result of violence, 13 percent vehicular, and 13 percent home recreation. Freeark reported a range of annual TU admissions of 6,000 to 3,000 from 1966–1981.[6]

The varying admission rates to the CCHTU reflected the prevailing crime rates and efforts toward more trauma regionalization in Chicago: the predominance of blunt injury of approximately 50-70 percent from 1989–2007.

## Trauma Unit Research Programs

The CCHTU provided a friendly environment for the triad of patient care, training, and research. Excellence in patient care, effectiveness in professional education and training, and basic and applied research not only co-existed but prospered. Residents, students, and nurses learned new treatment principles by practice and from the various ongoing clinical and bio-medical investigations. Lessons were learned in real time while managing patients and formulating protocols. A computerized trauma registry provided an accessible database for additional clinical and systems studies. An important theme of inquiry that soon became a hallmark of the CCHTU was the organizational concepts and systems methods that would have major impacts beyond the county hospital. These research activities were in large part performed by residents who became intimately involved and co-authored many of these studies. Some, for the first time, were exposed to academic surgery and made career changes, others gained an appreciation of the importance of clinical investigations in improving surgical and critical care.

Clinical and applied basic research is difficult to conduct in a busy and complex trauma unit setting. Trauma patients are in critical condition with a myriad of presentations and ill-defined pathology. The advance of science in this field was greatly facilitated by establishment of designated trauma units, the multidisciplinary approach to patient care, and collateral investigations. The CCHTU provided a laboratory for better understanding of the natural history of injuries, the biological basis of survival, best practices of diagnosis, surgical and intensive care, and rehabilitation and prevention. These and other advances became possible with the concentration and intense observations of trauma patients.

## Biomedical Investigations

William C. Shoemaker, MD, was a general surgeon trained at Hahnemann Hospital in Philadelphia and in physiologic research as a Damon Runyon Research Fellow (1958) at Harvard University. He came to CCH from Chicago's Michael Reese Hospital in 1965. He was appointed director of surgical research at the Hektoen Institute and established a robust research program on the trauma unit. Shoemaker's investigations evaluated the clinical manifestations of the shock syndrome in terms of morphologic, physiologic, biochemical, hemodynamic, and microcirculatory determinants, and described the manifestations of stages in progressive circulatory deterioration.

Shoemaker and his dedicated resident researchers developed pre-arranged plans for the emergency management of profound shock with indications, contraindications, and precautions in the use of transfusions; dextran and other plasma expanders; vasoconstrictors; vasodilators; mannitol; fluids; buffers; alkalies; antibiotics; cardiotonic agents; and steroids. Measurements of cardiac output were made to evaluate the pattern of changes in trauma, hemorrhage, and shock, sepsis, airway obstruction, and acute respiratory conditions. This research program was based on the concept that early recognition and vigorous therapy are essential to decreased morbidity and mortality in the prompt management of shock. The researchers proved that shock is caused by circulatory events that can be monitored hemodynamically to identify and treat underlying problems early and more effectively. Their descriptions of the evolving sequential hemodynamic patterns provided new dimensions for understanding the pathophysiology of traumatic shock. Shoemaker and his resident investigative team's interests were broad, productive, and highly respected.

The surgical residents who actively participated in this research group were Joseph J. Amato, David R. Boyd, Robert S. Brown, Charles W. Bryan-Brown, Joseph S. Carey, Richard S. Corley, Patrick D. Guinan, S. I. Kim, L.K. ( Cozy ) Kho, , Takayoshi Matsuda, David O. Monson, Kenneth J. Printen, Conrad Tasche, Robert R. Taube, Robert M. Vanecko, and James S.T. Yao. The senior staff involved included Robert J. Baker, Robert J. Freeark, and Norma J. Shoemaker.

**Trauma Registry**

In response to an obvious deficiency in the capacity to record and document the multiplicity of factors relevant to the trauma patient and a recommendation of the 1966 National Research Council in the Death and Disability Report, a computerized trauma registry (TR) was developed by D.R. Boyd at the CCHTU, the Department of Surgery of the Abraham Lincoln School of Medicine, and the Research Resources Laboratory of the University of Illinois in Chicago. The TR was a new computer method for trauma evaluation[7] funded by an unsolicited grant to the National Institutes of Health, General Medical Services, and Epidemiology Sections. The TR utilized currently available technological advances in data processing, a unique information storage and retrieval system that made possible a detailed, multifactorial analysis of the trauma problem. The TR recorded important details of the injured patient by accurate description of anatomical injury, physiologic status, clinical management, and from data on demographic, epidemiologic, and health care delivery factors.

The TR was developed to serve the following objectives:

1. to facilitate and improve patient care by rapidly locating and accurately reproducing significant amounts of clinical information ger-mane to the patient's present clinical problem
2. to provide on-line clinical summaries of diagnostic and therapeutic methods
3. to establish a data source for developing at-risk factors for accidental events
4. to define the variables on which patient morbidity and mortality depend
5. to determine logistical and manpower requirements for a given community's trauma needs
6. to estimate cost expenditures for certain injuries and their comprehensive care requirements, and
7. to provide continuous monitoring of project planning for the care of the critically injured.

These TR data would have a wide variety of both short- and long-term uses. The trauma registry was awarded the 1971 Billings Silver Medal by the American Medical Association.[7]

The TR was subsequently utilized in all 40 Illinois trauma centers connected on-line to the University of Illinois' computer center. Data entry was accomplished via remote terminals utilizing data phone patching to transmit directly to the central computer. In addition, epidemiologic information included accident time, location, and mechanisms of collection. Registration of these factors allowed for the detection of high-risk locations on highways, industrial injuries, and a variety of other environmental factors, and facilitated the planning of future emergency care facilities, accident safety and prevention programs, trauma manpower, and medical specialist needs. Effectiveness of care in the pre-hospital, initial hospital, and during secondary transfers to advanced treatment centers could be analyzed.

The initial publications from the trauma registry approach included:

1. "A Critical Review of the Management of Right Colon Injuries" made recommendations on surgical methods, reported on anaerobic infections, and identified time of transport to the CCHTU as a critical factor. [8]
2. "The Negative Laparotomy for Abdominal Trauma" presented the risks involved with emergency surgery and made recommendations for the expectant approach.[9]
3. "Clinical and Epidemiologic Characteristics of Non-surviving Trauma Victims in an Urban Environment" was presented at the National Medical Association, where it caused a stir. These data subsequently energized the minority city-county aldermen for the elimination of the Chicago Police "Squadrol" as ambulances.[5]
4. A report on the first implemented and studied Rural-Metropolitan Regional Trauma System in a central 15-county region around Springfield, Illinois, documented a decrease in deaths from motor vehicular crashes, a redistribution of accident victims to designated trauma centers, and a significant change in time factors with more patients arriving at the hospital alive.[10]

A keen interest in the trauma registry approach was maintained at the CCHTU by other residents and attendings including Robert Lowe, John Fildes, Richard Fantus, and Charles Sheaff. Ms. Lynne Carlson, a CCHTU laboratory technician, became involved in the TR research and development. She is recognized as the first trauma registrar in the nation. She earned her PhD in epidemiology, married Charles Sheaff, and continues her work in trauma research. Sheaff recognized the need to better track CCHTU patient data. With a desktop computer, she modified the original TR format utilizing advanced computer technology and with trauma attendings' consensus established essential data points. A TR modeled after Sheaff's plan was mandated for use by all Illinois hospital trauma centers for data collection and reporting to the state health department.

As the value of trauma registries continued to rise, J. Fildes and R. Fantus were instrumental in establishing, and remain active in, the American College of Surgeons' National Trauma Data Base (NTDB). It is now the largest aggregation of trauma registry data from participating trauma centers, and it consistently publishes reports in the ACS Bulletin.[11]

## Clinical Investigations

The resulting number, breadth, and quality of the clinical research produced at the CCHTU describe the multiplicity of questions and the need for new approaches to improving trauma care. Researchable questions and problems demanding investigation became obvious to the senior staff and the surgical residents, and came into focus by the number and concentration of observable patterns. The special unit environment provided the opportunity to observe, formulate questions, hypothesize, and study designs. The impact of the establishment of the Section of Clinical Investigation in the Division of Research and Education under Dr. Kimberly Nagy is reflected in the volume and quality of ongoing research, including prospective and multicenter studies. The compendium of the published papers from, and directly related to, the CCHTU are categorized elsewhere in a separate appendix.

## Patient Management

The publications on the resuscitation, immediate care, and management of the critically injured patient became a hallmark. Some of these were firsts of that genre. The large volume of patients with penetrating wounds of the abdomen with visceral injuries identified important problems and produced many publications. These important papers established early experience of the CCHTU in the management of esophageal injury, intestinal disruption, colon and rectal injuries, the duodenum and massive pancreatoduodenal trauma, and the utilization of pancreatoduodenectomy for penetrating trauma. Experience with selective and conservative management of blunt and penetrating abdominal wounds, and the effects of the negative laparotomy for abdominal trauma were often quoted. Transmediastinal gunshot wounds, penetrating wounds of the heart, and cardiac tamponade were examined. Penetrations of the neck and the definition of the three zones for guiding operative management were described.

Experiences with peripheral vascular injuries including the occult or partially severed arterial injury extremities, missile embolization, and venous repair and reconstruction were reported. Two unique cases describing a temporary internal vascular shunt for retrohepatic vena cava injury and angiographic embolization for traumatic hemobilia made interesting papers.

## Diagnostics

The role of angiography and aortography in the management of arterial and blunt abdominal trauma was pioneered at the CCHTU, as were venographic studies for thrombophlebitis. Diagnostic peritoneal lavage (DPL) was evaluated for prediction of intra-abdominal injury requiring celiotomy. Computed tomography (CT) evaluation of blunt and penetrating abdominal, chest and cardiac injuries, and minimal head injury were reported. CT and DPL were compared for abdominal injury assessments during pregnancy. The use of ultrasound for truncal blunt and cardiac trauma and routine one-shot intravenous pyelography were reported. The role of echocardiography for evaluation of occult penetrating and myocardial contusion was compared to subxiphoid pericardiotomy for cardiac injury.

## Complications and Squelae

There are many publications on complications after injuries including organ failure, management of a septic patient, gastrointestinal anastomosis, reoperations for pancreatic pseudocyst and venous thrombosis, including the inferior vena cava. Pulmonary dysfunction and ventilatory support focused attention on the etiology of failure, assessment and monitoring of posttraumatic insufficiency, and controlled studies comparing the effects of resuscitation with crystalloid and colloid.

## Repair and Prosthetics

Splenic preservation, the use of absorbable mesh splenorrhaphy, the optimal prosthetic material in temporary abdominal wall closure, and staged abdominal wall reconstruction were reported.

## Laboratory Studies

Central venous oxygen saturation, arterial base deficit, lactate concentration, and the utilization of serum osmometry as a predictor of outcome in monitoring intravenous hyperalimentation therapy and complex fluid managements were studied. Red cell survival of preserved blood, plasma, and whole blood viscosity changes after dextran infusion, intravascular cellular aggregate dissolution, and the use of Diaspirin cross-linked hemoglobin during resuscitations came under study. Evaluations of hypertonic saline and hyperthermia fluid resuscitation were done in various shock models. The physiologic and morphology effects of Stun Gun TASER®, discharges and the potential for fatal ventricular arrhythmias in the swine model were published.

## Protocols and Practice Guidelines

From the onset, the CCHTU created new and important approaches for evaluation, management and prioritization of critical and multiple injuries, changing concepts of hypovolemic shock, and the role of physiologic monitoring and algorithms for resuscitation. The Trauma Registry provided a new approach for categorizing anatomical injuries along with other impacting clinical and epidemiologic information. Important practice management guidelines were developed including emergency thoracotomy, blunt aortic and cardiac injury, mild traumatic brain injury, and blunt abdominal and penetrating neck trauma. Demographic studies of civilian cranial gunshot wounds lead to effective injury prevention activities.

## Multicenter Studies

The CCHTU, in conjunction with national trauma organizations and the American Association for the Surgery of Trauma (AAST), participated in the following studies: blunt aortic injury, penetrating esophageal injuries, penetrating colon injuries requiring resection, diversion or primary anastomosis, penetrating esophageal injury, hand-sewn versus stapled anastomosis in penetrating colon injuries requiring resection, use of presumptive antibiotics following tube thoracotomy for traumatic hemopneumothorax in the prevention of empyema and pneumonia, and practice patterns and outcomes of retrievable vena cava filters in trauma patients.

## Public Health Impact

The CCHTU leadership established important extra-clinical components for improving trauma care. By describing the functions of trauma care units and the organization and implementing of systems, they stimulated development of methods for hospital emergency categorization, trauma center designation, regionalization of trauma care, and emergency medical services systems. New professionals were identified, including trauma medical directors, trauma nurse specialists, trauma RN coordinators, and trauma registrars. They led other trauma centers in methods for training residents, establishing shock research units and organ transplantation donation, and retrieval programs. The CCHTU produced many citizen trauma advocates that educated the public, engaged the media, and lobbied politicians. They established government responsibility for these new concepts, providing resources and funding and promotion of injury prevention programs. The CCHTU can be credited for an extensive popular literature and several national television programs that contributed in major ways toward public acceptance and the lexicon of trauma terminologies.

## The County Way and Protocols

Over time, CCH medical staff by repetition and improvement developed a myriad of locally accepted medical practices that became known as the County Way. These clinical practices were considered the best at the time and were the basis for bedside assessment, diagnostic intervention, medical therapy, operative interaction, convalescence, and ward operations. Interns quickly learned these rules, approaches, techniques, and practices, typically by word of mouth or by one demonstration (See one: Do one: Teach one). The County Way was accepted on the TU and was especially useful due to the time-critical nature of acute trauma care. These consistent practices were repeatedly performed, honed, improved, and modified by consensus experience. They became more formalized and were now called protocols, though few of the early ones were actually written down.

Increased demand by visiting residents and outside professional interests led to the publication of a number of "How We Do It at the County" articles describing its approach for the Resuscitation, Evaluation and Initial Management of the Critically Injured. They were freely provided to many other surgeons developing trauma centers within and beyond Illinois.

Probably the most widely distributed CCHTU protocol is the schema developed for Estimation of Blood Loss and Suggested Therapy.[12-14] This simple clinical method for evaluating the extent of hemorrhage and planning for fluid resuscitation described four categories of blood loss, typical clinical findings, common etiologies, and recommended treatments. This basic guide became a core teaching element of the Advanced Trauma Life Support (ATLS) course.[14] It is estimated that many thousands of physicians around the world have learned from this basic County Way protocol. The Illinois trauma program reprinted many of these early clinical, operational, and administrative protocols and distributed them widely to developing trauma centers and trauma agencies throughout Illinois, other states, and developing international trauma programs.

John Barrett further developed and formalized many of the trauma unit protocols. He commented:

*The protocols are in essence "practice guidelines" for the unit. They were developed and approved by the attending physicians on the service with the understanding that we would all follow them as guidelines, i.e., if we deviated from the guidelines, we would explain why, when the case was presented at morning report. It made for a uniform approach to the management of the trauma patient and also facilitated teaching. They outline the standard management of the trauma patient and were used to orientate the incoming staff - residents - as to what we expect in the treatment of the patients. They were included in the Trauma Unit Orientation Manual and were never "published" in the strict sense of the word.[15]*

## The University of Maryland Hospital[7]

The Cook County Hospital trauma unit is especially indebted to Dr. R. Adams Cowley, Director of the Maryland Institute of Emergency Medical Service Systems for the inspiration and training he provided to David Boyd, who became the driving force behind our unit's planning and implementation. Boyd brought the realization of the Golden Hour for successful treatment of severe injury from Crowley's Unit to Cook County Hospital.[7]

Dr. Boyd spent the most productive years of his professional life in relentless pursuit of his goal of a nationwide network of trauma centers as the hub of a sophisticated emergency medical care system. According to Dr. Freeark's recollections "for reasons best known to him [Dr. Boyd], he gave up his surgical career and used his not inconsiderable talents as a teacher, investigator, intensivist, and surgeon by traveling to every region of this country to sell trauma centers and the systems approach to emergency medical care to every physician, newspaper reporter, politician, and citizen he could reach. He made mistakes, acquired a platoon of critics, and lost his battle in Washington. But he has an army of those who believe him and some stunning victories. Most of all, I believe he won our war of regionalization, emergency services, and the trauma center concept."[17] Dr. Boyd was appointed National Director, Office of EMSS in the DHEW and DHHS (1975–1983). A trauma consultant afterward, he returned to clinical work in 1991 and was the general surgeon at the Blackfeet Community Hospital in Browning, Montana, until 2006. Currently, he is the national trauma systems coordinator for the Indian Health Service (IHS) in Rockville, Maryland.

Figure 8-4 shows the ICU trauma uit.

## Leadership Surgeons:-The Second Generation

The positive impact of the CCHTU on the general surgical and subspecialty residents was immediate and sustained. The new environment brought enhanced interest, improved knowledge, and skills into the spectrum of poorly understood complicated injuries and complex pathophysiologic case scenarios. There were remarkable changes in resident attitudes toward these patients. The junior admitting resident was no longer alone dealing with these most challenging cases. Senior residents and surgical consultants were readily available and supportive.

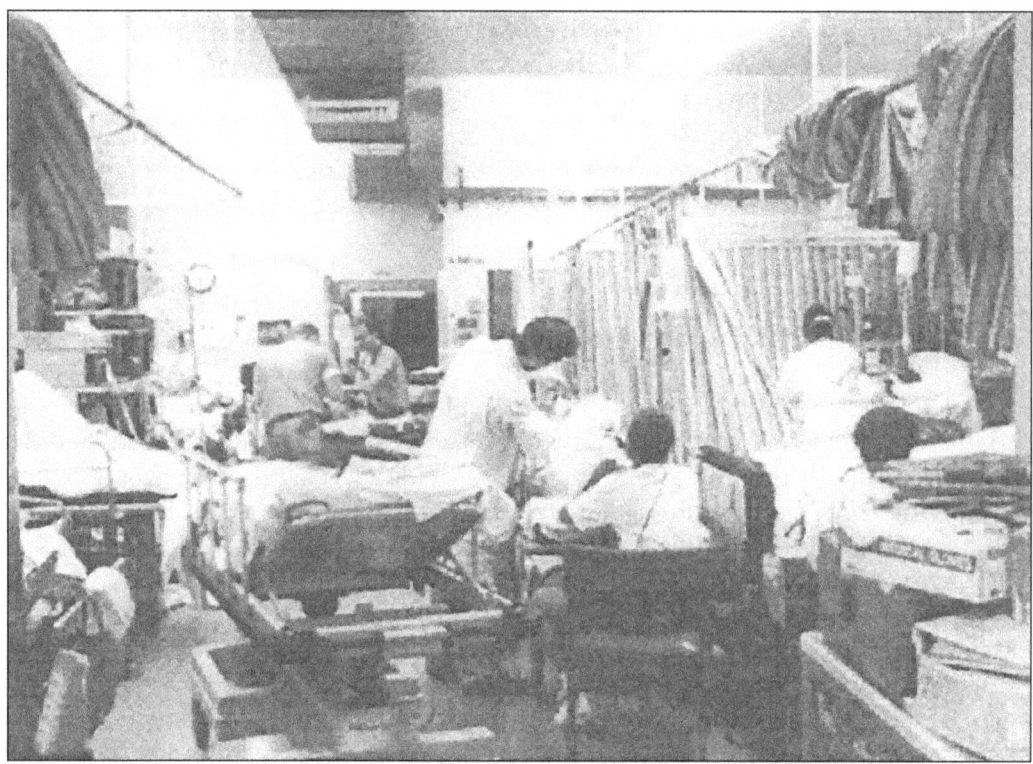

*Figure 8–4   ICU of trauma unit on the first floor of the old hospital*

Trauma nurses were a universally recognized enhancement and much appreciated. Laboratory, blood and X-ray support dramatically improved. Operating rooms were on a continuous first priority basis. Postoperative and critical care became more rational and consistent. Team-consensus case management provided a basis for learning new operative and intensive care techniques.

For residents with a special interest in trauma, this was heaven on earth. The natural competitiveness of young surgeons became evident with each great case expertly done and elevated the bar to new standards of expected performance. Those with less prior enthusiasm saw this as more tolerable, and many became "traumaphiles," at least while practicing in this new supportive environment.

Dr. John Saletta was the first junior resident and Conrad Tasche and Robert Vanecko the first two seniors assigned to the TU. Their first patient was a 12-year-old boy who fell 15 stories out of a tenement building and eventually survived. Saletta and Freeark performed a series of clinical investigations of vascular injuries of peripheral vessels describing the three zones of the anterior neck and best operative approaches for penetrating wounds. They pioneered the use of arteriography in extremity injury and aortography for abdominal trauma.

Successful treatment of major hepatic injury and control of massive hemorrhage was a particularly difficult management challenge. A perplexing technical problem was the vascular control and repair of the retro-hepatic inferior vena cava. The current literature described various by-pass shunts for return of caval blood without significant loss and diminished cardiac output, but none of these laboratory approaches seemed practical. The following CCHTU case report represents the first surviving retro-hepatic caval injury repair using an internal shunt.[16]

> CASE: A young male with a gunshot wound in the right chest was admitted, and clinical assessment of cardiac tamponade and intra-abdominal injury, with hepatic and vena caval injuries was made. At thoracotomy, a perforated right ventricle was repaired. Laparotomy showed blood and a large retrohepatic inferior vena cava laceration. An internal shunt with a modified #28 chest tube was placed in the right atrium bypassing this injury. The left hepatic vein and vena cava was repaired in a bloodless field. The postoperative course was complicated. The patient was presented to many visitors and became enchanted with his "first in the world" status. He would, on occasion, present his own clinical story. Some 35 days later, he left the CCHTU, a truly changed young man.[15]

## David R. Boyd, MDCM, FACS. General Surgery Resident (1967-1971) Attending Surgeon, Director of Trauma and Emergency Medical Services, Illinois Department of Public Health (1971-1975)

David R. Boyd (Figure 8-5) graduated in Medicine from McGill University, Montreal, Canada, with an expressed interest in trauma as a surgical specialty and academic career. He did a rotating internship at CCH in 1963. He was subsequently drafted for the Vietnam War and stationed in Baltimore where he started

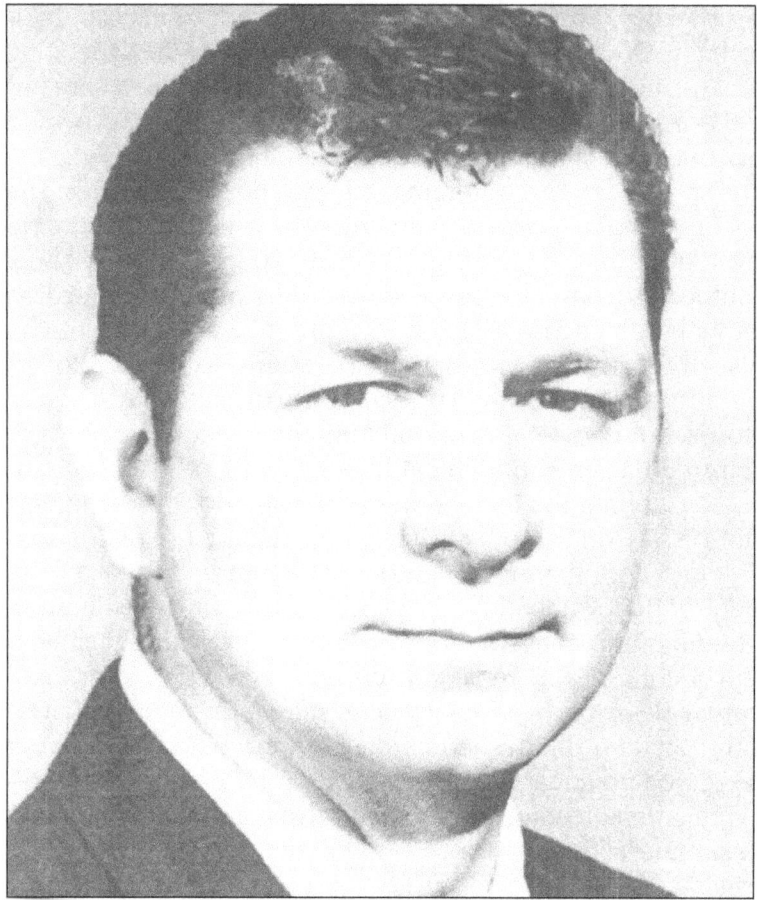

*Figure 8–5  David R. Boyd*

his surgical training at the University of Maryland. He decided early on "to do something about the trauma problem in the United States of America," and was recruited by R. Adams Cowley to be the first fellow at the University of Maryland Shock Trauma Program. Dr. Freeark invited him back to CCH to complete his surgery training with an emphasis on trauma. With a background in trauma resuscitation and shock research, he took a leadership role and exercised considerable influence on the early development of the CCHTU programs.

Boyd introduced several new approaches. From his McGill experience, he emphasized the Oslerian bedside teaching approach to the daily rounds and energized the clinical, surgical, and intensive care educational experience (Figure 8–6). These rounds became the place where open team discussions of the patient care, established practices, new approaches, protocol development, and the published literature met and meshed. Senior staff, general and subspecialty residents, nurses, and students were actively involved. Residents without a daytime surgery obligation spent time and intellectual energy discuss-

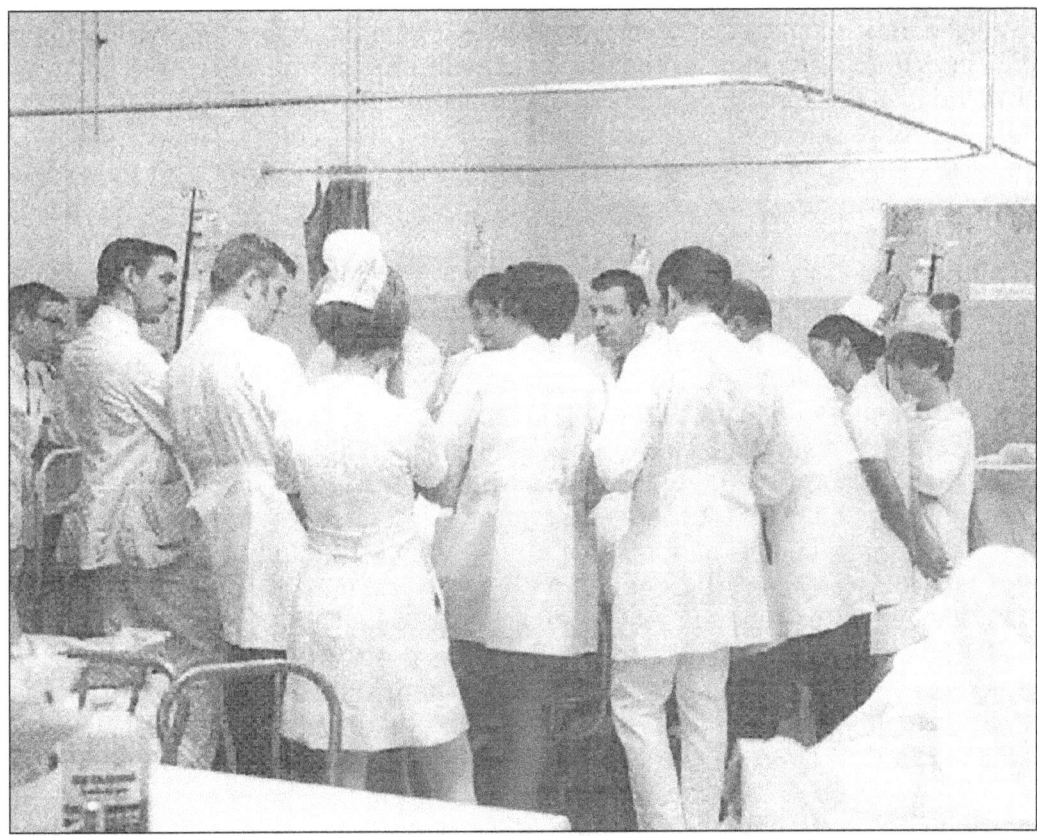

*Figure 8–6 Tauma rounds with Dr. David Boyd*

ing, arguing, and testing the best practices for a variety of clinical problems. The popularity of these rounds was evidenced by resident participation from other surgical services and neighboring institutions. Protocol practices became more standardized. Boyd established the practice of a single medical director being in charge with final sign-off authority on all cases. He transferred critical care and applicable research techniques learned at Maryland and upgraded the clinical laboratory with immediate blood gas analysis, osmometry by freezing point depression, and other standard tests.

The CCHTU was the place where a surgeon and often several others were always present, working, doing consultations, meeting colleagues, or posting contact information. Boyd saw the need to progress from a "unit" to a larger trauma center concept that would further emphasize excellence in trauma patient care, professional education, applied research, data management, and a variety of outreach practices. He was recognized as one of Chicago's Outstanding Young Men of 1970 by the Chicago Junior Association of Chamber of Commerce and Industry on September 21, 1970. (R.J. Freeark had received this award in 1960.) This caused a series of rapidly occurring and connected events that significantly changed Boyd's academic career plans and the future direction of trauma care in Chicago, the state of Illinois, and elsewhere. Illinois Governor Richard B. Ogilvie, a friend of the County Hospital since he was the Cook County Board President (1962–1968), took notice of this award and sent his public relations officer to interview Boyd. He recommended to the governor that organized trauma centers should be established downstate "so that lives could be saved as was routine at the CCHTU."

Two weeks later, the governor asked for a statewide trauma center plan. Boyd, along with Dr. Bruce Flashner, a former CCH general surgery resident and then with the Illinois Comprehensive Health Planning Agency, quickly wrote a rational plan based on their clinical and organizational experiences on the CCHTU. Their approach was to categorize all hospitals and to specifically designate some 40 new trauma centers in a Three Echelon System (i.e., regional, areawide, and local) in the nine administrative state regions. The selected hospitals would incorporate CCHTU concepts and practices. In addition, there would be several specialty centers designated for burns, spinal cord injuries, and pediatrics in Chicago. A prehospital program for an EMS system including ground and air ambulance transportation would be organized.

Governor Ogilvie asked Boyd to lead this program as the new Director of Emergency Medical Services and Highway Safety in the Illinois Department of Public Health (IDPH), and he announced the Illinois Trauma Center Plan on January 23, 1971. Boyd was assured that the IDPH trauma program would be under his direction, and he would maintain a clinical trauma surgical focus and office for this new trauma and EMS system (EMSS) at the CCHTU. Over the next four years (1971–1975), Boyd, Robert J. Lowe, and Theresa Romano, each in their dual capacities as attending surgeons and nurse on the CCHTU and employee or consultant with the state IDPH trauma program, conceptualized, described, demonstrated, and taught trauma care, trauma unit organization, trauma systems integration, and developed many of the essential EMSS operational components recognized today. These two trauma programs, juxtaposed on the third floor of the CCH, complementary in function and mutually led, can be considered the Menlo Park of trauma center and EMS systems for Chicago, Illinois, and the nation. Hundreds of interested physicians, surgeons, nurses, health care professionals, and their foreign counterparts visited these two programs.

The products of this phenomenon include most of the conceptualizations of trauma care as a system, the lexicon of new trauma terms, program definitions, and practical model approaches to trauma care delivery. An extensive body of trauma and EMS systems program information was produced. Numerous articles, newsletters, technical, and governmental documents were printed monthly and distributed widely on request to interested professionals and organizations starting up similar programs. Several TV documentaries featured the CCHTU and IDPH trauma programs, including NBC's *First Tuesday* and PBS' *Killers*, which introduced trauma and EMS systems to a national audience.

## Robert J. Lowe, MD, FACS. Resident General Surgery 1968, Director of Trauma Unit 1973–1982, Director of General Surgery 1974–1982.

Robert J. Lowe (Figure 8–7) graduated from Stritch School of Medicine at Loyola University, Chicago, in 1968. He took a rotating internship at CCH and worked with Boyd in general surgery on Ward 63. They established a strong personal and professional relationship in large part from a mutual interest in the care and study of the trauma victim. He devoted more than the usually assigned resident time to the trauma service. He was integrally involved with the development of the CCH trauma registry, the IDPH trauma program, and other ongoing teaching and investigative projects.

Lowe's scientific curiosity led him to seriously question himself and his colleagues, and he would ask, "Why are we doing it this way?" and "What can we do better to improve outcomes?" With Gerald Moss, he studied post-trauma pulmonary failure and whether the current standard approaches of resuscitation using generous quantities of Ringers lactate solution could be "one possible cause of pulmonary failure after trauma." He also questioned if laparotomy should be mandatory or selective in gunshot wounds and the effects of the negative laparotomy for abdominal trauma. With colleagues Moss and Saletta, he critically evaluated and presented indications for performing a pancreato-duodenectomy for penetrating pancreatic trauma and made recommendations for operative reconstruction.

In 1973, Lowe became the first full time director of the trauma service and a year later, also the director of General Surgery. He was popular, well respected and instrumental in the re-instatement of the general surgery residency program,

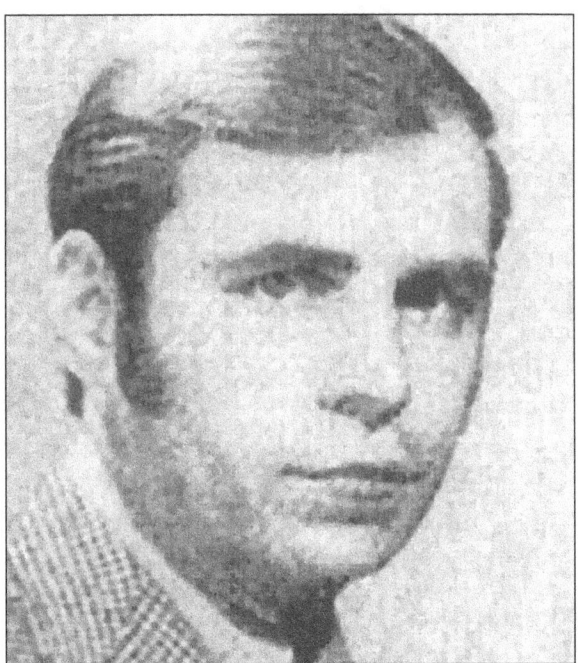

Figure 8–7  Robert J. Lowe

then on probation. He was diagnosed with cancer in 1975, only two years out of his residency. In a eulogy on February10, 1983, Dr. Baker described his unique attributes and contributions.

> *Bob Lowe was a thoughtful, dedicated resident and an impressive student of trauma, who threw himself into the maelstrom of an enormously busy and demanding Trauma Service, sometimes at considerable personal cost. His demeanor, in the resuscitation area, at the bedside or in the operative room, was invariably that of calm, collected clinical surgeon. He deeply cared about the welfare of the patient, and improving the quality of trauma care was the driving force in his professional life. He was an ideal choice to lead the Trauma Unit, as he proved time and again in the few years in which he served in that capacity. He was a quietly charismatic, highly effective trauma surgeon, in every sense of the term. Catastrophically, he became ill and ultimately succumbed to Ewing's sarcoma, primarily of his spine, when he was really in his prime. Despite his death at a young age, he left a strong legacy of leadership and of devotion to care afforded trauma victims which has persisted in the Cook County Trauma Unit to this day.*

### Max L. Ramenofsky, MD, FACS. General Surgery Resident 1967–1972

Ramenofsky graduated from th CCH general surgery residency in 1972, completed a fellowship in pediatric surgery at Pittsburgh Children's Hospital, and became the first pediatric trauma director at the Boston Floating Hospital and the Kiwanis Pediatric Trauma Institute, which he founded with the help of the New England Kiwanis Foundation. He wrote a national standard for pediatric trauma, which proposed a comprehensive set of standards and was published in the *Journal of Trauma* in 1982. The ACS-COT later incorporated these pediatric standards into the extant adult trauma optimal care document, where it has remained since. Ramenofsky's landmark paper has guided the development of pediatric trauma centers throughout the United States, Canada, Central and South America, Europe, Asia, the Middle East, and the Far East.[19]

### D.John Fildes, MD, FACS, FCCM. Fellow in Trauma and Critical Care1988–1989, Attending Surgeon Trauma and General Surgery 1989–1996

John Fildes earned his Bachelor of Science degree in biomedical engineering at Union College in Schenectady, New York, in 1977 and graduated from the University of Santo Tomas Medical School in Manila, Philippines, in 1982. He was an intern (1982–1983), resident (1983–1986), chief resident (1986–1987), and fellow (1987–1988) in general surgery at Bronx-Lebanon Hospital in Bronx, New York. Following his work at Bronx-Lebanon, Dr. Fildes received fellowship training in surgical critical care and trauma (1988–1989) at Cook County Hospital. Fildes began his academic career as an assistant professor of surgery at the University of Illinois College of Medicine-Chicago (1989–1995), at which time he was also a lecturer (1990-1992) and visiting assistant professor in general surgery (1992–1995) at Rush Medical College in Chicago. He is currently (1996–present) a professor of surgery at the University of Nevada. Dr. Fildes reflects, "I am often amused by the fact that the fellowship in 1988 was nearly identical to the curriculum developed for the new specialty of acute care surgery. Acute care surgery requires the trainee to complete an ACGME-approved surgical critical care year and an additional year of advanced surgical training to include, but not be limited to, trauma, burns and emergencies in general, and thoracic and vascular surgery. In retrospect, the fellowship program at Cook County provided all of these elements."

Dr. Fildes has received the White House Medical Unit Certificate of Appreciation (1998), the Las Vegas Chamber of Commerce's Community Achievement Award (1998), and the 2006 Physician of the Year by the Nevada State Medical Association.

### John Barrett, MD, M.Ch, FRCS. General Surgery Resident 1976–1981, Attending Surgeon, Director of Trauma Department 1982–2003

Dr. John Barrett (Figure 8–8) attended medical school and began his surgical training in his native city of Cork, Ireland. He received his master of surgery (M.Ch.) from the National University of Ireland and the FRCS Ireland in 1975. He followed this training with a surgical residency at Cook County Hospital. After

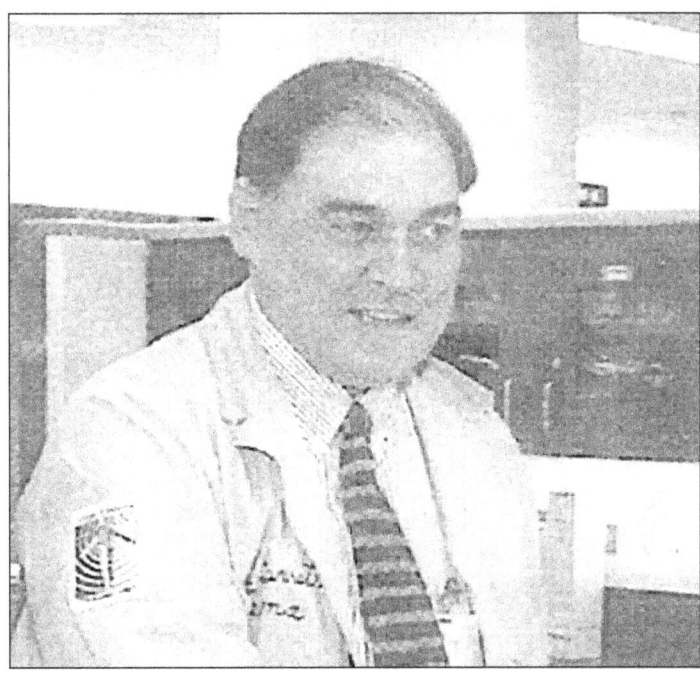

*Figure 8–8 John Barrett*

completing his training, he joined the trauma service at Cook County Hospital and became the director of the trauma unit in 1982. Under his leadership, the trauma unit flourished and grew into a separate department in 1994. He was promoted to professor of general surgery at Rush University in 1999.

During his professional career, Dr. Barrett was an active teacher, researcher, and clinician. He has received awards for both his teaching skills and his basic science research. His work on various hospital committees culminated with his election to president of the hospital's executive medical staff. At the city and state levels, he helped to advance trauma centers and trauma systems, primarily through his work with the Chicago Fire Department and the Illinois Department of Public Health. He was a member of several national trauma and surgical organizations. He was a charter member of the Eastern Association for the Surgery of Trauma.

Dr. Barrett has published extensively on his work with pulmonary effects of blood transfusion, resuscitation from hemorrhagic shock, splenic preservation, efficacy of safety belts, and importance of regionalization of trauma centers. Dr. Barrett took a major role in designing the new Cook County Hospital (Stroger Hospital), which opened in 2002. He retired shortly thereafter. He is currently enjoying his retirement in the Chicago area.

**Kimberly Ormsby Nagy, MD, FACS. General Surgery Resident 1992, Trauma and Critical Care Fellow 1994, Chair Research and Education 1995, and Vice Chair of Trauma 2003**

Dr. Kimberly Ormsby Nagy (Figure 8–9) received her Bachelor's degree from the University of Toledo and her Medical Doctorate from Ohio State University. While on her clinical rotations at Ohio State, she discovered a love for trauma surgery. She was attracted to the University of Illinois surgical residency because of its component of trauma at Cook County Hospital. She started her residency in

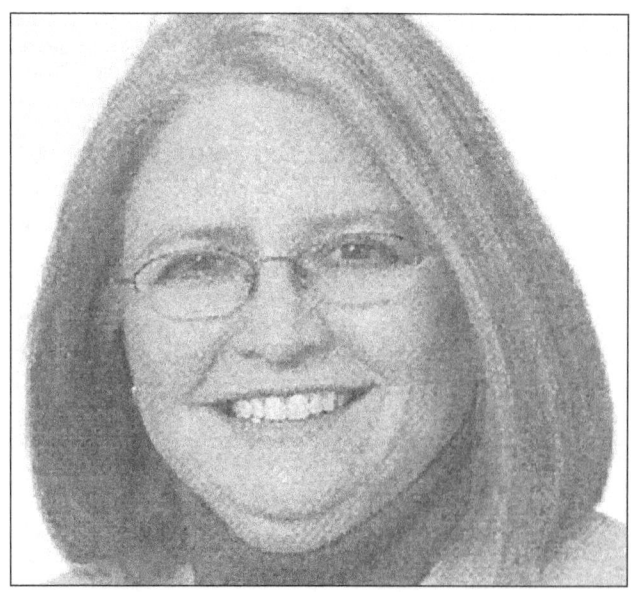

*Figure 8–9  Kimberly Ormsby Nagy*

1986 and spent about 50 percent of her clinical rotations at County.

Dr. Nagy had assisted in a surgical critical care laboratory in medical school and expanded on her research interests by spending a year as a trauma research fellow at Cook County, working with Drs. Marcel Martin and John Barrett to study the effects of hypertonic saline on resuscitation in both hemorrhagic and septic shock models. After completing her general surgery residency, she continued her training as the Cook County clinical trauma/critical care fellow.

Upon completion of her fellowship, she was offered a position on staff in the Trauma Department, where she rapidly was promoted to section chief of clinical investigations, then to division chair of research and education. When Dr. Roxanne Roberts assumed the chair of the department in 2003, Dr. Nagy was promoted to vice-chair for the department.

Dr. Nagy has been an active researcher for the Department, having presented and published her laboratory work on hypertonic saline resuscitation, hyperthermic resuscitation and temporary abdominal wall closure. Clinical research has focused on assessment of the trauma patient with publications on topics such as diagnostic peritoneal lavage, blunt and penetrating cardiac injuries, minimal head injury, and trauma in the elderly. She is professor of general surgery at Rush University.

Dr. Nagy serves on the editorial board of the *Journal of Trauma* and has served on committees for the American Association for the Surgery of Trauma. She was the first female president of the Eastern Association for the Surgery of Trauma, She was recently appointed to the prestigious Committee on Trauma of the American College of Surgeons.

## Continuing History of the World-Famous Trauma Unit ( WFTU) (1982–2008)

### Department Overview

The trauma unit entered another era in 1982 when Dr. John Barrett became the trauma director. Under his direction, trauma evolved from a subspecialty of general surgery to a fully functional department that is recognized as a center of excellence, both within Cook County as well as nationally and internationally.

In 1994, trauma became a separate department within the hospital, giving the department chairman equal stature with other department chairmen. This gave trauma the ability to control its own budget, make its own hiring decisions, and deal directly with hospital administration. Dr. Barrett accomplished this restructuring by showing that trauma is a unique disease that encompasses many types of injury resulting not only from the commonly thought of blunt and penetrating mechanisms, but also including burn mechanisms. The division of burn surgery and the division of trauma surgery share common goals relating to the care of the injured patient and naturally fit together to form one department.

Since 1993, we have had a physiatrist in our department who makes rounds regularly with our team. He is a valuable resource to help patients begin their rehabilitation before leaving our unit. This aids in the transition to the rehabilitation or nursing facility. Patients are also seen as outpatients in the trauma clinic or occasionally in the trauma resuscitation area by the same group of physicians.

## Training and Education

In 1986, our primary academic affiliation was with the University of Illinois surgical residency. The hospital changed its primary affiliation to Rush University In 1994. Since then, we have expanded to train residents and students from a number of programs. General surgical residents rotate from Rush University, University of Chicago, and Chicago College of Osteopathic Medicine. Emergency medicine residents rotate from three area programs in addition to the Cook County Emergency Medicine Residency. Residents rotate on the service from other specialties such as anesthesia, family medicine, and oral surgery, and frequently, residents from Canada train on our service. We train fellows from the disciplines of surgical critical care, pulmonary critical care, and pediatric emergency medicine as well. Students come to us from a variety of schools within the city, as well as from across the country and internationally.

The formal trauma fellowship started in 1987 as a one-year clinical fellowship designed to prepare surgeons to assume a leadership role in trauma care. The program contains instruction in the essential skills required of a trauma center director to include extensive clinical training in resuscitation, critical care, operative intervention, rehabilitation and administration, as well as exposure to injury prevention, trauma systems planning, education of prehospital personnel and trauma registry functions. One fellow is selected each year, and 17 trauma fellows have been trained. The program directors have been Drs. Barrett, Martin, Fildes, and Nagy, in that order.

Prior to the development of the organized fellowship program, there were several excellent surgeons who functioned in this role. The first was Constantinos "Dino" Chilimindris (1968), an accomplished and popular general surgeon who stayed on the CCH surgical teaching staff before returning to Baltimore. Fred Rodgers was another "first" trauma research fellow (1982), who went on to become head of the trauma service at University of Vermont.

## Physical Changes in the Trauma Unit

The CCHTU started out in the renovated physician's dining room on the third floor of the main hospital. In 1994, CCHTU was moved to the first floor into a renovated area adjacent to the emergency room. This new trauma unit had a 10-bed resuscitation area with an adjacent 16-bed intensive care unit. Contained within the resuscitation area was a shock room for the most critically injured patients, as well as a radiology room that vastly improved the ease of obtaining radiographs. Although this unit was a great improvement, it was still full and occasionally overflowing on a busy Friday or Saturday night (Figure 8–10).

In 2002, the new Stroger Hospital opened. Once again, the trauma unit

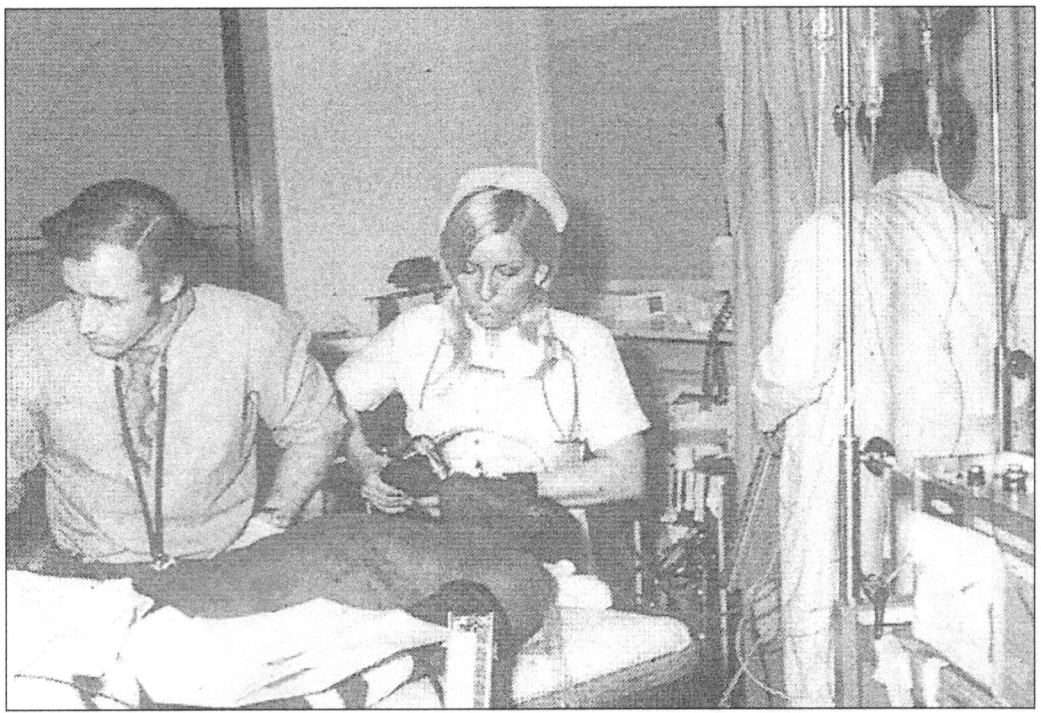

*Figure 8–10 Trauma unit on a busy Friday night*

moved into a new space. We now have a 15-bed resuscitation unit with two shock rooms, a 12-bed intensive care unit, and a 10-bed trauma observation unit. The observation unit allows staff to keep a close eye on patients who require neuro checks following blunt head trauma, patients who require cardiac monitoring to rule out blunt cardiac injury, and patients who are undergoing nonoperative management of a solid organ injury, all of whom were previously placed in the ICU. We frequently have postoperative patients or patients with chest tubes in the observation unit as well. The current trauma areas are located next to a CT scanner allowing for expeditious work-up of our patients. The entire new hospital is equipped with a digital radiographic system, as well as computerized order entry, and lab retrieval is in the process of becoming entirely paperless, all of which helps streamline our patient care.[18–20]

### The Famous and the Infamous

Cook County trauma unit has had its share of media attention. We frequently have patients with local renown such as police officers and victims of highly publicized events. We have had some national attention as well, some of which is recounted below.

In July 1966, Richard Speck murdered eight student nurses in Chicago. There was a nationwide manhunt to bring him to justice. A few days later, he was

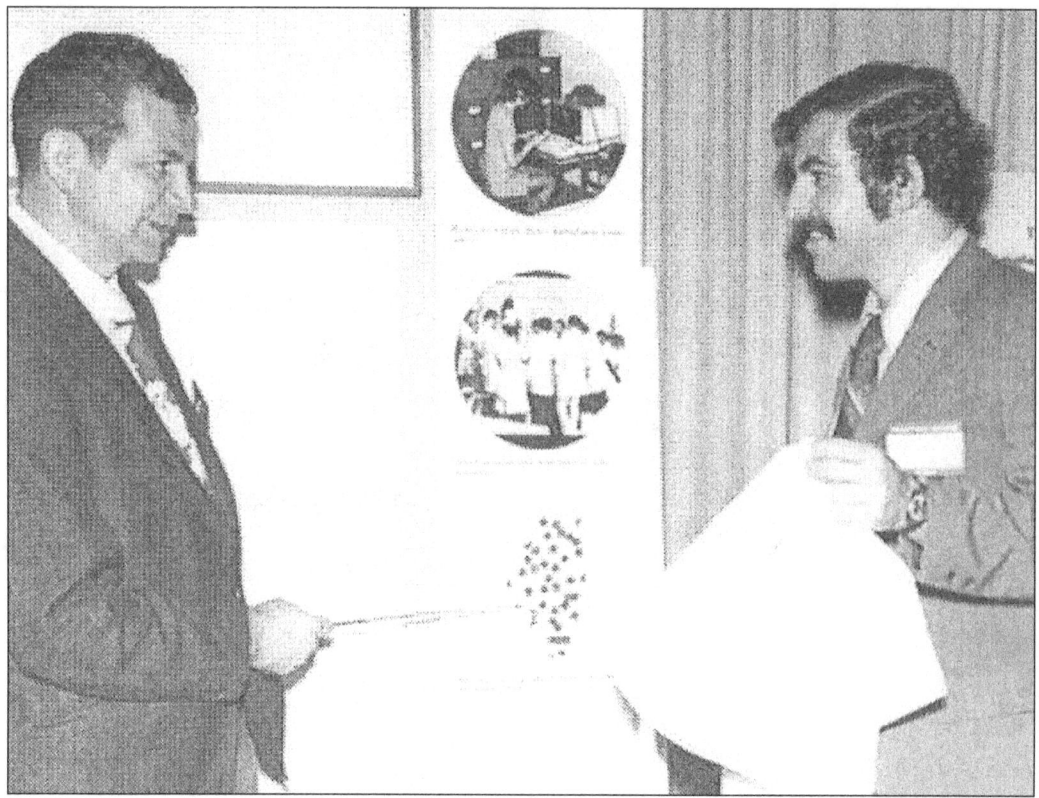

*Figure 8–11  David Boyd and Bruce Flashner*

brought to the trauma unit after a failed suicide attempt. The resident and nurse on duty recognized his "Born to raise hell" tattoo and turned him in to authorities.

In April 1994, nationally known singer Wayne Messmer was leaving a local restaurant when he was robbed at gunpoint. He was shot in the neck, sustaining an injury to his larynx. After treatment at our trauma unit, he was able to return to singing professionally.

In June 1996, Diana, Princess of Wales, was visiting Chicago. One of her stops was at our trauma unit where she visited with some of our intensive care patients.

Actor Harrison Ford visited our trauma unit prior to filming *The Fugitive* in 1993. Part of the trauma resuscitation area was recreated on a soundstage for a scene in that movie. Dr. Robert Smith served as a technical consultant for the film; several of our nurses appeared as extras, and Dr. Roxanne Roberts even had a small speaking role.

The NBC television series *ER* was loosely based on the emergency room and trauma unit at Cook County Hospital. In response to that show's popularity, several documentaries have been filmed to spotlight the unit, most notably *The Real ER* by the British Broadcasting Company in 1996 and a similar film in 2004 by a Japanese film company.

## Outreach Efforts

Clinical patient care is not the only focus of the attendings at Cook County trauma unit. We have a strong interest in injury prevention through linkages with substance-abuse intervention services, domestic-violence services, and child protective services. We have conducted our own injury prevention activities through elder abuse programs and education of Chicago elementary students in conflict resolution.

## Research Endeavors

With the wealth of clinical material to study, it is not surprising that the clinical research is based primarily in trauma resuscitation.

Previous oft-cited studies dealt with the consequences of negative laparotomies for trauma, and a new technique for splenic preservation, to name a few. We have published extensively on diagnostic peritoneal lavage and are known as the world-premiere site for this test. We have also published on penetrating thoracic trauma; the evaluation of both cardiac trauma and transmediastinal gunshot wounds. Blunt cardiac injury diagnosis and management were refined through several papers from our institution. We recently published a large series on the evaluation of the cervical spine.

Our research efforts are not limited to clinical studies. We have had ongoing basic science studies as well. Early research examined types of resuscitation fluid such as crystalloid vs. colloid, and hypertonic saline in resuscitation of both hemorrhagic and septic shock. We looked extensively at resuscitation with hyperthermic fluid in order to minimize the occurrence of hypothermia. Complex abdominal wall closure with fascial substitutes has been the subject of both animal and clinical studies. Recently, our laboratory has been studying the effects of electrical injury, specifically those arising from law enforcement devices such as the TASER®. The results of these studies have been published and presented nationally and internationally by our attending staff.

## Where We Are Today

Today, the Cook County Department of Trauma continues to provide comprehensive care to the injured patient. There are seven full-time trauma attending surgeons on staff who specialize in all aspects of trauma and critical care. Staffs are in-house 24 hours a day, seven days a week to provide care in our three clinical areas, as well as the operating rooms. We are frequently called on to respond in other areas of the hospital for immediate assistance with regard to airways, hemorrhagic shock, and critical care. The department also has two full-time burn attending surgeons, a nurse epidemiologist, a scientific officer, a chaplain, and a four-member surveillance team. Members of the department have had additional training and expertise in varied aspects of trauma care such as nutrition, complex wound care, emergency ultrasonography, injury prevention, disaster management, and surgical education. They are active at the national level by serving in various capacities for organizations such as Eastern Association for the Surgery of Trauma, American Association for the Surgery of Trauma, Society of Critical Care Medicine, American Society for Parenteral and Enteral Nutrition, and the National Medical Association.

The CCHTU maintains its public health leadership in Chicago, Illinois, Trauma and EMS deliberations, operations, and legislation.

In the mid-1980s, a logo was developed for the branding image of Cook County trauma unit by Randi Robin, a graphic artist and wife of trauma attending surgeon Dr. Arnold Robin. This image[21] is recognized worldwide by everyone familiar with the CCH trauma unit. It can be seen on scientific presentations from the Trauma Department on PowerPoint and posters, as well as hats, clothing, and lapel pins, just to name a few items. It remains a popular item representing the WFTU and its many contributions.

## Trauma Care as Public Health Policy

On October 14, 1972, Senator Charles H. Percy told his colleagues, "If you are going to get hurt, do it in Illinois."[22] Also that month, Elliot Richardson, then Secretary of the Department of Health and Human Services (DHHS), was invited to speak at the dedication of the St. Francis Trauma Center in Peoria. Richardson commented, "You and your associates, through planning and persistence, have converted a concept into productive reality." Later he wrote, "Since my return to Washington, I have been citing what I saw in Illinois."[23]

This recognition, other presentations, and testimony to Congressional Committees in 1972 influenced the passage of Public Law No. 93-154, Emergency Medical Services Systems Act of 1973 and as amended in 1976 (PL 94-573) and 1979 (PL 96-142). These Congressional Acts provided the recognition and grant funds for planning, implementation, and expansion of systems and technical assistance to develop a national program of regional trauma center and EMS systems.

In 1974, Dr. Boyd was appointed by President Gerald R. Ford to be the National Director of Emergency Medical Services Systems, Public Health Service (PHS), Department of Health and Human Services (DHHS), in Rockville, Maryland. Dr. Boyd soon convinced President Ford to host a White House Conference on trauma and EMS.

The EMSS legislation provided grant support ($304 million), technical assistance, and a national plan to establish some 303 contiguous Trauma/EMSS Regions covering every state and the four territories. Each of these regions implemented a trauma center and supporting EMS systems modeled on the CCHTU and Illinois Trauma/EMS System. Every state and large urban community was required to establish a lead agency for trauma/ EMS in their Public Health Departments as was done in Illinois. Over the next decade (1974–1983), this federal initiative provided extensive professional technical assistance, public, and political educational programs. Much of this was copied from the collaborating experiences of the CCH TU and IDPH Trauma/EMSS programs during that formative Menlo Park period on the third floor of CCH. Many governors and mayors, with Boyd's encouragement, followed Ogilvie's example and personally encouraged these chief executives to develop trauma programs for their states and communities. The progressive acceptance and extension of the trauma unit and EMS system concepts as governmental public health and safety policy changed thought and practices of trauma and emergency medical care everywhere. Trauma care became a national public health issue and one of high priority and visibility.[24]

Barrett and colleagues continued and expanded on these public health and safety responsibilities. They were in large part responsible for the passage of trauma systems legislation that regulates Trauma Center Designation and Verification in Illinois.

In 1972, Boyd and Stanley Zydlo, MD, an emergency physician from Arlington Heights, developed the Illinois paramedic programs in the several northwestern Chicago suburbs and worked together to secure statewide paramedic enabling legislation, operating regulations and new terminologies (i.e., medical control, offline and online supervision, and operational and treatment protocols).[25] These were effective, accepted, and subsequently folded into the federal EMSS program, and have been universally copied in developing paramedic programs. The CCH Trauma Department maintains an active role in oversight and medical direction of Chicago area paramedic services, and in the various state and local trauma and emergency department categorization programs.

## Summary

The Cook County Hospital's commitment and service to the Chicago community indigent population is legendary. Its long record and tradition of excellence in professional training is well recognized and greatly respected. The establishment of the new trauma unit was accepted by the lay and professional communities as another rational and practical innovation. From the beginning, the Cook County Hospital Trauma Unit demonstrated improvements in overall patient care resulting from an organized "team" approach of physicians and nurses working together in a continuum of care. This basic patient centered approach only got better and was extended further into the prehospital, rehabilitation, and prevention spheres over time. The CCHTU was the first civilian comprehensive trauma unit in the United States and continues as one of the largest, most active, and a leader in every category. The CCHTU has arguably treated more critically injured patients, being perpetually available and never on by-pass, providing essential and sophisticated state of the art care to all patients in need.

The worldwide impact of the CCHTU on trauma surgery, critical care, emergency medical services, and public health policy is incalculable. The CCHTU has generated more innovation for trauma, emergency medicine and emergency medical services systems, public health policy, and political recognition than any other. As predicted early on, the WFTU, or World Famous Trauma Center, is universally renowned, and its manifold contributions are acknowledged and profound.

## References

1. *NAS-NRC Death and Disability Report 1966*. Prepared by the Division of Medical Sciences, National Academy of Sciences, National Research Council. Washington, DC.
2. Private Notes of Robert J. Freeark. Contributed to this work by his daughter Kim Freeark.
3. Lowe RJ, Baker RJ. Organization and function of trauma care units. *J Trauma*. 1973: 13(4):285-290.
4. Romano T. Trauma nurse specialist. *Am J Nurs*. June 1973: 73(6):1008-1011.
5. Boyd DR, Flashner BA, Nyhus LM, Phillips CW. Clinical and epidemiologic characteristics of non-surviving trauma victims in an urban environment. *J Natl Med Assoc*. 1972: 64(1):1-7.
6. Freeark RJ . 1982 A.A.S.T. Presidential Address: The Trauma Center: its Hospitals, Head Injuries and Heroes *J Trauma*. 1984: 23 (3):173-179.
7. Boyd DR, Lowe RJ, Baker RJ, Nyhus LM. Trauma Registry. New computer method for multifactorial evaluation of a major health problem. *JAMA*. 22 1973: 223(4):422-428.
8. Chilimindris C, Boyd DR, Carlson LE, Folk FA, Baker RJ, Freeark RJ. A critical review of management of right colon injuries. *J Trauma*. 1971: 11(8):651-660.
9. Lowe RJ, Boyd DR, Folk FA, Baker RJ. The negative laparotomy for abdominal trauma. *J Trauma*. 1972: 12(10):853-861.
10. Boyd DR. A Symposium on The Illinois Trauma Program;a systems approach to the care of trhe critically injured introduction: a controlled systems approach to trauma patient care. *J Trauma*. 1973: 13(4).
11. *Bulltin of the Amer College Surgeons*.
12. Boyd DR. General Principles: Estimation of Blood Loss and Suggested Therapy. In: Condon RE, Nyhus LM, eds. *Manual of Surgical Therapeutics*. Boston: Little, Brown and Company; 1969: 1-65.
13. Boyd DR. Modern concepts in the care of the critically injured; Categories of Trauma-Hemorrhage Assessment and Treatment. In: McCredie JA, ed. *Basic Surgery*. New York: MacMillian Publishing Co., Inc.; 1977: 167-180.
14. Advanced Trauma Life Support® for Doctors. Chicago: American College of Surgeons -Committee on Trauma: 1997.
15. John Barrett, personal communication to Boyd, November, 2008.
16. Brown RS, Boyd DR, Matsuda T, Lowe RJ. Temporary internal vascular shunt for retrohepatic vena cava injury. *J Trauma*. 1971;11(9):736-737.
17. Ramenosfky: Standards of care for the critically injured pediatric patient. *J Trauma*. 1982: 22(11):921-923.
18. *Special Message on Health Care*. Richard B. Ogilvie, Governor of Illinois to the77th General Assembly, April 1, 1971.
19. Boyd DR. A total emergency medical service system for Illinois. *Ill Med J*. 1972;142(5):486-488.
20. Boyd DR, Mains KD, Flashner BA. A systems approach to statewide emergency medical care. *J Trauma*. 1973: 13(4):276-284.
21. http://www.cookcountyhhs.org/medical-clinicalservices/trauma/about-us/
22. Senator Charles H Percy. Congressional Record. October 14, 1972, S 18315, -Senate.
23. Boyd, D. Personal Communication.
24. Boyd DR. The history of emergency medical services (EMS) systems in the United States of America. In: Boyd DR, Edlich RF, Micik SH, eds. *Systems Approach to Emergency Medical Care*. Norwalk: Appleton-Century-Crofts; 1983: 1-82.
25. Boyd DR, Micik SH, Lambrew CT, Romano T. *Medical control and accountability of emergency medical services (EMS) systems*. IEEE Trans Vehicular Tech. 1979: 28(4):249.

# 9

# Evolution of Burn Surgical Service at CCH

*Marella L. Hanumadass, MD*
*Takayoshi Matsuda, MD*

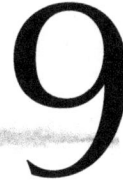

- *The Begining and the Early Years*
- *Unveiling and Development of the Sumner L. Koch Burn Center*
- *Era of Modernization, Investigation and Progress*
- *Entering into the New Century*
- *Conclusion*

Cook County Hospital held a vitally important place in the social and economic life of the City of Chicago and County of Cook as early as the 1920s and 1930s through its mission of rendering advanced clinical care to the indigent. Surgical specialties were not existent in those years. Nevertheless, general surgeons at Cook County Hospital took the lead in developing various specialized surgical services at this institution.

## The Beginning and the Early Years

Dr. Sumner L. Koch, 1888–1976 (Figure 9–1), is one of these surgical specialty pioneers. A graduate of Northwestern University Medical School, he interned at Cook County Hospital from 1914 to 1916. He joined the surgical practice and taught with Dr. Allen B. Kanavel, Professor of Surgery at Northwestern and Wesley Memorial Hospitals. With the U.S. entry into World War I, Dr. Koch left Chicago and served in France during the next two years. On returning from his tour of duty, he resumed work with Dr. Kanavel at Northwestern University Medical School. His association with Dr. Kanavel made him interested in hand infections and injuries. This interest led him to start a hand clinic and surgical service at Cook County Hospital in the early 1930s.

During that same period, Cook County Hospital saw many indigent children with severe burns. Because of his interest in soft tissue trauma, including burns,

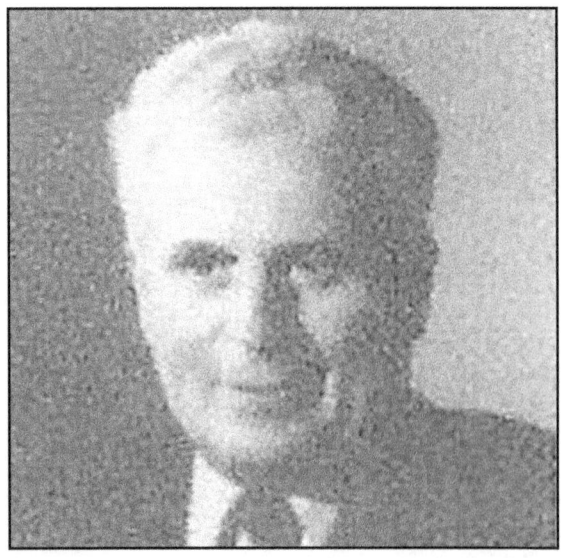

*Figure 9–1 Sumner L. Koch*

which he acquired during his experiences in World War I, he readily agreed to establish a burn surgical service at Cook County Hospital in 1938. Dr. Koch supervised the burn surgical service up until 1962.

In the 1940s, children younger than 12 years were treated in Ward 46 in the Children's Building. It was at this time that surgical specialties were evolving. Free to choose any one of many surgical fields, Koch chose to remain a general surgeon. He was one of this country's most outstanding surgeons whose influence was felt wherever wounds and burns were treated and injured hands were repaired. He was the first physician who suggested "Do No Harm" as the most important rule to consider in the first-aid treatment of open wounds, including burns. He advocated the open method of burn-wound care and grafting of granulating wounds. Dr. Koch served as a consultant to the Surgeon General regarding burn injuries and was a member of the National Research Council Subcommittee on Burns. He was awarded the President's Certificate of Merit for his contributions to the treatment of burn injuries.

In late 1946, Dr. Harvey Stuart Allen, 1906–1955 (Figure 9–2), also a graduate of Northwestern University Medical School, joined Dr. Koch. He had just returned from military service in Europe during World War II. He passed the competitive Civil Service Examination for the attending staff at Cook County Hospital and received the coveted appointment to the surgical staff. Soon after, he became the associate director of the hand and burn surgical services. Dr. Allen resolutely and persistently devoted his attention to the study and treatment of burn patients. The wards of Cook County Hospital offered unsurpassed opportunities for his superior work, which was supported generously by the National Research Council.

Dr. Allen popularized the use of petroleum (Vaseline) gauze dressings combined with pressure and strict immobilization. The use of pressure was soon abandoned because it was found ineffective in limiting fluid loss. However, absorptive occlusive dressings became very popular. In 1949, Dr. Allen advocated for the excision of full thickness hand burn eschar as early as five days postburn and for

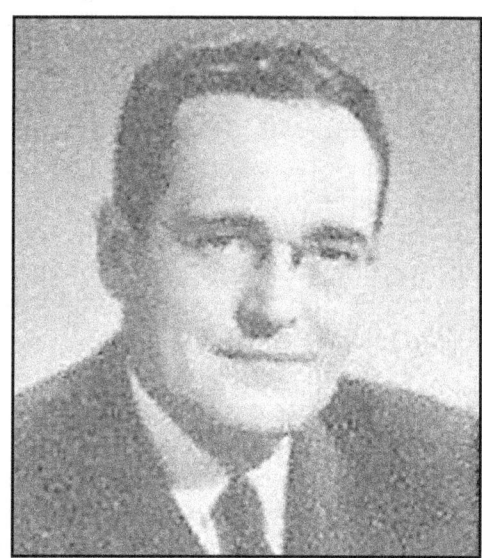

*Figure 9–2 Harvey Stuart Allen*

burn wound coverage with skin grafting as early as one week postburn. Together with Dr. Mason, a colleague whom he met in Italy during his tour of duty in World War II, Dr. Allen designed the so-called universal hand splint that permitted surgeons to carry out constant immobilization of the injured or burned hand in the position of function. These splints are popular even today. Dr. Allen was noted for his meticulous treatment of burn patients and his ability to harvest perfect skin grafts with a free-hand blade. In a tribute to Dr. Allen, Dr. Koch wrote:

> *Out of many contributions to the surgery, his outstanding one was his realization and repeated demonstration of the importance of clean surgical care, of compression dressings, of early excision of devitalized tissue, and of early grafting in the treatment of severe burns.*

The American Burn Association, which was established in 1969, recognized Dr. Allen's contribution with the Harvey Stuart Allen Distinguished Service Award at its annual meeting. In 1955, due to the untimely death of Dr. Allen and combined with increased responsibilities of Dr. Koch, the activity of the unit became essentially unsupervised for several years.

## Unveiling and Development of the Sumner L. Koch Burn Center

In 1960, Dr. Robert J. Freeark advanced from his position as director of surgical education to surgeon in chief at Cook County Hospital. He recruited new surgeons and new graduating residents who were interested in academic surgery. He also reorganized the surgical divisions.

In 1961, Dr. Freeark recruited Dr. John A. Boswick (1926–1999) as director of hand surgery and burn services. Dr. Boswick was a graduate of Loyola University Medical School and completed general surgery residency at Cook County Hospital. He also did a short fellowship in hand surgery at Northwestern University Medical School and at Passavant Memorial Hospital under the supervision of Dr. Koch.

In the early 1960s, adult burn patients were treated on the general surgical floors (Wards 60, 61, 63, and 64) in the main building of CCH with very little uniformity of care. In addition, it was impossible, in the extensively burned patients, to prevent infection from developing in their burn wounds, which eventually progressed to systemic infection. Because there was only a limited number of isolation rooms available on each surgical ward, surgeons and nurses were constantly afraid of the potential spread of infection from burn patients to other clean, elective surgical patients.

Pediatric burn patients were treated on the pediatric surgical floor, Ward 46, in the children's building. Between July and December of 1961, the daily census of pediatric burn patients was reduced from an average of 40 to 45 to between 20 and 25. Due to this reduction, it became possible to consolidate all pediatric burn patients into a separate section designated as the pediatric burn surgical service. Through 1962, due to a further reduction of the census of burned children and the consequential increase in bed availability in this section, several adult burn patients were admitted to the pediatric burn surgical service. The admission of adult burn patients continued to expand due to an increased number of referrals from other hospitals, and eventually it became necessary to accommodate adult burn patients on another floor in the Children's Hospital.

Dr. Boswick proposed to re-establish a consolidated Burn Unit (BU) for both adults and children at Cook County Hospital. After two years in preparation and some $250,000 in cost, a new BU was finally completed in 1964 on the fifth floor of the children's building at 700 S. Wood Street. The unit consisted of a 26-bed burn ward and a 24-bed hand ward, which was completely renovated and included air conditioning throughout the entire unit. Named after Dr. Sumner L. Koch, the first director of the hand and burn surgical unit and pioneer in these fields, this new unit was dedicated on May 27, 1964. In an 11:00 a.m. ceremony, Dr. Freeark, director of Department of Surgery, introduced Dr. Koch to the audience and reviewed his many accomplishments. Dr. Koch then spoke of the high degree of skill and devotion that Drs. Michael Mason, Harvey Allen, John L. Bell, William S. Stromberg, John A. Boswick, and others gave to the care of the patients with burn and hand injuries. Lieutenant Colonel John A. Moncrief, MD, director and commanding officer of the internationally renowned surgical research unit and burn center at Brooke Army Medical Center, delivered a speech entitled "The Current Management of Burns."

A major burn represents the greatest physical and emotional insult to which the human body can be subjected. Total care is both arduous and time-consuming, requiring special equipment and knowledgeable, skillful and

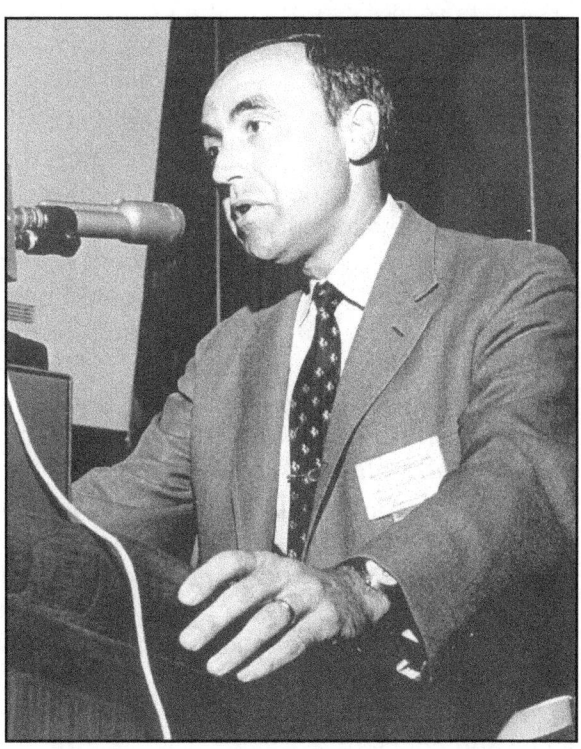

*Figure 9–3 John A. Boswick (1926–1999), Director, Hand and Burn Surgical Services, 1962–1972, welcoming the guests at the inauguration of Sumner L. Koch Hand and Burn Unit on May 27th, 1964.*

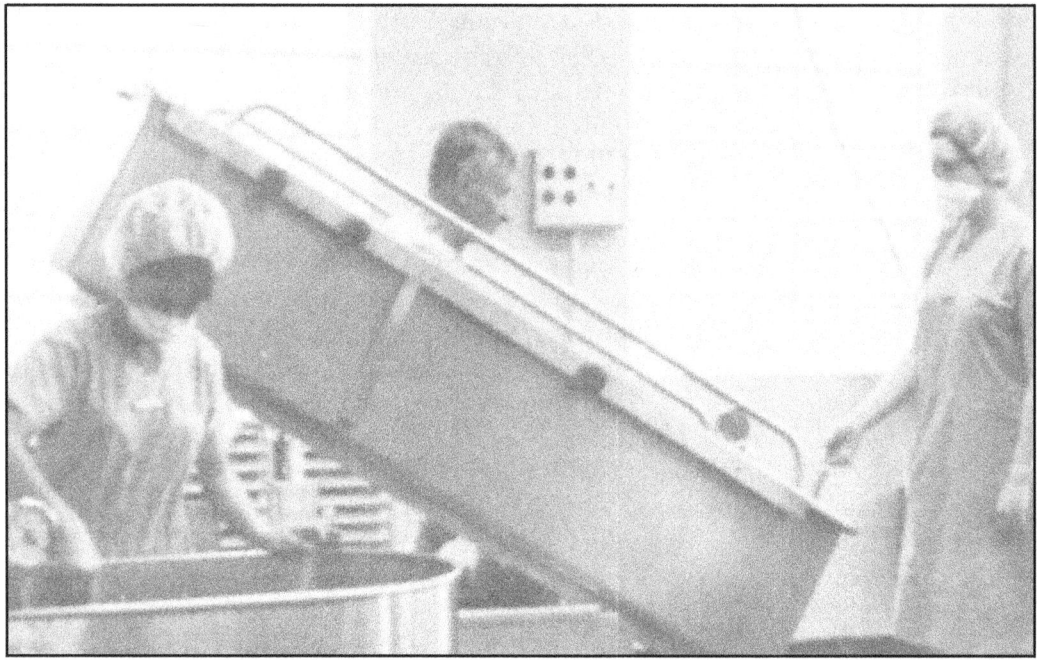

*Figure 9–4 Walk-in tub*

dedicated personnel including surgeons, anesthesiologists, nurses and other paramedical staff. The centralized and self-contained burn unit at Cook County Hospital was the first BU in the State of Illinois, and one of the 12 in existence in the United States at that time.

Dr. Boswick also organized an outpatient clinic for burn patients in Fantus Clinic every weekday afternoon that handled more than 700 new patients a year. Many of these people would have required hospitalization but were adequately treated in this expanded outpatient facility.

In a survey conducted in 1968 by the Illinois Department of Public Health, it was found that more than 80 percent of all patients with burns over 20 percent body-surface area and who were treated in the Chicago area received all or part of their care at the BU of Cook County Hospital.

Dr. Boswick recruited Dr. Nelson Stone as the associate director of the burn unit. Together, they organized a multidisciplinary team approach for the care of burn patients. Dr. Boswick was able to create various special-function rooms within the BU, including a hydrotherapy room, an operating room, two intensive care rooms, and a physical therapy room, in addition to the regular patient rooms for convalescing burn patients. In the hydrotherapy room, he had a special walk-in tub installed. This tub (Figure 9–3) was the first of its kind in this country. It tilted to a vertical position to allow the patient to step in, then reverted to a horizontal position to bathe the patient. To facilitate dressing changes, a "circle bed" was added to the intensive care area to painlessly flip burned victims from their backs to their stomachs and back again with a minimum amount of physical labor and contact.

Dr. Boswick also successfully negotiated and secured permanent paramedical staff including physical therapist(s), occupational therapist(s), a dietician, and a social worker. Each of these staff remained on the BU for a minimum of one year in order to maintain continuity of care. He was also successful in creating an office space within the BU for these paramedical staff. These physical accommodations promoted the acceptance of the paramedical staff members by the burn nurses as permanent members of the burn team rather than as "visiting" staff. In addition, a home-care program was established to provide home-care techniques and continuity of wound care after the patient was discharged from the hospital. He also created a position for a psychiatric nurse who provided psychological support for the burn patients and their families, as well as functioned as a liaison between the BU and the department of psychiatry.

Dr. Boswick successfully negotiated with the Chicago Board of Education to secure a school teacher who was regularly sent to the burn unit for children who were staying on the unit for a prolonged period of time. Also, the BU was an institutional host for the federally funded program, the Chicago Foster Grandparents Program, which was administered by the mayor's office for senior citizens. They provided special nonmedical, nurturing support to the burned children, including reading, feeding, playing, and the like. Thus, the BU became a self-contained burn center and functioned like an independent institution within Cook County Hospital.

Eventually, a formal rotation on the BU was established for surgical residents from the University of Illinois and Northwestern University. In addition, at any given time, six to eight burn and hand fellows from all over the world received advanced training at Cook County Hospital. Because of the magnitude of complex services provided within the BU, it was designated as a division within the Department of Surgery.

Because the Cook County Hospital burn unit was the only major burn-care facility in the state of Illinois, many extensively burned patients were transferred from all over the state, as well as from nearby states such as Wisconsin, Iowa, Nebraska, and Indiana. Partially supported by private donations, Cook County built a heliport named after Robin Dean, a child who was treated in the BU during the late 1960s. During this period, the American Burn Association was established in 1969, and in 1975, Dr. Boswick became its seventh president. He was also one of the founding members of the International Society for Burn Injuries and served as its secretary-general from 1978–1990.

In the early 1960s, the Brooke Formula was exclusively used for estimating the initial resuscitation fluid requirements for extensively burned patients. Central venous pressure monitoring became widely used as the new field of critical care medicine was being developed. Because the burn patients became known to be hypermetabolic, a nutritional support program was started for extensively burned patients, which began the third day postburn following successful initial fluid resuscitation. It consisted of a high-protein, high-calorie diet three times a day. In addition, the patients were given high-calorie milk shakes every two hours around the clock.

Burn wounds were treated using a "closed" method with the use of a

0.5% topical silver nitrate solution. Dr. Boswick was instrumental in some of the early trials using Silver Sulfadiazine (Silvadine®) as a topical antimicrobial agent. Full thickness burn wounds were treated in a conservative manner while surgeons waited for the separation of the dead tissue (eschar) from the underlying healthy tissue prior to skin grafting. It was a daily task for the surgical residents assigned to the burn unit to debride the dead tissue. This procedure was performed in the hydrotherapy room and was tedious and time-consuming. In addition, because it was not feasible to administer general, regional, or local anesthesia for the debridement on a daily basis, this procedure was very painful for the patient. This daily trip to the hydrotherapy room was agonizing and devastating for each patient. Some patients would even refuse to go to the hydrotherapy room. In general, removal of the eschar could be performed on only 2 to 3 percent of the body-surface-area each day. It usually took three to four weeks to complete the debridement process. Once debridement was completed, split-thickness skin grafting over the granulating wound was then performed to achieve wound closure.

During the second and third weeks postburn, most patients with large burns developed life-threatening infections. Generally, patients with burns over less than 20 percent of the total body-surface-area survived while those victims with burns greater than 30 percent total body-surface-area died. The gross mortality (number of deaths divided by number of total admissions) within the burn unit was approximately 25 percent in 1965 and decreased to approximately 18 percent by 1970. By 1975, this gross mortality rate had decreased further to approximately 14 percent. This improvement in mortality was reflective of the survival of patients with between 20 and 30 percent body-surface-area full-thickness burns. However, the mortality rate for those patients with more than 30 percent body-surface-area full-thickness burns remained extremely high. Early death was usually from inadequate initial fluid resuscitation. Subsequent death was generally attributed to burn-wound sepsis.

In 1972, Dr. Boswick left Cook County Hospital to assume the position as professor of surgery and chief of hand surgery at the University of Colorado in Denver. At CCH the hand surgery service was created in the division of orthopedic surgery, and thereafter, hand surgery patients were no longer admitted to the BU. Both the contracture clinic on the BU as well as reconstructive surgical procedures for former burn patients were supervised by the attending surgeons from the plastic surgery division. During the next three years, Dr. Conrad Tasche, Dr. Miguel Teresi, and Dr. Vijay Kumar were acting directors of the BU, consecutively. Without the presence of long-term leadership, continuity of care suffered, and it became impossible to maintain a standardized treatment protocol as new drugs and dressing materials became available. Also, it was difficult to maintain a cohesive burn team without a clearly defined responsibility assigned to each team member.

## Era of Modernization, Investigation, and Progress

In 1975, Dr. Gerald S. Moss, the chairman of the Department of Surgery at Cook County Hospital, recruited Dr. Takayoshi Matsuda (Figure 9–5) as the director of the burn center. Dr. Matsuda received his medical degree from Keio University in Tokyo, Japan. His internship (1965–1966) and surgical residency (1966–1971) were both at Cook County Hospital, during which time he was greatly influenced by Dr. Robert J. Freeark regarding clinical surgery, by Dr. Robert J. Baker regarding teaching, and by Dr. William C. Shoemaker regarding research. Dr. Shoemaker was also one of the pioneers in the development of the new field of critical care medicine. Consequently, Dr. Matsuda had the opportunity to witness the development of pulmonary artery catheterization, pulmonary capillary wedge pressure measurement, and cardiac output measurement. Under the guidance of Dr. Shoemaker, Dr. Matsuda published 11 papers in refereed journals during his residency.

From 1971 to 1975, Dr. Matsuda went back to his homeland in Japan as an assistant professor of surgery to help his father, who had recently established Kyorin University Medical School in Tokyo. In 1975, prior to his acceptance of the directorship of the BU at Cook County Hospital, Dr. Matsuda successfully negotiated with Dr. Moss and the hospital's governing commission in securing a funding commitment for a total upgrade of the intensive care section on the BU,

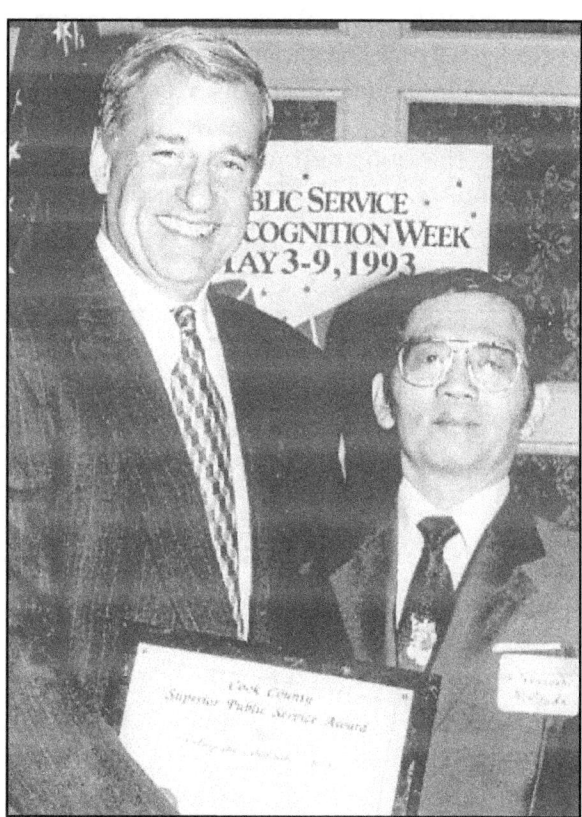

*Figure 9–5 Takoyoshi Matsuda received the Superior Public Service Award from County Board President Phelan.*

including the addition of comprehensive bedside monitors for arterial lines and Swan-Ganz catheters, equipment for cardiac output measurement, stat laboratory equipment (blood gas analyzer, electrolyte analyzer, osmometer, oncometer) and four laboratory technician positions, and four clinical burn fellowship positions.

In March of 1975, Dr. Matsuda began his work as director of the BU. At that time, the burn unit had a 32-bed capacity including an eight-bed intensive care section. There were approximately 450 to 500 admissions and more than 2,000 outpatients annually. In mid-1975, Dr. Marella Hanumadass (Figure 9–6), who had surgical and plastic surgical training in Ireland, was accepted as a clinical fellow in burn surgery. In 1976, Dr. Samuel Appavu, who also completed his surgical residency training at Cook County Hospital, joined as a full-time attending surgeon on the BU. Shortly thereafter, on completion of his burn fellowship, Dr. Hanumadass joined the unit as a full-time attending surgeon. In 1977, he was promoted to associate chairman of the division of burn surgery as well as clinical director of the burn center.

One of the initial goals of Dr. Matsuda was to establish standard operative procedures (SOP) for the BU by developing a policy and procedure manual for:

1. burn unit administration,
2. clinical patient care including medical care, nursing care, and paramedical care, and
3. the education of burn fellows, surgical residents and medical students.

This *Policy and Procedure Manual* for the BU was created with the participation of Dr. Hanumadass, Dr. Appavu, and all nursing and paramedical staff members. Clinical protocols were developed that standardized all aspects of burn treatment, and the responsibilities of each burn team member were clearly defined. The outpatient clinic was reorganized, and hours were decreased from every afternoon to three afternoons weekly on Mondays, Wednesdays, and Fridays. An emphasis on house staff education was formally established. Tuesday

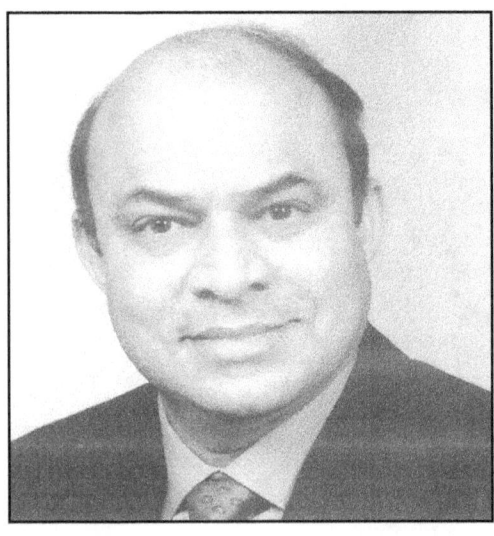

*Figure 9–6 Marella L. Hanumadass*

afternoons were designated for teaching conferences for burn fellows, surgical residents, and medical students. Thursday afternoons were reserved for multidisciplinary conferences. Dr. Hanumadass assumed responsibility for the contracture clinic and conducted this clinic every Wednesday morning. In addition, he supervised close to 70 reconstructive surgical procedures performed every year in the BU operating room.

In 1975, the national average for nursing turnover on burn units was approximately nine months. The average turnover rate on the Cook County Hospital Burn Unit was three months. In 1976, Mr. Lloyd Rockmore became the nurse coordinator (i.e., nursing supervisor) of the burn unit. He developed educational programs for the burn nurses and personally provided weekly in-services on the burn unit for each of the three shifts. Through his leadership and with the standardization of nursing burn care protocol, nursing morale improved and turnover dramatically decreased. In fact, the majority of nurses continued to work on the BU for many years. Mr. Rockmore also organized monthly burn support group meetings in which former patients of the unit gathered to discuss their problems and experiences. The former patients provided strength, hope, and encouragement to the recovering burn patients in the unit.

In order to further improve patient care, the BU needed a larger supply of homograft skin for the wound closure. There were two skin banks in the United States at that time. Dr. Baxter at Parkland Hospital in Dallas had a skin bank but was unable to provide other burn units with a consistent supply. The Shriners Burn Institute in Boston also had a small skin bank for the use of their patients only. Dr. Matsuda then assigned Dr. Appavu a project—to develop a skin bank program on the BU of Cook County Hospital. Negotiations were initiated with the Department of Pathology. It was agreed that the BU skin-bank team would harvest homograft skin in the autopsy room from patients who recently died in Cook County Hospital, who met certain criteria, and whose family signed a consent for skin donation in addition to an autopsy consent. The Department of Pharmacy agreed to produce a sterile solution to keep the harvested homograft skin during and after controlled freezing. A small freezer was procured and placed in the laboratory room for storing the frozen homograft skin. Thus, the first skin bank in the state of Illinois and in the midwest was established in September 1976. Dr. Appavu presented an exhibit on human skin banking at the American College of Surgeons' annual meeting in 1977.

In 1977, Dr. Olga Jonasson (1934–2006) became the chief of surgery at Cook County Hospital. She integrated the surgical residency program with that of the University of Illinois and established a new program called the University of Illinois–Cook County Combined Surgical Residency Program. In early 1979, Dr. Appavu left the BU to establish the surgical intensive care unit at Cook County Hospital. Then, in July 1979, Dr. Richard Kagan, a graduate of the University of Illinois Surgical Residency Program, joined the BU as an attending surgeon.

Throughout the 1970s, the field of critical care medicine continued to advance. The Society of Critical Care Medicine was created in 1970, and the *Journal of Critical Care Medicine* was established with Dr. William C. Shoemaker as the editor-in-chief. Dr. Shoemaker also became the third president (1973–1974) of the society. With personal advice and encouragement from Dr. Shoemaker, Dr. Matsuda was able to bring the essence of critical care medicine into practice on the BU. The intensive care section of the burn unit was upgraded with the installation of a bedside monitor for each intensive care bed. In addition, Dr. Matsuda was able to create a stat-laboratory equipped with a blood gas analyzer, an electrolyte analyzer, an osmometer, and an oncometer. In order to staff the stat-laboratory during the day shift, two laboratory technologists were hired in 1977, becoming the newest members of the burn team. They assumed the responsibility for drawing blood samples from the burn patients and for obtaining the test results from the central laboratory. This relieved the residents from much of the technical paramedical workload in the morning, thus improving their morale. Consequently, they were now able to devote their full attention to actually changing dressings, inspecting burn wounds, and scrubbing in for surgery.

With the installation of the bedside monitors and support from the stat-laboratory, routine use of central venous lines, arterial lines, and Swan-Ganz catheters became possible. Consequently, more precise hemodynamic monitoring, including the measurement of pulmonary capillary wedge pressure and of cardiac output, was utilized for critically ill patients with extensive burns and for burn patients with pre-existing cardiac conditions. For estimation of the initial resuscitation fluid requirement for the extensively burned patients, the Parkland Formula, established by Dr. Charles Baxter of Dallas, Texas, was designated as the formula of choice in the procedure manual for the BU.

Hyperalimentation, both central and enteral, was added to the nutritional protocol for the extensively burned patients. Peripheral venous hyperalimentation was not routinely utilized due to the high risk of infection and of thrombosis of the vein. Calories and nitrogen intake were calculated routinely by the dietician on the BU. The body weight of the patient was also routinely measured with the use of an in-bed scale. The burn unit participated in a clinical research trial to evaluate the efficacy of a new enteral feeding formula. The objective of the study was to evaluate the effect of calorie and nitrogen intake on nitrogen retention. A metabolic measurement cart was purchased, which enabled staff to determine the effects of the feeding regimen on a real-time basis, on the patient's oxygen consumption, and carbon dioxide production. As a result, the respiratory quotient was calculated, which allowed the staff to determine which substrate (dextrose, protein, or fat) was being metabolized. The study findings showed that better nitrogen balance was achieved with an increase in nitrogen intake and a concomitant decrease in dextrose intake when the total caloric intake was kept at a constant level. It also revealed that excessive caloric intake without adequate nitrogen intake would result in the production and deposition of fat (lipogenesis) instead of nitrogen retention. These research efforts resulted in the publication of several articles, which repopularized the concept of the calorie-to-nitrogen ratio in the national burn care community.

Burn wounds were treated either by an open method using Betadine® (povidone iodine) or by a closed method using 0.5% silver nitrate solution or silver Sulfadiazine® cream. With frequent observation of renal and hepatic failure in burn patients treated with Betadine®, Dr. Matsuda questioned the possibility of iodine absorption through the burned tissue, and if so, whether it could be the cause of detrimental renal and hepatic effects. Through a review of the literature, it was learned that intravenous injection of large doses of iodine into animals resulted in a very high serum iodine level, which in turn resulted in renal and hepatic failure and eventually led to the death of the animals. Thus, Dr. Matsuda conducted a study to examine the possible absorption of iodine in patients treated with Betadine® topical ointment. The results revealed that the burned patients treated with Betadine® showed a very high serum iodine level comparable to that shown in the animal studies in literature. The use of Betadine® on the BU was, therefore, discontinued, and the closed method using silver Sulfadiazine® cream as the topical antibacterial agent was then established on the unit as the standard method of burn wound care. Dr. Matsuda reported his research findings at the 1977 American Burn Association meeting.

With the extensive use of hemodynamic monitoring, almost all of the extensively burned patients on the BU now survived the initial few days of the resuscitation period. The problem, however, was that most of the patients with large burns did not survive despite receiving extensive nutritional support and diligent wound care using silver Sulfadiazine. The reason was very simple. Those patients with more than 30 percent body-surface-area full-thickness burns generally developed burn wound infections that progressed to systemic sepsis. Regardless of what types of systemic antibiotics were administered or what dosage was used, these septic patients could not be saved.

It was extremely painful for Dr. Matsuda and all of his staff to witness repeatedly the death of patients with more than 30 percent body-surface-area full-thickness burns. Everyone felt a sense of hopelessness and helplessness as they observed the burn patient slowly deteriorate over a short period of days to weeks, despite having done everything medically possible. Dr. Matsuda talked with many of the authorities in the American Burn Association only to confirm that this eventual death in extensively burned patients was a universal problem for which there was no apparent solution. In a desperate attempt to find a solution, Dr. Matsuda continued to analyze the chain of events leading to the death of the burn patients. He concluded that the death of the patient was caused by massive sepsis due to an invasive burn wound infection originating from the necrotic burned tissue. No systemic antibiotic was able to reach this necrotic burned tissue because it was avascular.

After a prolonged and soul-searching analysis, Dr. Matsuda concluded that the only possible solution would be to remove this necrotic tissue surgically before it became infected. When he talked with many leaders in the burn community regarding his proposed approach to use surgical excision therapy, nobody was willing to support his idea. Most burn surgeons said that it would cause too much blood loss to be a safe procedure. Additionally, some surgeons said that this excisional approach had been attempted in the past by other surgeons only to be abandoned because of extensive blood loss. Others simply discouraged such an approach due to lack of proven success. Then, Dr. Matsuda discovered that Dr. John Burke from the Shriners Burn Institute in Boston was routinely employing surgical excisional therapy on his pediatric patients with full-thickness burns. Dr.

Burke explained that he was able to perform up to 50 percent body-surface-area excision on a child during one surgical procedure. Dr. Matsuda knew that he would be unable to perform 50 percent body-surface-area excision on an adult because the total body-surface-area of an adult was so much larger than that of a child. Dr. Matsuda, however, reached a conclusion that it might be possible to perform up to 15 percent body-surface-area excision on an adult during one surgical procedure.

Dr. Matsuda brought home the concept of excisional surgery to the burn unit of Cook County Hospital. There was no institutional review board in the mid-1970s. Therefore, after careful consultation and discussion with the chairman of surgery, chairman of anesthesiology, director of the blood bank, director of pharmacy, and medical director of Cook County Hospital, a consensus was reached to try this potentially very dangerous surgical procedure only on three patients who were clearly dying from invasive burn wound sepsis.

The first case was an 11-year-old boy with about 20 percent body-surface-area full-thickness burns over his left arm, shoulder, and chest. The child was critically ill, and it was clear to everyone that he would not live beyond another day or two. In the operating room, the infected burn wounds were excised down to the healthy subcutaneous fat tissue using a free-hand knife. Complete hemostasis was achieved and homograft skin was applied. Everybody in the operating room breathed a deep sigh of relief when the child was transported out of the operating room in stable condition. He opened his eyes the next morning looking like a healthy postoperative patient rather than a dying burn patient. Encouraged by this miraculous result, surgical excision was performed on two other patients with successful results. A consensus was then reached among the hospital leadership that although the surgical excision was still a high-risk procedure, it was no longer considered experimental.

Over time, surgical excision became more frequently used, and the size of the burn wound that was excised during one procedure was gradually increased. Also, it was observed that with each day the excision was delayed, the patient became progressively more ill. Therefore, the timing of the surgical excision was progressively moved from the second week postburn to as early as the third day postburn when the wound was still without infection.

In the case of a circumferential wound on a leg, the leg had to be moved up and down numerous times during surgery because the surgeon required circumferential access to the leg in order to excise the wound, apply compression, and achieve complete hemostasis prior to applying the skin graft. It was rather easy to periodically elevate the leg of a child during such a surgical operation because the leg of a child was not too heavy. However, because an adult's leg is so much heavier, it was impossible to periodically elevate the leg of an adult during the surgical procedure. Initially, an attempt was made to maintain the leg in an elevated position by securing it to an IV pole. This was unacceptable because the leg could not be freely moved up and down as needed.

With cooperation from the Bioengineering Department, Dr. Matsuda devised a traction frame that was installed in the ceiling of the BU operating room in March 1977 (Figure 9–7). One end of a rope was secured to the ankle of the

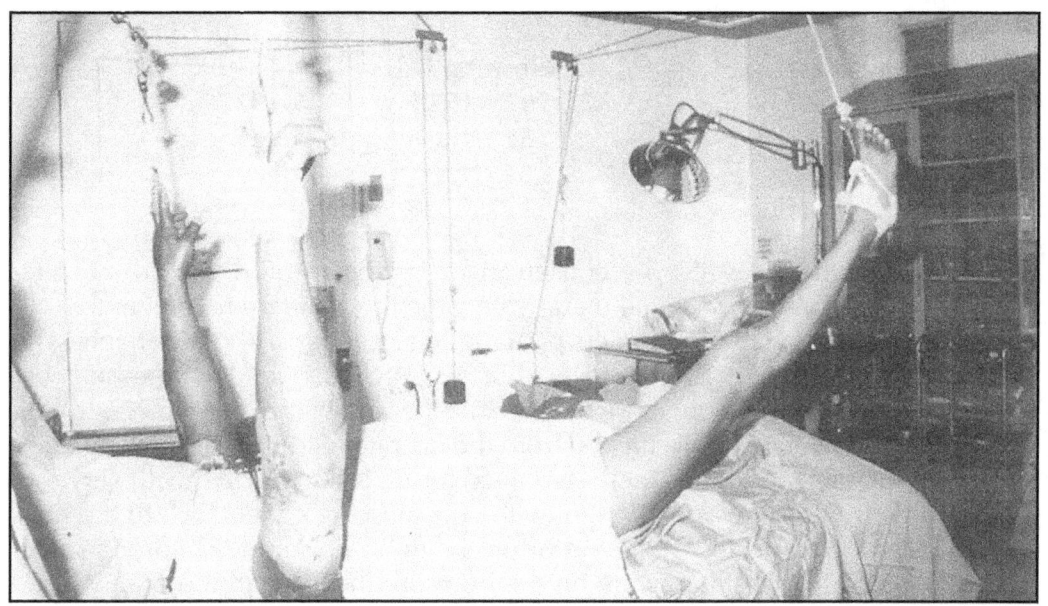

*Figure 9–7 Traction frame designed by Takayoshi Matsuda*

patient. The other end of the rope was passed through pulleys at a distance from the operating table and suspended along the wall of the operating room. A weight was attached to the end of the rope, and the leg could now be suspended in mid-air in an almost weightless condition. With this setup, the leg could be moved up and down very easily, and circumferential access was provided to the surgeon. The surgical procedures involving legs could now be performed with greater ease and in far less time. Because many patients had burns on both legs, it became routine for two surgical teams to scrub in so that each leg could be operated on simultaneously.

The biennial review (1976–1977) of the BU revealed a significant improvement in the survival rate as compared to the previous two years. The difference was solely attributable to the employment of surgical excision.

| Size of Burn (Full-thickness) | Survival Rate | |
| --- | --- | --- |
| | 1973-1975 | 1975-1977 |
| 11-20% | 83% | 95% |
| 21-30% | 24% | 63% |
| 31-50% | 6% | 29% |

Also, the length of hospital stay for the patient with smaller full-thickness burns was significantly shortened due to earlier wound closure with surgical excision.

| Size of Burn (Full-thickness) | Hospital Days 1973-1975 | 1975-1977 |
|---|---|---|
| 1-5% | 51 days | 29 days |
| 6-10% | 64 days | 45 days |

Based on these results, the conservative method of burn wound management was abandoned. Excisional therapy became the standard treatment for full-thickness burns as well as for deep partial-thickness burns. More patients with larger burns were now surviving instead of dying; consequently, more beds became necessary for their convalescent care. At the same time, more patients with smaller burns were being discharged from the hospital earlier, which, coincidentally, met the demand for this increased need for beds. Once filled with very sick patients, the burn unit was now filled with convalescing patients. Until the mid-1970s, when people exited the elevator on the fifth floor of the children's building, they could tell that they were on the burn unit because of the odor caused by the severely infected burn wounds from the numerous burn patients. Now, as a result of excisional therapy, that odor no longer existed. By the late 1970s, patients with up to 50 percent body-surface-area full-thickness burns were now routinely surviving.

In the early 1980s, the tremendous improvement in patient care on the burn unit at Cook County Hospital became widely recognized throughout Chicago. An article was published in the October, 1983 issue of *Chicago* magazine entitled "Doctors' Doctors: 40 of the Very Best," and Dr. Matsuda was selected among the top 40 doctors in Chicago. In this same year, *Business Week* published the article, "How to Pick a Good Hospital," selecting Cook County Hospital as one of the nation's top hospitals for burn care.

As a result of early excisional burn care, average hospital stays for patients with nonextensive burns were decreased from 40 days in the early 1970s to only 17 days in the early 1980s. As early excisional therapy for burn wounds became an established method of treatment, it brought many side benefits. For example, the number of dressing changes required decreased measurably. Full-thickness wounds were routinely excised and grafted between three and six days after the burn injury. The first dressing change following this surgery was done by the medical staff on the fifth postoperative day. Thereafter, dressing changes were done by the nursing staff. However, the wound underneath the dressing was, for the most part, a clean, grafted wound requiring much less time and supplies than a dirty, infected burn wound requiring a lot of supplies and extensive nursing time. This was a significant change when contrasted with the previous method of therapy when the dressing was changed three times a day for three weeks before the wound was even closed with a skin graft. Thus, early excision was significant in saving both nursing hours and supplies used in extensive dressing changes.

Another side benefit from early excisional therapy was a significant decrease in the need for later reconstructive surgery. Due to early excisional therapy, the number of reconstructive procedures decreased from approximately 70 cases per year in the 1970s to only 12 per year during the late 1980s. Dr. Matsuda and Dr. Hanumadass concluded that early excision and immediate skin grafting resulted in early wound healing. This facilitated early mobilization of joints preventing joint contractures.

As the early excisional therapy was performed on more and more extensive full-thickness burns, a new challenge appeared: how to achieve closure of the excised wound. For example, if the patient sustained a 60 percent body-surface-area full-thickness burn, there remained 40 percent body-surface-area of skin that was not burned. However, not all of this unburned skin could be used as a donor site because skin could not be harvested from the face, from the perineum, or from over the joint areas. Therefore, the size of harvestable skin was reduced to approximately 70 percent of the unburned area, or in this case, 28 percent of the total body surface area with the remaining 12 percent of the total body surface area of unburned skin unable to be used for harvesting. In this scenario, during the first surgical excision, the burn wound of about 30 percent of the total body surface area could be excised and closed with autograft skin. During the second surgery, which occurred about three to four days later, another 30 percent of the total body surface area needed to be excised. However, all of the available skin for autograft harvesting had been used for the first surgery. Consequently, homograft skin was needed to achieve wound closure. The application of dressing material or pig skin instead of autograft or homograft skin to an excised wound was not an option because its use would result in the wound not closing physiologically, and consequently, it would remain in the consistent progression toward a life-threatening infection. The only way to protect the freshly excised wound was to apply viable homograft skin. The wound heals temporarily before the homograft skin was rejected three to six weeks later. In the meantime, the donor site previously used for autograft harvesting healed within about 10 days and became available for a second harvesting by 14 days following the first surgery. So, two weeks following the first surgery, the homograft skin was removed and replaced with autograft skin obtained from the second harvesting. Now, all the excised wounds were closed using the patient's own skin. As more patients with extensive burns survived, the need for homograft skin became more critical.

As previously mentioned, Dr. Appavu established the first human skin bank in Illinois on the Burn Unit of Cook County Hospital in 1976. Several challenges quickly developed in this skin bank program. For example, there were not many autopsies performed because families refused to sign consent for autopsy. In addition, most patients did not meet the strict criteria for homograft skin donation, which included the absence of communicable disease and malignancy. Of those who met the strict criteria for skin donation, only a few families were willing to consent. Consequently, the skin bank program became inactive. For several years, Dr. Matsuda attempted to re-establish a skin bank program at the morgue of the medical examiner of Cook County, but without success.

Finally, in 1983, Dr. Matsuda was able to obtain the cooperation of Dr. Robert Stein, chief medical examiner of Cook County, who agreed to allow the burn unit personnel to harvest the homograft skin in the medical examiner's morgue. Prior to this re-activation of the skin bank, homograft skin had been purchased from another skin bank out of Dallas at a cost of $1,600 per square foot. Now, having its own skin bank, not only were many lives saved, but also thousands of dollars were saved every year for Cook County Hospital. At this time, Dr. Richard Kagan became director of the skin bank. During this same period, the burn intensive care unit was renovated to house 10 beds, each with complete hemodynamic monitoring capability. Four of these beds were also equipped with "clean air," bacteria controlled, laminar air-flow units (Figure 9–8). With an adequate supply of homograft skin, patients with up to 70 percent body-surface-area burns were now surviving much of the time, resulting in a gross mortality rate of less than 5 percent by the late 1980s.

During the 1980s, while very busy with patient care activities, the attending surgeons on the Burn Unit also engaged in a wide range of clinical research projects. These studies included pulmonary care (Dr. Matsuda), metabolic response and nutritional requirements (Dr. Matsuda), a motorized skin mesher (Dr. Kagan), infection (Dr. Kagan), axillary contractures (Dr. Hanumadass), electrical trauma (Dr. Hanumadass), groin flaps (Dr. Hanumadass), a new topical antimicrobial agent (Dr. Matsuda), and biosynthetic skin substitute (Dr. Hanumadass). These studies resulted in more than a dozen presentations at national and international conferences, followed by publications in major surgical journals. Dr. Matsuda also served on the editorial board of the *Journal of Burn Care and Rehabilitation* from 1987 to 1993.

In 1988, Dr. Kagan left the BU when he accepted the position of associate director of the burn unit at the University of Cincinnati and associate chief of staff at Shriners Hospitals for Children in Cincinnati. He was promoted to chief of staff in June 2004 and served as the president of the American Burn Association in 2007. Following Dr. Kagan's departure, Dr. Hanumadass assumed the additional responsibility for overseeing the skin bank. He also became certified as

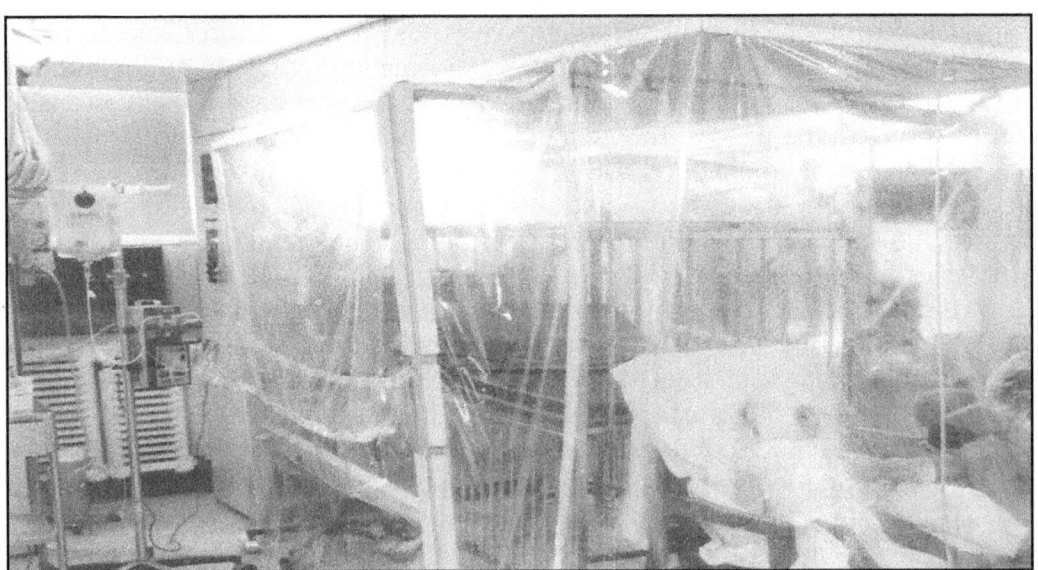

*Figure 9–8 Laminar flow unit*

an instructor in advanced burn life support course and taught several courses in Chicago and the midwest.

In the late 1980s, the City of Chicago enacted a city ordinance to mandate smoke detectors in residential housing, which dramatically reduced the incidence of burn injuries. In the 1990s, there were just under 300 burn victims of all ages admitted to the BU. The gross mortality rate had decreased to an average of 3 percent by this time.

In the early 1990s, Dr. Matsuda reviewed all the progress and improvements that had been made at the Cook County Hospital burn unit over the previous 15 years and was unable to identify any other clinical areas needing extensive improvement. Thus, he directed his attention toward the fundamental solution in clinical burn care, which was to discover or develop a pharmacological agent(s) that would minimize the postburn capillary permeability. At this time, there were no pharmacological agents available to test for efficacy against increased postburn capillary permeability. He was aware that a group in the Department of Pathology at the University of Michigan had clearly demonstrated that oxygen-free radicals were responsible for the increase in postburn capillary permeability. He was also aware that large doses of vitamin C (ascorbic acid) had been advocated as an effective antioxidant by Dr. Linus Pauling. As a result, Dr. Matsuda decided to spend most of his time conducting basic research projects in the animal research facility in Hektoen Institute while Dr. Hanumadass continued with the major clinical responsibilities on the burn unit.

Dr. Matsuda recruited several research fellows from Japan and conducted a number of animal studies. The results of these studies revealed that postburn administration of sodium ascorbate minimized the postburn increase in the capillary permeability. He also examined the efficacy of sodium ascorbate administered after the burn injury on the reduction of resuscitation fluid volume

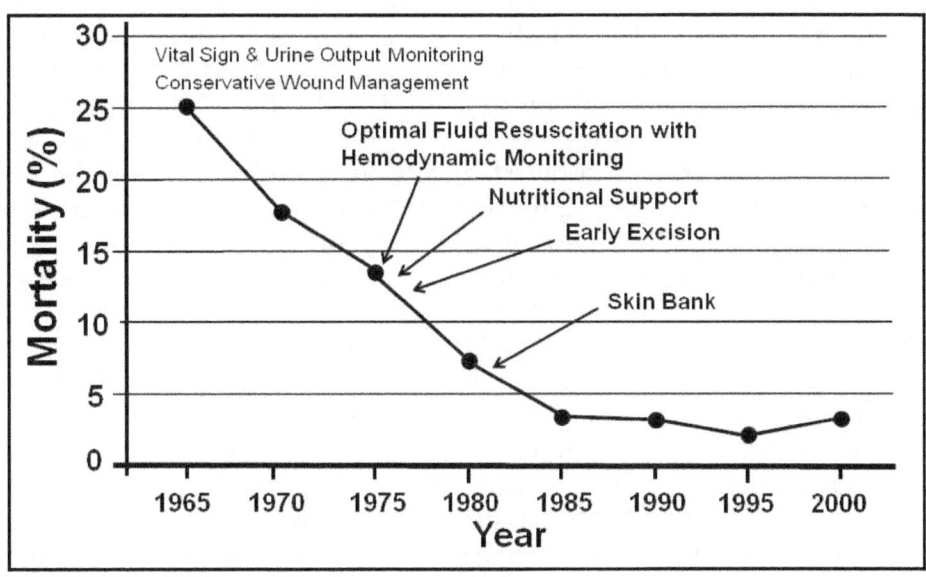

*Figure 9–9 Cook County Hospital Burn Center Mortality (1965–2000)*

requirements. His findings showed that continuous intravenous sodium ascorbate administration beginning one-half hour postburn definitely reduced the total volume of resuscitation fluid by 70 percent while maintaining adequate hemodynamic parameters. Dr. Matsuda's research efforts resulted in numerous national and international presentations and publications. One of his research fellows, Dr. Hideharu Tanaka, returned to Japan and conducted a clinical trial that confirmed the resuscitation fluid volume requirements in postburn patients were significantly reduced with the use of continuous high-dose vitamin C infusion.

Dr. Matsuda also collaborated with Dr. Robert Walter, director of surgical research, to develop skin substitutes. The goal of this project was to develop a permanent composite biological skin substitute to achieve permanent wound closure in extensively burned patients using minimum donor sites. As a first step, the study was performed with small animals. A small piece of skin was harvested from a guinea pig. Epithelial cells were removed to produce dermal tissue that contained no donor cells. Then a small amount of skin was harvested from a rat who would subsequently serve as the recipient. Epithelial cells from this skin were cultured. Once grown, these epithelial cells were then placed on the dermal tissue from the donor guinea pig. This composite skin equivalent material was then grafted back onto the recipient rat. The success of this project also resulted in several publications.

In April of 1993, Richard J. Phelan, president of the Cook County Board of Commissioners, honored Dr. Matsuda with the Cook County Superior Public Service Award for his outstanding performance and excellence as a public servant (Figure 9–5). Dr. Matsuda retired in May of 1993 but continued to participate in the educational program for the fellows, residents, and medical students in the burn center for several years.

In June of 1993, Dr. Hanumadass assumed the directorship of the burn center. In 1995, the division of burn surgery moved into the newly created Department of Trauma under the chairmanship of Dr. John Barrett. Under the direction of Dr. Hanumadass, the Cook County Hospital burn center attracted many area surgical programs for residency training. In the mid-1990s, general surgery and plastic surgery residents from Rush University Medical Center, the University of Illinois at Chicago and Peoria, Northwestern University, and Metro Group Hospitals sent their residents to Cook County Hospital for burn surgery education and clinical experience. In addition, medical students from Rush University Medical Center, the University of Illinois, and Chicago Medical School received their education in burn surgery at Cook County Hospital. Trauma surgeons were assigned to the burn service for nighttime attending coverage. Dr. Hanumadass was also able to recruit a full-time attending burn surgeon to help him fulfill his clinical responsibilities. In addition, he recruited two burn fellows from the local surgical programs each year who participated in patient care and research.

Dr. Hanumadass decided to accept and treat patients with extensive non-burn skin loss in the BU. Soon, many patients with toxic epidermal necrolysis, purpura fulminans, and necrotizing fasciitis, as well as patients with extensive soft tissue injuries, were referred both from other services at Cook County Hospital and from other local hospitals for intensive care and wound management. The burn center also started participating in the newly developed National Trauma Registry for burn patients initiated by the American College of Surgeons (TRACS).

Dr. Hanumadass also continued to work with Dr. Walter in animal and clinical research projects in the field of skin substitutes. They developed xenogenic (pig skin derived) acellular dermal matrix (ADM) and studied it in the rat animal model. They also prepared ADM from human cadaver skin from the BU skin bank. Dr. Hanumadass designed a method to use this material clinically in patients with freshly excised burn wounds by covering the wound with the cadaver-derived ADM and a very thin split thickness skin graft harvested from the patient during one stage. With this method, the donor site healed within a week with minimal scarring. These studies resulted in several presentations and publications. Dr. Hanumadass actively participated in the American Burn Association and served on several of its committees including the committee on organization and delivery of burn care, the committee on education, and the committee on rehabilitation.

After 23 years of uninterrupted service at the burn center in Cook County Hospital, Dr. Hanumadass retired in March of 1998. Dr. William Brownly, who Dr. Hanumadass recruited earlier as an attending surgeon, became the acting director for the next 14 months. Dr. Hanumadass continued his services at the burn center as a voluntary consultant surgeon, helping Dr. Brownly in the operating room and participating in the weekly teaching of residents and medical students.

## Entering into the New Century

Dr. Barbara A. Latenser (Figure 9–9) was recruited as the new director of the BU in March of 1999. She had been working as an attending surgeon in

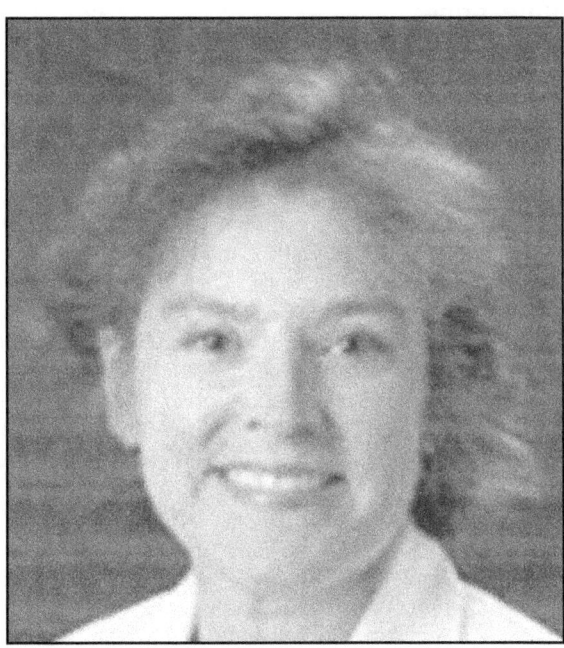

*Figure 9–10  Barbara A. Latenser*

the trauma and burn unit at Mercy Hospital in Pittsburgh, Pennsylvania. In May 1999, Dr. Brownly resigned from the burn unit.

Dr. Latenser recruited Dr. Areta Kowal Vern as director of tissue bank and burn research. She was board certified in pediatrics and pathology and worked in research on the burn center at Loyola University Medical Center. They worked together in setting up the in-house burn patient registry and continued participation in TRACS registry for burns nationally.

The burn intensive care unit was renovated to accommodate two isolation beds. During this time, harvesting of skin in the medical examiner's facility was abandoned, and the tissue bank became a skin storage facility. In 2001, the trauma section of the American College of Surgeons inspected the unit and certified the Sumner L. Koch Burn Center at Cook County Hospital as an accredited burn center.

In December 2002, a new County hospital was constructed and opened as the John H. Stroger Jr. Hospital of Cook County. The burn center was included in this relocation.

## Conclusion

As one of the first organized burn care centers in the United States, the BU at Cook County Hospital has faced many challenges in its more than 60 years of existence. Despite these challenges, continuous exceptional care based on expertise, devotion, and compassion has been provided to the burn victims throughout Cook County and beyond.

## References

1. Curtis P. Artz; History of Burns – A Team Approach, Edt. Artz; Moncrief and Pruitt, W. B. Saunders Co. 1979.
2. John G. Raffensperger; The old lady on Harrison Street, Cook County Hospital 1833-1995, Peter Lang Publishing. 1997.
3. Sydney Lewis; An Oral History of Cook County Hospital. The New Press: 1995.
4. In memorium; Sumner L. Koch: 1888-1976; The Jour. of Hand Surgery, 2, (4) PP, 328-329, July 1977.
5. Obituary; Sumner L. Koch: 1888-1976; Jour. of Plastic and Reconstructive Surgery, 60 (3) PP, 446-448, Sept 1977.
6. Daniel J. Nagle; The Chicago School of Hand Surgery, The Jour. of Hand Surgery 28A (5) Sept 2003.
7. Michaell L. Mason; Appreciations, Quarterly Bulletin, Northwestern University Medical School, 27 (4): 361-363 Winter 1953.
8. Tribute to Harvey Stuart Allen; Quarterly Bulletin, Northwestern University Medical School, 29 (3): 290-294 Fall 1955.
9. Richard Dozer; The Way-Out War Against Burns; Chicago Tribune, March 21, 1965.
10. David R. Boyd; Care of the Burn Patient in Illinois, Trauma Center Newsletter; 1 (5) March 1972.
11. Archives, Galter Health Sciences Library, Northwestern University, Chicago.

# 10

# Hand Surgery

*Sidney J. Blair, MD*
*John Elstrom, MD*
*James L. Stone, MD*

*"We must confess that it is in the human hand that we have the consummation of all perfection as an instrument."*

—*Sir Charles Bell, 1833*

- *Chicago School of Hand Surgery*
- *Infections of the Hand*
- *Acute Injuries of the Hand*
- *CCH Hand and Burn Services*
    - Michael L. Mason
    - Harvey S. Allen
    - John L. Bell
    - William B. Stromberg Jr.
    - John Schneewind
- *Modern Days in Hand Surgery*
    - John Boswick
    - Sidney J. Blair
    - John Bilos
    - Robert Hall Jr.
    - Mark Gonzalez
- *References*

## Chicago School of Hand Surgery

Hand Surgery at Cook County Hospital, also referred to as the Chicago School of Hand Surgery, has an illustrious history, and it played a pivotal role in the genesis of hand surgery as a specialty in the United States. As in other branches of surgery, the interest in hand surgery came about because of the poor care patients were receiving for their hand injuries and associated infectious complications before the introduction of antisepsis. When the original old Cook County Hospital (CCH, formerly City Hospital, corner of Eighteenth and Arnold Streets) opened in January of 1866, the first patient was a German girl transferred from the County poor farm (West Irving Park Road) with a palmar abscess of the hand.[1] She was likely cared for by surgeon George K. Amerman (1832–1867) who was largely responsible for the establishment of the hospital.[1,2]

Roswell Park (1852–1914), who had interned at the second CCH (1835 W. Harrison Street) in 1876, closely witnessed the adoption of antiseptic surgery at CCH:

> ...it happened that during my first winter's experience (1876–1877) — with but one or two exceptions — every patient operated on in that hospital, and by men who were esteemed the peers of any one in their day, died of blood poisoning, while I myself nearly perished from the same disease. This was in an absolutely new building, where expenditure had been lavish; one whose walls were not reeking with germs ...With the introduction of the antiseptic method, during the two years following, this frightful mortality was reduced to the average of the day, and in the same institution today is done as good work as that seen anywhere in the world.[3]

Park believed death from blood poisoning (sepsis) secondary to hand infections could be decreased by a more rational approach to incisional drainage and the use of antiseptics. In 1881, two years before his departure to Buffalo, Park presented a paper to the Illinois State Medical Society on the surgical anatomy of the palmar tendon sheaths studied after careful dissection and injection of plaster of paris or viscous wax, emphasizing the surgical importance of tendon sheath anatomy in the adequate diagnosis and treatment of hand and forearm infections.[4]

However, before the 20th century, most surgeons remained discouraged by the disappointing functional results following surgery for hand infections, nerve and tendon injuries, and deformities, so much so that these hopeless conditions remained largely neglected. Not until two immediate emergent situations could be reasonably addressed—acute hand infection and the acute injury—could the surgeon seriously turn his efforts to consideration of reparative and reconstructive surgery. The Chicago School of Hand Surgery was to be in the forefront of these critical developments.[5]

## Infections of the Hand

Allen B. Kanavel (1874–1938, CCH intern 1900–1901 and staff surgeon 1913–1919) was a Northwestern graduate stimulated to enter surgery by the ingenuity of Fenger and his trainees. Early in his career, Kanavel had a hand injury and witnessed progression of the infection before it subsided.[6] In those pre-antibiotic days, patients frequently died from hemolytic streptococcal septicemia several days after a seemingly minor soft tissue finger or hand injury. Acute cellulitis and ascending lymphangitis were prominent early symptoms. Doctors and nurses were especially prone after pricking a finger during surgery or a postmortem examination, especially if they continued working after the injury. These experiences encouraged Kanavel to comprehensively study the clinical and pathological aspects of hand infections.[7] Over a period of nearly 10 years, he thoroughly investigated the hand and forearm palmar sheath and tendon space anatomy by cadaver dissection with X-ray visualization after injection of radio opaque liquid contrast material. This resulted in a number of comprehensive papers beginning in 1905,[8,9] and culminated in his classic 1912 book *Infections of the Hand*[10] (Figure 10–1 ),which went through seven editions and was translated into many languages. The 6th edition in 1933 gave the results of 25 years' experience.[11]

Conservative therapy consisted of bed rest, elevation, hot moist dressings, promotion of local bacterial resistance by adequate diet and fluid intake, and avoidance of mechanical interference in the face of spreading infection. Prompt and well-placed incisional drainage of obvious pus, especially with the felon and tendon sheath infections, usually substantially reduced or obviated significant functional disability and even death. Drains were removed within 48 hours, dry dressings were used as soon as the infection was controlled, and hand and finger motion advocated within two days of incision. Later, more active physiotherapy and exposure to sunlight were believed to improve results.[7] Kanavel also introduced the important concept of placing the infected or injured hand

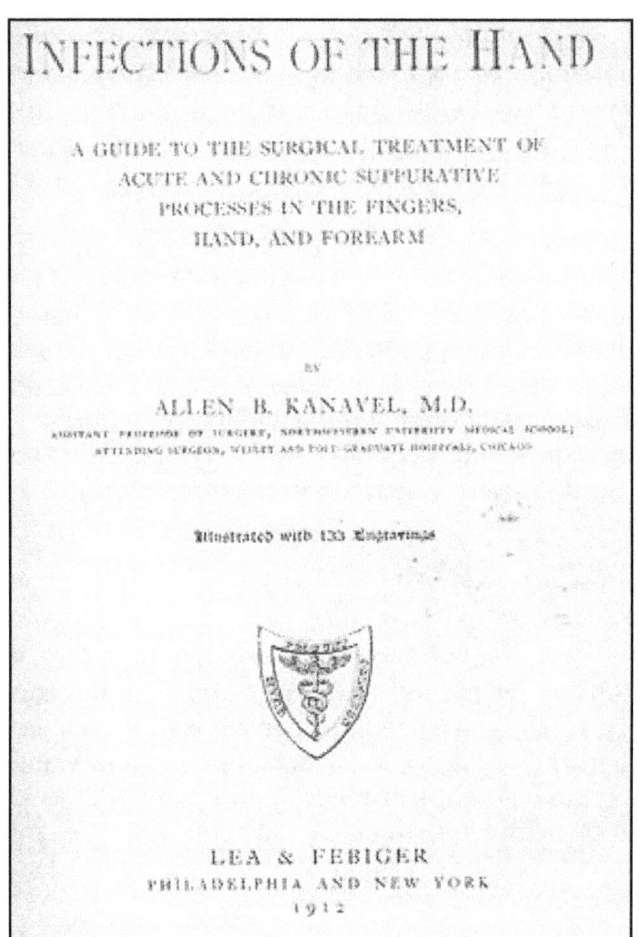

*Figure 10–1* Infections of the Hand *(1912) by Allen B. Kanavel*

in the now well known position-of-function with the wrist slightly extended and fingers flexed. This comfortable position afforded maximal power with the least effort, and even if recovery was incomplete, still facilitated the patient's use of his hand.[7,12]

In addition to his publications, Kanavel gave many talks all over the country emphasizing these points. Kanavel's clinical and experimental studies, when applied to clinical practice, did not just revolutionize the treatment of hand infections but ushered in a new and exciting interest in hand surgery such that the surgical subspecialty arose and flourished.[5] Kanavel was to remain America's foremost authority on infections of the hand and reconstructive hand surgery for the remainder of his life.[5,13–16]

Kanavel had a natural, simple, homely charm, unfailing courtesy, and shrewd common sense that appealed to his patients and made him a master of diplomacy. Second to the care of patients was his sincere concern for the welfare and education of his students, residents, and junior colleagues, and he was quick to recognize and reward merit. His formula for successful investigation in medicine, in which he believed all should participate, was simply the constant pursuit of intelligently directed thought. "During the early days, a soapbox in his apartment was the repository of notes and observations on infections of the hand. From this soapbox finally emerged the monograph that made its author world-famous."[17] Initiated into surgery at a time when few surgeons specialized, Kanavel was a master in a number of areas, including abdominal, gynecological, thoracic, neurological, and reconstructive surgery. He retired from surgery in 1932 and died secondary to an auto accident in 1938. "As with all great teachers, he lives on in those who studied under him and learned something of the kindliness, the humility and the idealism that were his outstanding characteristics."[16]

## Acute Injuries of the Hand

Once infections of the hand were better understood and their treatment came to the attention of experienced surgeons, not unexpectedly acute injuries of the hand began to receive better treatment. In the early 1920s, Kanavel encouraged Sumner L. Koch (1888–1976, CCH intern 1914–1916), a former student and general surgery trainee, to organize a hand surgery and burn center at Cook County Hospital. Koch, who joined Kanavel in practice in 1916 and served in World War I, was interested in trauma surgery, wound care, and burns in addition to the newly developing field of hand surgery.[15,18] Throughout most of WWI, pessimism regarding the development of hand infections resulted in most injuries being left open to drain and treated with an abundance of local antiseptic agents. The result was that tissues were often more damaged by antiseptics than were the bacteria for which the antiseptics were administered. Although near the end of WWI surgeons began to appreciate that excision of contaminated tissue could render a wound surgically clean and delayed primary closure was often successful, these lessons were not immediately carried over to civilian practice. In the mid-1920s Sumner Koch was among the first to speak and write about the logical care of open injuries of the hand.[19] This was an outgrowth of Halsted's teachings that tissue healing depended on healthy, well-vascularized tissues, undamaged by antiseptics, rough mechanical handling by sponges, heavy ligatures, large forceps, or postoperative hematoma formation. These principles practically revolutionized the care of open wounds of the hand. With reasonable assurance, primary debridement and closure after simple cleansing of wounds seen within six to eight hours was found to be as successful as delayed primary closure. Koch was also instrumental in setting earlier time limits after injury in which the primary repair of tendons could be undertaken.[5] In the 1920s, Koch and Kanavel also described the use of skin grafts and flaps for primary closure of hand wounds with loss of skin coverage.[20]

Kanavel and Koch pioneered the realization that particularly delicate techniques were required in hand surgery for a reasonable hope of securing primary healing with minimum scar formation, in addition to the careful suture of divided tendons and nerves. Kanavel, Chicago's best-known and most-capable neurological surgeon in the period before and after WWI and a founding member of the Society of Neurological Surgeons (1920), clearly recognized these technical issues and advantages, as did his close associate Koch. A few years later, Sterling Bunnell (1882–1957), a San Francisco hand surgeon and contemporary of Koch who was primarily interested in reconstructive hand surgery, introduced the phrase "atraumatic technique." Bunnell's early papers on hand surgery were published after WWI in *Surgery Gynecology & Obstetrics* (*SG&O*) under Kanavel's editorship. Many references to this era and the Chicago School are to be found in Bunnell's 1944 monograph "Surgery of the Hand."[21] The Chicago School never published a single comprehensive text on hand surgery but produced many extensive landmark articles in *JAMA, New England Journal, Surgery Gynecology and Obstetrics, Northwestern's Quarterly Journal of Medicine*, and others.

A notable CCH general surgeon and teacher from this period was Kellogg Speed (1879–1955, CCH intern 1904–1905, staff surgeon 1912–1933) who had done graduate work with both J.B. Murphy and the pioneering British orthopedic surgeon Sir Robert Jones. A University of Chicago athlete, Rush medical graduate, and decorated WWI surgical leader, Speed became an international authority on the treatment of fractures and dislocations, particularly of the upper extremity and hand.[22] He was a cofounder of the CCH fracture service, and following his motto "splint fractures where they are," he was instrumental in having first-aid equipment placed in Chicago ambulances and police cars.[23] Into the 1950s, as a Rush professor of surgery, he was still lecturing to medical students at CCH.[24]

## CCH Hand and Burn Service

The CCH hand and burn service with Sumner Koch as its founder and chief consultant was based at the Children's Hospital when that building opened in 1928. Hand surgery was then performed in a small operating room on Ward 46. In that room there was a sign that read "Not how quickly, but how well," indicating the importance that Koch put on precision and atraumatic and hemostatic technique in hand surgery.[15,18,24] "Due to Koch's religious upbringing and soft voice, he was affectionately known as 'whispering Jesus,' and when he was operating, a cathedral-like calm descended on the operating room. Woe betide anyone who disturbed it."[25] With the outbreak of WWII, Koch again emphasized the principles followed by our armed forces—that sound, healthy, well-vascularized tissues were the basic necessities for primary wound healing in a minimal period of time.[26] Carrying the educational torch handed to him from Allen Kanavel, Koch spent his long academic surgical career at Northwestern and CCH. In the 1940s, Koch taught a very popular weekly course to third-year Northwestern medical students in one of the eighth-floor operating amphitheatres emphasizing hand functional anatomy, physiology, pathology, and surgical wound care. An abundance of hand service patients were always available for demonstration. He contributed more than 50 articles on all aspects of hand surgery and was a founding member (1946) and president of the American Society for Surgery of the Hand (ASSH) in 1947. Koch continued working into his eighties and died in 1976 at age 88.[15,18,27]

## Michael L. Mason

Michael L. Mason (1895–1963, CCH intern 1924–1925—Figure 10–2) joined Kanavel and Koch in practice in 1926 at Northwestern Wesley and CCH. Mason, a Northwestern medical graduate with a PhD in anatomy, extensively studied the healing of flexor tendons over much of his career and was likely the world's authority on the subject. A prolific author and collaborator with a jovial personality, Mason wrote a number of comprehensive and oft-quoted hand surgery papers to include injuries, splinting, deformities, cysts, tumors, and nerve lesions. He was president of the ASSH in 1951.[5,15]

## Harvey S. Allen

Allen (1906–1955) was another Northwestern graduate who joined Koch and Mason in 1936 and worked closely with Mason on the investigation of tendon healing. Allen took charge of the Cook County hand clinic in 1936 and worked on the CCH Children's Ward 46 and fifth-floor burn unit. Mason and Allen together served overseas in WWII where they developed the Mason/Allen Universal Splint, a modification of which is still in use. Weather permitting, Allen would conduct his hand clinics outdoors on the Wood Street sidewalk in front of the Children's Hospital with patients seated on benches alongside tables. Allen used a "no touch" technique, and a fresh separate instrument set and sponges were placed along with each patient seen. A similar regimen has been followed in the hand clinic to the present time. Mason and Allen, like Koch, were founding members of the ASSH in 1946.[15,28]

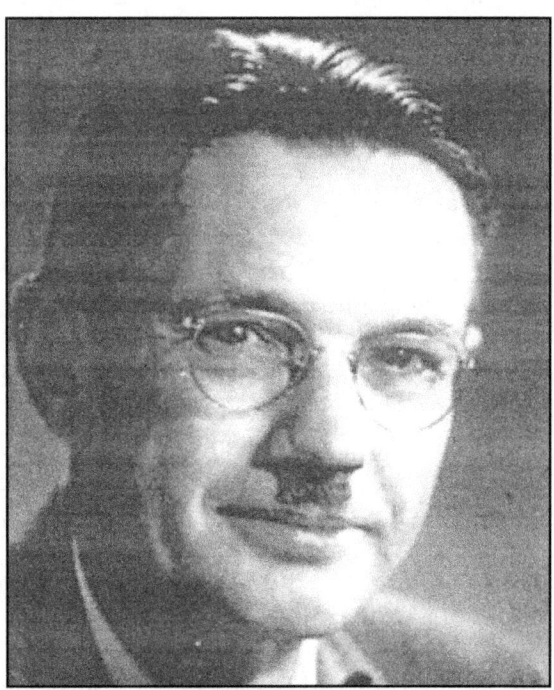

*Figure 10–2  Michael L. Mason*

## John L. Bell

John Bell (1920–1998) was trained by Koch, Mason, and Allen. He joined the practice in 1952, became a consultant at CCH, and like his teachers, became president of the ASSH in 1972.[15,29]

## William B. Stromberg, Jr.

Stromberg (1922–1991) was an orthopedic surgeon who joined the busy practice in 1957 after Allen's untimely death a few years earlier and Mason's incapacitating stroke shortly thereafter.[15,25] Nelson Stone also attended the CCH hand service at this time. The availability of Stromberg and Stone in the clinics and during operative procedures meant a great deal to the residents and fellows on the service.

## John Schneewind

Although most of the hand service consultants came from Northwestern, Schneewind (1916–1972, CCH intern 1950-53), a general surgeon by training and University of Illinois at Chicago (UIC) faculty, was an attending surgeon on the CCH hand service during this period.[24]

# Modern Days in Hand Surgery
## John Boswick

In 1963, John A. Boswick (1926–1999, CCH intern 1957), who completed his surgical residency at CCH and trained with Koch and Stromberg, was appointed chief of the hand service and director of the newly remodeled Sumner Koch Burn Unit on Ward 56 of the pediatric building. Boswick established a hand surgery fellowship that trained four to five fellows each year and continues to the present time. He was a difficult taskmaster and expected much from the hand fellows as well as the orthopaedic and general surgery residents who rotated to the service. In early 1972, Boswick relocated to the University of Colorado to be professor of surgery, chief of the hand service, and establish a burn unit at that institution. He extensively contributed to the study of hand problems, including infection (less of a problem with modern antibiotics), and nerve, tendon, and injection injuries. He was a founding member of the American Burn Association.[24,30]

Arsen Pankovich, who became CCH Orthopaedic Department chairman in 1972, requested the transfer of the hand service to orthopaedics that same year, with the burn unit incorporated into the Department of Surgery. Although by the later 1960s most elective hand surgery was performed in the Children's Hospital operating room at CCH, occasional cases under local anesthesia with sedation were performed in the Ward 46 treatment room through the 1970s. Throughout the 1970s and 1980s, residents and fellows on the hand service continued to come from the University of Illinois Chicago, Northwestern, and Loyola orthopaedic, plastic, and occasionally neurosurgery programs.

In the early part of the 20th century, most fractures and dislocations of the hand were treated by closed reduction and application of plaster of paris.[22] After WWII, because of the need of more accurate reduction and the necessity of starting early motion, more frequent use of open reduction and internal fixation (ORIF) with Kirshner wires or metal plates began. However many surgeons remained reluctant to open up fractures. In 1970, small, thin stainless steel plates were introduced that allowed more accurate reduction without the bulkiness that interfered with tendon function and obviated early motion. Improvement in X-ray image intensification in the operating room was taking place, and Pankovich, who arrived at CCH in 1972 from the University of Chicago, was pioneering long-bone intramedullary fixation techniques. Also in the 1970s and 1980s, the use of external fixation devices were adapted for the treatment of hand fractures with marked comminution as well as open fractures with a concern for infection obviating ORIF.

**Sidney J. Blair**

Sidney J, Blair (Figure 10–3), who was recruited by Pankovich to become chief of the hand service in 1972, initiated remarkable changes over the next four years that again placed the CCH hand service at the forefront of American programs. Born in 1923, Blair graduated from Loyola Medical School in 1948 and while a CCH Intern in 1948–49 was exposed to Harvey Allen and John Bell. Following military service, Blair completed orthopaedic residency at the Hines-Shriner's program in 1956 and a hand fellowship in Iowa with Adrian Flatt. In 1972, Pankovich, with Blair's support, initiated microsurgical animal laboratory training on the ninth floor of Hektoen for orthopaedic and hand service residents and attending staff. Utilizing the operating microscope, microsurgical

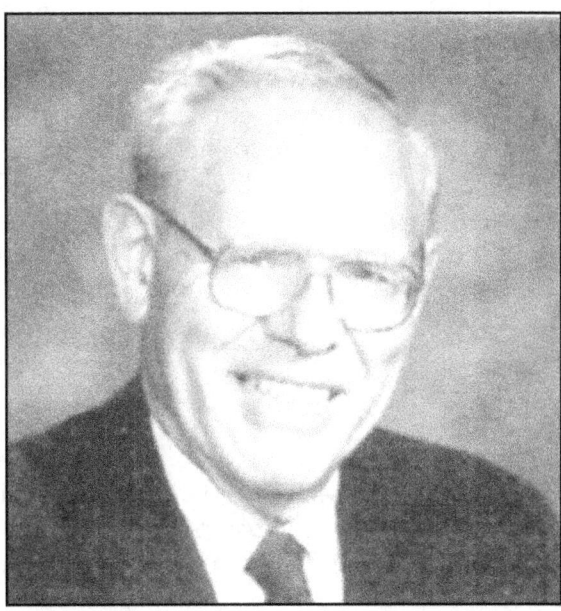

*Figure 10–3 Sidney Blair*

instrumentation, and the finest suture material available, the successful repair of smaller-than-1mm vessels in laboratory animals resulted. At this time, Pankovich also established an active regionalized upper extremity and digital replantation center at CCH, and patients were emergently sent from all over the midwest for replantation. Shortly thereafter, microsurgical techniques were applied to suturing fine veins and arteries in humans, enabling extremity and digit implants to be successful for the first time. The CCH hand program developed into one of the premier microvascular surgery services in the United States.[24] Edward Abraham, then a second-year UIC resident training in the microsurgical laboratory in 1972, successfully replanted a patient's index finger severed except for a tendon. This result was met with disbelief at the Saturday morning UIC orthopaedic conference and considered the work of Cook County "charlatans." Abraham was to become a pediatric orthopaedic attending at CCH for more than three decades and chairman of the Orthopaedic Department at UIC (1998–2007).

Boonmee Chunprapaph, who was a CCH hand fellow recruited by Boswick in 1971 and attending CCH hand surgeon to the present time, spent several years training in the microsurgery laboratory. In 1974, he was the first surgeon in the world successful in the replantation of four fingers. Ten-0 suture material was used for microvascular anastomoses of the digital veins, arteries, and nerves. The result was a functional hand that could feel, grasp, button and unbutton clothing, and write.[31] CCH received international acclaim for a medical milestone that many believed was not possible, and it signaled the future of microvascular techniques soon to be adopted in a number of surgical specialties. In addition to digital replantation, use of microvascular techniques in hand surgery led to digital transposition and microvascular free flaps, as well as compound flaps of tendons, muscle, subcutaneous tissue, and skin. Microsurgical techniques were also applied for the repair of peripheral nerves as well as revascularization of segments of bone that had undergone aseptic necrosis.

Dr. Blair additionally initiated a curriculum for the hand service residents, fellows, and attending staff to regularly visit the nearby UIC medical school gross anatomy laboratory and join him in performing especially instructive dissections of the hand, upper extremity, brachial plexus, and peripheral nerves. T. Shelly Ashbell was appointed to the service in 1973 and continued until 1982. In late 1975, Blair left to direct the hand section at his alma mater, Loyola, in Maywood. There he continued similar programs and mentored another generation of hand surgeons highly influenced by his careful attention to patients, meticulous ambidexterity, soft-spokenness, and humble but firm example. Blair was chairman of the Loyola Orthopaedic Department from 1986 until 1991.

## John Bilos

John Bilos, who completed orthopaedic residency at St Louis University in 1969 and a hand fellowship with the Kleinert Group in Louisville in 1972, became chief of the CCH hand service in late 1975 and carried on the programs initiated by his predecessor. In 1979, Bilos departed to Loyola and later formed a large, busy hand practice in the western suburbs. Peter Hui became a CCH attending hand surgeon in 1977, following a CCH hand fellowship, and remained on the staff until 1984. By the late 1970s, the regionalized CCH replantation program was discontinued due to Anesthesia Department constraints, and Loyola in Maywood began to provide such services. From the 1970s until the present time, the CCH hand surgery and orthopaedic residency programs became progressively affiliated and integrated with the UIC, although residents would occasionally come from Northwestern, Loyola, and within the most recent decade, Rush programs.

**Robert Hall, Jr.**

Dr. Robert F. Hall, Jr. (Figure 10–4) in 1979 became chief of the hand service, interim chairman of the CCH orthopaedic division in 1980 following Pankovich's departure, and in 1985, permanent chairman of the division until 1998. Hall was a Northwestern medical graduate, intern, and orthopaedic resident who spent much time at CCH before finishing his residency in 1976. After completion of a hand and microsurgery fellowship at Northwestern in 1977, he returned to CCH in general orthopaedics with emphasis on hand surgery. During his tenure, he pioneered the use of both locked and flexible intramedullary rods for fixation of long-bone fractures, including those of the hand.[32] Further improvements in X-ray image intensification in the 1980s, combined with innovative ideas and designs by Hall, led to an aggressive approach to fracture fixation for both closed and open hand injuries, including gunshot wounds, and he contributed to nearly 100 forums. Hall is remembered as an outstanding surgeon and teacher who tirelessly devoted six days a week to patient care in conjunction

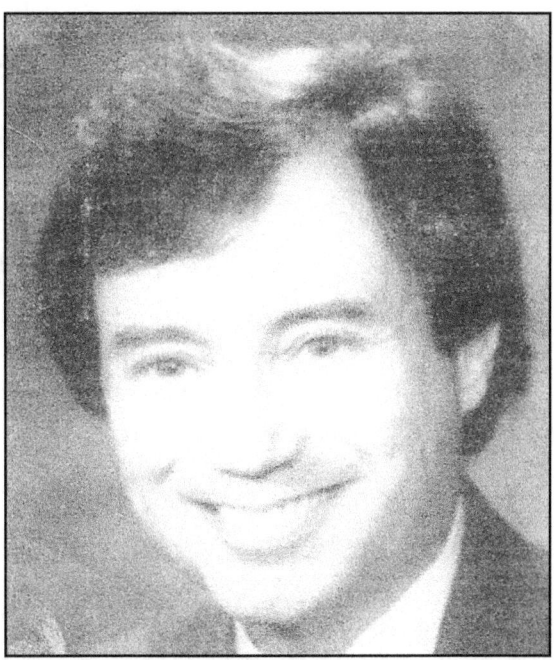

*Figure 10–4 Robert Hall*

with thoughtful and well structured resident training and supervison. He had little tolerance for wasted time or careless errors and displayed tremendous organizational skills over nearly two decades of leadership at CCH.

## Mark Gonzalez

In 1988, Mark Gonzalez (Figure 10–5) became the director of the section of hand surgery within the CCH division of orthopaedics. Gonzalez, who graduated from medical school at the University of Chicago in 1980 with an engineering degree, did internship and orthopaedic residency at UIC, finishing in 1985. Hand surgery fellowships were completed at Blodgett in Grand Rapids, Michigan, and the Kleinert Institute in Louisville, as well as a joint replacement fellowship before he was recruited back to CCH by Hall. Gonzalez continued particular interest in hand infections and fractures in addition to general orthopaedics and became CCH chairman of orthopaedics in 1998. Since March 2007, he advanced to chairman of the Orthopaedic Department at UIC. Dr. Gonzalez has made significant contributions by his research on biomechanics of the hand and original work on nerve regeneration with stem cells.[33] In addition, Hall and Gonzalez published several articles on intramedullary fixation of fractures and gunshot wounds of the hand. Under 20 years of direction by Mark Gonzalez, the hand service at CCH has continued to be a center for excellence for hand surgery in Chicago. They have continued to contribute extensively to the treatment of fractures, free tissue transfer, and atypical hand infections.[34,35]

Norman Weinzweig, trained as a plastic surgeon, was on the hand service since 1991 and with Gonzalez authored important articles on free tissue transfer and a very thoughtful monograph on severe hand injury. Alfonso Mejia II has been

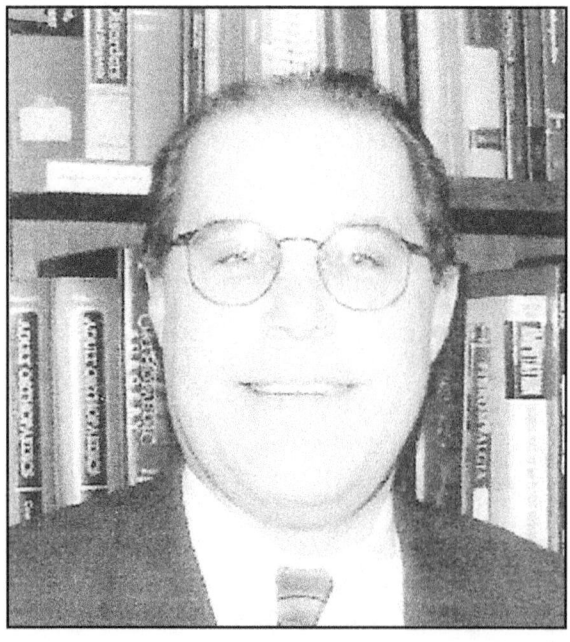

*Figure 10–5 Mark Gonzalez*

part of the CCH hand service from 1996 to the present after completion of the UIC orthopaedic program plus a hand and microsurgery fellowship at the Kleinert Institute in Louisville. Mark Grevious, a plastic surgeon fellowship trained in hand surgery, and senior hand surgeon Boonmee Chunprapaph, round out the present hand service attending staff. Many of the above named surgeons involved with the care at the CCH hand surgery service are members of the American Society for Surgery of the Hand.

In the Spring of 2009, the UIC Department of Orthopaedics rotated its residents out of CCH, and orthopaedic residents now come from the Rush and Northwestern programs. The hand surgery service is similarly in transition. A new era in the history of hand surgery at CCH is about to begin.

## References

1. Quine WE. Early history of the Cook County Hospital to 1870. *Bull Soc Med Hist Chicago*. 1911;1:15-24.
2. Lyman HM. A bit of the history of the Cook County Hospital. *Bull Soc Med Hist Chicago*. 1911;1:25-36.
3. Park R. *An Epitome of the History of Medicine*. New York: FA Davis; 1897:326-327
4. Park R. On the surgical anatomy of the sheaths of the palmar tendons. *Ann Anat Surg*. 1881;4:49-55.
5. Mason ML. Fifty years of progress in surgery of the hand. *Surg Gynecol Obstet* 1955;101:541-564.
6. Chipman W. A tribute to Allen B. Kanavel. *Surg Gynecol Obstet* 1939;68:424-428.
7. Sneddon J. *The Care of Hand Infections*. Baltimore: Williams & Wilkins; 1970:1-3.
8. Kanavel AB. An anatomical, experimental and clinical study of acute phlegmons of the hand. *Surg Gynecol Obstet*. 1905;1:221-260.
9. Kanavel AB. Tenosynovitis fo the hand. A clinical, experimental and anatomical study. *Surg Gynecol Obstet* 1909;8:49-64.
10. Kanavel AB. *Infections of the Hand*. Philadelphia: Lea & Febiger, 1912.
11. Kanavel AB. *Infections of the Hand*, 6th Ed. Philadelphia: Lea & Febiger, 1933.
12. Kanavel AB. Splinting and physiotherapy in infections of the hand. *JAMA*. 1924;83:1984-1988.
13. Kanavel AB, Koch Sl, Mason ML. Dupuytren's contracture. *Surg Gynecol Obstet*. 1929;48:145-190.
14. Kanavel AB. Congenital malformations of the hands. *Arch Surg*. 1932;25:1-53, 282-320.
15. Nagle DJ. The Chicago school of hand surgery. *J Hand Surg*. 2003;28:724-728.
16. Koch Sl. Allen B. Kanavel (1874-1938). *Clin Ortho*. 1959;15:1-4.
17. Elliott CA. The personality of Allen B. Kanavel. *Surg Gynecol Obstet*. 1938;67:163-165.
18. Bell JL, Boswick JA, Stromberg WB. Sumner L. Koch: 1888-1976. *J Hand Surg*. 1977;2:328-329.
19. Koch SL. The covering of raw surfaces with particular reference to the hand. *Surg Gynecol Obstet*. 1926;43:677-686.
20. Koch SL, Kanavel AB. Contractures due to burns; treatment with free full thickness grafts and pedunclulated flaps. *JAMA*. 1929;92:277-281.
21. Bunnell S. *Surgery of the Hand*. Philadelphia: JB Lippincott, 1944.
22. Speed K. *Traumatic Injuries of the Carpus*. New York: D Appleton, 1925.

23. Speed K. Kellogg Speed; 1879-1955. *J Bone Joint Surg Am*. 1956;38:245-246.
24. Raffensperger JG. *The Old Lady on Harrison Street*. Cook County Hospital, 1833-1995. New York: Peter Lang;1995:92-94,138,140,259,306-307,319,335.
25. Bolton H. The Chicago school of hand surgeons. *J Hand Surg*. 1991; 16B: 116-117.
26. Koch SL. Injuries of the parietes and extremities; The care of wounds under emergency conditions. *Surg Gynecol Obstet*. 1943;76:1-22, 189-196.
27. Kanavel AB, Koch SL. The treatment of infected wounds on a surgical service. *Bull Am Coll Surgeons*. 1930;14:19-27.
28. Allen HS, Koch SL. Treatment of patients with severe burns. *Surg Gynecol Obstet*. 1942;74:914-924.
29. Mason ML, Bell JL. The crushed hand. *Clin Ortho*. 1959;13:84-94.
30. Boswick JA, Schneewind J, Stromberg W Jr. Evaluation of peripheral nerve repairs below the elbow. *Arch Surg*. 1965;90:50-51.
31. Chunprapaph B. Replantation of portions of four fingers in one hand. *New Eng J Med*. 1974;291:460-461.
32. Hall RF Jr, Pankovich AM. Techniques of closed intramedullary rodding of diaphyseal fractures of the humerus. *Orthop Tran*. 1982;6:359.
33. Koldoff J, Amirouche F, Gonzalez M. A biomechanical study of the finger pulley system during repair. *Technol Health Care*. 2002;10:23-31.
34. Weinzweig N, Gonzalez M. Surgical infections of the hand and upper extremity. A county hospital experience. *Ann Plast Surg*. 2003;49:621-627.
35. Wynn S, Hassan B, Gonzalez M. Hand infection in the immunocompromised patient. *J Am Soc Surg Hand*. 2004;4:121-127.

# 11

# Breast Tumor Service

*Frank Folk, MD*

- *Introduction*
- *Louis River, MD—Breast Tumor Service at CCH*
- *The Fantus Clinic—Outpatient Care*
- *Breast Surgery—Inpatient Care*
- *Ward Rounds*
- *Continuing Medical Education*
- *Research*
- *References*

## Introduction

The first mastectomy for treatment of breast cancer was performed by American surgeon William Stewart Halsted of Baltimore.[1] The Halsted mastectomies are now considered archaic by today's standards because of the amount of tissue removed and the resulting long-term pain and disfigurement. However, they were considered standard practice until the 1960s. This practice changed, thanks to advances in mammography that began in the 1950s, about the same time chemotherapy became more popular and effective in the treatment of breast cancers. In the decade of the 1950s, surgeons began to develop multidisciplinary breast centers to more effectively treat breast cancer.

## Louis River, MD—Breast Tumor Service at CCH

In our present-day world of general surgical super-specialization, no one would think of establishing a service to deal with breast disease that did not meet the prerequisite standards to be certified as a comprehensive breast center. In the immediate post-WWII era, however, things were not quite as organized, and truthfully, there were not as many diagnostic tools available or many treatment options. During this timeframe and for many years after, there was an organized service at the County Hospital that dealt exclusively with breast disease, primarily tumors, which was led and personified by Louis P. River, MD, professor of surgery at Loyola's College of Medicine (Figure 11–1). Though he was in private practice, as were virtually all the Loyola faculty in the clinical disciplines, he usually spent two or three half-days per week at County for the usual stipend (here, insert the words "at no fee"). He established a County breast tumor service that mirrored as closely as possible his private practice at the Oak Park Hospital.

While there was, in general, a CCF-wide sense of loyalty and pride, the breast tumor service under the personal direction of Dr. River had a special attraction. The camaraderie was felt for years. Drs. Joe Silverstein (Figure 11–2), Dave Petty, Tom Samuels (up from Decatur), Ed Cruzat, Jim Kennedy (from Kankakee), Ellsworth Hasbrouck, Jack Tope, and Frank Folk (Figure 11–3) were among many long-term associates who regularly attended the clinics and operative sessions.

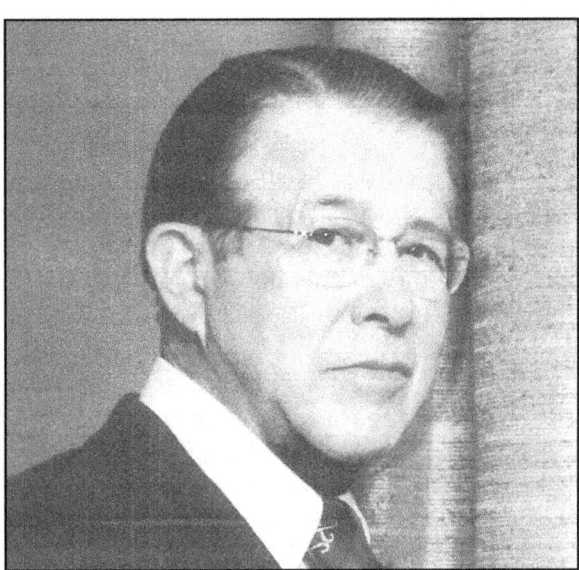

*Figure 11–1  Louis P. River*

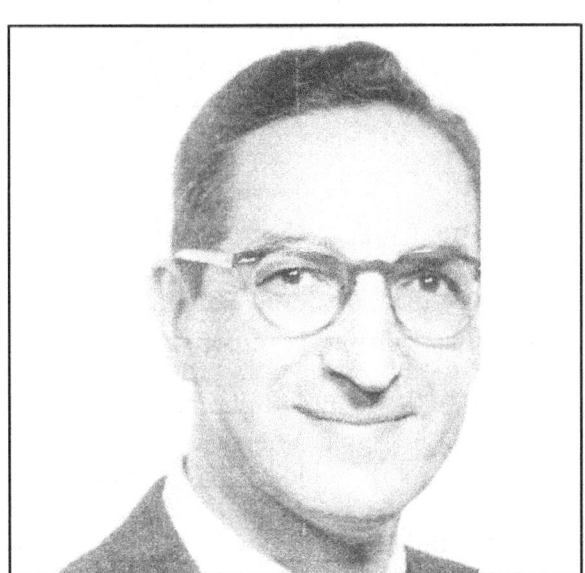

*Figure 11–2  Joseph T. Silverstein*

In the late 1940s, the breast clinic met with other outpatient clinics in the old University Hospital just west of the County Hospital. Those facilities had not yet been fully converted from hospital rooms and were significantly less than optimal. By the mi-1950s, the Bernard Fantus Clinic was located in what had been the old University Inn (an annex of "The Greek's") on the southwest corner of Harrison and Wolcott. With modest remodeling that provided space for examining rooms, a real conference room, and on-site radiology service, the new quarters were a marked and welcome improvement.

It wasn't long before Dr. River recognized that to provide the best in service, disciplines other than surgery needed to be involved on just as dedicated and regular a basis as the surgical consultations and treatments. Therefore, in the early 1950s, Dr. Marion Magallotti ("Mag" to us and his staff) was assigned to the clinic and provided great patient and educational service in the field of radiation therapy. Dr. Carlos Reynes, a diagnostic radiologist, gave us direct imaging support both for routine X-rays and also for advances in breast imaging such as mammography and newly developing techniques in localization biopsy. The trend toward multidisciplinary activity continued with the addition of Dr. Isaac Lewin, a medical oncologist, late of Mount Sinai in New York in the mid-1950s. We now had the makings of a comprehensive breast center, if not the first, certainly one of the first in the midwest. The breast center at Cook County Hospital was established far ahead of the UCLA breast clinic founded by Silverstein in 1973[2] (who later founded the free-standing breast center, the Van Nuys Breast Center in 1978 that included all medical specialties relating to breast cancer: surgical oncology, medical oncology, radiation oncology, diagnostic imaging, psycho-oncology, and plastic and reconstructive surgery[3]).

Dr. Tapas Dasgupta, a noted surgical oncologist, arrived on the scene in the early 1960s as a staff regular in the activities of the breast service and added notably to both the research and patient care activities of the group. In 1973, as the director of the division of surgical oncology, he amalgamated the breast service into this larger division.

## The Fantus Clinic—Outpatient Care

Once the outpatient activities had been transferred to the Fantus Clinic, new patient and nonoperative follow-up visits were scheduled for Friday afternoons. Patients were initially examined by the house staff and students, then reviewed with the attending responsible for the case. During the clinic, each patient not only underwent a complete history and breast-directed physical exam but also was instructed in the techniques of self-examination of the breast and the importance of continued follow-up. The attendings, residents, and students all interacted with the patients with the latter two groups experiencing firsthand the importance of dealing with the concerns of women with breast masses and, later, abnormal mammograms. Above all, the women were treated with a dignity that was rare in the large public hospitals of the day. There was minimal exposure of the affected breast and generally, the examination was conducted with minimal intrusion from parties not directly involved in the patient's care. Dr. River was insistent that if the women were treated with the same dignity as private patients, they would listen to the advice that was given, and above all, would continue to return for follow-up whether or not they were found to be operative candidates. He was, of course, correct, and follow-up was much less problematic on the breast service than on routine general surgical services. Once registered, all patients were scheduled for follow-up. Those with suspect malignancy were classified according to the Haagensen criteria, and all new patients, as well as those of special interest (e.g., inflammatory carcinoma), would be presented to the entire group for evaluation. After the patients were dismissed, the clinic group entered into a general discussion of the patients seen that day.

These informal conferences were part patient review, part journal club, and part discussions on various ethical issues. The decision about the second side, the remaining breast in a cancer patient, was a frequent subject, as was the possibility or necessity of breast reconstruction on the operated side. Needless to say, with the advent of newer techniques and changing attitudes toward operative preferences, our outlook had to be updated. There were also discussions about hormonal ablation therapy, changes in treatment criteria, and utilization of newer and more powerful chemotherapeutic agents. Sometimes, the discussion centered around more mundane topics, such as whether to perform a mastectomy on a 94-year-old woman with stage II disease. We did it, and she did well, proving again that age is no contraindication to cure.

A postoperative clinic was held on Tuesday mornings, generally by the resident staff who had taken care of the patient during her operative experience, and there was regularly an attending present. This again mirrored the private hospital experience since the patient was seen by her doctors who had taken care of her in the hospital. Once the wound was healed satisfactorily, the patient was returned to the main breast clinic.

## Breast Surgery—Inpatient Care

While the Fantus Clinic was the center of the outpatient activity of the breast service, the inpatient hub was Ward 31, a general surgical ward on the east end of the main hospital building. As was quite common in those days, the ward had three attendings: Dr. River, Dr. Manuel Lichtenstein, and Dr. Leo Zimmerman, each from a different medical school, Loyola, Northwestern, and Chicago Medical School, respectively. This meant that in addition to the normal rotation of general surgical admissions, the house staff on this ward were also responsible for those patients with breast disease diagnoses from the ER or the clinic who were admitted out of rotation directly to the River service.

There were two scheduled operating periods a week for the breast patients, one primarily for biopsies and the other for definitive procedures. In the early days, it was almost always a radical mastectomy along the classical Halstedian lines. Residents assisted at their first procedures, and thereafter they usually performed the operations with attending assistance, or at the very least, attending presence. Biopsies were almost always excisions under general anesthesia, with admission the previous night and discharge on postoperative day 1. By the early 1960s, we decided that it was acceptable to do some, and then almost all, as same-day procedures, many under local anesthesia. A driving force behind this change was Dr. Edward Saltzstein who went on to become the chief of surgery at the Texas Tech Medical School in El Paso, Texas, where as of 2015 he continues as the head of the breast service.

The use of the classical Halsted mastectomy demanded meticulous attention to detail in constructing paper-thin skin flaps, complete pectoral muscle excision, skeletonization of the axillary vein, and preservation of the long thoracic nerve. These were all carried out in a manner that has to be characterized as ritual. The resultant defect in the skin and substance of the chest wall was closed with a split thickness skin graft from the opposite thigh. Woe to the enterprising resident who proudly showed that he could close the wound primarily. He was always reminded that he had probably not removed enough tissue and had likely compromised the patient's chances of survival. Overall, the patients seemed to do well, but with varying degrees of arm lymphedema, which was considered a normal side effect of the operation and not a complication unless it reached the stage of requiring treatment with compression devices or in rare cases, one of the operative procedures that were tried to deal with this condition.

In the mid-1960s, the operative pendulum swung to the much less mutilating modified radical mastectomy as proposed by Patel. This procedure provided nearly as complete as axillary dissection, while sparing the pectoral muscles, providing better wound healing, and almost totally negating the necessity of skin grafting the chest wall. More and increasing attention was paid to breast reconstruction, both immediate and delayed, and as more limited excisions and the use of needle biopsies increased, there was a concomitant increase in breast-sparing procedures with axillary dissection and more adjunctive radiation therapy to both the breast and axilla. Chemotherapy increased both in use and in the variety of agents that were available.

## Ward Rounds

Formal ward rounds with attending were conducted about twice a week. All patients were examined and the records reviewed at bedside conferences. For the house staff and students, there was an added dimension in the sharing of experiences and sometimes autocratic opinions of the attending or senior residents. These generally took the form of injecting bits of personal philosophy into the discussions. Manny Lichtenstein, NU professor and attending on the ward though not on the breast service, occasionally joined in the rounds. He once stated, cynically, "Guys, I wouldn't go into medicine these days for nothing, with all the tissue committees, credentialing, and insurance forms." Mind you, that was 60 years ago. Little could he know that the future would hold an exponential increase in these administrative pieces of our daily practice life, but I'm sure he would agree that it's still the best job in the world!

While medical students from Loyola were the main undergraduates on the service, the ward rounds, clinical activities, and surgical procedures provided fine learning opportunities, and no interested student from any of the County-affiliated schools was ever turned away from participation. The regular presence of the same attending staff on this as well as many of the other specialty services added a measure of real world practice to the experience.

## Continuing Medical Education

The breast service was a regular contributor in the field of graduate medical education as well. Operative clinics were regularly performed for the Cook County Graduate School of Medicine. These events were either held in the large surgical clinic on the eighth floor of the main hospital building or in one of the regular ORs that had two rows of elevated side seating. It was also not uncommon to have visitors hovering around the operating table either asking questions or providing their own opinions about the surgical procedure. The procedures selected varied from needle or sample biopsies to total excisional biopsies and curative procedures of all types. For lesser procedures, it was common to operate on several patients during the same session. The cases, as was the normal practice, were performed either by the staff or by senior residents assisted by an attending. On at least one occasion, the operation, a mastectomy, was performed by Dr. Raymond McNealy in his usual dramatic fashion: very slick, but not the same operation that would have been performed by one of the breast service attending.

The breast service also contributed the "wet" clinics for the video clinics of the American College of Surgeons when they met in Chicago. On one occasion, a bilateral adrenalectomy for palliation of metastatic breast carcinoma was performed. Other groups also attended these operative clinics, including the Illinois Academy of Family Practice, the Chicago and Illinois Surgical Societies, the National Medical Association, and the Western Surgical Association. Once, when a touring French surgical group attended, our linguistic abilities were put to a severe test, but everyone seemed to understand at least the basics of what was going on, even the host surgeon. The breast service team also participated in nonoperative lecture and conference sessions with these organizations. At one meeting of the Illinois Surgical Society, George Block, a noted University of Chicago surgeon—while serving as a moderator during a mastectomy—chided the operator (with tongue in cheek) for not making the skin flaps thin enough, alluding to our notorious fixation on this technical aspect of the procedure.

## Research

Research activities from the service were almost entirely based on clinical observations until additional staff, both clinical and support, became available in the 1960s. Studies of the results of diagnosis and treatment of benign and malignant disease were presented at various local, regional, and occasionally national meetings. In the mid-1960s the service began to reach into investigational research. We participated in cooperative studies, including one chaired by Drs. Warren Cole and Gerald McDonald of the University of Illinois. By 1966, we presented a paper entitled "Synthetic Steroids in the Treatment of Advanced Breast Carcinoma" in Tokyo at the International Cancer Congress.

Research on the breast service had matured, and the goals of constantly increasing the level of good patient care, skilled surgical treatment, and research continually advanced.

In 1973, the separate breast service was amalgamated into the larger division of surgical oncology. Chaired by Dr. Tapas Dasgupta, it continued to provide first-rate care for the patients of CCH.

The secret of the care of the patient is in caring for the patient.[4] That has always been the guiding principle followed by our predecessors and mentors at Cook County Hospital, especially so of Dr. Louis River on the breast service. When asked by Dr. Ed Goldberg, a resident, why honors went to so many other less-dedicated County physicians, River replied, "Do your best work, take care of your family, and anything else that comes along is gravy."

## References

1. Burket WC. Halsted WS: *Surgical papers by William Stewart Halsted*. Baltimore. Johns Hopkins Press: 1934.
2. Silverstein MJ: The UCLA multidisciplinary breast clinic. A new approach. *UCLA Cancer Bulletin* 1:5: 1973.
3. Silverstein MJ. The Van-Nuys breast center: the first free-standing multidisciplinary breast center. *Surg. Oncolog.Clin*.N.A. 2000: 9:159-175.
4. Peabody, Francis W. The care of the patient. *JAMA* 1927: 88:877-882.

# 12

# Bernard Fantus and Development of the World's First Blood Bank

*James L. Stone, MD*
*Richard J. Fantus, MD*
*Henry H. Fantus, MD*

- *The History of Blood Transfusion*
- *The Cook County Hospital Blood Bank*
- *References*

Dr. Bernard Fantus (Figure 12–1) founded the world's first blood bank in 1937 at Chicago's Cook County Hospital. It was a testament to his medical prowess, ingenuity, administrative abilities, and foresight. One cannot begin to calculate the thousands of lives saved by the conceptualization followed by solution of multiple technological, methodological, and practical considerations that led to a self-sustaining blood bank. The obvious necessity for timely blood transfusion was grounded in the essence of CCH, a busy urban surgical and medical teaching hospital with large numbers of traumatized and critically ill patients. It was Fantus' inspiration to improve the inefficient, cumbersome blood-donor system then in existence. He even predicted future national and regionalized systems for blood transfusion distribution. Shortly thereafter, his methods significantly impacted World War II injury treatment and future developments in blood product preparation and administration.[1-3]

Bernard Fantus was born on September 1, 1874 in Budapest, Austria-Hungary, and received his early education at the Real-Gymnasium in Vienna. After arriving in Chicago in 1889, he worked in a drug store and studied pharmacy. He was fortunate to attend the College of Physicians and Surgeons (P&S, later the University of Illinois) in Chicago as his father, a printer, agreed to handle the school's printing needs in exchange for his son's first-year tuition. After graduation in 1899, he

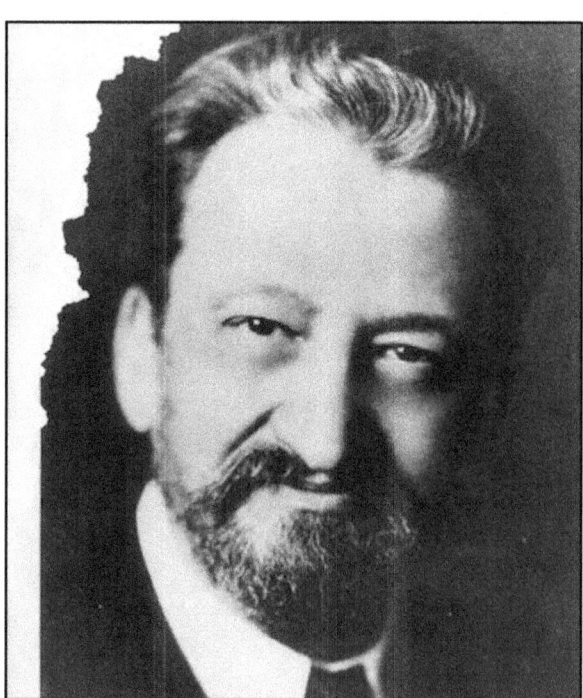

*Figure 12–1 Dr. Bernard Fantus (1874-1940)*

interned at CCH until July 1901, studied pharmacology in Strasbourg (1906) and Berlin (1909), and obtained a master's degree in pharmacology and therapeutics from the University of Michigan (1917).

During his career, Dr. Fantus held advancing faculty positions at Rush and particularly the University of Illinois College of Medicine and Pharmacy. He was an attending medical staff member at CCH (1901–1940) and the University of Illinois Hospital, and the founder and director of the CCH Department of Therapeutics (1932–1940). Dr. Fantus was actively involved in medical research and wrote a number of articles and books. His work on making medicines more palatable, especially for children, resulted in the innovative *Candy Medication* for children in 1915 and other books and papers on medication, prescription writing, and community medicine. He was a member of the U.S. Pharmacopoeia and National Formulary and for many years edited the *Merck Manual* and *Yearbook of General Therapeutics*.[4-7] He urged the medical students and house staff to carefully listen to the patient's complaints, perform a thorough examination, and emphasize compassionate care at all times. Fantus was always the kindly gentleman who loved people and had a contagious zeal for selfless service. His lectures earned him the attention, respect, and confidence of students and colleagues alike.[8] Affectionately nicknamed JC (Jesus Christ) by the CCH nurses and house staff, Fantus' appearance and gentle demeanor gave the distinct impression of a higher calling. He maintained a private practice on the near west side of Chicago as a necessary source of income, and it also provided inspiration and practical experience. Fantus was more concerned with helping his patients than what they paid him, and he freely treated the poor and multiple family members. Money was of little importance to him, and his fee was kept at one dollar when others charged five times that amount or more. He was not included in lucrative drug-company patents taken out on his *Candy Medication*, and Dr. Fantus and his wife struggled through the Great Depression. At his wife's insistence, higher lecture honorariums and editorial fees managed to sustain them.

In the early 1930s, Fantus founded the Medical Center District and proposed the Medical Park in Chicago to generate community spirit and investigative collaboration between CCH, Rush-Presbyterian, and the University of Illinois with establishment of a large park to serve the patients and staff. Sponsored bills failed to pass in the Illinois General Assembly, but he later convinced Cook County to purchase the block immediately across the street from CCH as a convalescent park, later named Pasteur Park. In recent years, a collaborative West Side Medical Center research endeavor—Technology Park—was established as Fantus envisioned decades earlier. Professor Fantus was honored by the American Therapeutic Society in 1933, and his biography was listed in American Men of Science that same year.[4,5,7]

## The History of Blood Transfusion

For thousands of years, blood was considered the essential life force. In the 17th century, the injection of blood from animals to humans was attempted as a possible therapeutic procedure but was soon abandoned because violent, fatal reactions almost invariably followed. In the early 19th century, occasional efforts to perform transfusion with human blood usually resulted in a severe and sometimes fatal reaction.[9]

The first scientist to carefully study and report a convincingly successful transfusion was James Blundell (1790–1877), a London obstetrician and physiologist. His basic deductions were that death from hemorrhage can be prevented by transfusion of blood, but the blood must be from the same species (only human blood for human transfusions); passage of blood through a syringe does not deprive it of its life-saving properties; and either venous or arterial blood is satisfactory for transfusion. Successful transfusions from donor(s) to recipient by means of a syringe were reported in 1818 and a life-saving postpartum case in 1829.[9] Others who attempted Blundell's method had occasional success, but usually serious reactions or death occurred.

In the United States, transfusion was rarely attempted before the 20th century. In the early 1860s at the first Cook County Hospital, a blood transfusion was given during a leg amputation. Blood from the incision was caught in a bowl, stirred to remove fibrin clots, and given back to the patient with a syringe and needle.[6] During the Civil War, one of only two reports of blood transfusion is believed to have saved a soldier's life, but the latter is questionable in that only two ounces of blood was transfused. In the other case, the patient died of hemorrhage despite a 16-ounce transfusion.[9] William Halsted from New York and later Johns Hopkins in Baltimore successfully transfused blood from himself to his postpartum sister in 1881.[10] Interest in transfusion of blood diminished in the 1890s as intravenous infusion of physiological salt solutions came into usage in the Spanish-American War to support circulation without severe reactions.[1,9]

The riddle of why blood transfusion was so successful in a few cases and so disastrous in others would only be solved in 1900. Before this, it was learned that when animal serum is mixed with human blood, the human red blood cells disintegrate and release their hemoglobin. S.G. Shattock of England in 1900 noted that the blood serum of some individuals caused the red blood cells of other individuals to clump together or agglutinate. Karl Landsteiner from Vienna in that same year discovered agglutination groups (types A, B, and O, the universal donor). A fourth blood type, AB, was discovered a few years later, and it became apparent that to avoid severe reactions, it was necessary to transfuse an individual with blood that matched his or her own type. In 1930, Landsteiner was awarded the Nobel Prize in medicine for his discovery of the blood groups. Later, he discovered the Rh blood factor so important in obstetrics.[1,9]

Nevertheless, other obstacles had to be overcome before blood transfusion would become a fully practical procedure. Two troublesome problems were the donor's blood clotting in the aspirating syringe or tubing, and uncertainty as to how long donor blood would keep before hemolysis.[3] By 1914, the first problem was overcome with the discovery that addition of a citrate solution to the blood acted as an anticoagulant to prevent such clotting. A few years later, it was found that with glucose added as a preservative, the blood could be stored in a refrigerator for use up to several days later. Importantly, with the addition of citrate and glucose, blood could then be stored in larger glass containers and injected slowly, further reducing the incidence of severe reactions.[2,11] In the later years of World War I, blood transfusion was extensively used to treat the wounded and likely saved thousands of lives as the citrate/glucose method was improved and standardized for more widespread use.[1,2] Following World War I, civilian hospitals began to keep a roster of typed blood donors to be called when needed or possibly needed, but this often proved unsatisfactory, especially in emergencies or for those with less common blood types. By 1929, S. S. Yudin in Moscow discovered that although blood clotted in the vessels after death, an hour or two later it reliquefied and within 6-8 hours, several sterile liters of blood could be withdrawn, citrated, and transfused to type specific patients. Only cadavers who died from sudden death were suitable for this technique, and the blood was refrigerated for later use before hemolysis about three weeks later. In 1935 Yudin reported satisfactory use of cadaver blood in over 1,000 human patients.[3,9]

## The Cook County Hospital Blood Bank

In 1932 when Fantus became director of therapeutics at CCH, the most pressing problem was the preparation of fluids and blood for parenteral use without a high rate of adverse reactions. His establishment of a solutions laboratory at CCH led to specially prepared and sterilized, standard parenteral fluids to be given intravenously with much greater safety in an era before commercially available fluids. However, the problem of preparing and storing whole blood was more difficult to solve.

> *Previously, when blood transfusion was required, donors had to be called for. The response sometimes would be a horde of excited, noisy, "volunteers." A little blood had to be drawn from half a dozen or even more of these "volunteers" to find one of the blood type to match that of the patient. Should this blood unfortunately give a positive Wassermann reaction, which occurred in about 10% of cases, then the whole process had to be repeated. The patient not infrequently expired before blood suitable for transfusion was obtainable... Death sometimes occurred also in the case of those unfortunate persons who, being friendless, could obtain no donor, as the hospital had no means of paying professional donors.[12]*

Fantus' first step was the use of a closed tube system that made it possible to collect a donor's blood directly into a bottle containing citrate solution. A second major innovation was administration of donor blood to a patient by slow but continuous IV drip instead of the traditional but much more dangerous direct syringe injection. Although the problem of an efficient means of blood collection and administration seemed to have been solved, there was still a pressing need to have blood immediately available for emergency cases.[3] When Fantus learned of Yudin's work in Moscow it was evident to him that the use of cadaver blood would not be acceptable in the United States, nor would the amounts of blood be sufficient to meet the needs of CCH. Instead, he decided to obtain blood from suitable living donors to which was added a sodium citrate solution without glucose, and after proper testing for syphilis, malaria, and blood group typing, the blood was stored in a refrigerator at low temperature (4° C) for up to 10 days. Many specific details had yet to be addressed and studies were necessary in regards to the preparation, storage, and administration of whole blood.[3,12,13]

Organization of the CCH Blood Preservation Laboratory, as it was initially called, took place during the years 1935 and 1936. Many conferences and discussions were hosted by Dr. Fantus with various administrative and physician staff members at CCH, notably Medical Superintendent Karl A. Meyer, Ole C. Nelson, Frederick Tice, Harry Richter, Richard Jaffe, Samuel Hoffman, and many additional interested CCH physicans and those from surrounding universities, especially the University of Illinois. The details to be worked out included problems of collection, storage, and administration of blood, including prevention of hemolysis; the optimal temperature and maximum time for blood storage; methods of administration to patients; precautions observed before administration; indications for transfusion; the amount of blood to be given; and the temperature at which it should be given.[3] Necessary financial support was provided by a grant facilitated by Dr. Irving Muskat and Mr. Louis Feinberg, and later the Rebecca Muskat Memorial Fund. This made it possible to employ Dr. Schirmer

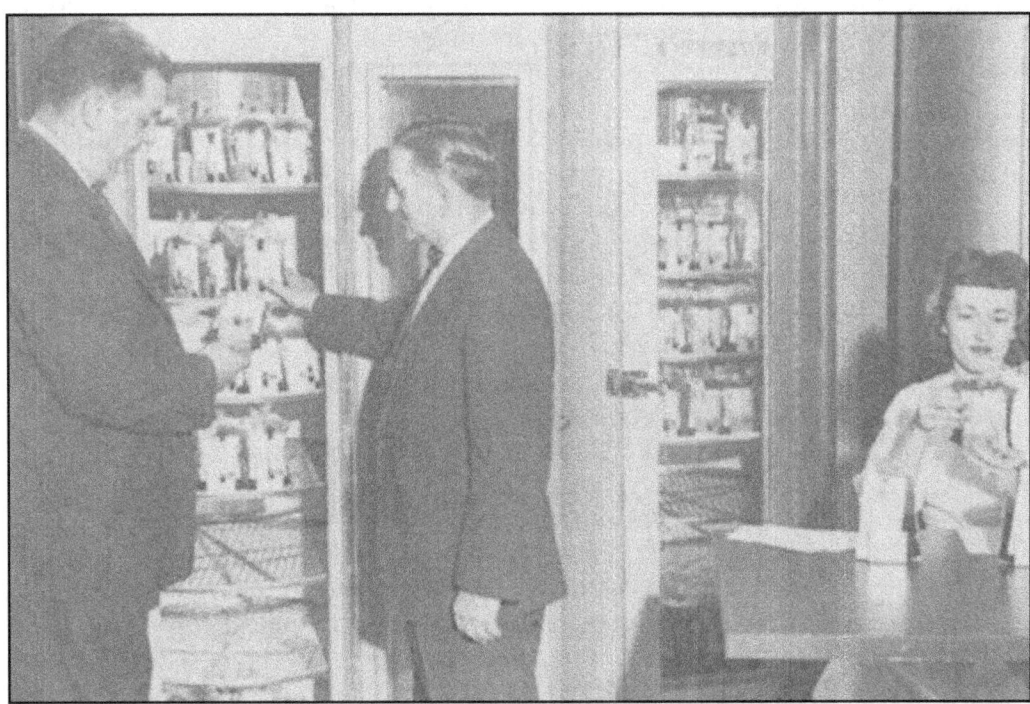

*Figure 12–3 First blood bank in America was established by Dr. Bernard Fantus at Cook County Hospital in 1937. Laboratory inspection in the late 1950s by (from left) Dr. George C. Blaha, Medical Director since 1953, Warden Fred A. Hertwig, and laboratory technician, Ms. Patricia Hayes.*

as director to supervise the practical application of the various methods discussed during the meetings and also employ a technician. The Fantus group—associates Drs. Fantus, Schirmer, Barnard and Steigmann—systematically studied the various problems related to blood preservation in 1936. The hospital furnished suitable space and equipment that included a refrigerator, centrifuge, small incubator, microscope, glassware, tubing, stoppers, and needles. Blood was to be stored and refrigerated in pint bottles to which an appropriate amount of citrate and glucose had been added to prevent coagulation and enhance storage. A label on each bottle showed the date on which the blood was obtained, the blood group, and other important data.[3,12,13,14]

The Blood Preservation Laboratory was almost complete in early 1937, and while discussing the proposed methods of obtaining blood donors, Dr. Fantus coined the term "blood bank."[3,9,11] He realized that to maintain an adequate supply of blood for emergency usage, a responsible credit system for deposit and withdrawal must be established and rigorously followed, similar to a bank. The name "bank" signified saving dozens of units of all four blood types in a place from which it could be quickly obtained whenever needed. Patients for whom blood transfusion was possibly needed or expected in the future—those requiring major elective operations or pregnant women—were instructed to send relatives or friends as donors to the blood bank in order to establish credit for that particular hospital service, such as surgery, medicine, obstetrics, or pediatrics. Thus, the blood bank functioned like any other bank with regular accounts from which withdrawals could be made. Blood was immediately available for emergencies, even though some patients had no credit in the bank, by sending friends and relatives to replace the blood.[3,12,13,14]

The CCH blood bank opened on March 15, 1937 on the third floor of the main hospital at an initial cost of $1,500. Staff consisted of a medical director, two technicians, and a dishwasher. With the assistance of Dr. Fantus and several other attending staff members, the laboratory could be kept open 24 hours a day. Dr. Lindon Seed chaired the important administrative committee on blood transfusion with representatives from all involved hospital services. The blood bank received tremendous support and enthusiasm from the CCH personnel and the City of Chicago, and it created national and worldwide headlines. Many people came to CCH to observe the methods used in the first blood bank, and numerous inquiries came from all over the globe.[3,12,13,14,15,16]

The blood bank has been a tremendous asset in the treatment of surgical and medical emergencies, and in many other cases. The year before the blood bank opened at CCH, there were 649 blood transfusions. There were more than twice as many, 1354, the following year. The incidence of transfusion reactions simultaneously decreased from 33 percent to 8 percent. In its earliesst years, the blood bank was essentially a trial-and-error laboratory where physicians observed the advantages of transfusion and the reactions that occurred in recipients who had received carefully preserved blood. The Fantus team carefully studied all the various good and bad phenomena and reactions, always searching for causes, correcting responsible techniques, and improving transfusion results.[8] The therapeutic value of whole-blood transfusions subsequently became recognized throughout the world.[2,3,9] In the late 1930s, after the two-year struggle for completion of the blood bank, Dr. Fantus began to tire easily and came less often to the hospital. He died of apparent heart disease in his Oak Park home on April 14, 1940 at age 65.[8] Later that year, the CCH outpatient clinic (then located at the old P&S - West Side Hospital across from CCH on the NE corner of Harrison and Wolcott), was named the Fantus Outpatient Clinic of CCH.[17] Today the Fantus Clinic remains one of the busiest clinics in the world.[17]

During World War II, the blood bank principle was extensively used by the Army and Navy. The American Red Cross collected 13 million pint bottles of blood between 1941 and 1945. Some of this refrigerated whole blood was used in combat-zone hospitals, but a considerable amount was processed into dried blood plasma. Dried plasma did not require refrigeration and was stored in lightweight packets. After reconstitution with sterile solutions, it was used as a volume expander to treat shock in the field or in military hospitals.[1,2,9]

After the war, many civilian hospitals organized their own blood banks.[2,9] In 1946, the CCH blood bank was enlarged, renovated, and moved to the seventh floor of the main building.[15] Ten years after the County blood bank opened, approximately 1,200 blood transfusions per month were administered at CCH.[3] Members of the medical staff were among the first to recognize the value of blood transfusions in a number of nonsurgical conditions as well.[3] In 1947, the American Red Cross began to establish regional blood centers and teams to collect donor blood in the cities and small communities. By 1962, every part of the United States was covered, and five to six million pints per year were collected by 55 Red Cross centers, in addition to 4,400 hospital blood banks and 153 nonhospital blood banks. Improved methods of blood preservation in recent years have extended the life of refrigerated (1-6° C) donor blood from four to six weeks, and chemical and physical techniques have been developed for separating out the various cellular and protein fractionations from donor whole blood.[1,2,9] Today, the American Red Cross collects about 50 percent of the blood supply in the United States. The rest is collected by local or regional blood banks. About 15 million blood transfusions are given each year. The American Association of Blood Banks has honored Dr. Fantus on multiple occasions, and in 1987, it coined a gold medal after him presented to those scientists contributing the most to blood banking.[6]

It is clear that many lives have been saved by the immediate availability of blood for transfusion, and the blood bank serves as a memorial to the vision and energy of Dr. Fantus who made it a reality. It has been said that chance favors the prepared mind, but it was no accident that Fantus was at CCH. He unselfishly dedicated much of his long professional career to this grand institution that fostered the practical reality of a blood bank. Had Bernard Fantus lived longer, CCH may well have had its first Nobel laureate.

## Acknowledgements

The authors wish to thank the following individuals for their assistance with this chapter: Mr. Terrence S. Norwood, former CCH Archivist; Ms. Susan Glover from the Special Collections Archives of the University of Illinois at Chicago Medical Center; and Ms. Debra Welch, BS, MT (ASCP, SBB) from the blood bank at Carle Clinic Hospital, Urbana, Illinois.

## References

1. James B, McGehee HA. *Two Centuries of American Medicine 1776-1976*. Philadelphia: W.B. Saunders; 1976: 310-314.
2. Diamond LK. History of blood banking in the United States. *JAMA*. 1965: 193:128-132.
3. Meyer KA. The history of the Cook County Hospital blood bank. *Q Bull Northwestern Univ Med Sch*. 1949: 23: 318-320.
4. Cattell JM, Cattell JC. American Men of Science. *A Biographical Directory*. New York: Science Press; 1933: 345.
5. Sloan LH. Dr. Bernard Fantus - Obituary. *Ann Int Med*. 1940: 13:2371-2372.
6. Raffensperger JG. *The Old Lady on Harrison Street. Cook County Hospital, 1833-1995*. (International Healthcare Ethics, V. 3) New York: Peter Lang; 1997: 13, 89-90, 430-431.
7. Coogan TJ. Bernard Fantus - Obituary. *Trans Am Ther Soc*. 1940: 40: 12.
8. Steigmann F. Inspiration from the past – Medical giants from County's golden age will never be forgotten. *Chicago Med*. 1991: 94: 12-16.
9. Hutchin P. History of blood transfusion: A tercentennial look. *Surgery* 1968: 64: 685-700.
10. Crowe SJ. *Halsted of Johns Hopkins. The Man and His Men*. Springfiled, Illinois: Charles C. Thomas; 1957: 21.
11. Sebastian A. *A Dictionary of the History of Medicine*. New York: Parthenon; 1999: 131, 303.
12. Fantus B. Cook County's Blood Bank. *Modern Hosp*. 1938: 50: 57-58.
13. Fantus B. The therapy of the Cook County Hospital. *JAMA*. 1937: 109: 128-131.
14. Fantus B, Seed L, Schirmer E. Reactions to Blood Transfusions. *Arch Path*. 1938: 26: 160-164.
15. Telischi M. Evolution of Cook County Hospital Blood Bank. *Transfusion* 1974: 623-628.
16. Perkins HA. Blood Transfusion. *JAMA* 1983: 250: 1902-1904.
17. Johnson CB. Growth of Cook County. *A History of the Large Lake-Shore County that Includes Chicago*. Chicago: Cook County Board; 1960: 183,199-200,231-232.

# 13

# Hektoen Institute for Medical Research

*Patrick Guinan, MD*

- *Ludvig Hektoen and Cook County Hospital*
- *Incorporation of the Hektoen Institute*
- *Early Years: 1943-1968*
- *More Recent Years: 1969 –present*
- *Current Status*
- *References*

The Hektoen Institute for Medical Research is a not-for-profit corporation founded on July 23, 1943 to support clinical research at Cook County Hospital. The institute is unique for at least four important reasons: it supported medical research when others did not; it investigated the more common clinical problems; it served economically disadvantaged patients; and it has worked collaboratively with local government.

## Ludvig Hektoen and Cook County Hospital

In a real sense, the Hektoen Institute is the direct result of the humanitarian efforts of the doctors who trained or were staff attending physicians at one of the great hospitals in the United States, Cook County Hospital.

Opened in 1866, the mission of the hospital was to care for patients in Cook County who lacked the means to pay for their medical care. Of necessity, the hospital was the product of the medical-education and health care system of the 19th century. In the 1800s, before the release of the Flexner Report, many medical schools were mere diploma mills. Medical education, such as it was, was by preceptorship or by internship in such large charity hospitals as Chicago's Cook County, New York City's Bellevue, Philadelphia's General, or New Orleans' Charity Hospital.

Because of their large volume of patients and unregimented atmospheres, these public hospitals attracted medical men of unusual talent and personality. To CCH came such giants as Drs. Christian Fenger, Nicholas Senn, John B. Murphy, Gideon Wells, and Frank Billings. These physicians cared for patients and taught students and also made original clinical observations, studied disease processes, and developed new medical and surgical treatments. In a word, they conducted medical research in both the basic science and clinical venues.

Of these legendary pioneers, perhaps the greatest was Dr. Ludvig Hektoen (Figure 13–1), who interned at Cook County Hospital in 1887. His mentor was Dr. Fenger, acknowledged in Chicago as the father of pathology. Dr. Hektoen succeeded Dr. Fenger as the hospital's pathologist in 1895, and for the next 30 years he encouraged and guided the clinical research at the hospital.

Born in Wisconsin in 1863, Ludvig Hektoen attended the University of Wisconsin in 1883–1884 and earned his medical degree from the College of Physicians and Surgeons in Chicago in 1887. Hektoen did well and was elected valedictorian at the graduation in 1887. He placed first in the Cook County

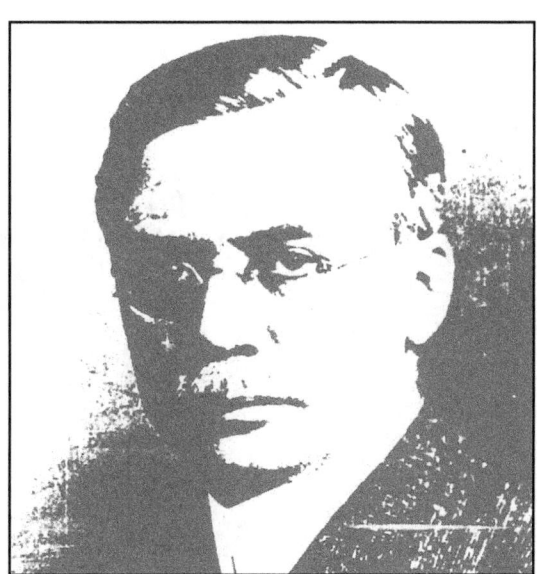

*Figure 13–1  Ludvig Hektoen*

Hospital intern examination and was an 18-month intern from 1887 to 1889. After succeeding Dr. Fenger in 1895, he remained active until his death in 1951.[1]

Dr. Hektoen was an outstanding clinical investigator who appreciated the need to integrate the basic sciences into the study of pathophysiology of disease. He also understood that the pursuit of the science of medicine should be protected from the pressures of day-to-day clinical care and administrative duties.

The idea of a research institute was conceived by several leaders. Besides being a great surgeon, Karl Meyer was also a good administrator. He always listened carefully to any suggestions for improvement in the hospital, whether of a clinical, therapeutic, or laboratory nature. Meyer invited members of the staff to discuss such problems with him. In the early 1940s, Drs. Hans Popper and Frederick Steigmann had a regular meeting with him every Friday evening beginning at 8 p.m. and lasting until 9:30 or 10. These meetings continued until Dr. Popper left for New York in 1957. It was at these conferences that many new therapeutic and laboratory procedures were discussed and implemented. At one of the meetings, the plan for the Hektoen Institute for Medical Research was discussed with Dr. Meyer, and with the additional support of Dr. Samuel Hoffman, the Hektoen Institute was established.[2]

In 1942, the County Board acquired the old McCormick Institute for Infectious Diseases and the Durand Hospital (Figure 13–2). The McCormick Institute building was converted into a laboratory building and housed the expanded laboratories of biochemistry, bacteriology, parasitology, and serology. It also housed the newly organized Hektoen Institute for Medical Research. The Institute (Figure 13-3) was organized in the 1940s as a private nonprofit corporation, solely supported by contributions from individuals and private research foundations and by grants, as the research facility of the Cook County Hospital. The old Durand Hospital (Figure 13–2) was taken over by the Hektoen Institute when Karl Meyer Hall was completed.

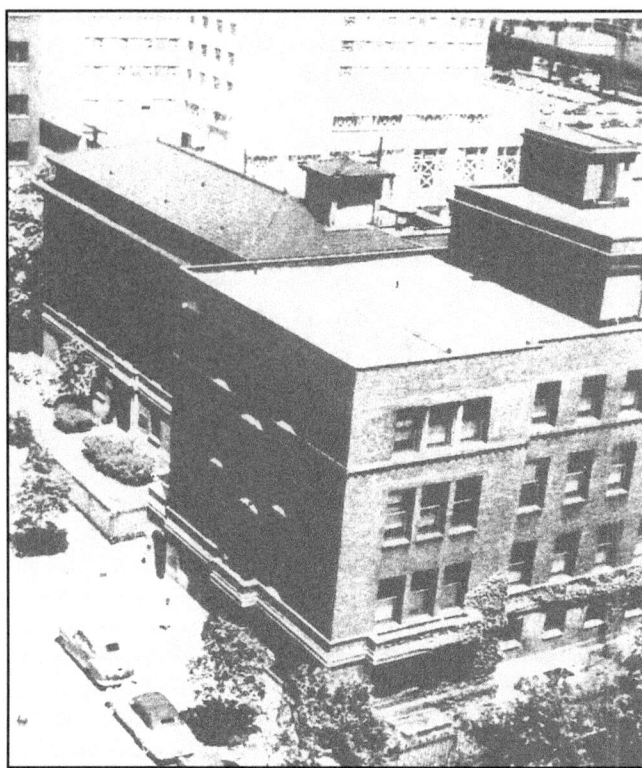

*Figure 13–2  1951, Durand in the foreground, original Hektoen behind and farther back.*

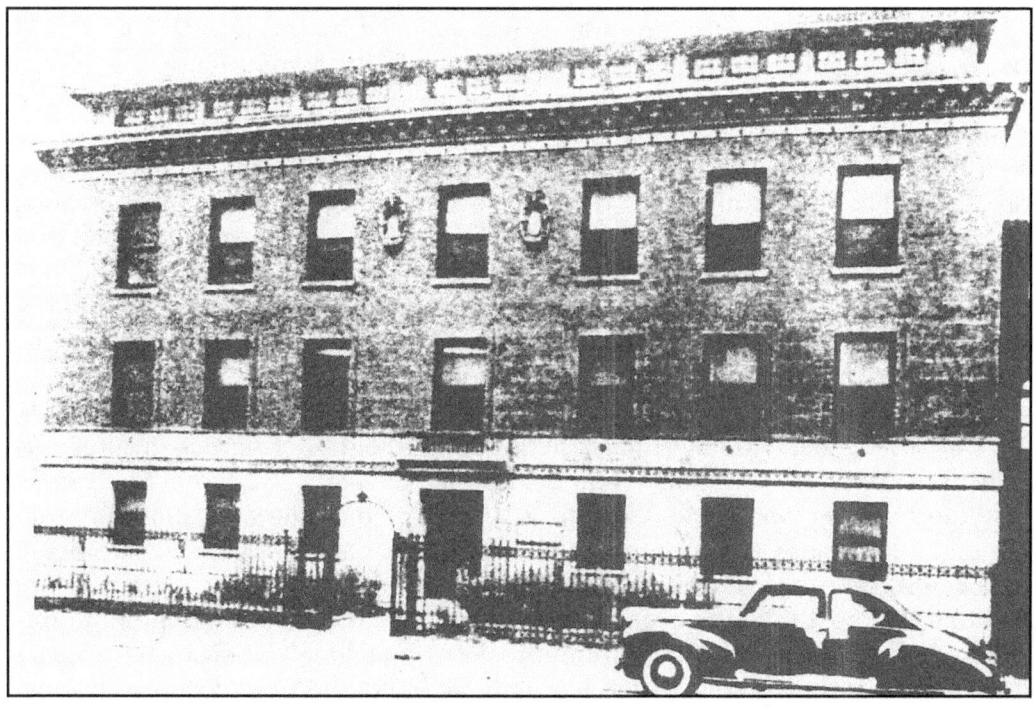

*Figure 13–3  Hektoen Building, 1940–1963*

Besides Meyer, Popper, and Steigmann, other leading physicians at County who lent significant support for the Hektoen Institute were Morris Fishbein, Samuel J. Hoffman, Morris T. Friedell, and Robert J. Freeark (Figure 13–4 ). The bylaws of the Institute clearly express its missions, as shown in Table I (below). Table II on the next page shows the area of scientific accomplishments by Hektoen Institute, including the publication of more than 2,700 scientific papers (Table III).[3] The Institute has had a number of scientific exhibits at various medical conventions, some of which have won prizes.[4]

**Table I  The Mission of Hektoen Institute**

| | |
|---|---|
| 1. | To organize, develop, and support laboratories for research and surgery |
| 2. | To extend the boundaries of science whereby measures will be found to combat disease in general and to improve the care of the sick |
| 3. | To utilize the clinical material of Cook County Hospital for the extension of the advances in diagnosis and treatment |
| 4. | To further develop the clinical laboratories and Cook County Hospital by providing better facilities for diagnosis and treatment of the indigent sick of Cook County |

## Early Years: 1943–1968

The first 50 years of the Hektoen Institute can be divided roughly into two eras, 1943–1968 and 1969–1994. The early years were driven by the energies of such early investigators as Drs. Frederick Steigmann, Howard Armstrong, Morris Friedell, Steven Schwartz, Maurice Lev, Alvin Dubin, and Paul Szanto. During

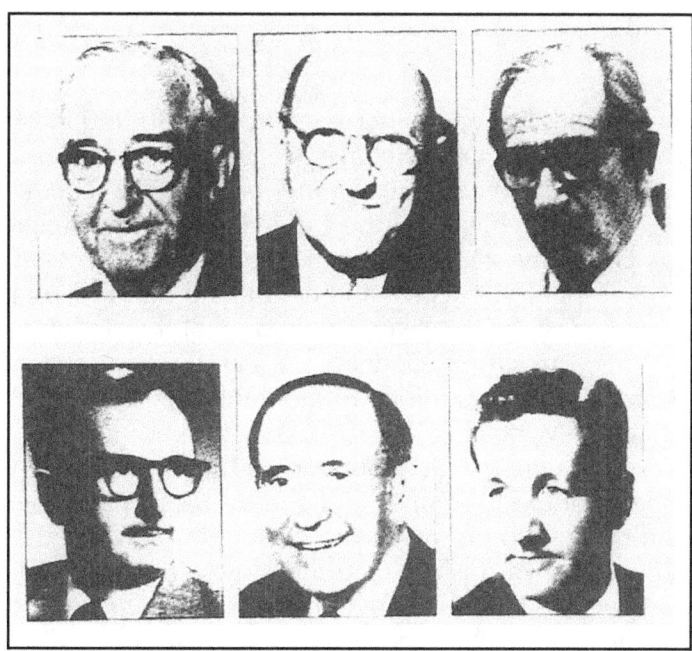

*Figure 13–4* Left to Right, Top Row: *Karl Meyer, Morris Fishbein, Frederick Stiegmann* Bottom Row: *Samuel Hoffman, Morris T. Friedell, Robert J. Freeark.*

### Table II  Areas of Scientific Accomplishments

| |
|---|
| AIDS |
| Blood Replacement |
| Cardiology |
|     Congenital Anomalies |
| Medicine |
|     Peptic Ulcer |
|     Hepatitis |
| Nephrology |
| Oncology |
|     Steroidal Receptors |
| Prostate Cancer |
| Radioactive isotopes |
| Surgery |
|     Vagotomy |
|     Shock |

### Table III  Scientific Publications

| Decade | Publications |
|---|---|
| 1943–1952 | 331 |
| 1953–1962 | 392 |
| 1963–1972 | 351 |
| 1973–18982 | 651 |
| 1983–1992 | 823 |

that period, its budget increased from $430,000 in 1958 to $1,937,000 in 1968. The high point may well have been the construction of the new Hektoen Building in 1964, with the help of $5 million from the federal government (Figure 13–5).

Some highlights of the early years are: Dr. Steigmann and his gastroenterology group investigated hepatic coma and the use of liver function tests, pioneered work in peritoneoscopy, and conducted research on peptic ulcers. He often collaborated with Dr. Meyer on diseases of the stomach.

Dr. Armstrong conducted research on various aspects of renal diseases, especially the immunology of glomerulonephritis, often in collaboration with Dr. Abraham Mark.

The hematologic group, under the direction of Dr. Schwartz, studied various aspects of the leukemias and anemias, especially sickle cell disease. Dr. Szanto and the division of pathology collaborated with other groups on many projects, especially liver disease and the effect of alcohol on various organ systems. Dr. Lev pursued numerous investigations in the area of congenital heart disease, particularly its effect on the conduction system.

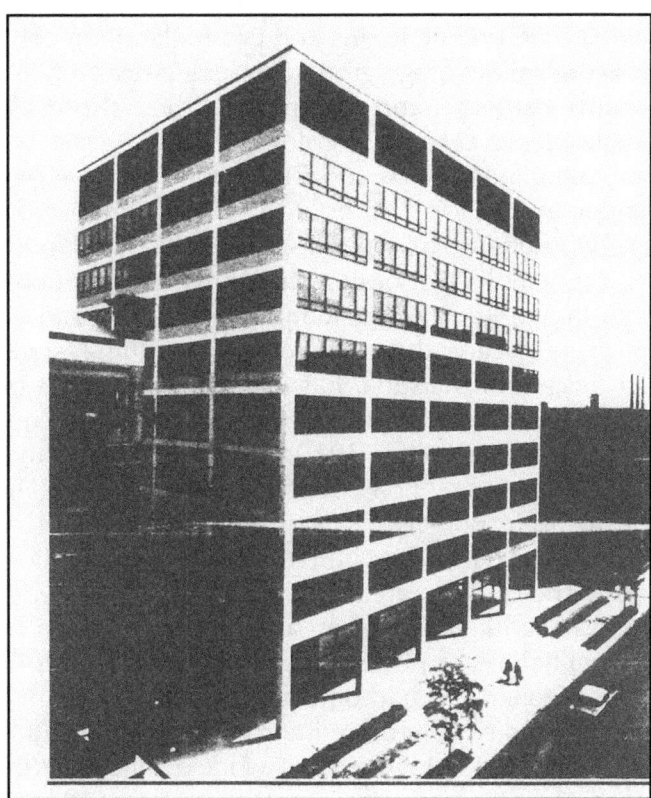

*Figure 13-5 New Hektoen Building, 1964*

## More Recent Years: 1969–Present

During the 1960s, funding for clinical research projects was generous, particularly from the federal government as part of the Great Society programs. In the mid-1970s, however, during the Nixon era, this support diminished. The Institute became less able to support all clinicians and directed its efforts mainly in the Department of Research Biochemistry.

Institute funding declined, but individual investigators continued the research work of the Hektoen Institute. A bridge between the two eras was provided by surgical research. Dr. William Shoemaker, with the support of Drs. Robert Freeark and Robert Baker, pursued research into the hemodynamic effects of shock. It is during this period that surgical residents were, for the first time, exposed to surgical research. Under the leadership of Shoemaker and aided by Joseph Carey, senior surgical resident, junior residents were involved in study of cardiac dynamics in shock, cardiac tamponade in penetrating heart injuries, and the effect of Dextran-40 on viscosity. The volume-expanding effects of Dextran was also studied later by Gerald Moss. More recently, under the direction of Dr. Harry Richter III, the division of surgical research investigated the pathophysiology of the gastroenterologic tract.

Dr. George Dunea and the nephrology group have continued investigations on dialysis and renal problems. In collaboration with research biochemistry, they worked on uremic toxins and prostaglandin receptors. Dr. Tapas Das Gupta and his surgical oncology group conducted research into hormone receptors in breast cancer, sarcoma, and melanomas. They also evaluated the role of monoclonal antibodies in surgical oncology.

Drs. Irving Bush and Patrick Guinan have worked on problems of urologic oncology, especially prostate cancer. The present coordinator of research is Dr. Marvin Rubenstein, who has reorganized and modernized the laboratory. His division of molecular biology has thrust the research efforts of the Hektoen Institute into the forefront of contemporary science, and his molecular antisense studies promise to carry the institute well into the 21st century. The burn group, led by Dr. Takayoshi Matsuda, has evaluated the effect of administering large doses of vitamin C to reduce fluid loss in extensively burned patients.

In the mid-to-late 1970s, in conjunction with studies Dr. Moss was conducting on shock and hemodilution in the baboon (Figure 13–6), Dr. Robert Moody of the Neurosurgery Division introduced novel neurophysiological stimulation and recording studies utilizing the first generation of signal averaging computers in the Chicago area. This work was expanded into the first intensive study of increasing intracranial pressure leading to brain herniation in a cat model with sequential electrophysiological brainstem monitoring. Throughout the 1980s, Dr. James Stone, who had been a resident participant in the earlier work, performed similar studies with more improved instrumentation in a primate model.

Dr. Moss continued his work on the best method to provide volume expansion in the critically ill patient and moved beyond the use of Dextran to the solubilized hemoglobin product (Polyheme), which is still in the study phases of clinical care as a substitute for blood in acute hemorrhagic shock. Though Dr. Moss left County in the later 1970s, his successor, Dr. Olga Jonasson, continued the legacy of surgical research at County, both in the area of critical care and by

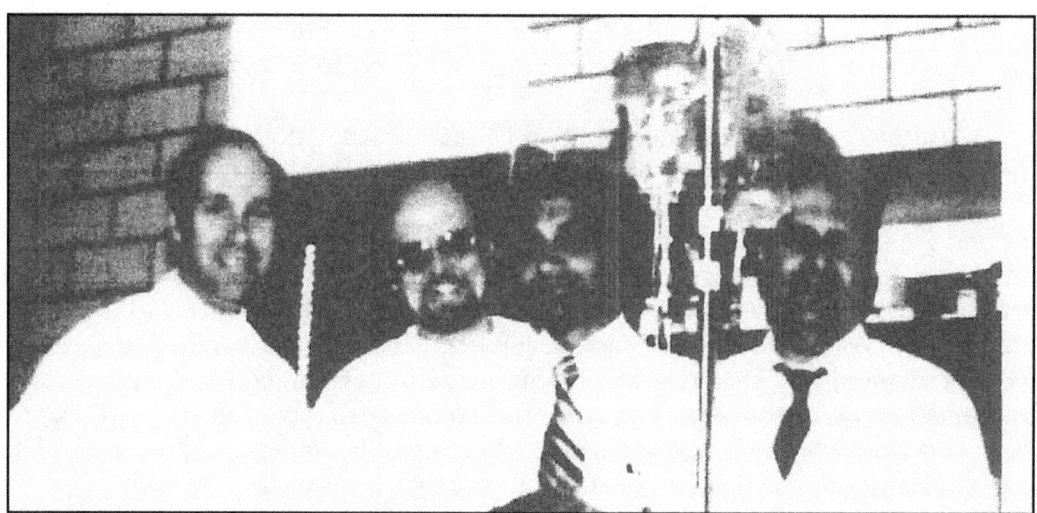

*Figure 13–6 Baboon experiment by Gerald Moss and his team at the Hektoen Institute.*

encouraging other faculty members from the University of Illinois, among them Drs. Thomas Bombeck, Hernand Abcarian, and Philip Donohue, to increase their activity in the field of fiberoptic endoscopy. This effort led to the establishment of an esophageal laboratory at the U of I Hospitals and provided a starting place for the instruction of surgical residents in the nuances of endoscopy and esophageal manometry, as well the performance of and early research work in the development of the floppy Nissen procedure for the treatment of esophageal reflux. It was so successful that Drs. Bombeck, Abcarian, and Donohue were all privileged to become founding members of SAGES.

## Current Status

Dr. Samuel J. Hoffman, who had directed the Institute since its founding in 1943, died in 1989. He was succeeded by Professor Alvin Dubin who died suddenly in 1991. Dr. Patrick Guinan is the present chairman of the board of trustees. The current chief executive officer is Dr. George Dunea. The Institute has continued as a unifying force for clinical investigations by Cook County Hospital's attending physicians in caring for the indigent sick of Cook County. This mission will continue to guide the Institute into the 21st century.

## References

1. Beatty WK. Ludvig Hektoen—Scientist and Counselor. *Proc Inst Med Chicago*. 1982: 35: 7-9.
2. Steigmann F. Karl Albert Meyer, in: Steigmann F, Lantz J. *Cook County Hospital: Institute of Learning*. Chicago:University of Chicago,1990.
3. Meyer KA. Historical background of Cook County Hospital. *Q Bull Northwestern Univ Med Sch*. 1949: 23: 271-274.
4. Guinan P, Friedell MT ,Steigmann F. Cover Story/Research giant celebrates 50 years. *Chicago Med*. 1994: 97: 12-15.

# Section IV

## *Specialty Surgery at Cook County Hospital*

# 14

# Cardio-Thoracic Surgery

*Frank J. Milloy, MD, MS*
*Milton Weinberg, MD*
*Walter Barker, MD*
*Constantine Tatooles, MD*

- *The Beginning*
- *Contributions by J.B. Murphy and E. Wylie Andrews*
- *Thoracic Surgeons at CCH*
- *Cardiac Surgery—Dr. Egbert Fell*
- *Cardio-Thoracic Program—Dr. Milton Weinberg*
- *University of Illinois and Rush Affiliation*
- *References*

## The Beginning

In the early 1800s, surgical procedures were quite unpleasant events. Speed was of the essence for the surgeon, but even at that, wound infections were nearly inevitable. The introduction of general anesthesia in the 1840s and the basics of sterile technique in the 1860s made abdominal operations more feasible and greatly increased the acceptance of surgeons into the mainstream of medical practice. Operations on the contents of the chest, however, posed an additional set of problems. Unless the lung was adherent to the chest wall, once the chest was opened, the lung deflated, collapsed, and the mediastinum shifted toward the opposite side with resultant compression of the opposite lung. If allowed to progress, this condition was incompatible with life. This problem of pneumothorax with lung collapse would have to be solved before routine thoracotomy could be added to the armamentarium of the surgeon. However, the management of pus in the pleural space had been successfully treated operatively since the time of Hippocrates. When pleural pus forms adjacent to an infected lung, it most often becomes encapsulated, and with time, the adjacent lung becomes adherent to the pleura. This circumstance allows drainage of the pus through an opening in the chest wall with or without removal of a segment of rib.

This open drainage of emphysema and resection of chest wall tumors were likely the most common chest operations performed at County during the late 1800s and early 1900s. They were done by general surgeons and were a part of their standard surgical techniques. However, in Europe, notably in France, surgeons like Tuffier had already begun to operate directly on the lung.

## Contributions by J.B. Murphy and E. Wylie Andrews

In 1884, Dr. J.B. Murphy returned to Chicago after an 18-month sabbatical spent at the leading medical centers of Europe. He began an active private practice with Dr. Lee and was promptly appointed to the attending staff of County Hospital.[1] As Murphy gained recognition through his teaching activities and scientific publications, he was asked to speak at more and more medical meetings. In those days at the annual meeting of the American Medical Association, a prominent surgeon was chosen to give an "oration" on progress in the field of surgery during the previous year. Murphy was chosen to deliver this speech in 1898, a distinct honor, especially at the relatively young age of 41. Rather than review the entire field of surgery, Murphy chose "The Surgery of The Lung" as his subject.[2] This lengthy oration was reported in four consecutive weekly installments in *JAMA*.[3,4,5,6] Murphy detailed his own experiences, including a lung operation to drain a bronchiectic cavity performed at CCH. He solved the problem of lung collapse by grasping the lung with an instrument and drawing it into the incision. The cavity could then be incised and packed open with favorable results. In what Murphy considered a minor aside, he also told of inserting nitrogen gas into the pleural spaces of five tuberculosis patients in order to create pneumothoraces, causing the tuberculosis cavities to collapse, close, and heal. At that time, TB was a dreaded scourge in America, striking young adults and frequently serving as the leading cause of death in the industrial cities. Collapse of these cavities had previously been done by thoracoplasty. The therapeutic pneumothorax promoted by Murphy was much less invasive and, therefore, welcome news, which was widely publicized in the press. Dr. Murphy went on to scale other heights in academic and clinical surgery, which are described in other chapters of this history, but in historical retrospect, the 1898 surgical oration was arguably the most significant surgical event of his early career in Chicago.

After Dr. Murphy's death on Mackinac Island in 1916, Dr. E. Wyllys Andrews succeeded him as both chairman at Northwestern and Cook County Hospital. In the following year, the American Association for Thoracic Surgeons (AATS) was founded, and 40 surgeons from North America were invited to the inaugural meeting. Of all the surgeons in the Chicago area, Dr. Andrews was the sole invitee.[7] This was most likely in deference to his association with Dr. Murphy, since Andrews' expertise as demonstrated in his published work was primarily in hernia surgery and abdominal operations.[8]

## Thoracic Surgeons at CCH

Thoracic surgery was mostly performed by general surgeons, and according to Dr. Malcolm Todd, one of the first surgical residents appointed in 1938 and a past AMA president, it consisted mostly of empysema drainage and chest wall procedures with only a few lung resections. During the period leading up to and including World War II, the surgery department—and later (1940 on) the whole hospital—was under the guidance of Dr. Marshall Davison, who was also listed as the attending thoracic surgeon. Dr. Davidson was born in 1896 in Chicago[9] and graduated Alpha Omega Alpha from the University of Illinois College of Medicine in 1919. He took first place in the 1937 examination for appointment to the attending staff at Cook County Hospital. Later he became chief of the County surgical staff and was made medical director of the hospital in 1940.

Again, according to Dr. Todd's recollection, because of Dr. Davison's severe angina, which was to contribute to his death of coronary atherosclerosis in 1946 at age 50, most of the thoracic surgery was performed by his associate Dr. John M. Dorsey, a 1930 graduate of Rush trained at the Mayo Clinic. Dr. Dorsey maintained a very active practice at Presbyterian Hospital where he was president of the medical staff in 1946. In 1951, he left the West Side Medical Center to become chief of surgery at the Evanston Hospital, where he remained until his retirement. He was the first of the County surgeons to be certified in both general and thoracic surgery.[10]

The era of the specifically trained thoracic surgeons began at County after the Second World War. Dr. Saul Mackler, a 1937 graduate of the University of Chicago Medical School, served his internship and residency in general surgery at the Michael Reese Hospital and served as a thoracic surgery fellow under Evarts Graham at Barnes Hospital in St. Louis. After a four-year stint with the Army Medical Corps in North Africa and Italy, he returned to Chicago in 1946 and was appointed as attending thoracic surgeon at County and Michael Reese Hospitals, where he remained active for the next 20 years. He maintained a life-long interest in the diseases and surgery of the esophagus, designing the Mackler tube as a way to palliate patients with nonresectable carcinoma of the esophagus. At about the same time that Dr. Mackler was appointed to County, Dr. George Holmes, a 1937 Rush graduate who had interned at the Washington Park Hospital and gotten his thoracic experience at the Chicago Municipal Tuberculosis Sanitarium and the Hines Veteran's Hospital, was also appointed to the attending staff at County. Since general endotracheal anesthesia had now become commonplace, it was obvious that more operations on the lung were possible and would likely be done. To that end, Drs. Mackler and Holmes were given patient beds on Ward 54. Since they confined their private practices to thoracic surgery, this timeframe ended the practice of general surgeons performing noncardiac thoracic surgery at Cook County Hospital. This position was strengthened later when Dr. Joseph SaintVille, also a trained thoracic surgeon from Michael Reese, was added to the staff.

## Cardiac Surgery—Dr. Egbert Fell

By the end of World War II the noncardiac portion of the thoracic cardiovascular equation was largely solved, but the cardiac portion was just beginning. Operations directly on the heart had been rare and mostly limited to the occasional traumatic injury that could be controlled by simple suture or pericardectomy/otomy. The first recorded case of this type in Chicago occurred at the Provident Hospital, now a part of the County Hospital System. It was performed by Dr. Dale Williams, a member of a family that provided several generations of surgeons and obstetricians to the city. In a prelude to direct operations, both Dr. Edwin Miller—a County intern of 1914 and a veteran of both world wars who served as a County attending surgeon from 1934–1954—and Dr. J.B. Herrick were doing animal experiments on the effect of specific cardiac vessel occlusions on EKG patterns. The modern era of heart surgery began on August 27, 1938, when Dr. Robert Gross of Boston ligated a patent ductus in a planned operation. In 1944, Dr. Clarence Crawfoord of Sweden resected the first coarctation of the aorta. Then in 1945, Dr. Blalock of Baltimore anastamosed the inominate artery to the right pulmonary artery in a child with Tetralogy of Fallot.[11] This progress in pediatric cardiac surgery prompted Dr. Meyer to set the wheels in motion to start a cardiac surgical program at County. His choice to direct the program was Dr. Egbert Fell (Figure 14–1) who along with Dr. John Keeley was an attending on the pediatric surgical service on Ward 46 in the County Children's Hospital. Dr. Harvey Allen, a noted hand surgeon, was the other attending on that ward.

While the choice was well-received by the surgical community, Dr. Fell's name was not widely known among the younger physicians of the County community, at least not at that point. As Dr. Milloy recalls, "In January 1948, I was assigned to Dr. Fell's service on Ward 46, but I didn't know anything about him. I did know of Dr. Harvey Allen from Northwestern, and I offered to trade services with the intern assigned to him, but my offer was refused. So I was Dr. Fell's intern. This was the most decisive event of my life and began my career in thoracic surgery. I was shortly informed that Dr. Fell was planning to start a heart surgery program and that he and his associate, Dr. Carl Davis Jr., had been performing operations in the animal laboratory at Presbyterian Hospital in preparation for that program."

The first patient admitted to Cook County Hospital for operation on the heart was admitted by noted cardiologist Dr. Benjamin Gasul. The patient was a cyanotic six-year-old with Tetrology of Falllot. Dr. Raymond McNealy, the president of the medical staff, performed a Blalock shunt on the child, who unfortunately expired over the course of the next several days, but the autopsy showed the shunt to be patent. The next patient[12] had coarctation of the aorta and was operated on by Dr. Fell with Drs. Davis, Albi, and Milloy as assistants. Over the remaining weeks of the first quarter of 1948 Dr. Fell did four more cardiac cases. All five of these patients did well and left the hospital improved. There was also an active heart surgery program at the Children's Memorial Hospital. It is interest-

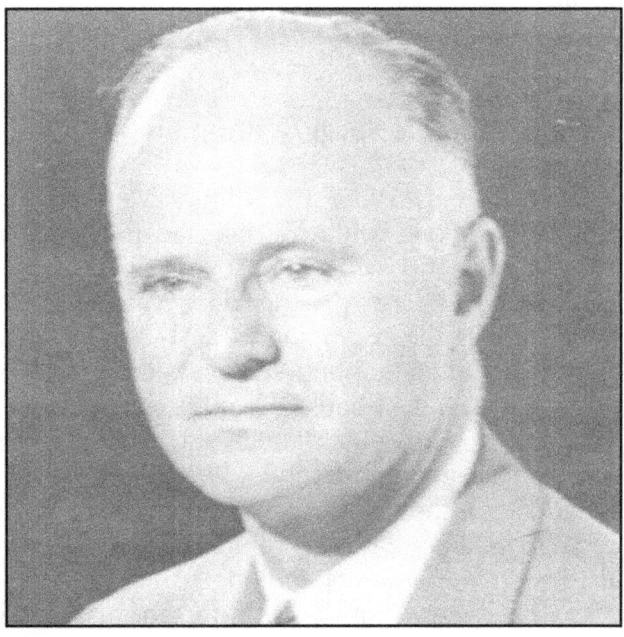

Figure 14–1 Egbert Fell

ing that at this time (the late 1940s), the two most active heart surgeons were Dr. Fell and Dr. Willis Potts, both pediatric surgeons, not thoracic surgeons, while the third busiest heart surgeon, who had been trained at Children's Memorial by Dr. Potts, was Dr. Arthur DeBoer who was starting the cardiac surgery program at Northwestern's Wesley Hospital.

By the early 1950s, cardiac surgery was becoming more focused on methods to bypass the heart to allow for cardiac surgery under direct vision. Dr. John Gibbon, Jr. had for years worked on a cardio-pulmonary bypass machine and used it successfully on May 6, 1953.[10] This ushered in a whole new era of possibilities for operating on the heart. The surgical training for this subspecialty was still rather relaxed, and, as Dr. Milloy recalls, in his final year of surgical residency he asked Dr. Fell if he could spend the year with him assisting with heart procedures. Dr. Meyer agreed with the proposal, and for the last year of Milloy's surgical residency, he was vascular fellow at the Presbyterian Hospital and a general surgical resident at County. He had a mailbox at Presbyterian and ate meals there but slept in his room at Karl Meyer Hall at County. At the end of the academic year in July 1956, Dr. Milloy was able to make another unconventional move by visiting with Dr. William Adams, professor of surgery at the University of Chicago and chairman of the board of thoracic surgery and asking him directly what more training he (Dr. Milloy) would need to take to sit for the thoracic boards. The answer was immediate: six months of tuberculosis experience and six months of general thoracic experience. Not only was the answer swift, but Dr. Adams picked up the phone and called Dr. Hiram Langston, the head of the only approved thoracic program in the area, to make an appointment for the aspiring surgeon.

A year later, in July of 1957, Dr. Milloy was a newly minted board-eligible thoracic surgeon, having spent six months at the State of Illinois Tuberculosis Sanitarium in the Medical Center and another six months at the Hines VA Hospital in Maywood.

## Cardio-Thoracic Surgery Program—Dr. Milton Weinberg

On July 1, 1955, Dr. Milton Weinberg (Figure 14–2) arrived in Chicago from Charleston, South Carolina, to join Dr. Fell as a cardiovascular fellow at Presbyterian and County Hospitals. Since the heart-lung machine was all the rage, Dr. Weinberg's primary duty was to develop this apparatus for use on patients. It was the beginning of a 30-year affiliation with Cook County Hospital from which literally hundreds of residents, fellows, and students benefited.

While Dr. Fell had done numerous cardiac procedures—patent ductus and coarctation, Potts and Blalock shunts, aneurysms, closed valvular procedures, and open heart surgery under hypothermia and limited cardiac arrest—the red-letter day for the first open-heart procedure done with a heart-lung machine was in 1956 for a complicated ventriculo-septal defect (VSD). Unfortunately, the child died shortly after the operation.

The second pump-assisted case, also a VSD in a child, was successfully

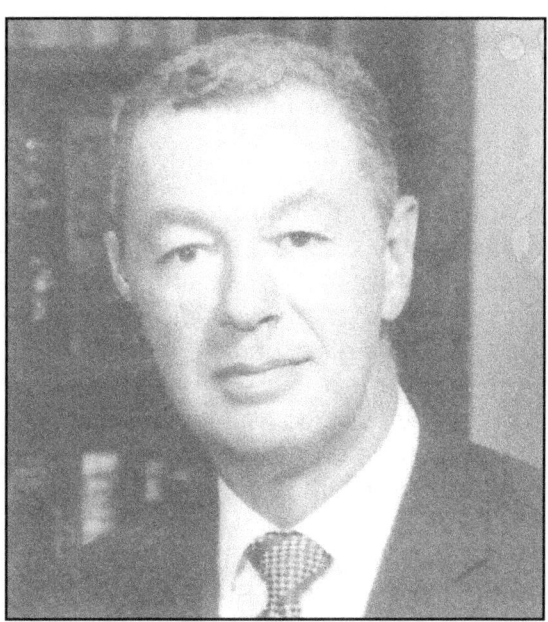

*Figure 14–2  Milton Weinberg*

done later that year. This was probably the first successful such procedure done in Chicago, and by 1958 Dr. Weinberg was able to present the first series of successfully completed open-heart procedures in the city to the Chicago Surgical Society. These cases were from both Cook County Hospital and Presbyterian Hospital and included children and adults.

It was not all sweetness and light in getting the County heart program up and running. Dr. Weinberg recalls that the first heart-lung machine was donated by a private foundation for use at both County and Presbyterian, but it was stored at Presbyterian and had to be carted across Harrison Street every time it was needed at County.

When the team started to set up for the first case in the Children's OR, they contacted the hospital electricians to ask them to help ensure the electrical connections were secure. The medical professionals were amazed when the electricians refused to help out. It seems that the electricians at Presbyterian were nonunion and the staunchly union County electricians wouldn't touch any equipment worked on by nonunion labor. When it was explained that a patient could die if a connection came apart during the operation, they predictably replied, "that's too bad," and walked away.

The upshot of this was that from that time on, each evening before an open-heart was on the schedule for the next day, the surgical team taped all the plugs to the electrical outlets and all other lines to the floor of the OR with either adhesive or duct tape. The tape didn't help in the moving, but it did help to ensure that the connections remained as they were at Presbyterian where they were known to work. This mostly seemed to solve the problem, but even at that, the all-powerful nursing supervisor of the Children's OR, the indomitable Miss Gressitt, would get there before the surgical team and pull up all the tape from her cleaned floor. In spite of this, cases were done in what now seems clearly to have been satisfactory fashion.

## University of Illinois and Rush Affiliation

Dr. Weinberg became the head of the division of cardio-thoracic surgery in 1964 and petitioned the American Board of Thoracic Surgery for a training program, which was approved and begun in 1965 with one trainee per year in a two-year program. Beside the formal trainees, Drs. Tom Murphy and John Raffensperger also received a major part of their eligibility for thoracic boards from CCH. There was an influx of new faces with the addition of Drs. Walter Barker (Figure 14–3), Penfield Faber (Figure 14–4), and Hiram Langston in the area of noncardiac thoracic surgery. Dr. Dino Tatooles (Figure 14–5) was added to the staff in cardiac surgery. In addition, to support the fellowship, a rotation through the Chicago Municipal Tuberculosis Sanitarium under Drs. William Lees and Robert Fox was established. The Saturday morning chest conference was re-established with participation from County and Presbyterian attending including Leon Love, the chief of radiology at County, and Dr. Harold Levine, the top teaching pulmonologist at County. This was a period of intense academic activity in the division since besides the fellows, there were a number of general surgery residents who would enter Cardiothoracic or vascular training programs rotating through the service as both junior and senior residents. Drs. Joe Carey and Dave Monson, with their interest in hemodynamics of cardiac injury and the physiology and mechanics of hemopericardium in both the animal model and the traumatized patient, produced a number of papers, as did Dr. James S.T. Yao with his ever-present camera and nose for interesting cases. Dr. Bob Vanecko many times seemed more like a movie producer than resident, and he put together several films for the ACS Surgical Spectacular Series during this time. And during this period, Dr. John Raffensperger provided liberal offerings of his surgical expertise in the treatment of pediatric chest disease.

Dr. Weinberg left the chairmanship of the division in 1968 and was replaced by Dr. Tatooles. After several years, Dr. Walter L. Barker was added to the paid

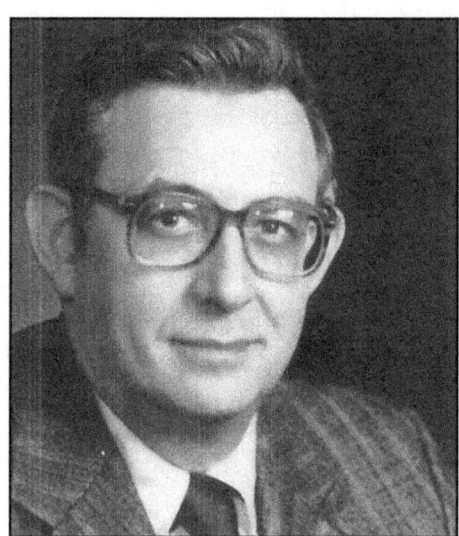

*Figure 14–3 Walter Barker*

CARDIO-THORACIC SURGERY

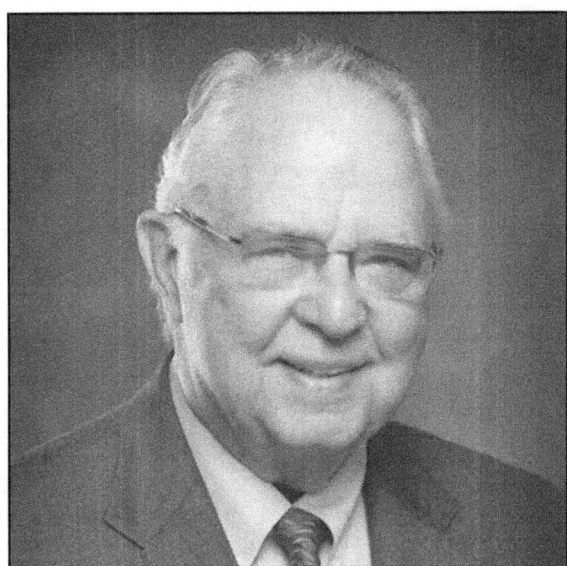

*Figure 14–4  Penfield Faber*

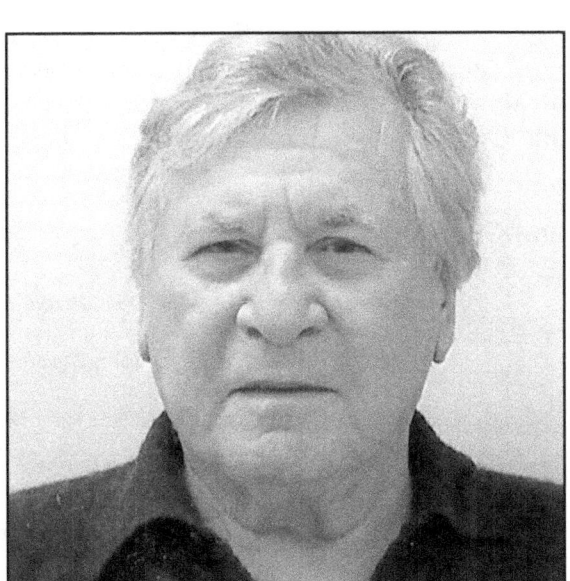

*Figure 14–5  Constantine Tatooles*

staff as a part-time assistant director of the division. He remained active at County until his retirement in 1993. In 1978, a unified cardio-thoracic program was instituted between Cook County Hospital and the University of Illinois with Dr. Sidney Levitsky of the U of I as chairman. All County patients requiring elective cardiac operations were routinely transferred to the U of I. Thus, the program in heart surgery instituted by Dr. Fell in 1948 and maintained and expanded by Drs. Weinberg and Tatooles was ended. For a period of 13 years, only emergency heart operations were done at County. In 1989, pediatric heart cases from County continued to be performed by Dr. David Monson, Dr. Weinberg's associate.

After the end of Dr. Levitsky's chairmanship, several surgeons performed adult heart operations at County beginning in 1991. Dr. Vincent Kucich performed about 50 cases in that year and continued to operate at County until he entered private practice with Dr. Tom Murphy in 1993. Dr. Cyrus Seery became the chairman at County and was able to do 50 cardiac operations that year despite maintaining a busy private practice. Dr. Robert March, a graduate of the Presbyterian-St. Luke's program, joined the staff in 1992. By 1994, the U of I and County had mutually terminated their association, and arrangements were made to replace the U of I residency programs and institute Rush-Presbyterian-St. Luke's programs. This was actually done in one year without any major administrative problems. Under the leadership of the new academic affiliation and the hard work of Dr. Edward Savage, the number of cardiac cases done at County rose to nearly 300 by the late 1990s. The bulk of the work done in the later 1990s and 2000s was under the direction of Drs. William Warren and Ozura Okoha. Dr. Milloy returned as an attending in 1983 and remained active until his retirement in 1997.

The program, which began as a close affiliation between the County and Rush and survived a transition as an independent service with distinction, is still healthy after providing learning experiences to the residents and students of both the University of Illinois and the revitalized Rush College of Medicine.

## References

1. Schmitz RL and Oh,TT. *The Remarkable Surgical Practice of John Benjamin Murphy.* Urbana:University of Illinois Press,1993.
2. Milloy F. The Contribution of John B. Murphy to Thoracic Surgery. *Surg Gynecol Obst.* 1990;171:421-32.
3. Murphy JB.Surgery of the lung. *JAMA.* 1898;31:151.
4. Murphy JB.Surgery of the lung. *JAMA.* 1898;31:281.
5. Murphy JB.Surgery of the lung. *JAMA.* 1898;31:341.
6. IBID 341
7. Speed K. Edward Wyllys Andrews (1856-1927) *Proc Chicago Inst Med.* 1927;6:263.
8. Andrews EW. A future for pulmonary surgery. *JAMA.* 1885;261:261.
9. Meyer KA. In Memoriam, Marshall Davidson (1896-1940), *Transact West Surg Assoc.* 1940;55:298.
10. Coffey RJ: John Dorsey In Memoriam , Transact *Am Surg Assoc.* 1993;45:380.
11. Shumacker H,B Jr, *The Evolution of Cardiac Surgery.* Indianapolis:University of Indiana Press, 1992.
12. Milloy FJ. Fell EZH. Coarctation of the aorta. *Arch Surg.* 1959;78:759.

# 15

# Evolution of Pediatric Surgery at CCH

*Hernan M. Reyes, MD, FAAP, FACS*
*Jayant Radhakrishnan, MD, FAAP, FACS*

- *Introduction*
- *The Beginning*
- *The Era of John Raffensperger*
- *Combined Pediatric Surgical Service with University of Illinois*
- *The Era of Hernan Reyes*
- *Rush University Medical Center and CCH*
- *Epilogue*
- *References*

## Introduction

The development of Pediatric Surgery at Cook County Hospital as a surgical subspecialty parallels much of what has taken place in surgical practice throughout the country after World War II, more specifically during the sixth decade of the 20th century. Prior to that era and despite the pioneering work of Drs. William Ladd and Robert Gross of Boston, very few surgical practitioners devoted their full-time practice to the surgical care of children. The concept that special skills, knowledge, and training were essential in the practice of pediatric surgery slowly gained ground. Full-time pediatric surgeons were, for the most part, concentrated in children's hospitals throughout the country where complex surgical cases were referred for care. General hospitals with pediatric departments depended on general surgeons to perform common procedures. It was not until the middle of the 1960s that trained pediatric surgeons started to practice in general hospitals with pediatric intensive care units and Level I neonatal intensive care units staffed with appropriately trained personnel.

The growth of pediatric surgery in this country was slowed by general surgeons who were threatened by the establishment of a separate subspecialty. In many major Institutions, department heads of surgery were of the opinion that a competent general surgeon was sufficiently trained to provide adequate care to children with surgical problems.

By 1950, there were 18 approved training programs in pediatric surgery. While the American Academy of Pediatrics established a surgical section in 1948, and the *Journal of Pediatric Surgery* started publication in 1966, it was not until 1970 that the first president of the American Pediatric Surgical Association was elected. The American Board of Surgery granted official recognition of the specialty in 1975 when the first Certificate of Special Competence in Pediatric Surgery was issued following a written examination given in 1974. Recertification required successful passing of a written examination every 10 years.

## The Beginning

When the old Cook County Hospital was opened in January 10, 1866,[1] the first surgeon, Dr. George K. Ammerman, a well-known surgeon and politician instrumental in establishing CCH, performed his first operation at this institution. It was a limb amputation. Among the early operations was the removal of a bladder stone in a three-year-old female child.[2] At the turn of the 20th century, Dr. John B. Murphy is reported to have removed a kidney tumor (most likely a Wilm's tumor) in a child, and his early work on appendicitis included the first intestinal anastomosis at County using a button.[3] Surgery in infants and children was performed by general surgeons without any special training in pediatric surgery, doctors who also took care of adult patients with burns, fractures, and urologic and neurosurgical problems. Prior to 1963, direct patient care at the institution was relegated to interns and residents under the supervision of volunteer senior attending physicians and their respective associates; thereafter, full-time, in-house attending surgeons assumed this responsibility.

Pediatric patients were admitted to a separate ward in the hospital, and in 1900, Dr. Isaac Abt, an attending physician at County who would later become the chairman of pediatrics at Northwestern University Medical School, described the children's ward at the institution as "a dark, unattractive place cut up by big columns which shut out light and air."[4] To rectify the unmet needs of pediatric patients, a three-story children's hospital with 120 beds was built in 1904 (Figure 15–1). The facility was subsequently replaced in 1927, with a new eight-story children's hospital built at the Cook County Hospital site on the west side of Chicago (Figure 15–2). By then, Cook County Hospital was a medical complex with several buildings housing 2,700 beds. All pediatric activities were moved into the new building on April 1, 1928. While pediatrics was already a recognized specialty, there were no surgeons at County who devoted their entire practice to the care of pediatric patients with surgical problems. Pediatrics was

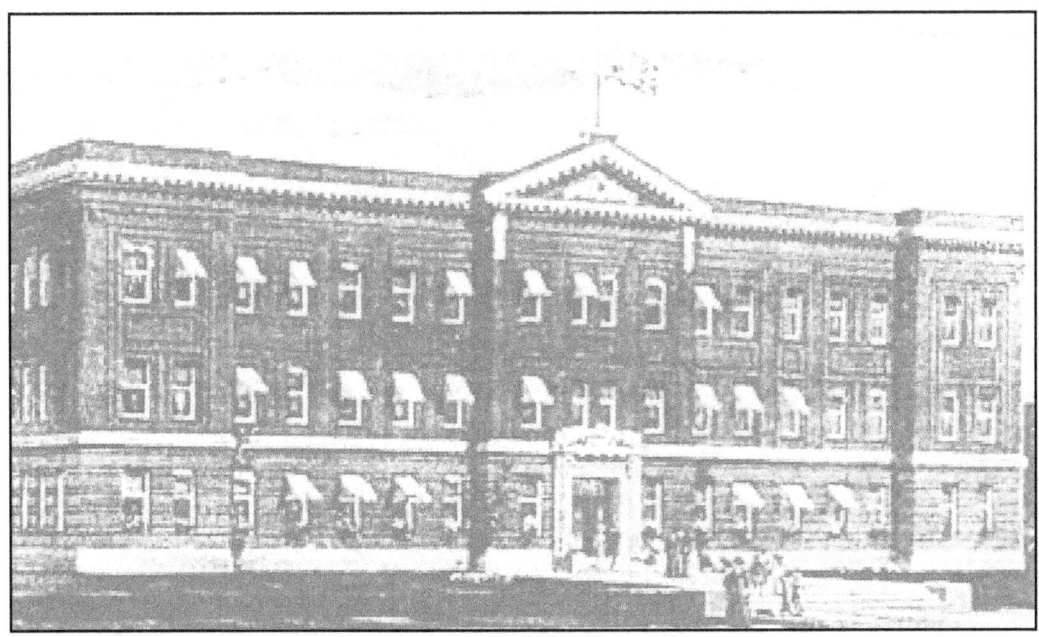

*Figure 15–1 The first Children's Hospital built in 1904*

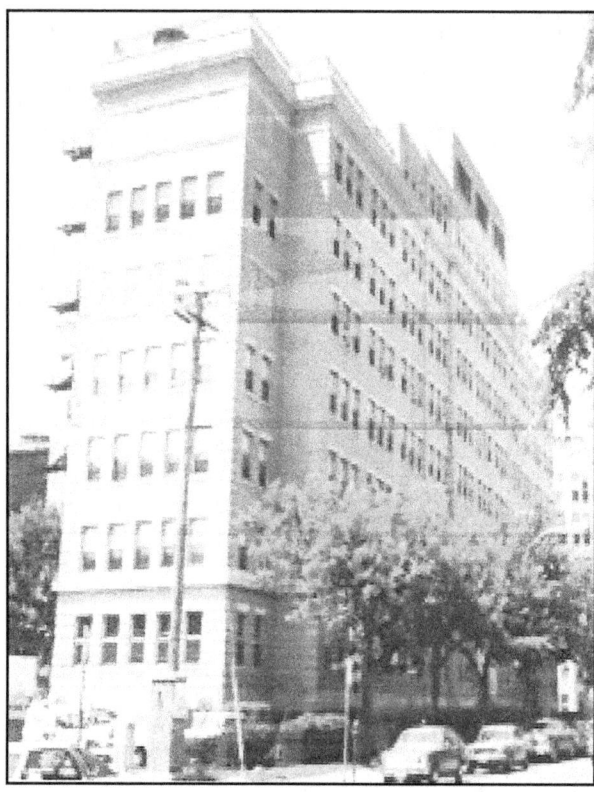

*Figure 15–2 New Children's Hospital built in 1927*

administratively a children's section of the hospital with Dr. Julius H. Hess as the chief of staff from 1920 to 1927. Dr. Hess and Dr. Arthur H. Parmelee, another member of the children's section, introduced the use of covered incubators and special clinics for premature infants and the diagnosis of diseases in newborn infants.[5] Dr. Maurice L. Blatt became chief of staff of the children's division from 1928 to 1944, and Dr. Samuel Hoffman, the first pediatric resident at the Children's Hospital in 1927, was the chief of staff from 1955 to 1956. Dr. Joseph Greengard, a County intern who practiced pediatrics at Michael Reese Hospital, became the full-time director of pediatrics at Cook County Children's Hospital in 1958. Although the Children's Hospital had a separate emergency room and operating room for pediatric patients, most diagnostic facilities were shared with adult patients in the main hospital.

Other surgeons during the early half of the 20th century, such as Drs. Harry I. Oberhelman and John Keeley (who successively served as chairman of surgery at Loyola's Stritch School of Medicine) were on the pediatric surgery service. Dr. Keeley, who had observed Dr. Robert Gross at the Boston Children's Hospital, did most of the newborn surgery at County. While serving as an associate of Dr. Oberhelman in 1941, Dr. Keeley was prevailed upon by Dr. Karl Meyer (the much-admired and respected medical warden appointed in 1914, later becoming chief of surgery and, in 1940, medical superintendent of all County institutions up until his retirement in 1967) to perform a uretero-sigmoidostomy, a new and innovative treatment on a newborn infant with an extrophy of the bladder.[6] A distinguished and skillful general surgeon, Dr. Meyer himself performed the first successful repair in Chicago of an esophageal atresia with fistula in a newborn infant at Columbus Hospital.[7]

From 1935 to 1946, the two most important surgeons with responsibility for the children's surgical ward were Drs. Edwin Miller and Sumner Koch. Although both surgeons had been members of the surgical staff at CCH since 1926, their specific assignment to the children's surgical ward was not made until 1935. Dr. Miller, a fine general surgeon, was known for his traction treatment for supracondylar fractures of the humerus that eliminated the nerve and vascular complications of this injury.[8] He performed the full spectrum of pediatric surgery including newborns with intestinal atresia,[9] intussusceptions, and the conservative treatment of a giant omphalocoele. He reported a reduction in the mortality rate from appendicitis in children with use of intravenous fluids.[10] Mark Ravitch is purported to have commented that much of his inspiration for the barium enema treatment of intussusception, which he advocated, came from Dr. Miller. Dr. Miller remained a voluntary attending consultant in pediatric surgery even after his retirement in 1960.

Dr. Sumner Koch was famous for his treatment of hand injuries and burns. The burn unit at Cook County Hospital bears his name in honor of his early contributions to the treatment of burns. He and Dr. Harvey Allen established a clinic designed to treat hand injuries, burns, and infections based in the Children's Hospital. Dr. Allen presented his experience in the management of a thousand cases of burn patients from one to 14 years of age admitted to Cook County Children's surgical service between 1947 to 1951 at the annual meeting of the American Surgical Association in April 1951. Emphasis was on blood volume replacement, recognizing the unique difference between adults and children, immediate burn wound debridement, thin layered vaseline impregnated dressing replaced after six days with fine mesh gauze, burn wound excision, and early coverage with skin graft.[11] This pioneering work revolutionized the care of children with burns and led to more research and refinement in the management of these patients that characterized the burn unit subsequently established at Cook County Hospital.

When Dr. Miller relinquished his responsibilities for the children's surgical ward in 1946, his assistant at Rush, Dr. Egbert Fell, took over this assignment. A true general surgeon and role model for surgical trainees, Dr. Fell provided most of the pediatric surgical coverage at Cook County Hospital, although most of the onsite supervision of work by trainees was provided by associates of senior attending surgeons, most of whom knew very little about pediatric surgery. Dr. Fell also had a variety of surgical interests, including the treatment of pediatric fractures that he authored for a chapter in *Christopher's Textbook of Surgery*. Eventually, he became better known for developing cardiac surgery at County. He was the only surgeon who was allowed by Dr. Meyer to develop the evolving surgical specialty of cardiac surgery. Together with Dr. Benjamin M. Gasul, a pediatric cardiologist, and Dr. Maurice Lev, cardiac pathologist at the Hektoen Institute, he established the cardiac surgery program and performed the first cardiac operations on children with patent ductus arteriosus and coarctation of the aorta. He and Dr. Milton Weinberg performed the first open-heart operation in Chicago at Cook County Hospital.[12]

Pediatric surgical care at the institution was associated with an unacceptably high mortality rate. Dr. Raffensperger relates his experience as a surgical resident in the mid 1950s while assisting on the surgery of an infant with bowel obstruction by a night surgeon who closed the abdomen as a negative laparotomy. The infant subsequently died, and the autopsy revealed aganglionic bowel as the cause of the bowel obstruction. The obstruction could have been relieved by a simple colostomy that the resident suggested, but he was turned down repeatedly by several of the attending surgeons. In 1964, Dr. Raffensperger published a paper, co-authored by Drs. Freeark and Fell, illustrating the sad state of affairs regarding infant surgery between 1954 and 1958 at the institution where the mortality rate in babies with intestinal obstruction was 72 percent and 14 percent in babies with pyloric stenosis.[13]

During much of the 1950s and 1960s, routine pediatric surgical cases were supervised by volunteer part-time attending surgeons such as Dr. Paul Fox, an attending surgeon at the Chicago Children's Memorial Hospital, and other general surgeons, principally Drs. Edwin Sinaiko and Robert Condon. A senior general surgery resident, a junior resident, and an intern completed the surgical team responsible for the care of pediatric surgical patients. Emergency cases at night and weekends were cared for by the chief general surgery resident on call who, for the most part, relied on the senior attending surgeon or his associate for coverage.

The state of surgical care at the hospital was such that in the late 1950s Dr. Joseph Greengard, chair of the Department of Pediatrics, strongly recommended to the Department of Surgery that pediatric surgery be organized as a full surgical subspecialty division within the Department of Surgery, staffed by a full-time pediatric surgeon. This goal was soon fulfilled when Dr. Robert J. Freeark was appointed as the first full-time salaried attending surgeon at County, director of surgical education in 1958, and later chief of surgery in 1963. More than anyone else, he radically restructured the Department of Surgery. He gradually changed the supervision of interns and residents and ultimately shifted responsibility for patient care at the institution from a group of part-time volunteer attending staff to a full-time, on-site salaried attending physician. Experience eventually proved that the full-time system was far superior to a part-time, volunteer attending staff, regardless of the latter group's honest motivation and dedication.

## The Era of John Raffensperger

As part of Dr. Freeark's plan to establish full-time, salaried attending surgical coverage in all surgical specialties at Cook County Hospital, he appointed Dr. John Raffensperger, who was then the surgical associate of Dr. Fell at the Cook County Children's Hospital, to become the full-time pediatric surgeon and chief of the service in 1964. Fell was further made the acting chair of the division of thoracic surgery when Dr. Milton Weinberg resigned from the volunteer attending staff, although to this day he does not remember whether he was officially appointed to that position.

Dr. Raffensperger single-handedly provided attending coverage for all major cases, including pediatric thoracic surgery. He elevated the surgical care of infants and children to its highest level with competence and dedication, and for the first time, surgical care of the pediatric patients at County was comparable to other children's hospitals in the country, which were similarly staffed by full-time trained pediatric surgeons. He was virtually on call every night for all emergencies including trauma, the volume of which was quite large considering that at the time, Cook County Hospital was the recipient of most patients in the city, both adults and children, who were suffering from severe trauma. Traumatic injuries included gunshot wounds, stab wounds, falls from heights, burns, vehicular accidents (either pedestrian or passenger), and victims of child abuse. Occasionally, Dr. Olga Jonasson, a general and renal transplant surgeon from the University of Illinois Hospital, would likewise attend to some major cases.

Dr. Raffensperger initiated clinical research and organized teaching sessions with students and surgical residents. He published his clinical experiences in surgical journals, and together with general surgery residents presented them at meetings of the surgical section of the American Academy of Pediatrics and local surgical associations. While he was a stern and strict taskmaster, he was nonetheless an excellent teacher with superb surgical skills and clinical judgment. He required observance of proper professional demeanor in the classroom (on a number of occasions, he was noted to have thrown a penny to wake up a student who had fallen asleep during one of his lectures), the operating room, and the wards while making patient rounds. His biggest emphasis during clinical rounds and in the operating room was a rigid discipline in decision-making, good surgical skills, and careful application of good postoperative care. Any deviation, however minor, from what was expected of the house staff was rewarded with a strong reprimand. He became a role model and mentor to a great number of surgical residents, pediatric surgical trainees, and medical students, some of whom went on to become chiefs of pediatric surgery at various children's hospitals and full-time pediatric surgeons at medical centers in this country.

In 1964, Dr. Hernan M. Reyes, who had just completed his general surgery residency in the program, stayed on as a research fellow in the Department of Surgery at Hektoen Institute of Medical Research with Dr. Abe Marks, an immunologist. Dr. Freeark assigned him as the senior resident in pediatric surgery during that entire period under the supervision of Dr. Raffensperger, whose influence directed Reyes to a career in pediatric surgery rather than the then-emerging specialty of transplantation surgery. Without any doubt, Dr. Raffensperger brought the institution to the forefront for the excellence of pediatric surgical care during his tenure. Dr. Raffensperger left County in 1970 to assume the position of professor of surgery at Northwestern University Medical School, director of the division of pediatric surgery, and later as surgeon-in-chief of the Children's Memorial Hospital of Chicago. He eventually returned to County as a volunteer surgeon in 2003 to substitute for the incumbent chair of the division of pediatric surgery, Dr. Katherine Bass, during her pregnancy.

At the time of Dr. Raffenperger's tenure as full-time chief of pediatric surgery at County, surgical patients were admitted to the fourth floor of the Children's Hospital (Ward 46). General pediatric surgery patients were assigned to a section of the ward; orthopedic patients usually attached to various traction devices went to a separate section, and burn patients to another. During any given day, there were from 10 to 12 patients in traction and six to 10 patients with burns undergoing daily dressing changes. The total bed census of the ward was 60, although additional beds were opened whenever required. Neonatal patients with surgical problems remained on the third floor (Ward 36), which was designated as the neonatal ICU (NICU) and neonatal step-down unit with a total of 66 beds. Patients with medical problems were admitted to the second floor (Ward 26) and sixth floor (Ward 66), and the seventh floor (Ward 76) housed the pediatric ICU and pediatric cardiology service. The fifth floor of the pediatric hospital was reserved for adult surgical patients under Dr. Karl Meyer's service. On Dr. Meyer's retirement in the late 1960s, Ward 56 was converted into a burn unit for adult and pediatric patients with its own operating rooms, separate ICU, and hydrotherapy sections. The adult hand service, previously a part of the burn unit, was eventually incorporated with the orthopedic and plastic surgery services in the main hospital. The operating room and recovery room of the Children's Hospital was on the eighth floor of the building. This floor was connected to the main hospital operating room by a covered bridge. The children's operating room was used for pediatric patients by the various surgical specialties except for one room that was used exclusively for adult patients, which was housed on the fifth floor of the Children's Hospital under Dr. Meyer's service until his retirement. The house staff assigned to the pediatric surgery service consisted of an intern and a junior and senior general surgery resident from the free-standing CCH general surgery residency program. In 1978, the residents assigned to the service were from the University of Illinois-Cook County Hospital integrated program. Starting in 1994, a gradual transition of residents took place from the University of Illinois program to the Rush University Medical Center-Cook County Hospital integrated residency program in general surgery.

## Combined Pediatric Surgical Service with University of Illinois

Dr. Hugh Firor, who trained with Professor Jan Louw at the Red Cross Hospital in Capetown, South Africa, was recruited in 1971. He took over as chief of the division of pediatric surgery and continued to provide the leadership for the surgical care of pediatric patients. Dr. Firor established a combined parallel pediatric surgery service at County and the University of Illinois Hospital with a unified attending surgeon coverage but separate residents assigned from each institution's general surgery residency program. Outpatient clinics and regularly scheduled operations were conducted at both institutions. Pediatric surgical patients continued to be admitted to Ward 46 of the Children's Hospital, and consultations were made in the medical wards. At the University of Illinois Hospital, Pediatrics was on the 13th floor, and the slow-moving elevators (slower than those at County) were a constant source of aggravation to the surgical residents who had to start pediatric surgery rounds early in the morning in order to b able to get to the operating rooms on time. In 1973, Dr. Firor recruited Dr. Art Besser, who trained in pediatric surgery at different periods with Drs. Orvar Swenson and John Raffensperger at Children's Memorial Hospital in Chicago, as a part-time salaried attending pediatric surgeon in the division. At that time, Dr. Besser had a full-time private pediatric surgery practice at Lutheran General Hospital in Park Ridge, Illinois. In January 1976, when Dr. Firor unexpectedly left County on very short notice, Dr. Besser became the de facto pediatric surgeon for the division of pediatric surgery, even though he was a part-time physician. Additional coverage was provided by full-time general surgeons on the staff, particularly Dr. Miguel Teresi, and on occasion, by volunteer attending surgeons who remained on the staff to cover routine pediatric surgical cases.

The minor crisis fortuitously benefitted Dr. Jayant Radhakrishnan. He had come to the United States with the express purpose of obtaining pediatric surgery training. At the time, he was on the verge of completing retraining in general surgery at County, having completed a full residency in general surgery including pediatric surgery training as a senior registrar following his graduation from medical school in India. In June of 1976, Dr. Herand Abcarian, Dr. Gerald Moss, then chief of surgery at County, and Dr. Jack Saletta, general surgery residency program director and chief of general surgery, persuaded him to stay on at County as fellow/surgical attending in pediatric surgery. After careful soul searching, he decided to remain at County and turned down an offer for a pediatric hyperalimentation fellowship at the Medical College of South Carolina, Charleston, with Dr. H. Bieman Othersen, the distinguished head of pediatric surgery at that institution who would have assisted him in obtaining a pediatric surgery fellowship. Dr. Radhakrishnan came to the conclusion that the wealth of experience at County could not have been duplicated anywhere else, and to this day, he has no regrets whatsoever of his decision. At the very outset, he was on call every day and covered all pediatric surgical work with assistance from Dr. Miguel Teresi. For neonatal problems, Dr. Raffensperger was available for consultation and/or coverage. Dr. Radhakrishnan relates that throughout his entire career, the only occasion he interacted with Dr. Raffensperger in a civil fashion was in 1976 when the latter came to County to help him irrigate the colon of a newborn infant with meconium ileus obstruction.

## The Era of Hernan Reyes

In 1976, Dr. Hernan M. Reyers ( Figure 15–3) was a half-time attending surgeon at Wyler Children's Hospital (now defunct) of the University of Chicago and associate professor of surgery at the medical school with a busy private practice in the southwest suburbs. He was recruited by Dr. Gerald Moss, chief of surgery at County (who later become dean of the College of Medicine at the University of Illinois) and Dr. Lloyd Nyhus, the Warren Cole Professor of Surgery and head of the Department of Surgery at the University of Illinois College of Medicine, to become the chairman of the division of pediatric surgery at Cook County Hospital and simultaneously professor of surgery and chief of the section of pediatric surgery at the University of Illinois College of Medicine and the University of Illinois Hospital. By this time, there was a close academic relationship in the Department of Surgery between Cook County Hospital and the University of Illinois College of Medicine in Chicago. He joined both institutions on September 16, 1976, and maintained an organizational structure of a combined pediatric surgical service at County and the University of Illinois Hospital with parallel programs, a unified faculty and educational program and separate set of general surgery residents covering each institution.

With Dr. Radhakrishnan (Figure 15–4) on board and Dr. Besser remaining as a part-time salaried attending surgeon, clinical coverage in pediatric surgery of both institutions was effectively provided, including the organization of a weekly pediatric surgery conference and teaching of medical students from the University of Illinois. Routine surgery was scheduled three times a week at County, once a week at the University Hospital, and emergency surgery at both institutions was fully staffed. Most major operations were performed by both Drs. Reyes and Radhakrishnan at County and by Dr. Reyes at the University of Illinois Hospital. Having recognized a deficiency in the pediatric urological coverage at both institutions, the opportunity to better provide this care was realized when Dr. Radhakrishnan indicated his interest in this subspecialty. He secured a pediatric urology fellowship with the famous Dr. W. Hardy Hendren at Boston Children's Hospital from July 1977 to June 1978. During their first meeting, Radhakrishnan was informed by Dr. Hendren that he was often called "hardly human" for reasons that would be apparent in due course.

With Dr. Besser's 1977 departure for Henry Ford Hospital in Detroit,

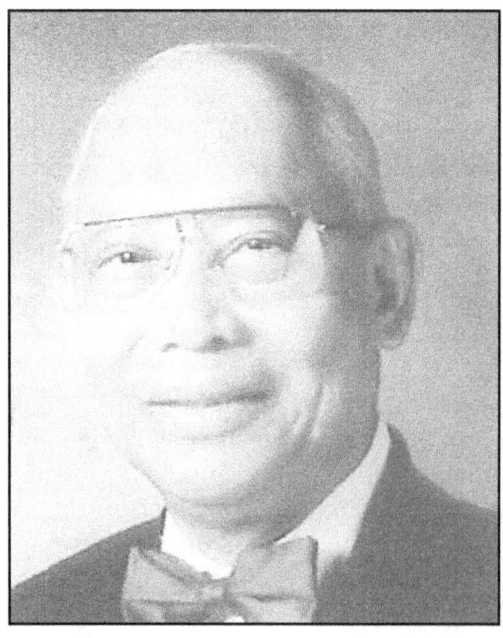

*Figure 15–3 Hernan M. Reyes*

Michigan, to assume the position of chief of pediatric surgery, Dr. Art Rettig, an associate of Dr. Richard Goldstein at Lutheran General Hospital, was persuaded to join the staff at County as a part-time, salaried attending pediatric surgeon. Trained in pediatric surgery at Children's Memorial Hospital, Dr. Rettig religiously stayed on at County, and provided much-needed assistance in both teaching and clinical practice until he left for Rockford, Illinois, in 1980 to establish his own practice in that city.

Several faculty recruitments soon followed. Dr. Kevin Pringle joined the full-time staff in pediatric surgery on July 1, 1978. A graduate of the University of Otago Medical School in Dunedin, New Zealand, he obtained his surgical training at the Dunedin Hospital and a pediatric surgery fellowship at the Royal Children's Hospital in Melbourne, Australia. He then joined Dr. John Burrington at the University of Chicago for a year prior to joining the pediatric surgery service at the University of Illinois and Cook County Hospital. His primary responsibility was to cover the clinical work and teaching at the University of Illinois in addition to continuing his research on fetal surgery and therapy.[14] He was a tremendous asset to the service, but in 1981, he was recruited to join the pediatric surgery faculty at the University of Iowa where he remained for six years. After this, he returned to New Zealand as a senior pediatric surgery consultant, and in 2001, he was appointed professor of surgery and chairman of the Department of Surgery, Obstetrics, and Gynecology at his alma matter. He continued his research activities, and at one time served as president of the International Fetal Medicine and Surgery Society.

Soon after Dr. Radhakrishnan returned from Boston Children's Hospital, he was appointed chief of the section of pediatric urology at both Cook County Hospital and the University of Illinois Hospital. This was in addition to his participation in the clinical care of general pediatric surgery patients and teaching of residents and medical students. He remained full time up until 1984 when he de-

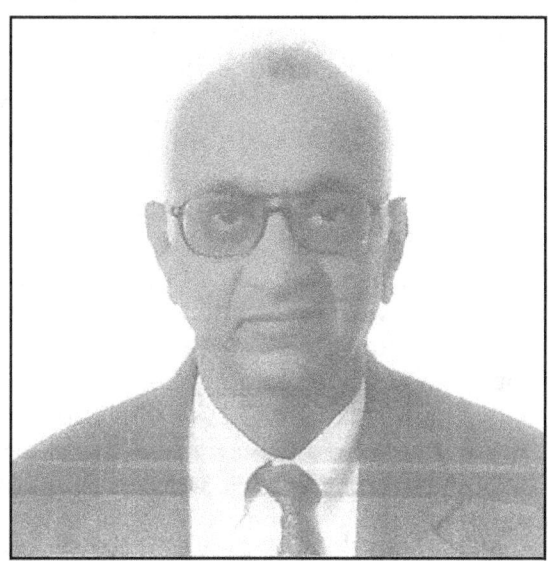

*Figure 15–4 Jayant Radhakrishnan*

cided to start a private practice in pediatric surgery at Lutheran General Hospital. He continued to provide voluntary coverage for pediatric urology and general pediatric surgery until 1985 when he left Cook County Hospital completely. The departure of Dr. Radhakrishnan from the West Side Medical Center was a tremendous loss to both County and the University of Illinois because the division chair of pediatric surgery relied on him to take full charge of the service at both institutions during his absence. A patient and soft-spoken man, he was deeply admired by all his colleagues, peers, residents, and students, not only because of his teaching, superior surgical skill, and excellent clinical judgment, but also the caring attitude he always had for his patients. In 1991, Dr. Jayant Radhakrishnan returned to the West Side Medical Center as professor of surgery and urology and chief of the section of pediatric surgery and pediatric urology at the University of Illinois College of Medicine and the University of Illinois Hospital, after being recruited by Dr. Gerald S. Moss, dean of the college of medicine, and Dr. Herand Abcarian, professor and chairman of the department.

On July 1, 1981, Dr. Zafer Skef joined the full-time staff in pediatric surgery with responsibilities at both institutions. He received fellowship training in plastic surgery and a fellowship in pediatric surgery at Children's Memorial Hospital following graduation from Damascus University College of Medicine, Syria. His major interest was in the development of an artificial rectal sphincter utilizing the gluteus maximus muscle in patients who were incontinent following pull-through operation for imperforate anus.[15] He was also interested in plastic surgery and contributed a great deal in the clinical coverage of pediatric surgery at both institutions. Unfortunately, he was unable to return to the United States after he left to visit his family in Syria, his native country, in 1983.

Following the departure of Drs. Pringle and Skef, Dr. Janet Meller, a graduate of the Chicago Medical School who completed her general surgery residency at the University of Chicago and a year of pediatric surgery fellowship with Dr. Dennis Shermeta at the same institution, joined the full-time attending staff as an associate surgeon at County and the University of Illinois. This was followed a few years later by the recruitment of Dr. Deborah Loeff who received her pediatric surgery fellowship at The Hospital for Sick Children, Toronto, Canada, with Dr. Robert Filler. By 1985, three full-time pediatric attending surgeons continued covering Cook County Hospital-University of Illinois Hospital in addition to the Rush-Presbyterian St. Luke's Medical Center. The proximity of these three institutions with each other at the West Side Medical Center allowed relatively easy coverage by the three members of the attending staff. Dr. Loeff confined her clinical activities at County and Rush, while Dr. Meller was primarily at County and the University of Illinois. Dr. Antonio Chaviano, a pediatric urologist, soon joined the attending staff in the divisions of urology and pediatric surgery. Dr. Angel Bassuk received appointment as a voluntary consultant in the division. Dr. Bassuk obtained his fellowship in pediatric surgery at St. Christopher Children's Hospital in Philadelphia and had a thriving private pediatric surgery practice at the Advocate Christ Hospital in Oak Lawn, Illinois, and at Little Company of Mary Hospital in Evergreen Park, Illinois.

With the continued increase in pediatric trauma admissions, especially after the designation of Cook County Hospital as one of the five Level I Pediatric Trauma Centers in metropolitan Chicago in 1987, Dr. John R. Hall was recruited into the divisions of general surgery and pediatric surgery at County. He assumed a dual role as a full-time attending surgeon in general surgery and surgical critical care, and section chief of pediatric trauma and pediatric surgical critical care. Dr. Hall was a graduate of Stanford University and the University of Arizona College of Medicine and a board-certified general surgeon who completed a pediatric trauma and critical care fellowship at the Shock Trauma Institute, University of Maryland, Johns Hopkins University, and the Zurich Children's Hospital

With the appointment of Dr. Reyes as chairman of the Department of Surgery at Cook County Hospital in December 1986 in an acting capacity and full chair on January 7, 1987, Reyes found that the new load of administrative responsibilities limited his participation in the clinical work and teaching in the division of pediatric surgery, leaving the major coverage of the clinical service to Drs. Meller and Loeff, and in trauma to Dr. Hall. Reyes remained an active member of the pediatric surgery attending staff, however, rotating regularly with the rest on the call schedule and operating one day a week at Cook County Hospital, in addition to covering emergency cases during the absence of the other members of the attending staff. He also remained available to his colleagues for immediate consultation. In 1990, he relinquished his position as chief of the section of pediatric surgery at the University of Illinois although he remained on the active attending staff and associate director of the integrated residency program in general surgery. In a similar fashion, he gave up his position as chairman of the division of pediatric surgery at County in 1992 and appointed Dr. Janet L. Meller to the position.

The pediatric surgery service at both Cook County Children's Hospital and University of Illinois Hospital provided the full spectrum of surgical care including complex general surgical problems in infants and children, in addition to thoracic noncardiac and urologic surgery. For several years, the annual operative case load at County was close to a thousand. Approximately four hundred cases were operated at the University of Illinois Hospital. There were two half-day outpatient clinics at County and one half-day at the University of Illinois. Referrals were generated from outlying hospitals, especially those in the west and south sides of Chicago. The wealth of pediatric surgical experience at one time convinced the faculty to apply for a fellowship program in pediatric surgery, but the deficiency in solid tumors and Dr. Reyes' commitment to the training of the general surgery residents quashed this plan altogether.

Together with the oncology service at both County and the University of Illinois, the pediatric surgical service participated with National Cancer Study protocols in the treatment of solid tumors in children. During the last quarter of the 20th century, new developments and new technology further improved the surgical care of infants and children, not only at Cook County Children's Hospital but throughout the country. Surgical practice conformed to the latest accepted standards and techniques in the management of complex surgical problems in children and was likewise guided by ongoing clinical experience of the attending staff and research protocols conducted in the service. For example, the surgical treatment of imperforate anus transitioned from the abdominoperineal approach advocated by Kiesewetter to that of a posterior anorectoplasty procedure described by Pena. The old concept of immediate and emergent surgical repair of a congenital diaphragmatic hernia was replaced by a preoperative medical management of respiratory failure followed later by repair of the defect. At County, we can count on a number of innovative treatment modalities conducted by the attending staff that has reduced the mortality of patients with complex surgical problems. A few include the following:

A series of infants with gastroschisis were treated with an 85 percent success rate in achieving primary closure utilizing full thickness abdominal wall stretching with only 25 percent requiring an artificial silo that was removed sooner with secondary closure of the abdomen than previously described without any significant morbidity and no mortality.

A series of patients with Hirschprung's disease underwent a two-stage operation (first stage, rectal biopsy with frozen section biopsy and diverting colostomy followed six to 12 weeks later, with a second stage consisting of colostomy resection and primary modified Soave pull-through operation) in contrast to what was the standard practice at the time, a four-stage operation (first stage, rectal biopsy; second stage, diverting colostomy; third stage, pull-through operation; and fourth stage, colostomy closure) with no postoperative morbidity or mortality and on long-term follow-up, a 7 percent fecal incontinence rate, a complication similar to other medical-center experience reported in the literature.[17] Additional studies showed a reduction in the infectious complications of perforated appendicitis in a large series of patients treated in a prospective fashion with appendectomy, generalized peritoneal lavage, and no drains without primary skin closure.[18] To prevent a tight wrap from a Nissen fundoplication with serious consequences in patients treated with intractable GE reflux, the staff advocated and routinely inserted an appropriate sized intra-esophageal bougie orally prior to performing the fundoplication.[19]

The experience and practice of the entire staff in pediatric trauma care was significantly increased and refined, especially after the recruitment of Dr. John R. Hall and the designation of the Cook County Children's Hospital as one of Chicago's five Level I Pediatric Trauma Centers in 1988, a few months after the designation of Level I Adult Trauma Centers. It was the consensus that seriously injured children should be treated at a center with personnel and facilities dedicated only for children. The ICU experience demonstrated a greater than 50 percent higher mortality rate in severely injured children transferred to Cook County Children's Hospital after prior treatment elsewhere as compared to a similar cohort of patients treated as direct admits to County. This study was widely used to justify the development of Level I Pediatric Trauma Centers in the city.[20] The pediatric surgical staff with their resident and the radiology department were among the first in the country who demonstrated the accuracy of using CT scans to evaluate organ injury from blunt trauma of the abdomen; they were among the first to recommend that CT scans can supplant the use of peritoneal lavage, an invasive procedure in the evaluation of blunt abdominal injury.[21] More importantly, the first year experience of the Level I pediatric trauma center at County had a mortality rate that was lower than what was predicted when compared to other Pediatric Trauma Centers in the Country, according to a formula devised by the National Pediatric Registry. County had one of the top-three outcomes in head injury in North America, as recorded in the same registry data. County was the only unit where the outcome of infants with severe head trauma was as good as that of older children. All three hospitals followed similar strict protocols that mandated ICP measurement for patients with a Glasgow Coma Scale (GCS) <8.[22] The pediatric trauma center at County, together with others, reconfirmed that children with blunt trauma have a significantly better outcome at designated pediatric trauma centers as compared with adult trauma centers with pediatric capacity or no trauma center at all. Additionally, not only was survival increased, but also the incidence of nonoperative management of liver and spleen injuries was significantly ($p < 0.0001$) higher.[23] As early as 1979, the attending staff advocated the nonoperative treatment of clinically stable patients with solid organ injuries following blunt abdominal trauma.[24]

The use of strict protocols for all injured children admitted to Cook County Children's Hospital pediatric trauma center was ahead of its time due to the leadership of the department chair of surgery and the division heads of neurosurgery and orthopedics. This dynamic protocol allowed changes to practices that did not work and the immediate use of those that did without the random changes of the physician on duty that day. This protocol allowed County to present the first major review of nonoperative management of penetrating neck injuries as well as of penetrating abdominal stab wounds: both are now standard practice at all trauma centers in the world. Additionally, County was at the forefront in demonstrating that penetrating extremity injuries did not require angiography for proximity alone. In terms of advances, the pediatric trauma center was one of the first hospitals in America to use internal fixation for children with femur fractures, allowing early mobilization instead of keeping them in bed in traction. This treatment was especially useful in those suffering from multiple injuries who required early mobilization and ambulation. The staff also presented its data showing that falls were the seventh leading cause of death in all children and third in the one- to four-year-old age group, and that "minor" falls could cause death. This study, along with other pediatric trauma centers in Chicago, prompted a campaign to develop a "kids can't fly program" by the city mandating the use of bars in all high-rise windows to successfully help prevent this cause of death and injury. The pediatric trauma center at County also had a full-time pediatrician who dealt with the courts on a daily basis as an advocate for abused children.

In pediatric urology, complex urologic reconstructions were carried out for bladder and cloacal extrophy and persistent cloaca[25,26,27] and trauma.[28] A large series of patients (the largest in the Chicago area) with Prune Belly Syndrome were treated with early, complete reconstruction of the genitourinary tract. The results in this series of patients were superior to those reported in the literature. This approach was taken at a time when many important centers felt that Prune Belly Syndrome should be managed nonoperatively since these patients are a high operative risk.[29,30]

On the nonmedical side, numerous anecdotes have been written about residents' experiences at Cook County Hospital. A number of these incidents at the Children's Hospital illustrate the awe-inspiring rewards of medical practice.

- *Once, the members of the staff worked feverishly to save the life of a six-year-old girl. She had been stabbed 48 times, two of which wounds were potentially fatal, to the heart and aorta. The girl survived and on her return for a postoperative visit several months later, she related to the group that she was going to pursue a career in criminal justice.*
- *Then there was the sad tale of a sandwich vendor in front of the Children's Hospital on Wood Street who was shot and killed by two gunmen while waiting for the hospital elevator to escape his assailants. Evidently, he had never entered the hospital before, or he would have realized how slowly the elevators moved.*
- *And there was the time a Roma family patriarch demanded to see the head of the hospital when he was told by Dr. James Stone, chairman of the division of neurosurgery, that his son needed an operation for a brain tumor. He agreed to the procedure only after a conference with Dr. Reyes, the chairman of the Department of Surgery, Dr. Stone, and himself. It became clear that he wanted to hear from the "head honcho" the information regarding the surgical treatment being simultaneously given by Dr. Stone. A minor disruption in the hospital and the neighborhood occurred when the king and his clan put up several tents in an empty lot across the street from the hospital and remained there until his son had his operation and was subsequently discharged from the Hospital.*

Basic research projects were conducted at the Hektoen Institute of Medical Research and the University of Illinois research laboratories. In 1978, Dr. Eugene Ostrovsky, a native of Russia and a trained general surgeon who had recently immigrated to this country, joined the division of pediatric surgery at Cook County Hospital as a surgical research associate. He was responsible for conducting and supervising the research projects in the animal laboratory and a number of the clinical research projects of the division until his departure several years later. As part of the overall restructuring of the Department of Surgery at County, Dr. Robert J. Walter was appointed in 1987 to supervise, assist, or initiate all research activities at the Hektoen Institute of Medical Research conducted by the department, including those of the division of pediatric surgery.

A summary of some of the more important basic and clinical research projects conducted in the Division of Pediatric Surgery from 1976 to 1997 include the following:

- *Pleural effusion in rabbits and model for short gut in piglets (1976)*

- *Esophageal manometry and continuous intra-esophageal pH monitoring in normal and symptomatic infants and children*
- *Gastroenterology laboratory, division of pediatric surgery, Cook County Children's Hospital (1979-1981)[32]*
- *Antibody response in partially splenectomized rats (1979 – 1981)*
- *Technique of splenic biopsy and hemisplenectomy for hematologic disease, University of Illinois Hospital (1980)[33]*
- *Phase III study, clinical evaluation BL-S786R in the treatment of bacterial peritonitis, University of Illinois Hospital*
- *Observations on the gubernaculum during descent of the testis[34]*
- *Absorption, bacteriological, and pressure studies of the small intestine in small bowel syndrome with construction of an Ileo-cecal valve (1981-1982)[35]*
- *A critical review of urban pediatric trauma (1981-1985)*
- *Computerized tomographic study in the evaluation of blunt abdominal trauma in children (1985)*
- *Mortality of childhood falls (1989)*
- *Traumatic deaths in children (1993)*
- *Arteriography in the evaluation of penetrating pediatric extremity injuries (1994)[36]*
- *Vascular trauma and reconstructive approaches (1994)*
- *Penetrating neck injuries ((1989)*
- *Outcome of blunt trauma management in children (1996)[37]*
- *Management of perforated appendicitis in children based on a prospective protocol (1978-1985)*
- *Mechanism of chemotaxis defect in leukocytes from patients with head and neck tumors (1988)*
- *Evaluation of Janeway gastrostomy as optimal method of achieving enteral access in neurologically impaired children (1988-1990)*
- *Perforated appendicitis: Randomized prospective study of one- and two-drug antibiotic therapy (1988-1989)[38]*
- *Survival of pancreatic islet homotransplants following immunosuppression of donors (1990)*
- *Newcastle disease virus*
- *Tumor specific, anti-neoplastic effects (1990–1997)[39,40,41]*
- *Treated acellular dermal matrix as a dermal substitute in rats (1997).[42]*

Educational programs conducted included two weekly conferences with mandatory attendance, a pediatric surgery clinical conference that lasted two hours where all admissions, discharges, operations, complications, and deaths in the service were thoroughly discussed, and an hour lecture given to medical students and surgical residents on various topics in pediatric surgery. The surgical staff also joined a combined weekly tumor conference conducted by the oncology service and the weekly morbidity and mortality conference conducted by the Department of Surgery every Saturday morning. Daily teaching rounds and operative teaching sessions were a major component of the teaching program. Except for complex surgical procedures, the attending surgeon served as the teaching assistant to the senior resident or junior resident. All emergency operations were performed only after the approval of the attending surgeon on call and pending his or her presence in the operating room.

All members of the attending staff were invited to give lectures outside of the institution, wrote articles that were published in peer-reviewed journals, and gave presentations at local and national surgical-association meetings on a variety of clinical subjects. These included:

- *Neonatal surgery*[43,44,45]
- *Surgical emergencies in infants and children*
- *Solid tumors in children*
- *Common pediatric surgical conditions*
- *Urologic problems and complex intersex conditions*
- *All aspects of pediatric trauma, especially the need for centralized care of the severely injured child*
- *Evaluation of blunt abdominal trauma in children*
- *Nonoperative treatment of solid organ injuries following blunt trauma*
- *Perforated appendicitis*
- *GE reflux*
- *Role of an artificial autologous Ileo-cecal valve in short gut syndrome in animals*
- *Fetal surgery in animals, specifically the creation and closure of a diaphragmatic hernia*

This trend in clinical care, research, and academic productivity at Cook County Children's Hospital that prevailed until the turn of the century positively influenced the care of pediatric patients with surgical problems, and the reduced mortality and morbidity of patients undergoing complex operative procedures was comparable to, and in some instances better than, those observed in major teaching children's hospitals in the country. This period represented the golden age of pediatric surgery at CCH. It was also during this time that a significant number of the general surgery residents in the general surgery program decided on a career in pediatric surgery and successfully entered post-residency fellowships in highly competitive and limited pediatric surgery programs.

The divisions of neurosurgery, plastic surgery, dentistry and oral surgery, otolaryngology, ophthalmology, and orthopedic surgery joined in upgrading the care of pediatric patients with full-time, trained pediatric surgical specialists utilizing state-of-the-art diagnostic equipment and surgical therapy.

The achievements in surgical care of the pediatric patient certainly were the result of a confluence of events that included advances in neonatal care; newer diagnostic procedures such as CT scan, MRI, ultrasound, and other biologic scans; and the advent of total parenteral nutrition. More important was the commitment and invaluable contribution of a group of overworked and highly dedicated nurses and other health care providers along with the presence of a well-organized Department of Pediatrics at County. Nurses and other health care workers who stayed on past their shifts to complete unfinished work in the wards, intensive care unit, and operating rooms because of an insufficient staff was simply remarkable and a testament to their compassion and genuine love for their patients.

The Department of Pediatrics was headed in succession by Dr. Ira Rosenthal who succeeded Dr. Joseph Greengard. He was followed in turn by Dr. Robert Miller, the chief of pediatric cardiology, Dr. Rosita Pildes (interim chair), and Dr. Philip Ziring toward the end of the century. They were a group of knowledgeable leaders, compassionate children's health care advocates, and sincere educators. The Department of Pediatrics had a very strong and dedicated faculty with highly recognized subspecialties, notably the world-famous neonatalogy intensive care unit that Dr. Rosita Pildes developed and organized at Cook County Hospital.

Similar units were developed by Drs. Ruth Seeler, Emily Pang, and Sudha Rao in pediatric hematology and oncology; Dr. Norman Jacobs in infectious diseases; Dr. Billie Adams, a well-respected teacher and general clinician; Dr. Demetra Soter, an excellent general pediatrician with a deep interest in child abuse and trauma prevention; a well-run intensive care unit headed by the much-admired Dr. Natesan Janakiraman, followed by Dr. William Haden; a group of pediatric anesthesiologists headed by Dr. Alfonso Wong, a highly qualified and excellent pediatric anesthesiologist; Dr. Jose Ramilo and Dr. Vivian Harris in radiology who were always available for immediate consultation; and a host of others in the Department of Pediatrics too numerous to individually include in this chapter.

At the University of Illinois, Dr. Darmapura Vidyasagar, a trainee of Dr. Pildes at County, organized a well-respected NICU, and together with the new members of the pediatric staff who were recruited by Dr. Rosenthal on assuming the chairmanship of the Department of Pediatrics following his departure from County, strengthened the program at the University of Illinois.

Dr. Reyes played a major role in establishing pediatric trauma centers in Chicago as vice president of the Board of Health and chairman of the Pediatric Trauma Oversight Committee of the Board of Health in 1986, which led to the designation of pediatric trauma centers in metropolitan Chicago in 1987, apart from the adult trauma centers.

A significant contribution of Drs. John R. Hall and Reyes to pediatric trauma care at County was the coordination of care among the various surgical specialties. Strict protocols for care were instituted for all patients with severe injuries including orthopedic, neurosurgery, and critical care, which allowed data/performance-delivered care. Dr. John R. Hall was responsible for the critical care of all injured patients admitted to the pediatric intensive care unit regardless of the nature of their injuries. This collaboration of care with Drs. Robert Hall, chairman, division of orthopedic surgery and James Stone, chairman, division of neurosurgery, made possible the achievement of better survival rates and reduction of long-term morbidity despite the severity of injuries suffered by these patients.

The decade of the 1990s saw a decline in the number of neonatal surgical cases referred to the pediatric surgical division. This can be attributed to the diminishing rate of deliveries at the hospital, reduction in the number of high-risk pregnancies due to more comprehensive prenatal care, fewer numbers of teen-aged pregnancies, and advancements in antenatal diagnosis. By this time, most major medical centers in the city and the suburbs were staffed with fully trained pediatric caregivers and equipped with facilities for even the sickest neonate. Trauma cases, especially those suffering from penetrating injuries, increased.[46] The pediatric trauma centers previously designated in 1987 were still active under the auspices of the state emergency medical system. The operative volume of common pediatric surgical conditions such as hernias, undescended testicle, lumps and bumps remained unchanged, only this time, operations were performed as outpatient procedures under the same-day surgery program that the institution embraced. Patients were admitted the day of surgery and discharged following an adequate postrecovery observation. The number of admissions to the surgical ward declined as a result of the outpatient program, and the length of stay for other conditions was drastically reduced. The outpatient volume, however, continued at the same level as in previous years.

During this period and toward the end of the 20th century, the academic productivity of the staff was concentrated on trauma, solid tumors in children, and the advances in neonatal surgical care. Dr. John R. Hall and the resident staff evaluated and reported their experiences with the management of children injured from falls, penetrating zone II neck injuries, and nonoperative management of penetrating lower extremity injuries with minor vascular trauma.[47,48,49] Dr. Janet Meller continued her clinical research interest in the diseases of neonates,[1] and after completing a course on the Extracorporeal Membrane Oxygenator (ECMO) management of neonatal respiratory failure at the University of Michigan, Ann Arbor, with Dr. Robert Bartlett, she initiated the development of a similar program (among the first in the city) at County. Of the three neonates initially treated (two with meconium aspiration syndrome and one with diaphragmatic hernia), all of whom had intractable respiratory failure, two survived with ECMO treatment for a period of three to seven days. This program was eventually discontinued due to the extensive resources required to maintain the program, including a full-time perfusionist and other medical personnel who stayed with the patient virtually 24 hours a day until the treatment was completed. It was not only taking a toll on Dr. Meller and her colleagues but was also taking a considerable amount of her time away from her other responsibilities in the division.

Basic research continued on the viral treatment of various tumors, more specifically, neuroblastoma as a tumor model in experimental animals. These were conducted primarily by Drs. R. M. Lorence, Kirk Reichard (a surgical resident at the now integrated University of Illinois-Cook County Hospital residency program), and Dr. Robert J. Walter.

## Rush University Medical Center and CCH

In 1993, at the direction of the hospital administration and the executive medical staff of Cook County Hospital, an overall inter-hospital academic affiliation with Rush-Presbyterian-St. Luke's Medical Center and Rush Medical College was initiated after approval by the Cook County board. Pediatric surgery attending coverage at Cook County Hospital, Rush, and University of Illinois remained unchanged despite the academic disaffiliation with the University of Illinois. The new overall institutional academic affiliation between Cook County Hospital and Rush University Medical Center was, in essence, a renewal of a relationship that started with the establishment of Rush Medical College and the beginnings of a county hospital that lasted until the middle of the 20th century.

In 1996, Dr. Kathryn D. Bass was recruited by Dr. Richard Prinz (professor and chairman, Department of General Surgery, Rush University Medical Center) and Dr. Hernan M. Reyes (chief of surgery at Cook County Hospital) to become the full-time chair of the division of pediatric surgery at both Cook County Hospital and Rush University Medical Center. This appointment included the section of pediatric trauma. Dr. John R. Hall had, by this time, left County for a position as professor of surgery at East Tennessee State University School of Medicine. Dr. Janet Meller remained chief of the section of general pediatric surgery on a part-time salaried basis. She and Dr. Loeff eventually became associated and formed a partnership in the private practice of pediatric surgery at Advocate Christ Hospital in Oak Lawn, Illinois, and Lutheran General Hospital in Park Ridge, Illinois, although they remained as part-time attending pediatric surgeons at Cook County Hospital. A husband and wife team of pediatric surgeons were recruited at the University of Illinois, and Dr. Bass remained as chair of the division of pediatric surgery at County until the turn of the 21st century. Dr. Reyes took an early retirement as chairman of the Department of Surgery at Cook County Hospital on September 1, 1998 but remained on the voluntary consulting staff in pediatric surgery until September 2, 2001.

## Epilogue

With the opening of the John Stroger Jr. Hospital of Cook County to replace the old Cook County Hospital in 2002, the clinical services of the Department of Pediatrics underwent a change. The Department is now housed on a floor of the general hospital, as was the case when the first Cook County Hospital was established in 1866. The Cook County Children's Hospital that was built in 1904 and replaced with a larger facility in 1927 was never an independently administered and managed children's institution. Now that the Department has been physically folded back into the general hospital, some of the clinical gains delivered by the CCH pediatric service may be promoted less vigorously, but the dedication and commitment of those delivering care is the same as it has always been.

## References

1. Holmes EL, Lackey RM, Lyman HM. Hospital Reports. *Chgo Med J.* 1866;23:91.
2. Raffensperger JG. *The Old Lady on Harrison Street. Cook County Hospital, 1833-1995. (International Healthcare Ethics, V. 3)* New York: Peter Lang;1997:13-14.
3. Murphy JB, Medical Round, vol. 42:665, 1892. In: A. Scott Earle, ed. *Surgery in America.* Philadelphia:W.B. Saunders and Co, 1965:235.
4. Abt IA. *Baby Doctor.* New York: McGraw Hill, 1944: 134-154.
5. Hess JH, *Diaphragmatic Hernia, Eventration, True and False Hernia in Infants and Children.* MedClinNorth Am, 1924 (Sept).
6. Raffensperger, John, The Old Lady on Harrison Street; Cook County Hospital, 1833 – 1955, (International Healthcare Ethics; v. 3, page 195
7. Raffensperger JG. *The Old Lady on Harrison Street. Cook County Hospital, 1833-1995. (International Healthcare Ethics, V. 3)* New York: Peter Lang;1997:108.
8. Miller E, Fell E., Brock C. Progress in Treatment of Supracondylar Fractures of the Elbow. *Proc Inst Med Chgo.* 1940-1941;13. Presented to the Chicago Surgical Society, March 1, 1940.
9. Miller, E. Congenital Bowel Obstruction. *Surg Clin North Am,* 1927;7:649-655.
10. Miller E, Turner E. Appendicitis in Children. *Proc Instit Med Chgo,* 1936-1937;11:139. Presented to Chicago Medical Society, May 1, 1936.
11. Allen HS. Treatment of the Burned Wound Based on 1000 Hospital Patients. *Ann Surg.* 1951;134:566-573.
12. Fell E H, Gasul B M, Weinberg M, Gordon A, Johnson, FR, Heckel E. Experience with Open Cardiotomy Using a Heart Lung Machine. *Proc Instit Med Chgo.* 1958;22:99.
13. Raffensperger JG, Freeark R J, Fell EH. Neonatal Surgery at the Cook County Hospital. Review of Period 1954 – 58" Am J Surg. 1964,107:712-801.
14. Pringle KC, Reyes HM, Bennett EJ. Preoperative and postoperative care of the pediatric surgical patient. *Crit Care Med.* 1980;8:10,554-58.
15. Skef Z, Radhakrishnan J, Reyes HM. Ano-rectal continence following sphincter re-construction utilizing the gluteus maximus muscle. *J Pediatr Surg.* 1983:186; 779-781.
16. Meller JL, Reyes HM, Loeff DS. Gastroschisis and Omphalocele. Clin Perinatol. 1989;March:113-122.
17. Reyes HM. Transperitoneal Extramucosal rectal biopsy and Proximal Colonic Biopsy and the Soave Procedure for Hirschprung's Disease. In: Nyhus LM and Baker RJ(eds): *Textbook of Mastery of Surgery.* Boston, Little Brown and Co; 1984: 955-964.
18. Samuelson S, Reyes HM. Management of Perforated Appendicitis in Children – Revisited. *Arch Surg.* 1987;122.
19. Reyes HM, Ostrovsky E. Diagnosis and Treatment of Gastroesophageal Reflux in Infants and Children, in Nyhus (series ed). *Surgical Annual.* New York:Appleton: Century, Crofts; 1983: 61-71.
20. Holmes MJ, Reyes HM. A Critical Review of Urban Pediatric Trauma. *J Trauma.* 1984;24:253-55.
21. Mohamed G, Reyes, HM, Fantus R, Ramilo J, Radhakrishnan J. Computed tomography in the assessment of pediatric abdominal trauma. *Arch Surg.* 1986;121:703-707.
22. Hall JR, Reyes HM, Meller JL, Stein RJ. Traumatic Death in Urban Children, Revisited. *Am J Dis Child.* 1993;147:102 – 107.
23. Hall JR, Reyes HM, Meller, JL, Loeff DS, Dembeck R. The Outcome for Children with Blunt Trauma is Best at a Pediatric Trauma Center. *J Pediatr Surg.* 1996: 31:72 -77.
24. Hall JR, Reyes HM. Blunt liver injury in childhood: Evolution of Therapy and

Current Perspective. Invited Editorial. *Curr Surg*. 1988;January-February:41-42.
25. Radhakrishnan J, Reyes, HM. Unilateral Renal Agenesis with Hematometrocolpos: Report of two cases. *J Pediatr Surg*. 1982;17:749-750.
26. Radhakrishnan J. Colon interposition Vaginoplasty: A Modification of the Wagner-Baldwin Technique. *J Pediatr Surg*. 1987;22:1175-1176,.
27. Hendren WH, Radhakrishnan J. Pediatric Pyeloplasty: *J. Pediatr Surg*. 1980;15:33-144.
28. Radhakrishnan J, Mouli KBC, Reyes HM. Genitourinary Injuries in Urban Children. *J Trauma*. 1982;22:633.
29. Radhakrishnan J. Urologic defects in Prune belly syndrome: An operative Approach. 5th Annual Illinois Chapter Conference of the American Academy of Pediatrics. Chicago, June 21, 1981.
30. Radhakrishnan J. Editorial Comment, Current Surgery 39:4, 261-262,1982. Surgical Correction and rehabilitation for children with "prune belly" syndrome. *Ann Surg*. 1982;193:757-762.
31. The Hektoen Institute for Medical Research Biennial Report, 1976 – 1997. Clinical Studies, Cook County Children's Hospital Division of Pediatric Surgery published in peer reviewed surgical journals.
32. Reyes HM, Ostrovsky E, Radhakrishnan J. Diagnostic accuracy of a 3-hour continuous intraluminal pH monitoring of the lower esophagus in the evaluation of GE reflux in infancy. *J Pediatr Surg*. 1982;17:625-31.
33. Radhakrishnan J, Reyes HM. Technique of Splenic Biopsy and Hemi-Splenectomy for Hematologic Disease. *Proc Instit Med Chgo*. 1980;32:68.
34. Radhakrishnan J, Morikawa Y, Donahoe, PK, Hendren WH. Observations on the Gubernaculum during descent of the Testis. *Invest Urolog*. 1979;16:366-368.
35. Grieco GA, Reyes HM, Ostovsky E. The role of a modified intussusceptions jejuno-colic valve in short-bowel syndrome. *J Pediatr Surg*. 1983;18:354-59.
36. Reichard KW, Hall JR, Meller JL, Spigos D, Reyes HM. Arteriography in the Evalu-ation of Penetrating Pediatric Extremity Injuries. *J Pediatr Surg*. 1994;20:19-22.
37. Hall, JR, Reyes HM, Meller JL, Loeff DS, Dembek R. The Outcome For Children with Blunt Trauma is Best at Pediatci Trauma Center, *J Pediatr Surg*. 1996:31:72-77.
38. Meller JL, Reyes HM, Loeff DS, Federer L, Hall JR. One-drug versus two-drug antibiotic therapy in pediatric perforated appendicitis: A prospective randomized study. *Surgery*. 1991;110:764-768.
39. Reichard KW, Lorence RM, Cascino CJ, Peeples ME, Walter R, et al. New Castle Disease Virus Selectively Kills Human Tumor Cells. *J Surg Res*. 1992;52, 448-453.
40. Lorence RM, Reichard KW, Katubig BB, Reyes HM, Phuangsab A,et al. Complete Regression of Human Neuroblastoma Xenografts in Athymic Mice after Local Newcastle Disease Virus Therapy. *J Natl Cancer Instit*. 1994; 86:1228-1233.
41. Reicard KW, Lorence RM, Cascino CJ, Peeples ME, Walter, RJ, et al. Newcastle Disease Virus Selectively Kills Human Tumor Cells. *J Surg Res*. 1992;52:448-453.
42. Walter J, Jennings L, Matsuda T, Reyes HM, Holian O. Dispase/Triton Treated Acellular Dermal Matrix as a Dermal Substitute in Rats. *Curr Surg*. 1997;54:371-374.
43. Reyes, HM. Neonatal Necrotizing Enterocolitis, Nelson RL and Nyhus L (ed). *Surgery of the Small Intestines*. Norwalk, CT: Appleton& Lange; 1987: 111-115.
44. Reyes, HM, Meller, JL, Loeff D. Management of Esophageal Atresia and Tracheoesophageal Fistula. *Clinics in Perinatol*. 1989;16:79-84.
45. Reyes, HM, Meller, JL, Loeff D. Neonatal Intestinal Obstruction. *Clin Perinatol*. 1989;16:85.
46. Hall JR, Reyes HM, Meller, JL, Loeff DS & Dembek R. The New Epidemic in Children: Penetrating injuries. *J Trauma*. 1995;39:487-491.

47. Hall JR, Reyes HM, Horvat M, Stein R. The Mortality of Childhood Falls. *J Trauma*. 1889;29:1273-275.
48. Hall JR, Reyes HM, Meller, JL. Penetrating Zone II Neck Injuries in Children. *J Trauma*. 1991;31:1-4.
49. Reichard KW, Reyes, HM. Vascular Trauma and Reconstructive Approaches. *Sem Pediatr Surg*. 1994:3:124-132.
50. Meller JL, Loeff DS, Reyes HM. Restorative Proctocolectomy in Infants and Children. *Curr Surg*. 1997;54:307-311.

# 16

# Neurological Surgery

*James L. Stone, MD, FACS*
*George R. Cybulski, MD, FACS*

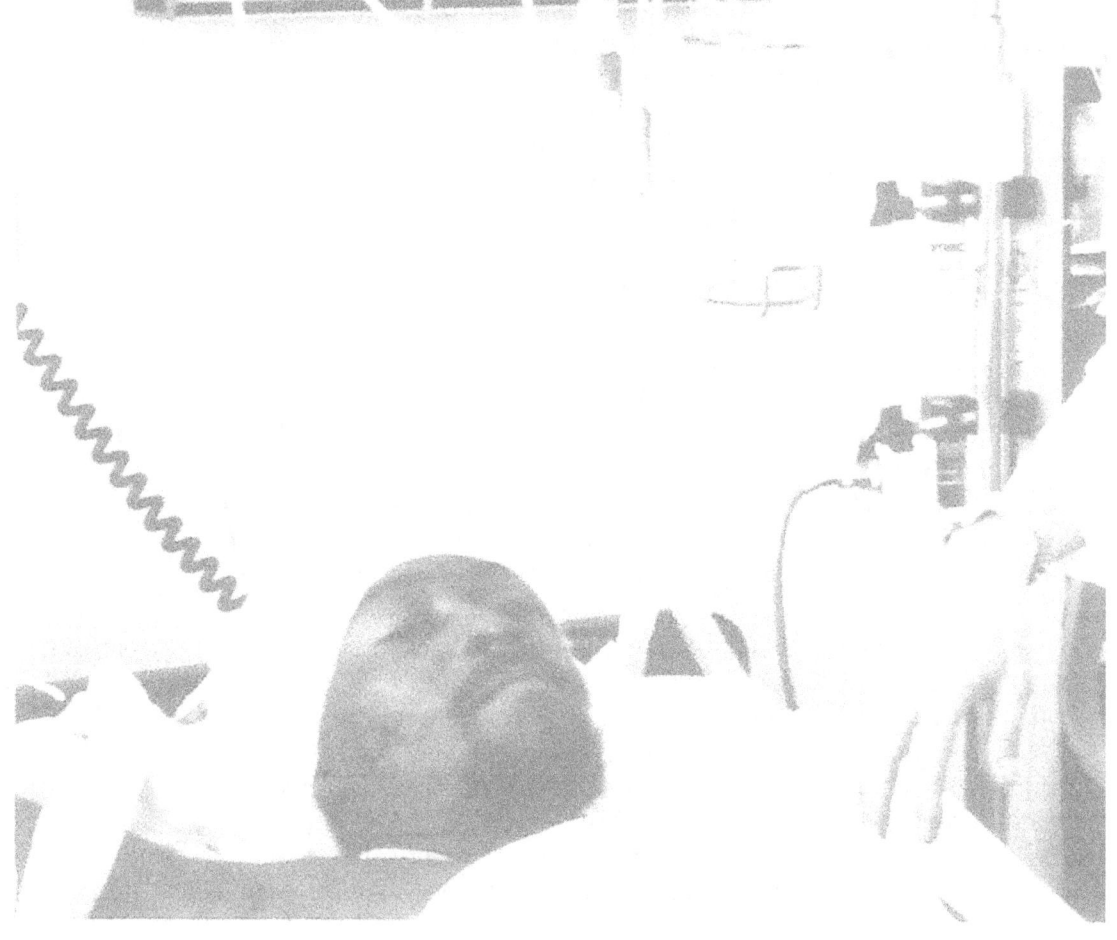

- *Introduction*
- *Neurosurgical Contributions by Fenger and Early Trainees*
- *Allen B. Kanavel, A.E. Halstead, and Dean Lewis*
- *Program Development*
- *Education and Present Service*
- *References*

## Introduction

In the last decades of the 19th century, as Chicago rapidly grew it also rose to surgical pre-eminence. The predominant stimulating activity was centered at Cook County Hospital and corresponded to the arrival of the Danish-born and European-trained Christian Fenger (1840–1902) in 1877 and his CCH staff appointment in 1878. Fenger was a master pathologist who had performed thousands of autopsies, an innovative surgeon, and an inspiring teacher. He is credited with introducing modern medicine to Chicago and the Midwest. A capable bacteriologist and early supporter of Lister's methods, Fenger introduced antisepsis to Cook County Hospital and went on to create a "midwestern school" of surgical progress and teaching comparable to the greatest centers in Europe and the United States. Those truly interested in the modern progress of medicine and surgery could not help but be attracted to and stimulated by Fenger, who was essentially a developer of notable surgeons, pathologists, and internists.[1-5]

A slow and deliberate surgeon frequently stopping to make teaching points, Fenger approached every operation as a challenge to diagnosis in correlating the surgical pathology with the clinical picture.[6] Christian Fenger's surgical determination was exemplified in an operation at CCH in the early- to mid-1890s that was observed by Dr. William Mayo:

> *Fenger had made a brilliant diagnosis of a fibroid tumor of the brain and operated to remove it. Although as he was closing the wound the patient died. "Dr. Fenger, the patient is dead," said the anesthetist quietly. There was no answer. Again, more clearly, "Dr. Fenger, the patient is dead." Still not a word. Carefully the surgeon sewed up the incision and as carefully wound the bandages around it. Then he said softly, "You damned fool, to die just as you were cured."[6]*

The first group of Fenger-taught surgical instructors were noteworthy for their far-reaching surgical expertise. It included Arthur D. Bevan, Franklin Martin, Charles and William Mayo, L. L. McArthur, John B. Murphy, Albert J Ochsner, Roswell Park, Charles T. Parkes, and Nicholas Senn. Senn and Murphy, in particular, were to become the foremost surgeons in the United States around the turn of the 20th century, but neither had the personality to create a local following or school of surgery. By forceful example and fear of competition, their direct surgical descendents were to resist surgical subspecialization and surgical residency training in Chicago for three decades to come.[4,7,8] If an apprentice was given a period of training by a senior surgeon, it was usually agreed on in advance that he must leave the Chicago area after training (E. Oldberg personal communication, 1983).

Neurosurgical training programs began in the early years of the 20th century by Harvey Cushing (1868–1939) in Baltimore and later Boston. Before World War I, programs were formed in New York, Philadelphia, St. Louis, and Los Angeles. Although two charter members of Cushing's original Society of Neurological Surgeons (1920) were Chicagoans (general surgeons self-trained in neurosurgery but not limiting their work to that specialty), it may seem surprising that until the mid-1930s, a number of general surgeons in Chicago believed they could perform neurosurgery as well as trained neurological surgeons (L. Davis, personal communication, 1979). Not until 1925 did Chicago (CCH, 1926) have its first "trained" neurological surgeon, and by 1935, there were perhaps a half-dozen neurosurgeons in Chicago. The fact that no surgeon in this large city limited his practice to neurosurgical cases until 1925 resulted in general surgeons performing neurological surgery for some time after this date. The development of neurosurgery in Chicago and CCH in the late 19th and first quarter of the 20th centuries is thus unique in terms of contributions made by a number of notable general surgeons confronted with neurological patients.[5,8,9] This aknowledged, we will highlight a number of Fenger's 19th century "neurosurgical firsts" performed at CCH, neurosurgical accomplishments by Fenger's earlier and later CCH surgical trainees, and trace Chicago's subsequent neurosurgical program developments beyond these early roots.

## Neurosurgical Contributions by Fenger and Early Trainees

Fenger, assisted by Edwin W. Lee, J.B. Murphy, and L.L. McArthur in 1881, treated a young man at CCH who had an enlarging traumatic vertebral artery aneurysm at the C1 level near the base of the skull, secondary to a gunshot wound. The pulsatile mass was enlarging and painful. During surgery, the patient became apneic and pulseless from blood loss and was revived with intravenous whiskey and blood transfusion. The aneurysm was trapped, and the vertebral artery was ligated above C1. The patient fully recovered. In retrospect, Fenger believed that the operation might have been facilitated by "securing the proximal vertebral artery with a loop to be used for compression during operation."[10] This is likely the first successful case of an aneurysm surgically obliterated at this level.

In early 1883, Fenger was assisted by Edwin W. Lee and John B. Murphy in the exploration and drainage of an abscess of the frontal lobe of the brain in a police officer shot at close range in the supraorbital region.[11] Local debridement of the entrance wound was initially performed. Six days later, increasing headaches, fever, and wound drainage led to re-exploration with further removal of orbital roof bone fragments and a small localized extradural abscess. A drainage tube was placed after irrigation with carbolic acid. About five weeks after injury, the patient became lethargic, compatible with increased intracranial pressure. The opinion of Fenger was that "the normal state of the temperature pointed rather to an abscess than to meningitis... (and) increasing coma accompanied by a slow pulse clearly indicated augmented intracranial pressure." Fenger operated on the comatose patient without need for anesthesia, and the bone, dura, and brain appeared normal but no pulsations were noted. The frontal lobe was systematically explored with a long hypodermic needle and syringe. He reached the abscess at a depth of about 2.5 inches and opened it with a forceps to drain about 1.5 ounces of odorous pus. A rubber drain was dusted with iodoform, placed in the cavity to be irrigated with a boric acid solution twice a day, and gradually advanced out over two weeks. The patient improved dramatically, but three weeks later the headache and semicomatose state recurred. Fenger operated for a fourth time. He aspirated half a teaspoonful of thick yellow pus from the brain abscess cavity and used a rubber drain to irrigate the cavity with a solution of carbolic acid over a period of about one week. The patient recovered fully and returned to work despite an occasional seizure and a small fistulous tract at the trephine site. This is considered one of the first successful cases of brain abscess drainage in the era of antiseptic surgery and the first reported case in which a hypodermic needle was used to systematically explore and localize a brain abscess. A rubber drain was inserted for postoperative drainage and irrigation of the brain abscess cavity with an antibacterial solution.[11] As of 1881 and 1882, Dr. William Macewen of Glasgow—often labeled the "father of cerebral surgery"—had not mentioned use of an aspirating needle or employment of a drain in the treatment of brain abscess. Macewen subsequently used decalcified chicken bone drains and joined Fenger in using antiseptic solutions to wash out the abscess cavity.[11] Fenger additionally appreciated that a slow pulse indicated increased intracranial pressure, approximately 20 years before that finding was well documented by Cushing.[11,12]

Another one of Fenger's remarkable operative cases at CCH was a 38-year-old man referred by an internist in 1890 with a one-year history of back pain and progressive weakness of both legs.[13] Tactile sense was greatly diminished and temperature sense almost absent on the chest, trunk, and lower extremities below the level of the fourth rib. Fenger performed a laminectomy of T4 and T5, opened the dura, and exposed the spinal cord. When he inspected the cord, he could appreciate a slight dorsal enlargement and palpated a dorsal hard mass. He incised the posterior column in the midline, which revealed a conical tumor nearly two inches long. Following excision of the central portion, it was easily enucleated and seemingly without hemorrhage. After surgery, the patient had a complete paraplegia, ran a febrile course, and died five days after surgery. An autopsy performed by Fenger showed a gross total removal of the sarcoma with a small transverse hemorrhage within the spinal cord just distal to the inferior tumor cavity. Other than this, "the anterior two-thirds of the cord was intact, the gray matter seemingly was compressed, and the tumor had been in the posterior third of the cord covered with a thin layer of the white columns." Fenger commented that although it was unknown why an infection of such severity developed despite antiseptic precautions, it was conceivable that a spinal cord tumor entirely within the cord substance could be removed and the patient recover, except for some sensory loss from opening the posterior columns.[13] This represents the first recorded case of gross total removal of an intramedullary spinal cord tumor. Although the first successful case of removal of a spinal cord tumor within the dura, but outside of the spinal cord, was performed in 1887 by Horsley, it was not until 1905 that Cushing incised the posterior column in a case similar to Fenger's and was surprised by his patient's partial recovery. In 1907, von Eiselsberg of Vienna is believed to be the first to successfully remove an intramedullary spinal cord tumor and obtain a good outcome.[12]

In 1891, Fenger reported the successful excision of a sphenoethmoidal encephalocele in a 29-year-old man with hypertelorism who presented to CCH with nasal obstruction.[14] A compressible mass filled the left post-nasal space above the soft palate and was believed to be a polyp. An intranasal biopsy revealed brain tissue reported by Fenger as "cerebral cortical mantle with numerous small round and large multipolar ganglion cells supported by fine fibrillated neuroglia tissue." Subsequent to the biopsy, cerebrospinal fluid leakage began from the left nares. Fenger performed a one-stage osteoplastic transmalar elevation of the superior maxilla to expose the base of the skull. The pedicle was ligated with a silk suture about 1 cm posterolateal to the left cribiform plate to seal off the leakage and avoid meningitis. The patient recovered with only moderate cosmetic deformity and returned to work. This, again, was in all likelihood the first sphenoethmoidal encephalocele definitively treated, and it would be a difficult operation to perform even today. Fenger also wrote an important paper describing fat embolism of the brain and lungs following long bone fractures.[8]

Nicholas Senn (1844–1908) was a CCH intern in 1868–1869, a contemporary and friend of Fenger, and probably the most prolific academic American surgeon of his time.[4] Although well known as a pioneering abdominal and experimental surgeon, Senn's practical experience included several reviews on neurological surgery and gunshot wounds to the head and neck in the Spanish American War (1893).[15,16] Roswell Park (1852–1914) obtained his medical education in Chicago, interned at CCH, and came under the stimulating influence of Fenger and associates before his departure to Buffalo, New York, in 1883. While in Chicago, he had successfully sutured a sciatic and radial nerve,[17] and by 1886 and 1887 became one of several American surgeons to apply the principles of cerebral localization in attacking intracranial tumors and epilepsy problems.[18] Another nationally recognized Chicago surgeon influenced by Fenger's surgical experience and internship at CCH was Lewis L. McArthur (1858–1934, Figure 16–1). He pioneered many important advances in general surgery, and contributed to the surgery of trigeminal neuralgia and cerebral tumors.[9] His lasting contribution to neurosurgery was introduction of the supraorbital, subfrontal craniotomy approach to the pituitary region, and in 1908, he was the first to perform this approach with tumor removal.[19] Over the next 10 years, he further modified his approach with supraorbital ridge removal.[20] The last of this exceptional group of late 19th and early 20th centuries CCH-trained surgeons was John B. Murphy (1857–1916), considered by many the greatest surgical teacher of that era. Murphy was an intern (1879–1880), attending surgeon (1882–1905), and consultant surgeon (1905–1916) at CCH. A flamboyant and fiery demonstrator, he had been greatly stimulated by the surgical ingenuity of Fenger. Murphy wrote an important review on neurological surgery

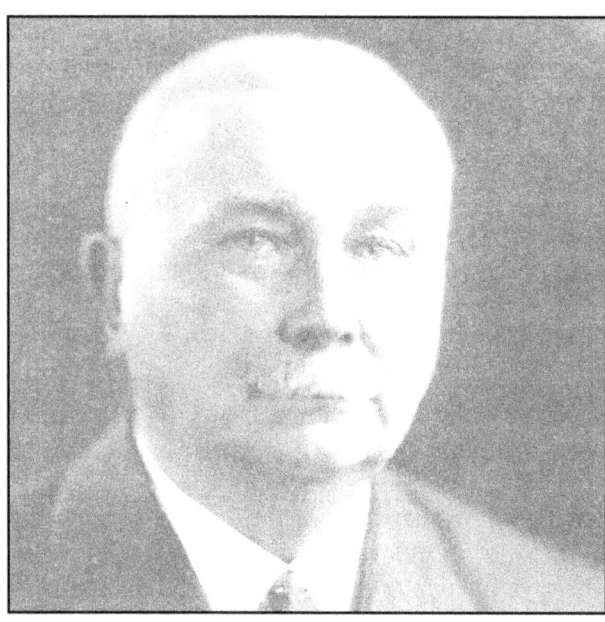

*Figure 16–1  Lewis L. McArthur (1858–1934)*

in 1907 and made notable contributions to spinal surgery, trigeminal neuralgia and peripheral nerve surgery.[21,22] The popular Surgical Clinics of J.B. Murphy became the Surgical Clinics of Chicago after his death, and several years later, the Surgical Clinics of North America. Other notable CCH surgical interns or attending staff surgeons performing neurosurgical cases in the early decades of the 20th century included E. Wyllys Andrews, Daniel Eisendrath, Albert E. Halstead, Allen B. Kanavel, Dean D. Lewis, Karl A. Meyer, Dallas B. Phemister, Harry Richter, Kellogg Speed, and Roger T. Vaughn.

## Allen B. Kanavel, A.E. Halstead, and Dean Lewis

Although many general surgeons in Chicago handled neurological cases in the first quarter of the 20th century, Allen Buckner Kanavel (1874–1938) did more to develop neurological surgery in Chicago than any other individual.[5] This was accomplished by his surgical contributions as well as his ability to stimulate young surgeons and encourage them to subspecialize in the various fledgling fields, including neurosurgery. A product of turn-of-the-century Chicago, Kanavel as a Northwestern student (MD 1899) and CCH intern (1900–1902) had as role models the then-active Fenger, Senn, and Murphy.[5,9]

Following his early training, Kanavel returned to Northwestern and CCH to build his academic career, remaining a CCH staff surgeon through 1919. Kanavel also began work with Franklin Martin (1857–1935), an industrious surgeon, teacher, and experimental animal surgeon who quickly recognized his potential. Martin appointed Kanavel scientific editor when he founded the journal *Surgery, Gynecology and Obstetrics* (*SG&O*) in 1905 to work closely with Senn, Murphy, and W.J. Mayo. In 1913, Kanavel joined Martin in founding the American College of Surgeons (ACS) in Chicago). Kanavel went on to become chairman of surgery at Northwestern (1920–1929) and president of the ACS (1931–1932). Although most of Kanavel's contemporaries addressed all aspects of surgical practice, and Kanavel himself never limited his surgical activities to neurological or any other surgical subspecialty, he had the foresight to realize surgical specialization was necessary and inevitable in light of medical progress. Kanavel was best described as a specialist in many fields of surgery, and his opinion was frequently sought out in the most difficult patients. Soft-spoken, humble, and always one to avoid attention or controversy, Kanavel was Chicago's foremost scientific surgeon and teacher over much of the first 40 years of the last century.[5,9]

Very early in his career, Kanavel was confined to bed with a serious hand infection. He studied the course of his infection, the haphazard conventional therapy, and recalled the many poor functional outcomes from hand infections observed during his internship. Over a period of 12 years, using bismuth paste injection techniques in cadavers at CCH, Kanavel worked out the tendon sheath and fascial space anatomy of the forearm and hand. This painstaking experimental and clinical investigation revolutionized the preantibiotic surgical drainage of hand infections and resulted in the classic textbook, *Infections of the Hand* (1912), which was widely translated and went through seven editions. Always interested in practical research, he was to remain America's most noted authority on reconstructive hand and limb surgery for the remainder of his life.[23,24]

In June of 1909, Kanavel saw a patient suspected of harboring a pituitary tumor. Signs and symptoms included headaches, visual loss, and an enlarged sella turcica on skull X-ray. The referral to Kanavel was based on both the advisability of operation and partly for the purpose of stimulating research into the best methods of approach to the pituitary region. In the autopsy room of CCH, he studied the relations of the various approaches, and in November 1909, published a novel infranasal, transsphenoidal approach to the pituitary.[25] That same month, Kanavel, assisted by his close associate Harry M. Richter, operated by this method on his first patient at the old Wesley Hospital.[26] Today, the infranasal transsphenoidal technique remains the standard, most frequently used approach to a pituitary tumor.[9] Besides his writings on pituitary tumor surgery, Kanavel wrote additional papers and chapters on brain tumors and made advances in spinal surgery, congenital disorders, and facial pain.[9] A particularly notable work is a 75-page chapter from *Ochsner's Surgery* (1920) on tumors and abscesses of the brain that provided a sophisticated appreciation of neurologic diagnosis, cerebral localization, and surgical treatment.[27]

In 1917, Kanavel reported the case of a youth who, several weeks earlier, was shot in the neck, with the bullet localized on X-ray at the C1-C2 junction anteriorly.[28] The boy had severe neck pain whenever he moved his head. Kanavel operated on the boy at CCH by a transoral approach, with intraoperative localization by X-ray fluoroscopy, and removed the bullet. The boy fully recovered. This remarkable case is believed to be the first instance of using the transoral approach for a spinal problem at the C1-C2 junction, other than infection, and one of the first to employ intraoperative fluoroscopy.[8]

Although Kanavel turned much of Northwestern's neurosurgical work over to his trainee, Loyal Davis (1896–1982), even into the early 1930s—before retirement was prompted by radiation dermatitis of his hands—Kanavel's routine surgical day at Northwestern might include a brain tumor, abdominal surgery, orthopaedic or plastic surgery, and gynecologic patients (L. Boshes, personal communication, 1982).

Albert Edward Halstead (1868–1926, Figure 16–2) was another notable surgeon from CCH with particular interest in neurological and head and neck surgery. He graduated from Northwestern in 1890 and interned at CCH the following year. Early in his career, Halstead became a professor of anatomy at Northwestern and headed the anatomy department for several years (1899–1901). He was an attending surgeon at CCH from 1893 to 1917 and rose to professor of surgery at Northwestern and the University of Illinois. He was a bibliophile with a large medical library including many French and German texts.[9] In July of 1909, Halstead called on Kanavel, one of his former students whose then unpublished work he knew well, to assist him with the world's first infranasal transsphenoidal pituitary tumor removal. The operation was performed at the old St. Luke's Hospital on South Michigan Avenue. Halstead modified Kanavel's suggested method by making his incision under the upper lip in the gingiva above the mucocutaneous gum line, leaving no external scar on the patient.[29] The Kanavel/Halstead approach was soon extensively utilized by Cushing (1910) and greatly popularized in the 1970s with the use of the operative microscope.[9]

Halstead presented several of his early pituitary tumor patients at the 1910 meeting of the American Surgical Association with Cushing, Kanavel, Lewis, and others present. Halstead also published on trigeminal neuralgia, hydrocepha-

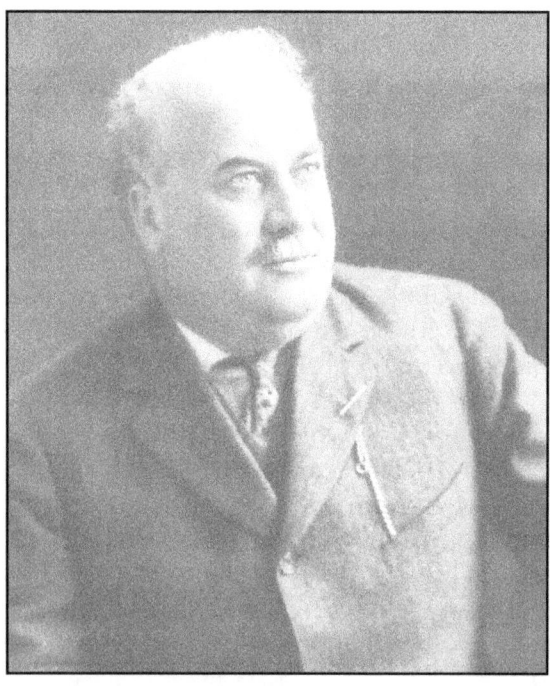

*Figure 16–2  Albert E. Halstead (1868–1926)*

lus, and in 1913 wrote a very practical and extensive chapter on surgery of the brain and spinal cord[9] with a junior CCH associate and friend Roger T. Vaughan (1878–1950). During this period Halstead and Vaughan wrote neurosurgical papers. Vaughan became CCH night surgeon for many years under the tenure of Karl Meyer and positively influenced a great number of surgeons in training.[30]

Dean DeWitt Lewis (187–1941), a contemporary of Kanavel, graduated from Rush Medical College in 1899 and interned across the street at CCH the following year. Dean Lewis enthusiastically taught surgical anatomy and clinical surgery at the University of Chicago and Rush Medical College, and he actively investigated the histology, pathology, and physiology of the pituitary gland. This brought him into association with the pioneer neurological surgeon Harvey Cushing (1869–1939) who was similarly interested in the pituitary. Lewis histologically examined most of the pituitary tumors removed by Kanavel and Halstead's infranasal approach in the years before World War I. Lewis and Kanavel together wrote an important chapter in *Keen's Surgery* on surgery of the pituitary (1916). Dean Lewis also developed extensive experience on regeneration, and surgery of peripheral nerve injuries and reconstructive extremity surgery.[5] In the pre-World War I era, Kanavel and Lewis were said to be the only neurological surgeons in the Mississippi Valley, and unlike most qualified neurosurgeons of this period, both were largely self-taught, and neither devoted himself exclusively to neurosurgery.[9] On a national basis, World War I significantly promoted the specialty of neurological surgery, and Armed Forces neurosurgery courses were given at CCH by Kanavel, Lewis, and others. Kanavel and Lewis were each closely associated with Harvey Cushing and joined as original members of the Society of Neurological Surgeons (1920). Dean Lewis rose to professor of surgery at Rush, and in 1925 he was appointed chief of surgery at the Johns Hopkins Medical School in Baltimore, several years after the death of William S. Halsted. Walter Dandy was the predominant neurosurgeon at Hopkins during this period. Dean Lewis' interest in medical education and writing led to the popular multivolume text *Lewis' Practice of Surgery*, and he also edited the *Archives of Surgery*. He was president of the American Medical Association in 1933.[9]

## Program Development

In 1920, Kanavel encouraged Loyal Davis (1896-1982, CCH intern 1918) to pursue neurosurgical training under his guidance.[5,31] Davis spent his first year learning neurology from Lewis J. Pollock at the CCH Psychopathic Hospital and was assigned to the neuroanatomy laboratory at Northwestern. This was followed by three years' operating with Kanavel on neurosurgical cases at Northwestern, the old Wesley, and a number of Chicago-area hospitals. In 1924, Kanavel arranged a 9- to 10-month period of intensive training for Davis as a fellow under Harvey Cushing in Boston, before requesting his return to Chicago. Loyal Davis returned from Boston in 1925.[5,8]

Davis, who was always to consider Allen Kanavel his mentor and chief, was Chicago's first formally trained neurological surgeon and the first surgeon in

Chicago to limit his work to neurological surgery. His primary appointment was at Northwestern in 1925, and the following year, Karl Meyer appointed him at CCH after a civil service examination. However, at CCH, the general surgeons refused to refer cases to Davis, believing they could do neurosurgery just as well. Although Davis came over to CCH on a few occasions and wore his personalized scrubs, shortly thereafter he resigned from the CCH staff (L. Davis, personal communication, 1979).[31] The most stubborn of these CCH general surgeons regarding neurosurgical capability was Dr. X (attending surgeon 1920–1931). A few years later, Dr. X became immortalized in CCH history by declaring he could perform an appendectomy with "one hand behind his back." The operation had begun when Karl Meyer, chief of surgery at CCH, was summoned to the operating room and ejected Dr. X from the surgical attending staff. Dr. X died a short time later, and it was apparent he had acquired central nervous system syphilis (luetic paresis of the insane; S. Hoffman, personal communication, 1987).

The second neurosurgical training program in Chicago was established at the University of Chicago in 1928 by Percival Bailey (1892–1973), a notable Cushing resident who had obtained both his MD and PhD in 1918 at Northwestern and the University of Chicago, respectively. Bailey spent 10 months in 1920 at the CCH Psychopathic Hospital learning neuropathology from G.B. Hassin, at that time America's foremost authority on the subject. Bailey was to spend nearly 10 years as a trainee of Cushing, mostly in neuropathology. This culminated in the landmark Bailey and Cushing histological classification of primary brain tumors, which is very similar to the scheme still used today.[5,8]

The third neurosurgical training program in Chicago was established at the University of Illinois in 1931 by Eric Oldberg (1901–1986). Oldberg, who had been a medical student under Kanavel and Davis at Northwestern, was recommended by Kanavel to Cushing for residency training. Oldberg's neurosurgery residents from the nearby Illinois Research and Education (R&E) Hospital were occasionally rotated to the nearby CCH.[5,8]

Adrien VerBrugghen (1899–1985), a Mayo Clinic trained neurosurgeon, joined the CCH and Rush-Presbyterian Hospital staffs in 1932. In 1934, VerBrugghen was joined at CCH by neurosurgeon Harold C. Voris (1902–1980), also a Mayo Clinic trainee. VerBrugghen established a neurosurgery training program at the Rush-Presbyterian (later Rush-Presbyterian-St. Luke's) Hospital, and Voris headed the newly organized Loyola-Mercy Hospital program.[5,8] Both programs were then adjacent to CCH and sent neurosurgical residents to CCH for training. Voris and VerBrugghen formally established the CCH neurosurgical service on October 1, 1938. Ward 22 was a 50-bed unit used predominantly for head injuries, although a certain number of patients with tumors, trigeminal neuralgia, and spinal disorders were treated there as well.[8]

Harold Voris was the essential director of neurosurgery at CCH until 1948. Milton Tinsley was an attending staff neurosurgeon from 1948 to 1958, as were Joseph "Burr Hole Joe" Cascino from 1948 to 1962, and Charles E. Corcoran and David Voris in the 1950s. Paul R. Rosenbluth was appointed chief of CCH neurosurgical services from 1958 to 1962. Sanford Larson (Figure 16–3) and Harold Keegan were active attending staff members in the early 1960s, but until this

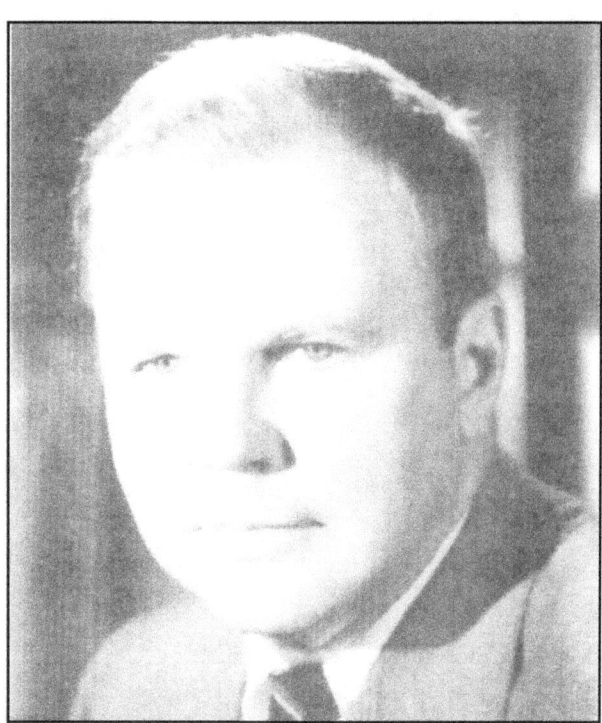

*Figure 16–3 Sanford J. Larson (1930–2012)*

time, no attending staff members were full-time and most were voluntary. In addition to the CCH general surgical house staff, neurosurgery residents who rotated from the Rush-Presbyterian (until 1952), Loyola, and occasionally the University of Illinois programs, managed the busy neurosurgical service.[5,8]

The first full-time, salaried chairman of neurosurgery at CCH was Anthony J. Raimondi (1928–2000, Figure 16–4), a University of Chicago trainee appointed in March 1963. The adult neurosurgical service was housed on Ward 30, and a large pediatric neurosurgical unit was housed on Ward 46. Oscar Sugar (1914–2008, Figure 16–5), a trainee of Bailey and Oldberg and expert on cerebral angiography, came over from the University of Illinois to conduct a Wednesday X-ray review and case presentation conference (from 1962 until 1987).[5,8]

Raimondi, by the mid-1960s, was able to build a successful, independent residency training program at CCH and pioneered developments in pediatric neurosurgery and neuroradiology. Hernando Torres, who completed the Unversity of Chicago program one year after Raimondi, along with David Yashon from Illinois, were also neurosurgical attendings. Raimondi relocated to Children's Memorial Hospital in 1969 and in 1972 became chairman of neurosurgery at Northwestern. Torres became acting head in late 1969 until Roy Selby, an Illinois trainee, was appointed chairman of the CCH neurosurgery division from July 1970 until the spring of 1974. By 1973, the CCH independent neurosurgical resident training program had been disbanded and became an affiliate of the University of Illinois program, then led by Oscar Sugar. After Selby, Harvey Henry

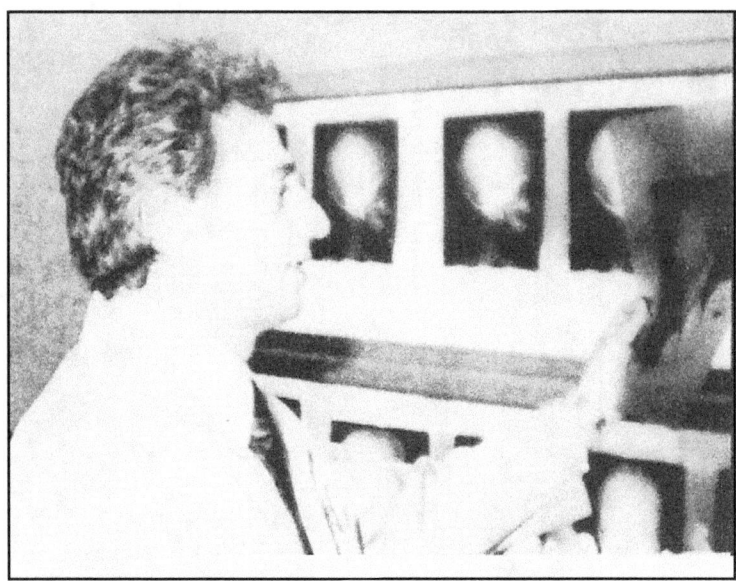

*Figure 16–4
Anthony Raimondi
((1928–2000)*

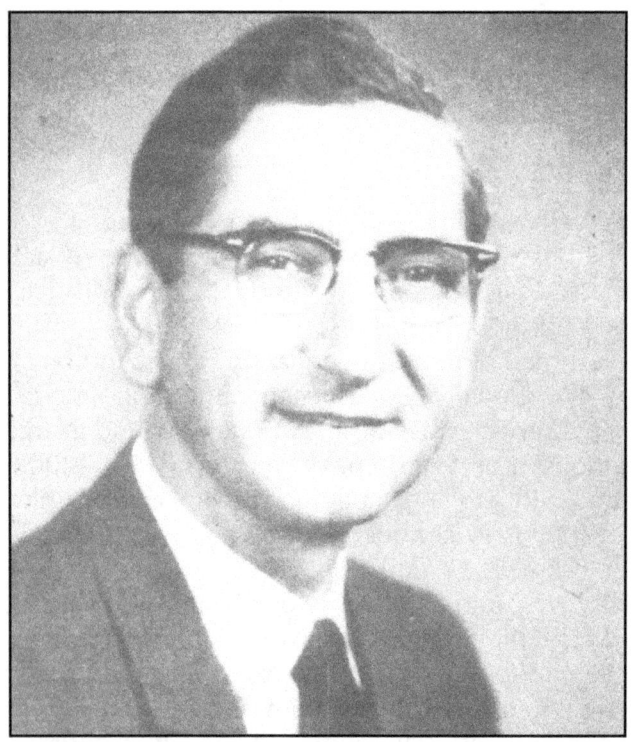

*Figure 16–5 Oscar Sugar
(1914–2008)*

was acting head until Robert A. Moody was appointed chairman of neurosurgery at CCH in September 1974 and professor of neurosurgery at Illinois. Moody, a product of the University of Chicago, trained at Vermont and the Lahey Clinic before several additional years as a staff member at the University of Chicago. Under Moody's direction, the neurosurgical services were expanded, intracranial pressure monitoring was introduced, the benefit of large decompressive craniotomy in head injuries was established, and the first fully dedicated neurosurgical intensive care unit in Chicago was opened in 1978 (nine-bed, three Unit East).

At the Hektoen Laboratory, Moody, with the assistance of Japanese-trained neurosurgical fellows, embarked on extensive translational experimental work on brain injury in the cat and a shock model in baboons, both utilizing highly advanced electrophysiological monitoring techniques. Moody left in January 1981, and John B. Oldershaw, a Voris trainee from Loyola with special interest in peripheral nerves, assumed the chairmanship from 1981 through 1986. A very active period of research continued at Hektoen under the support and stimulation of the surgical department head Olga Jonasson (1934–2006), with collaboration of Robert J. Lowe and later John Barrett from trauma. The animal work with intracranial pressure and cerebral blood flow monitoring strongly supported vigorous resuscitation with hypertonic saline, predicting its current usage in head-injured patients.

James L. Stone (Fig 16-6), a trainee of Moody and Sugar, and CCH neurosurgical attending since 1980, presented a large series of acute subdural hematoma patients to the Chicago Surgical Society and local health officials, showing that direct admission to the Trauma Unit resulted in statistically improved outcomes, compared to those transferred (JAMA 256;#11,p1439). This work in collaboration with trauma, Robert Baker, and Cook County Medical Examiner- Robert Stein was instrumental in the May 1986 implementation of the Chicagoland Trauma System mandating serious trauma be brought directly to a Level 1 center. Stone became CCH chair of neurosurgery division at CCH (1987-2004), and remains a volunteer.

In 2004, George R. Cybulski, a Rush-Presbyterian-St. Luke's trainee who had been a CCH neurosurgical attending (1986–1988), came over from Northwestern

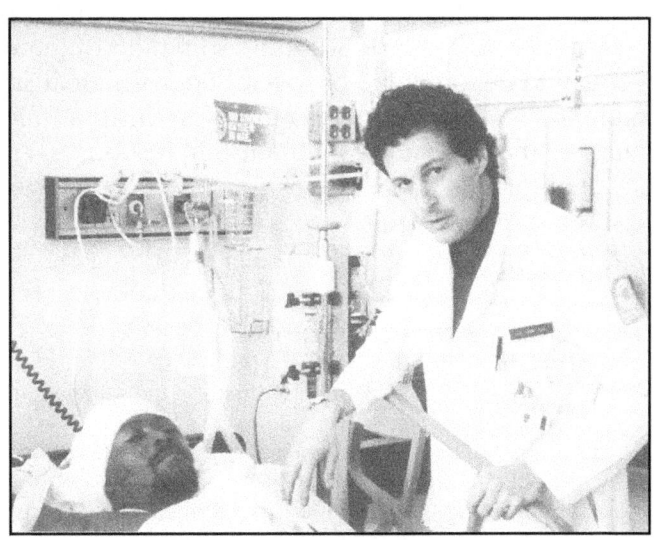

*Figure 16–6 James L. Stone in the Neurosurgery ICU, 1985*

where he had developed a successful teaching and clinical practice to assume the chairmanship at CCH until 2013.

## Education and Present Service

From 1973 until 1992, the neurosurgical service at CCH was closely affiliated with the University of Illinois at Chicago Department of Neurological Surgery under Oscar Sugar and later Robert M. Crowell. Crowell, trained largely at Harvard, imparted a high degree of expertise in microscopic cerebrovascular and tumor surgery, and he regularly took call and performed surgery at CCH. In later 1992, neurosurgery at CCH became an affiliate of the expanded Loyola University Department of Neurological Surgery under Howard Reichman and later Thomas Origitano. By 1996, additional affiliation occurred with the Rush-Presbyterian-St. Luke's program, headed by Walter Whisler, an Oldberg trainee. The two residency programs at CCH initially set up integrated and later separate clinical services. In recent years, osteopathic residents receive training on the CCH neurosurgical service. The present neurosurgical service at CCH includes four full-time attending neurosurgeons and a 10-bed dedicated neurosurgery intensive care monitoring unit with a stable, highly experienced nursing staff. Yogesh Gandhi, an Illinois trainee with special expertise in spinal neurosurbgery is the present Division chair.

Over the past several decades, the attending staff has been fortunate to include Roberta Glick, Don Penney, Terry Lichtor, Patricia Raksin, and Diane Sierens. Of the approximately 550 neurosurgical operations performed yearly, about 25 percent are trauma related, and the remainder consist of adult and pediatric general neurosurgery (brain, spinal, and peripheral nerve) and neurovascular surgery. Over 100 patients with severe head injuries are admitted yearly, and neurotrauma fellowships have been offered. Research initiatives over the past 30 years have included cat, dog, and primate models of head injury and increased intracranial pressure, clinical reviews of penetrating and closed brain injury, pioneering motor-evoked potential studies in primates and humans, brain tumor receptor biology, and MRI scan estimation of intracranial pressure. Plans are underway to become one of several neurosurgical sites worldwide to initiate novel noninvasive bedside monitoring of brainstem function and intracranial pressure utilizing modified auditory brainstem responses. From 1979 until the present, our invaluable neurosurgery divisional administrator is Ms. Ernestine Daniels.

## References

1. Bonner TN. *Medicine in Chicago*. 1850-1950. Madison, WI: The American History Research Center; 1957.
2. Dragstedt LR. Christian Fenger and the Midwestern school of surgery. *Bull Guthrie clinic*. 1963;33:13-24.
3. McArthur LL. Christian Fenger as I knew him. *Proc Inst Med Chgo*. 1922-23;4:42-48.
4. Sperry FM. *A Group of Distinguished Physicians and Surgeons of Chicago*.

Chicago: JH Beers; 1904:15-31,34-42,73-76,189-194.
5. Stone JL, Cybulski GR, Bailey OT. The history of surgical neurology in Chicago. *Proc Inst Med Chgo.* 1983;36:62-67.
6. Clapesattle H. *The Doctors Mayo.* Minneapolis: The University of Minnesota Press; 1941:279-292,426,764.
7. Davis DJ. *History of Medical Practice in Illinois.* Vol II - 1850-1900. Chicago: Illinois State Medicall Society; 1955:183-205.
8. Stone JL. The development of neurological surgery at Cook County Hospital. *Neurosurgery.* 1994;34:97-102.
9. Stone JL, Meglio G, Laws ER. Development of pituitary surgery: The Chicago contributions. *J Am Coll Surg.* 2005;201:784-805.
10. Fenger C. *The Collected Works of Christian Fenger, MD.* Philadelphia: W.B. Saunders, 1912, Vol 1, pp 1-5, 308-315, 463-465.
11. Fenger C, Lee EW. On opening and drainage of abscess cavities in the brain. *Am J Med Sci.* 1884;88:17-30.
12. Walker AE. *A History of Neurological Surgery.* Baltimore: Williams & Wilkins, 1951.
13. Church A, Eisendrath DW. A contribution to spinal cord surgery. *Am J Med Sci.* 1892;103:403-405.
14. Fenger C. Basal hernias of the brain. *Am J Med Sci.* 1895;109:1-17.
15. Senn N. Surgery of the brain and nerves. In Sajous CE, ed. *Annual of the Universal Medical Sciences.* Vol 3. Philadelphia: FA Davis;1889: A1-A86.
16. Senn N. Gunshot wounds of the skull and neck; fractures of the skull. In Senn N. *Practical Surgery.* Philadelphia: WB Saunders;1901:255-261,486-505.
17. Park R. Ssuture of the sciatic and radial nerves, restoration of function. *Chgo Med J and Exam.* 1884;48:635-635.
18. Park R. Surgery of the brain, based upon the principles of cerebral localization. *New York Med J.* 1888;48:479-484, 514-519, 539-546.
19. McArthur LL. An aseptic surgical access to the pituitary body and its neighborhood. *JAMA.* 1912;58:2009-2011.
20. McArthur LL. Tumor of the pituitary gland: Technic of operative approach. *Surg Clin Chigo.* 1918;2:691-699.
21. Murphy JB. Neurological surgery. *Surg Gynecol Obstet.* 1907;4:385-500.
22. Murphy JB. Tumor of the spinal cord. *Surg Clin. J.B. Murphy* 1912;1:695-697.
23. Davis L. Allen Buckner Kanavel (1874-1938). *Proc Inst Med Chgo.* 1938;12:186-188.
24. Martin FH. Allen B. Kanavel, MD. *Surg Gynecol Obstet.* 1934;59:1-2.
25. Kanavel AB. The removal of tumors of the pituitary body by an infranasal route. A proposed operation with a description of the technic. *JAMA.* 1909;53:1704-1707.
26. Kanavel AB., Grinker J. Removal of tumors of the pituitary body with a suggestion as to a two-step route, and a report of a case with a malignant tumor operated upon with a primary recovery. *Surg Gynec Obstet.* 1910;10:414-418.
27. Kanavel AB. Diagnosis and treatment of tumors, inflammations and abscesses of the brain. In: Ochsner AJ, ed. *Surgical Diagnosis and Treatment.* Vol 1. Philadelphia: Lea & Febiger, 1920:327-405.
28. Kanavel AB. Bullet located between the atlas and the base of the skull: Technic of removal through the mouth. *Surg Clin Chgo* 1917;1:361-366.
29. Halstead AE. Remarks on the operative treatment of tumors of the hypophysis with the report of two cases operated on by an oro-nasal method. *Surg Gynecol Obstet* 1910;10:28;73-93.
30. Beatty WK. Roger Throop Vaughan – Diagnostician and teacher. *Proc Inst Med Chgo.* 1987;40:117-128.
31. Davis L. *A Surgeon's Odyssey.* Garden City, New York: Doubleday;1973:336.

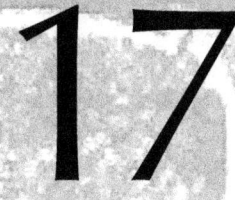

# Vascular Surgery

*Richard Keen, MD*
*James S.T. Yao, MD, PhD*

- The Beginning
- The John B. Murphy Era
- 1900s–1946—The Era of Indirect Surgery
- 1950s—The Breakthrough Decade of Direct Arterial Surgery
    Chicago Artery Bank at Cook County Hospital
- 1960s—Specialized Care for Civilian Vascular Trauma: The Trauma Unit at CCH
- 1970s—Vascular Surgery as a Surgical Specialty
    Vascular Surgical Service at Cook County Hospital
- 1990s—The Decade of Endovascular Surgery
- The New Millennium
- References

## The Beginning

Vascular surgery began with the first attempt to control a bleeding vessel. Sushrita, the great surgeon of ancient India, was the first to practice ligation of a blood vessel.[1] In antiquity, ligation and cauterization were the common practice. In 1759, William Hollowell, a surgeon from England, first repaired a lacerated artery using a figure-eight sutures[1] (Figure 17–1). This was the beginning of reparative vascular surgery. In 1877, Nicolas V. Eck, a Russian surgeon, first performed a vascular anastomosis between the portal vein and the vena cava to study the effect of diverting blood from the liver, a procedure that became known as Eck's fistula.[2] The procedure was the first documented anastomosis of two blood vessels. Since then, there has been an increasing interest in vessel suturing and anastomosis by

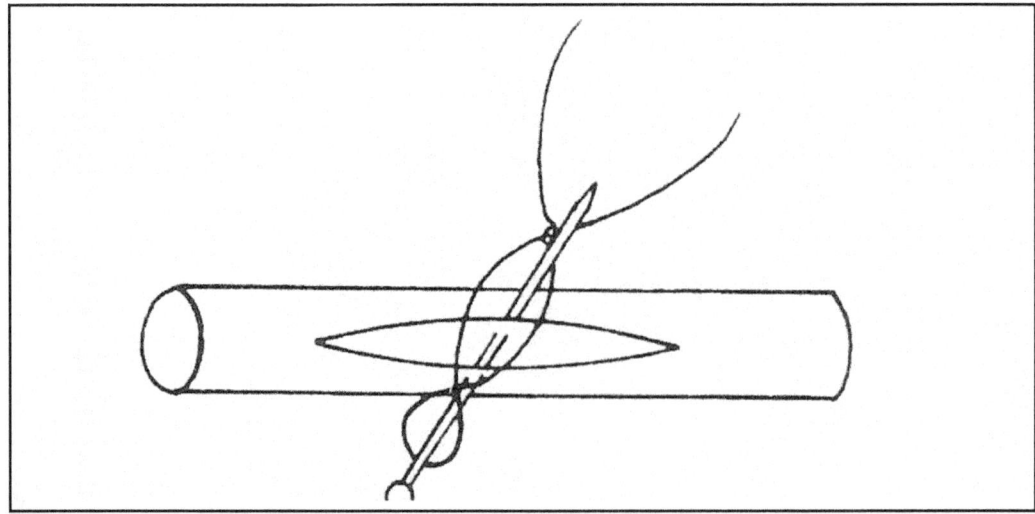

*Figure 17–1* The Hallowell-Lambert repair of a lacerated artery with a figure eight suture

many surgeons, among them Jassinowsky, Von Horoch, Abbe, Payr, and Jaboulay.[1] All these operations, however, were done in animals. The first successful arterial end-to-end anastomosis in a human was performed by John B. Murphy, an attending surgeon at Cook County Hospital for 18 years and the third chairman of the Department of Surgery at Northwestern University Medical School. He performed the surgery on October 7, 1896.[3] This was the first recorded case of an artery being united successfully by suture after circumferential resection of the injured portion, and is considered the beginning of modern vascular surgery.[4]

## The John B. Murphy Era

After completion of his internship at Cook County Hospital in 1880, John B. Murphy joined the staff as attending surgeon. Although he changed academic appointments several times, the appointment at County Hospital remained constant, and he served for 18 years. Murphy was the first surgeon to repair a damaged femoral artery due to a gunshot wound at CCH in 1896.

Murphy's interest in blood-vessel surgery was stimulated by an experience while he was associated with Dr. Edward W. Lee, an attending surgeon at CCH.[5] A case of aneurysm of the internal carotid artery was mistaken for tonsillar abscess. Incising what he believed was the abscess; Dr. Lee had actually opened the aneurysm. As Murphy described it,

*First a few clots of blood slowly wriggled their way out, and, later, faster, a few more, then came the rush of the arterial current with full force of the spurting blood. The patient strangling in his own blood, struggled wildly, and his friend ran away in panic, an abject deserter. Before Dr. Lee could gain control of the patient the latter had bled to death, and the office was in a shambles from the struggle.*

This made a strong impression on Murphy, and he decided to do something about it. He vowed that no surgeon should start the active practice of blood vessel surgery until he had done a considerable amount of experimental work on arteries and veins in animals. Later, he went on to study vessel anastomosis and to describe different forms of aneurysm.[3]

Prior to his historic operation on a human artery, Murphy performed extensive experimental surgery on arteries in search of a satisfactory technique for end-to-end anastomosis. He made many contributions in surgery and always had a laboratory at hand for experimental work. The animal laboratory was in his barn. For arterial work, he used 34 animals in his landmark article entitled "Resection of Arteries and Veins Injured in Continuity—End-to-End Suture: Experimental and Clinical Research" in *Medical Record* on January 16, 1897.[3] Of 34 experiments, 13 were on arterial anastomosis, and only three were successful. The first animal study was conducted on the carotid artery of a male dog on March 4, 1896. The study was to test whether it was feasible to repair a lacerated artery. Murphy first made an oblique incision dividing one-third of the circumference of the artery, then closed with continuous silk suture. The repair proved to be successful, and postmortem examination 21 days later revealed a patent artery, albeit of a slightly diminished caliber. He repeated the same experiment on a second dog but this time made a longitudinal incision. The anastomosis of a divided artery was attempted on March 7, 1896 (Experiment No. 4) on the femoral artery of a hunting dog. He described the invagination technique, which he applied to humans later: "Two double-needled silk sutures were used to draw the intussusceptum one-third of an inch into the intussuscipiens. Several interrupted sutures bind the end of the intussuscipiens to the circumference of the intussusceptum" (Figure 17–2). Postmortem examination eight days later found the artery to be infected and thrombosed. He then performed end-to-end suture of a divided artery without invagination. This was also infected and thrombosed. It was not until Experiment No. 9, on March 26, 1896, that he achieved successful end-to-end anastomosis with the invagination technique on a divided carotid artery. He then repeated the technique on a femoral artery, aorta, and vein in a series of animals using calves, sheep, and dogs. On November 10, 1896 (Experiment No. 33), he refined the technique by placing three internal sutures and seven external sutures. The invaginating suture was inserted differently than in previous experiments. They included only the adventitia and media of the invaginated portion, and when tied, were not exposed in the lumen of the artery. The sheath of the artery was then sutured with catgut. By this method, the size of the artery was not diminished to the same degree that it had been before. Also, there was no foreign body left in the lumen of the artery, as had been done in the previous method of invagination, and, therefore, there was less likelihood of thrombosis.[3]

The first human patient was an American salesman who at Cook County

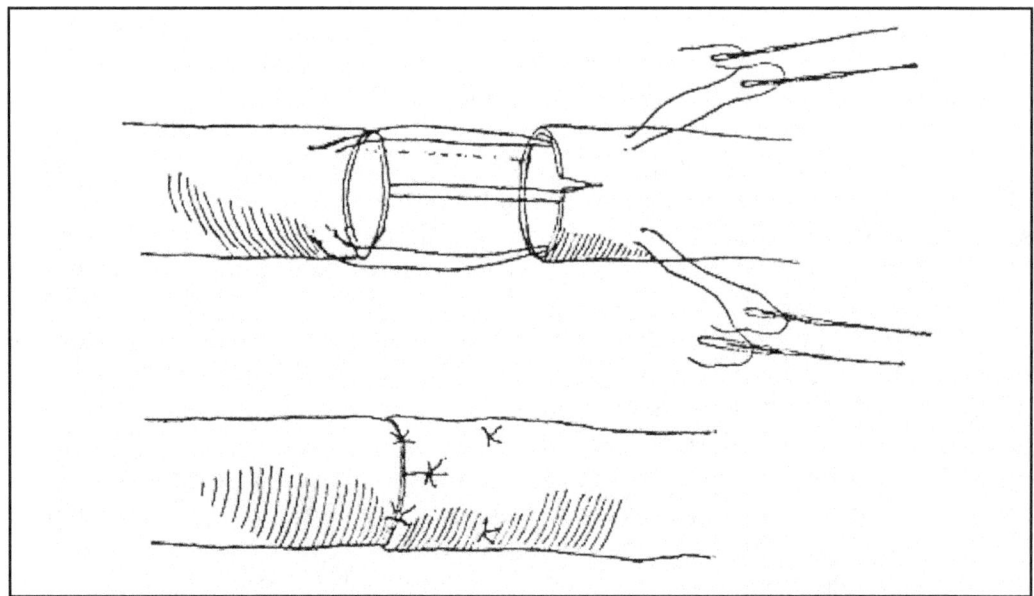

*Figure 17–2 The invaginated technique of end-to-end anastomosis pioneered by John B. Murphy*

Hospital in 1896 underwent ligation of a vein injured by a bullet wound. Later, the patient was re-explored for an infected hematoma, and the eroded artery was ligated. In the second case, Murphy reported the arterial anastomosis in great detail. The patient was described as a peddler of Italian descent, age 29, who had sustained a gunshot wound to the right groin on September 19, 1896. On October 4 he was found to have a loud bruit and palpable thrill along the femoral artery. On October 7, 1896, Murphy exposed the femoral artery and found an aneurysm sac connecting the artery to the vein. The artery was perforated by the bullet (Figure 17–3) and was subsequently transected for preparation of end-to-end anastomosis. The invagination technique was then applied. The following was described by Dr. Murphy:

> *The adventitia was peeled off the invaginated portion for a distance of one-third of an inch; a row of sutures was placed around the edge of the overlapping distal end, the sutures penetrating only the media at the proximal portion: the adventitia was then drawn over the line of union and sutured. The clamps were removed. Not a drop of blood escaped at the line of suture. Pulsation was immediately restored in the artery below the line of approximation and it could be felt feebly in the posterior tibial and dorsalis pedis. The sheath and connective tissue around the artery were then approximated at the position of suture with catgut, so as to support the wall of the artery.*

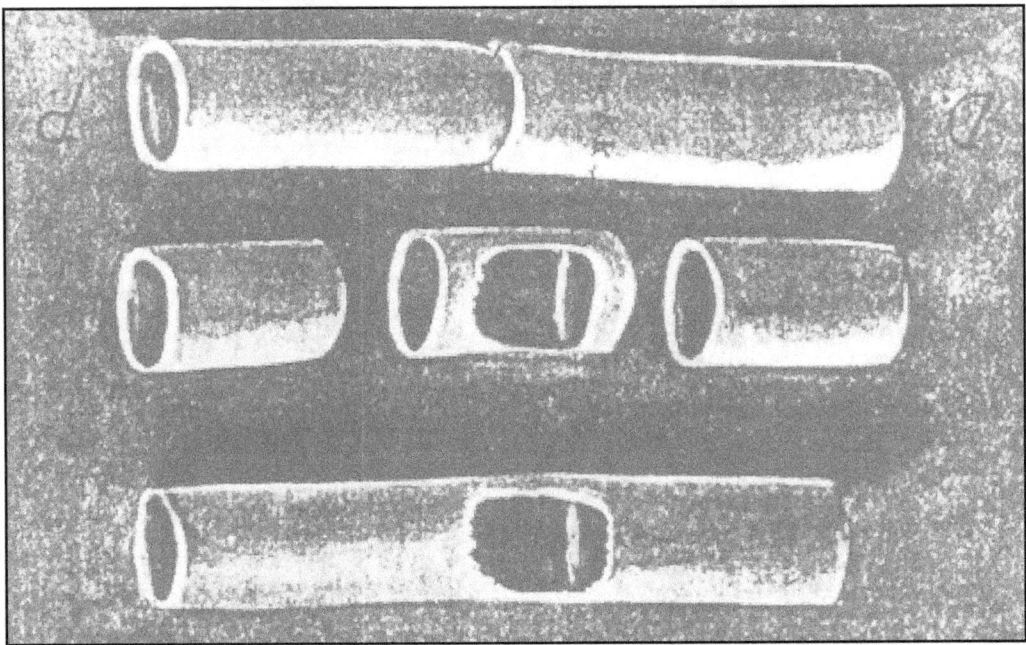

*Figure 17–3  Resection of a damaged artery (center) followed by end-to-end anastomosis using the invaginated technique (top)*

Three months following surgery, the patient was ambulatory without any circulatory symptoms. These two cases represent the first arterial repair in a human.[3]

After Murphy's invagination technique, many surgeons attempted different techniques. At this period, most surgeons concentrated on the importance of confining the thread used for suturing to the outer coat, believing that if the suture material passed through the inner coat (intima) and came in contact with the flowing blood, thrombosis would be promoted. In 1899, Dorfler suggested the use of continuous suture embracing all coats of the vessels with a fine round needle, which became the main feature of the methods that are now generally used.[6] The significance of Murphy's contribution in surgery was not realized until Alex Carrel won the Nobel Prize for his work in arterial anastomosis in 1912.[7,8] Central to Carrel's technique was Murphy's concept of triangulation for the efficient end-to-end anastomosis of two blood vessels. In 1902, a brief article written by Carrel, "Surgical Technique of Vessel Anastomosis and Transplantation of Organ," described in detail what has become known as the triangulation technique (Figure 17–4). In 1905, working with C.C. Guthrie at the University of Chicago, Carrel performed 13 experimental arteriovenous anastomoses without any failure.[8] In describing direct vascular anastomoses, Carrel notes the essential

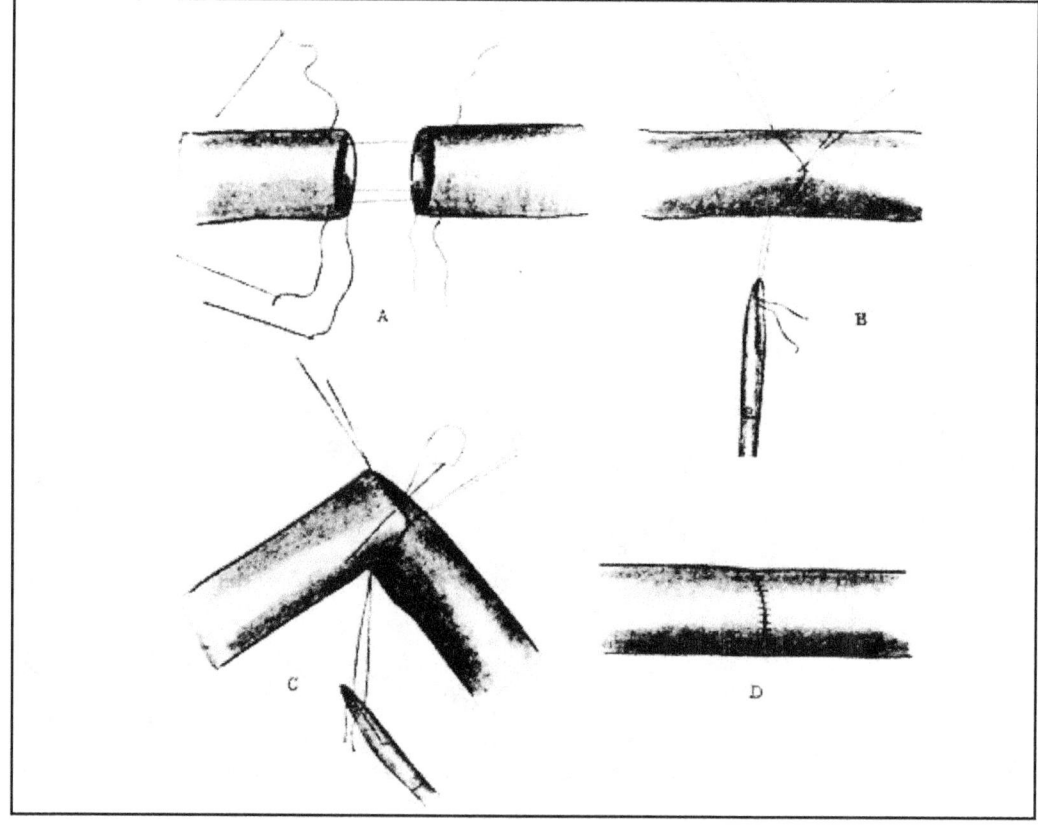

*Figure 17–4 Triangular technique by Alex Carrel*

aspects of the triangulation technique introduced by Murphy.

> *The termino-terminal anastomosis is probably the most valuable. The most important stage of the operation is the approximation of the ends of the vessels by three threads applied in three equidistant points of the circumference of the vessels. Traction on each thread transforms the circumference into a triangle. While the sides of the triangle are stretched a continuous suture is made along each of them. The end-to-end suturing of the carotid artery of a dog can be performed in four to five minutes.*

Murphy's interest in vascular surgery went far beyond arterial anastomosis. In November 1904 he reported a case of subclavian artery aneurysm due to cervical rib to the meeting of the Chicago Surgical Society. Subsequently, he published the case in *Annals of Surgery* in 1905.[9] The patient was a 34-year-old farmer with a one-and-a-half-year history of having tingling and numbness of the left index finger. The left forearm and hand were always cold. On examination, Murphy felt a pulsatile mass above the clavicle and also the cervical rib, which he described as a hard, unyielding mass that could be traced backward to the lateral process of the seventh vertebrae. The brachial and radial pulsations were normal with the arm extended but with the shoulder depressed, there was a pronounced diminution of arterial pulsation. The patient was admitted to Mercy Hospital and underwent surgery. A supraclavicular incision was made, and the subclavian artery was exposed and found to be somewhat enlarged. The entire cervical rib was removed. Murphy did not resect the aneurysm, and follow-up examination one month later revealed that the vessel had contracted to almost the normal size with no further ischemic symptoms of the hand. In 1906, Murphy reported a patient with goiter associated with a cervical rib with similar hand symptoms. Murphy removed first the goiter and then the rib. The arm symptoms were relieved. In the Surgical Clinic series, Murphy gave a detailed review (112 references) of the surgical significance of cervical rib. He described two distinct sets of symptoms; those from arterial pressure and those from brachial plexus pressure.[9]

In 1909, Murphy reported a remarkable operation for removal of an embolus from the common iliac artery.[10] The patient, a 41-year-old woman, presented with pain in the left lower chest and upper part of the abdomen. Later, the pain shifted to her pelvis and legs. At first, both legs were cold, but the right one warmed up while the left one became blue from the thigh down and blebs began to appear. It wasn't until the fourth day of the illness, when she was admitted to Mercy Hospital, that Murphy saw the patient. He took her to the operating room immediately. He described the procedure: "An incision one-inch long was made in the femoral artery, which was found to be completely thrombosed. With a delicate forceps, the clot (a bifurcated plug an inch-and-a-half long) was drawn from below upward, when fresh arterial blood came from below...." Cleaning out the proximal clot proved more difficult but Murphy persisted with forceps, spoons, and various catheters until finally an arterial sound, an "intense arterial flow, carrying with it a lot of embolic debris and fresh bright blood," was obtained

(Figure 17–5). In his summation of this experience and his experimental works on thrombi, he suggested that even cerebral ischemia from emboli lodged in the common or internal carotid arteries should be amenable to extraction. He suggested that aspiration through a catheter would probably be made away from the area of the thrombus to minimize rethrombosis. Suffice to say his concept of removal of embolus from a common iliac artery is appropriate even today as we practice with the Fogarty catheter technique.

Murphy also carried out experimental work on aneurysm repair and devised his own method of endoaneurysmorrhaphy, which he reported at a New Orleans meeting of the American Medical Association.[11] The work, however was not published, perhaps because, as Murphy admitted "I think Matas' suture method is better than the plan I had advocated previously."[11] Murphy recorded an operation on a false aneurysm on a syphilitic axillary artery that had caused brachial plexus paralysis by pressure. The aneurysm was ligated above and below the aneurysm and relied on the collateral circulation to supply the arm. The patient gained excellent recovery of muscular function afterward. While performing endoaneurysmorrhaphy on an endarteritic aneurysm of the brachial artery of the mid-arm, he gave a magnificent overview of aneurysmal disease, including histology, etiology,

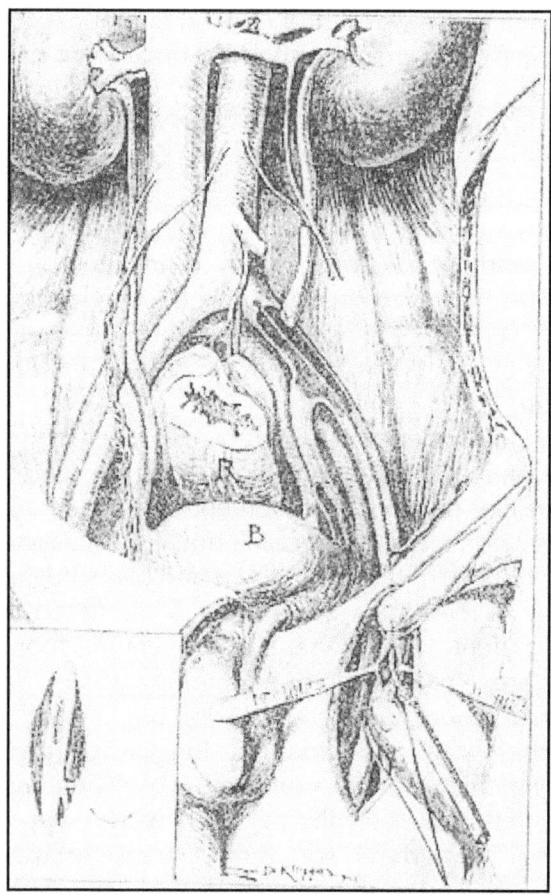

*Figure 17–5 Femoral embolectomy in a patient with left iliac embolus: a ureteral catheter was used to break up the clot.*

classification, and treatment. For proximal control, he used a little spring forceps commonly used in operations on the muscle of the eye. In his landmark article in *Medical Record* published in 1897 he gave detailed descriptions of various forms of aneurysms including fusiform, vascular, and arteriovenous aneurysms[3] (Figure 17–6). Murphy also wrote extensively about etiology and different types of aneurysms.

Venous problems were no strangers to John B. Murphy. He spoke on "varicose veins and varicose leg ulcers," although they were "old and hackneyed subjects, still they form a large percentage of one's practice, and the mere fact that so much is constantly being written about them goes to show that there are many knotty problems." He went on to describe multiple venous resections in the thigh and leg for varices. For leg ulcers, he devised a lace-on "leg corset" of heavy-grade linen or silk from the ankle to the head of the tibia. He also used it to relieve the "leg fatigue" that accompanies varicose veins. It is interesting to note that his concept of compression support remains the mainstay for treatment of venous insufficiency.[12]

For his many contributions in surgery, John B. Murphy was elected president of the American Medical Association in 1911. He was a founder of the American College of Surgeons. In 1904, a conversation between Murphy and Franklin H. Martin of Chicago resulted in the creation of a new surgical journal entitled *Surgery, Gynecology and Obstetrics* (*SG&O*), and for a few years, Murphy was chief editor of the journal (now known as the *Journal of American College of Surgeons*). He was one of the charter members of the Chicago Surgical Society and served as its third president. The book *J. B. Murphy, Stormy Petrel of Surgery* by Loyal Davis aptly summarized the life and times of this unique surgeon. The

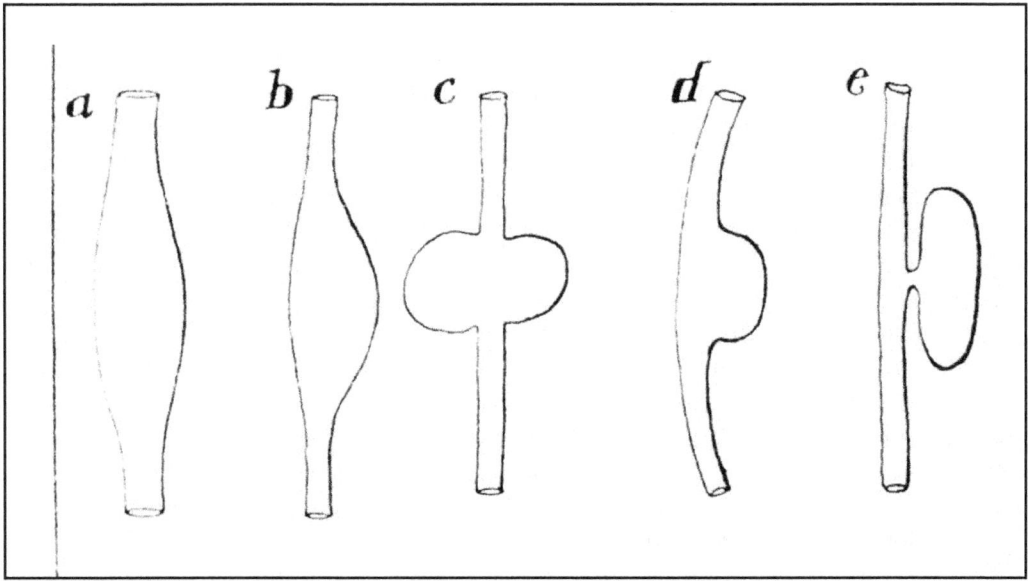

*Figure 17–6 Types of aneurysms described by John B. Murphy*

stormy petrel is a small sea bird that sailors traditionally have considered to be a sign of an approaching storm.[5] It certainly appeared to be an appropriate term to characterize the man and the nature of this truly remarkable part of vascular surgical heritage at Northwestern and Cook County Hospital.

## 1900s–1946—The Era of Indirect Surgery

From Murphy's arterial anastomosis to the early part of 1940s, there was no direct surgery on arteries. Surgical treatment was often by ligation, either proximal, distal, or both. For ischemic extremities, sympathectomy was often employed to improve blood flow. The clinical practice of vascular surgery, in most instances, was limited to ligation and stripping of varicose veins. At County Hospital, besides John B. Murphy, there were only a few surgeons interested in vascular surgery. Among the early surgeons was Dr. Albert Halstead, a graduate of Northwestern. He joined CCH as attending surgeon in 1891 and served until 1914. He was on the academic faculty at Northwestern in 1898 and was appointed professor of surgery from 1907 to 1914. He first presented his work on the treatment of gangrene of the leg by femoral arteriovenous anastomosis to the American Surgical Association on June 19, 1911. Together with Dr. Roger Vaughn, attending night surgeon at CCH, he presented arterioplasty for aortic aneurysm to the American Surgical Association. Additionally, Halstead presented his experience in ligation of subclavian aneurysm in 1902 and then in 1920, on innominate aneurysm to Chicago Surgical Society meetings.

One surgeon who shared many of John B. Murphy's characteristics—his flamboyance and theatrical presence—was Raymond McNealy, attending surgeon and chief of staff at CCH. He was also chief of surgery at Wesley Memorial Hospital. McNealy was acknowledged to be a premier surgeon who could operate on everything including blood vessels. From 1922 to 1934, he published 15 articles on various topics in vascular surgery, including treatment of aneurysms of the axillary artery, femoral artery and aorta, sympathectomy, amputation criteria, vein ligation and phlebitis, the use of fascia strips as a bypass graft, and therapy of injuries to large vessels. In 1943, he addressed the Midwest Clinical Society in Omaha on *Advances in Blood Vessel Surgery* and gave an in-depth review of arterial surgery of that time period.[13] He discussed sympathectomy, a very popular technique at that time; the surgical technique of repair of injured artery; the use of sulfa drugs and Heparin; and postoperative care by splint and elevation, cotton dressing, and nursing care. McNealy concluded that successful blood vessel surgery requires clinical experience, good judgment, excellent technique, and extremely efficient nursing care. All these elements remain true today. McNealy was well known for his surgical skill. He worked with tremendous concentration, which enabled him to operate very quickly while giving close attention to every minute detail. His hands actually moved slowly, an economy of motion, which he passed on to many trainees. He was an amazingly intelligent, truly gifted person, and a superb technical operator.

In May 1926, Dr. Allen Kanavel, chairman at Northwestern and attending surgeon at CCH, presented to the American Surgical Association on cervical and lumber sympathectomy for Raynaud's disease and other vascular lesions.

Several faculty members of University of Illinois (Rush) who were attending surgeons at CCH also had interest in vascular surgery. They were John Reynolds, Carl Beck, and Frank Theis. All were leading surgeons in Chicago. Based on their experience at CCH, these three surgeons reported on surgical management of acute embolic occlusion, a challenging surgical problem. The first report was by Koucky, Beck, and Hoffman in 1940,[14] followed by Reynolds and Jirka in 1944,[15] and then Klingensmith and Theis in 1952.[16] All these procedures were done before the introduction of the Fogarty catheter with direct arteriotomy to remove the embolus inside the femoral or iliac artery. Frank Theis also had interest in aneurysms, and in 1937, he presented on the treatment of popliteal aneurysm to the Chicago Surgical Society.

Kidney transplantation requires a precise arterial anastomosis. Carl Beck, attending surgeon at CCH (1894–1917) and a close friend of Alexis Carrel, had performed some of the first experimental kidney transplantations in 1903 within two years after the first kidney transplantation by Ulmann and before Carrel had published his technical adaption of Murphy's technique.[8] Beck undoubtedly encountered difficulties with arterial thrombosis in his first transplantation and this problem of arterial thrombosis interested him throughout his career. Carrel's adaptation of Murphy's technique led to the first technically successful experimental transplantation.

In 1946, 31 surgeons with interest in vascular surgery founded the Society for Vascular Surgery to promote the exchange of scientific information and surgical experience. This was the beginning of a giant step to make vascular surgery a surgical specialty. In the 1940s, the practice of vascular surgery still was limited to indirect surgery on arteries. Venous surgery such as ligation and stripping of varicose veins dominated the clinical practice.

Direct surgery became possible in 1946 when Dos Santos first reported disobliteration of an artery by thromboendarterectomy.[17] The technique was later popularized by E. J. Wylie of America.[18]

## 1950s—The Breakthrough Decade of Direct Arterial Surgery

The breakthrough of direct surgery on arteries came in the decade of the 1950s, thus beginning the era of reconstructive surgery. In this decade, Jean Kunlin of France first introduced the autogenous saphenous bypass graft in 1951.[19] This was followed by Jacque Oudot of Paris who performed the first successful resection of the aorto-iliac bifurcation and replacement with arterial homograft.[20] In 1951, Schafer and Hardin of Kansas City[21] and Dubost of France[22] reported the use of homograft to repair aortic aneurysm. In 1953, DeBakey,[23] and in 1954, Eastcott and Rob, reported on carotid endarterectomy[24] in treatment of carotid stenosis. These landmark procedures ushered in a period of rapid growth of reconstructive surgery. In Chicago, Ormond Julian and his colleagues first repaired an aortic aneurysm at the Hines Hospital with a homograft.[25]

In the late 1950s, there also was great interest by surgeons in the development of prosthetic graft. In 1954, Arthur Voorhees and his colleagues reported their experience in repairing 17 aortic aneurysms and one popliteal aneurysm with Vinyon-N tube.[26] Research in prosthetic grafts by Edwards, DeBakey, Szilagyi, and others resulted in the emergence of the Dacron graft (woven and knit) as the graft of choice as a substitute for the aorta and also as a bypass graft for limb arteries.

## Chicago Artery Bank at Cook County Hospital

In 1953, one of the leading cardiovascular surgeons in Chicago, Dr. Ormand Julian, wrote to the Chicago Heart Association about his experience with an artery bank for use of homografts in several patients at University of Illinois. He suggested a wider use of the artery bank to benefit patients with aortic aneurysms. In response to this request, the Chicago Heart Association appointed an advisory committee of the Chicago Artery Bank to look into the establishment of some sort of central source for providing arterial segments to Chicago surgeons. The committee consisted of Geza de Takats (chairman), Oglesby Paul, Willis Potts, John Olwin, J. Garret Allen, and S. Howard Armstrong. Under the leadership of de Takats, a new advisory committee of the Chicago Artery Bank was formed in 1954 to explore ways to distribute funding support from the Chicago Heart Association to participating hospitals. The committee consisted of William Adams, Edward Avery, William Grove, Saul Mackler, Willis Potts, and Egbert Fell. Dr. Fell was attending surgeon at CCH. In the ensuing period, the committee encountered administration problems with allocation of funds among various hospitals. It was then decided to establish a central artery bank to be housed at Cook County Hospital. The Municipal Artery Bank of the Chicago Heart Association was organized according to a plan submitted by Dr. Fell. The plan was approved on December 2, 1954, and Fell was appointed coordinator of the bank. The concept of a central artery bank for the city of Chicago gained enthusiastic support from all medical schools. The great volume of autopsy material at one location—the Cook County Hospital and Cook County coroner's laboratory—was unique. Most importantly, the project enjoyed the full cooperation of Dr. Karl Meyer, medical superintendent of the County Hospital. With funding support from the Chicago Heart Association, the first specimen was obtained on January 1, 1955, under sterile conditions at the Cook County morgue. The artery bank was opened formally on October 11, 1955, with Fell as the medical director without compensation and Frank Milloy as assistant medical director. In 1956, Milton Weinberg succeeded Fell as the medical director.[27,28] Harold Laufman established a branch of the artery bank at Passavant Memorial Hospital.

In the late 1950s, nylon and later Dacron emerged as a durable substitute for a diseased aorta. Gradual refinement of synthetic graft material made the use of homograft obsolete. In the last advisory committee meeting on April 29, 1960, it was decided to close the bank and dispose of the equipment. In the four years of its existence, 380 vessels were used in 353 patients. Not only did the patients benefit from bank-supplied vessels but also from the group of vascular surgeons that had come together in Chicago, which was equal to any in the country.[28]

Dr. Egbert Fell contributed to the artery bank and was a distinguished pediatric cardiac surgeon who practiced at St. Luke's Hospital as well as CCH. He maintained an interest in surgery of arteries and reported the creation of autogenous vessel grafts by a combined use of vein and fascia as a conduit.[29] Fell and Weinberg also performed surgery on thoracic aortic aneurysms (syphilitic or atherosclerotic) at CCH. Weinberg recalled that the vascular clamps used were the Potts-Smith clamp and sutures were 5-0 silk lubricated with mineral oil. At this period, four attending surgeons at CCH were members of the Society for Vascular Surgery: Frank Theis (1949), Harold Laufman (1949), Egbert Fell (1957), and Milton Weinberg (1964).

The decade of the 1960s was a period of further expansion of direct surgical techniques. The introduction of the Seldinger catheter arteriographic technique allowed surgeons to understand the pathology of visceral ischemia and renal artery pathology causing renovascular hypertension.[30] For cerebral ischemia, catheter arteriography allowed detailed examination of the vertebral artery and documented the subclavian steal phenomenon. Pathology defined by arteriography has made possible direct surgery either by endarterectomy or bypass graft in every vascular bed. A wide spectrum of vascular procedures was made available for revascularization.

As young attending surgeons at CCH both Robert Freeark and Robert Baker were interested in vascular surgery, and they attended all cases with vascular problems at County Hospital. During the 1960s, portal hypertension was common, and porto-caval shunt became a frequently performed vascular procedure. Another attending surgeon interested in vascular surgery in the 1960s was Dr. David Movitz of the Chicago Medical School faculty. Movitz had done a feasibility study of catheter arteriography in dogs. In 1968, Freeark recruited Otto Trippel and John J. Bergan, two leading vascular surgeons of the Northwestern faculty, to staff vascular cases. This recruitment greatly improved the training in vascular surgery for surgical residents.

## 1960s—Specialized Care for Civilian Vascular Trauma: The Trauma Unit at CCH

In March 1966, under the direction of Drs. Robert J. Freeark and Robert J. Baker, the first trauma unit in the country opened its door for specialized care of trauma patients.

Wars are notorious for providing the impetus for improvement on the management of the injured patient. World War II provided the opportunity for more experience on direct care of arterial injuries. DeBakey and Simeone in 1946 reported on World War II experiences with direct arterial reconstructions using both vein grafts and direct anastomoses. The result of arterial repair in World War II was not significantly better than the results for arterial ligation.[31] DeBakey observed that the delay in the time that a surgeon could care for an injured artery seldom was less than 12 hours and exceeded the reasonable amount of time under which any arterial reconstruction could be achieved. The standard for civilian injuries at that time was repair performed in less than six hours from the time of injury. According to DeBakey, the high amputation rate of World War II inspired many surgeons to develop vascular surgery as a specialty.[31]

The end of World War II saw the rapid development of arterial reconstructive surgery in the nonmilitary setting, and most importantly, the founding of the Society for Vascular Surgery (SVS). This advance made available a number of surgeons exposed to arterial reconstructive techniques who were able to apply these surgical skills in the Korean conflict.

The Korean War also coincided with the development of the Mobile Army Surgical Hospital (MASH) units that permitted a much more rapid evacuation and definitive treatment of arterial injuries. With more rapid surgical treatment available, combined with more widespread surgical training in arterial reconstructive technique, Jahnke reported results from the Korean conflict with amputation rates for femoral and popliteal artery injuries that were 75 percent lower than in DeBakey's World War II series.[32]

The wealth of trauma cases provided County surgeons an opportunity to contribute to vascular injuries under the direction of Freeark and Jack Saletta, who reported their experience in penetrating wounds of the neck and the definition of "three zones for guiding operative management." They also reported on various types of arterial injuries and missile embolization. They advocated the use of temporary shunt in retro-hepatic vena cava injury and the use of angiographic embolization for traumatic hemobilia. For venous problems, they reported on post-traumatic venous thrombosis including vena cava and the role of venography in the detection of deep vein thrombosis.

## 1970s—Vascular Surgery as a Surgical Specialty

In the decade of the 1970s, two reports called for better care for patients with vascular disease. The first was the report by DeWeese and his committee on vascular practice in hospitals in the United States,[33] and the second was the SVS presidential address by E.J. Wylie.[34] Both reports emphasized the inadequacy of vascular training for most surgical trainees and the poor care of vascular patients. Both reports called for the need for better training in vascular surgery. As a result of these reports, the leadership of the SVS started two initiatives; the first was to develop accreditation of vascular training programs, and the second was to seek Board Certification of vascular surgeons. A one-year fellowship in vascular surgery in addition to five years of general surgery training was proposed. At the same time, SVS formed a committee to approve centers for training of vascular surgeons, and many surgical programs started to form a vascular surgical service. These two initiatives began in 1972 and went on for 10 years before vascular surgery examination and certification was finally given by the American Board of Surgery (ABS) in 1982.[35]

The decade of the 1970s also saw many vascular surgeons interested in noninvasive studies. This led to the introduction of various types of plethysmography as well as Doppler ultrasound techniques. Further refinement of ultrasound technology by the University of Washington group, notably D. E. Strandness, resulted in the development of the duplex scan, a combination of B-mode imaging and velocity interrogation at a specific site. With this instrumentation, the noninvasive vascular laboratory was established to provide diagnostic testing for patients suspected of having carotid stenosis, arterial occlusive disease, and acute deep vein thrombosis. The vascular laboratory, founded and developed by vascular surgeons, enabled the surgeons to bring a special diagnostic service to hospitals in addition to operative care. As a result, noninvasive testing became an important component in the training curriculum of vascular surgeons. It is also an essential component in credentialing as a vascular surgeon in most hospitals in the United States.

## Vascular Surgical Service at Cook County Hospital

In 1972, Dr. Gerald Moss took over the chairmanship at Cook County Hospital. Recognizing the national trend of specialization in vascular surgery, a vascular surgery service was established, and in 1978, with Dr. Leo Lim as the chief and Rau Villasuso as a vascular attending surgeon, a noninvasive vascular laboratory was established to provide diagnostic test for patients at CCH. In 1980, Lim reported on the treatment of popliteal injuries, injuries that most modern civilian series still have a limb loss rate of 10 percent. Lim demonstrated that in cases of popliteal artery injury, when fasciotomy was the first very procedure performed before tackling the vascular injury, 100 percent limb salvage could be achieved even in injuries up to 24 hours old. Lim was a proponent of the medial approach for all popliteal injuries with taking down and tagging medical muscular structures because it provided wide exposure and facilitated rapid fasciotimy, something that the posterior approach for popliteal injuries does not offer.

Management of subclavian or innominate arteries is often challenging. Leo Lim, along with Joe Meyer, the chief of vascular surgery from 1984 to1986, reported their experience in the management of subclavian-innominate artery injuries. In patients with retrohepatic vena cava injury, Robert Brown advocated the use of a temporary shunt for management. R. Keen, J. Meyer, and J. Durham reported on the superior results of vein interposition grafts in the treatment of over 130 patients with extremity vascular injuries using specialized techniques such as paneled and spiral vein grafts.

While some vascular injuries were handled by the trauma service, the majority of vascular trauma cases outside of the abdomen were cared for by the vascular service, a practice that continues to this day. Vascular staffs provided expertise in patients who needed reconstructive vascular care.

Since 1978, four surgeons served as chief of vascular surgery: Leo Lim (1978–81), Joe Meyer (1982–91) Darwin Eton (1992–93) and Richard Keen (1994–present).

As we entered the decade of the 1980s, vascular surgeons continued to negotiate with ABS and the resident review committee to play an increasing role in the training and certification of vascular surgeons. The 1980s also saw many academic centers including an additional one year of basic science research. The study of endothelial cell seeding of grafts by many vascular surgeons resulted in expansion of bio-technological research in many academic centers. At present, basic science studies using molecular biology and gene-based techniques are common in many centers. In order to foster the research effort by vascular surgeons, SVS started to work with NHLBI/NIH and the von Liebig Foundation to initiate the KO-8 and K-23 grants for career development of surgeon-scientists and surgeon-clinical investigators.

Preston Flanigan and Jim Schuler from the University of Illinois vascular group participated in the growth of the County vascular service in the 1980s. Jim Schuler was Preston Flanigan's first vascular fellow at Illinois in 1981, providing the critical number of trained vascular surgeons so that the Illinois group could participate in the vascular care at County.

The initial combined mentorship of Flanigan and Schuler from 1981 to 1987 and Joe Meyer with Schuler from 1985 through 1990, was responsible for many residents from the combined Illinois-County surgery residency choosing to pursue careers in vascular surgery. These County, Illinois-trained surgeons who pursued specialty vascular training after County included Larry Williams, Bruce Dillon, Dan Douglas, Steve Schaefer, Jim Walsh, Chad Tober, Richard Keen, Marty Ellenby, Norm Cumins, and Marty Borhani. Deborah Lange, Tom Schwarcz, Jens Jorgensen, Joe Durham, and Henry Baraniewski also served as County vascular surgery attending surgeons in the late 1980s.

## 1990s—The Decade of Endovascular Surgery

The 1990s was the defining decade in vascular surgery. Sweeping changes in training and practice came to vascular surgery as a result of the technological development of endovascular surgery. The introduction of endovascular graft and stent drastically changed the face of practice in vascular surgery. At present, catheter-based endovascular techniques account for nearly half of operative cases in most centers.

Following completion of his vascular fellowship in 1989 at County and Illinois under Flanigan and Schuler, Darwin Eton completed the first minimally invasive vascular surgery fellowship in the country at UCLA under Wesely Moore. Eton then served as chief of vascular surgery at Cook County Hospital in the early 1990s and introduced endovascular technology to CCH.

After completion of a vascular surgery fellowship at Northwestern from 1992 to 1994, Richard Keen (Figure 17–7) joined CCH as chief of vascular surgery. Under his direction, endovascular surgery began to be incorporated into the surgical armamentarium in the treatment of vascular disease. Shortly thereafter, CCH renewed its affiliation with Rush Medical College and the surgical training program merged with Rush. Walter McCarthy, chief of vascular surgery at Rush, joined the CCH vascular service as a consultant.

As endovascular surgery emerged as a viable alternative to open surgery, SVS mandated a change of training curriculum for vascular surgeons. Training of

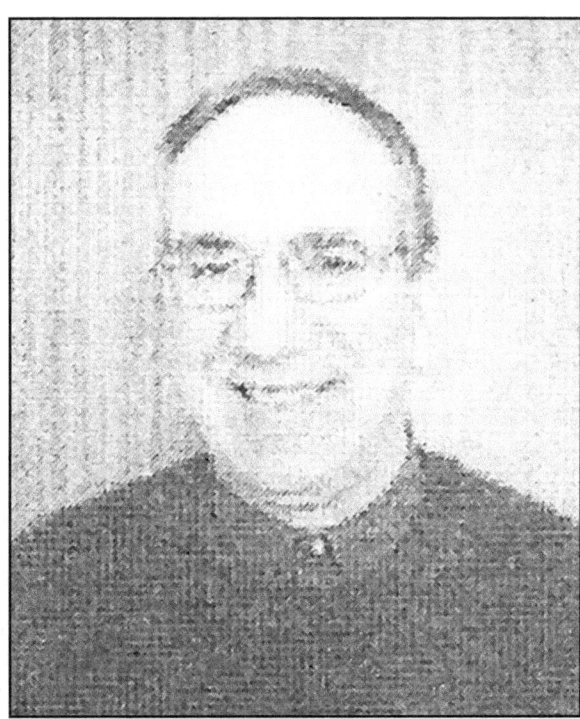

*Figure 17-7* **Richard Keen**

vascular surgeons is now extended to two years to include four major components: open surgery, endovascular surgery, noninvasive tests, and medical knowledge. With the approval of ABS and the American Board of Medical Specialties (ABMS), certification in general surgery is no longer a prerequisite for taking the vascular surgery examination. Also, the pathway to becoming certified as a vascular surgeon has changed. There are now three pathways to be certified as a vascular surgeon: five years of resident training in vascular surgery straight from medical school, four years of general surgery and two years of vascular surgery, or five years of general surgery and two years of vascular surgery to allow a combination of general surgery and vascular surgery certification. All these changes were targeted for shorter training time and better care for patients. The complexities of endovascular surgery have made it an impossible task for general surgeons to do occasional vascular surgery.

## References

1. Friedman SG. *A History of Vascular Surgery.* Malden MA: Blackwell-Futura, 2005.
2. Konstantinov IE. Eck-Pavlov shunt: The 120$^{th}$ anniversary of the first vascular anastomosis. *Surgery*. 1997;121:640-645.
3. Murphy JB. Resection of arteries and veins injured in continuity—end-to-end suture: experimental and clinical research *Medical Records (NY)*. 1897;51:73-88.

4. Yao JST. The first arterial anastomosis in a human by John B. Murphy: The 100th anniversary. *Cardiovasv Surg.* 1997;5:553-556.
5. Davis L. *J.B. Murphy: Stormy Petrel of Surgery.* New York: G.P. Putnam's Son, 1938.
6. Dorfler J. Uber arteriennaht *Beirr Klin Chir.* 1899;25:781.
7. Carrel A. La technique operatoire des anastomoses vasculaires et la transplantation des visceres. *Lyon Med.* 1902;98:859-864.
8. Carrel A. The surgery of blood vessels. *Johns Hopkins Hosp Bull. 1907;18:18*
9. Murphy JB. A case of cervical rib with symptoms resembling subclavian aneurism. *Ann Surg.* 1905; 41:399-406.
10. Murphy JB. Removal of an embolus from the common iliac artery, with re-establishment of circulation in the femoral. *JAMA.* 1909;52: 1661-1663.
11. Murphy JB. Aneurysm of the brachial artery—endoaneurysmorrhaphy. *The Clinics of John B. Murphy.* 1915;5:53-75.
12. Murphy JB. Talk on varicose veins and varicose leg ulcers. *The Clinics of John B. Murphy.* 1916;5:775-798.
13. McNealy RW. Advances in blood vessel surgery. *The Nebraska State M.J.* 1944;29:369-372.
14. Koucky JJ, Beck WC, Hoffman JM. Peripheral arterial embolism. *Am J Surg.* 1940;50:39-49.
15. Reynolds JT, Jirka FJ. Embolic occlusion of major arteries. *Surgery.* 1944;16:485-518.
16. Klingensmith W, Theis FV. Femoral and iliac artery embolectomy: Critical review of cases at Cook County Hospital from 1946 to 1951. *JAMA.* 1952;150:1393-1396.
17. Dos Santos. Lerich memorial lecture: From embolectomy to endarterectomy or the fall of myth. *J Cardiovasc Surg.* 1976;17;113-128.
18. Wylie EJ. Thromboendarterectomy for arteriosclerotic thrombosis of major arteries. *Surgery* 1952;32:275-292.
19. Kunlin J. Le traitement de l'ischeme arteritique par la greffe veineuse [Long vein transplantation in treatment of ischemia caused by arteritis]. *Rev Chir.* 1951:70:206-235.
20. Oudot J, Beaconsfield P. Thrombosis of aortic bifurcation treated by resection and homograft replacement: Report of five cases. *Arch Surg.* 1953;66:365-374.
21. Schafer FW, Hardin CA. The use of temporary polythene shunts to permit occlusion, resection, and frozen homologus graft replacement of vital vessel segments: A laboratory and clinical study. *Surgery.* 1952;31:186-199.
22. Dubost C. Resection of an aneurysm of the abdominal aorta: reestablishment of the continuity by a preserved human arterial graft, with result after five months. *AMA Arch Surg.* 1952;64:405-408.
23. DeBakey ME. Successful carotid endarterectomy for cerebrovascular insufficiency. Nineteen year follow-up. *JAMA.* 1975;233:1083-1085.
24. Eastcott HHG, Pickering GW, Rob C. Reconstruction of internal carotid artery in a patient with intermittent attacks of hemiplegia. *Lancet.* 1954;2:994.
25. Julian O.C. Chicago and the treatment of abdominal aortic aneuyrsms. *Proc Inst Med Chgo.* 1974;30:24-34
26. Voorhees AB Jr, Jaretzki A III, Blakemore AH. The use of tubes constructed from vinyon"N" cloth in bridging arterial defects. A preliminary report. *Ann Surg.* 1952;135:332-336.
27. Milloy F, deTakats G. The Chicago artery bank *Proc Inst Med Chgo.* 1976; 31:31-33,47.
28. Weinberg M. Jr, Fell EH, deTakats G, McElwaine N. Use of homografts dispensed by central artery bank of Chicago Heart Association. JAMA 1959;170: 2132-2134.

29. Chun N, Forney RA, Fell EH. Creation of autogenous vessel grafts: An experimental study. *Arch Surg*. 1954;68:574-590.
30. Seldinger SI. Catheter replacement of the needle in percutaneous arteriography: A new technique. *Acta Radiol*. 1953;39:368-376.
31. DeBakey ME. and Simeone FA. Battle injuries of the arteries in World War II ; An Analysis of 2471 cases. *Ann Surg*. 1946;123-534
32. Jahnke EJ. Howard JM. Primary repair of major arterial injuries. Report of 58 battle casualties. *Arch Surg*. 1953;66:646-649.
33. DeWeese JA, Blaisdell FW, Foster JH. Optimal resources for vascular disease. *Circulation*. 1972;46:A-305.
34. Wylie EJ. Vascular surgery: A quest for excellence. *Arch Surg*. 1970;101:645-648.
35. DeWeese JA. Accreditation of vascular training programs and certification of vascular surgeons. *J Vasc Surg*. 1996;23:1043-1053.

# 18

# Urological Surgery

*Patrick Guinan, MD*

- *Introduction*
- *The Beginning of Chicago Urology (1832–1880)*
- *Urology at the Cook County Hospital (1889–1900)*
- *Urology Becomes a Separate Specialty (1900–1950)*
- *Contribution of Medical Schools and Residencies*
  - *Medical Schools*
  - *Residencies*
- *Early Era*
- *Cystoscopy Era (1915–1965)*
- *Modern Era (1965–Present)*
- *Conclusion*
- *References*

The history of urology in Chicago involves pioneer surgeons and urologists as well as hospitals, particularly the Cook County Hospital, where many of the early urologic icons trained and practiced. Cook County Hospital, where modern surgery developed, was also where urology became a separate specialty in Chicago. As urologic specialists differentiated from general surgeons, they organized local and national societies, and the specialty of urology became organizationally independent. Urology then developed its own standards and board certification. As the need for uniform urologic training became apparent, residency programs were instituted and guidelines were promulgated and regulated by the Resident Review Committee for Urology. Medical schools, following the Flexner Report, were also governed by stricter criteria and gradually assumed oversight over graduate medical education across the board, including urology.

## Introduction

Modern surgery began following the development of general anesthesia in 1846[1] and antisepsis in 1865.[2] These discoveries facilitated control of pain and morbid infections related to surgery. The last two decades of the 19th century (1880–1900), as medicine built on these innovations, witnessed the development of remarkably gifted surgeons whose contributions to surgical technique have given 21st century society the benefits of modern surgery. Chicago was a focal point of these surgical developments. The appropriate mix of factors required for excellence in the development of surgery at Cook County was crystallized by Dr. Christian Fenger, a surgeon of wide and diverse interests who also served as chief pathologist of Cook County Hospital. Fenger primarily influenced general surgery, but his fingerprints can also be seen in other surgical subspecialties, including urology. Prior to about 1880, major urologic surgery was rarely performed.

## The Beginnings of Chicago Urology (1832–1880)

Chicago's first physician, Dr. Jean Rousseliere, treated Jacques Marquette in 1674.[3] Chicago was first settled in 1775, but it did not have a permanent physician until 1800. The first surgeon, Dr. William C. Smith, arrived in 1803 and was stationed at Fort Dearborn. The first recorded operation was a leg amputation performed by Dr. Edgar Harman in 1832.

The city was incorporated in 1837[4] but had an almshouse, a forerunner of the County Hospital, for the care of the sick five years earlier in 1832. As early as the 1840s, Illinois medical journals reported on urological procedures such as hydrocelectomy and stone surgery,[5] but there was little major urologic surgery and no urological specialization prior to about 1880 because of inadequate pain control, no reliable anesthesia, and high mortality rates from infections.

Daniel Brainard, an early Chicago physician and founder of the Rush Medical College, pioneered techniques in the management of urethral strictures. Edmund Andrews reported on numerous urologic cases and made several attempts to improve the endoscope, a forerunner of the cystoscope. In 1865 Charles Gilman Smith was appointed the head of the Cook County Hospital Department of Skin and Venereal Diseases, the first Urologic Department in Chicago. In 1895 Charles Wesley Purdy published *Practical Urinalysis and Urinary Diagnosis*.[6] Isaac Newton Danforth (Figure 18-1) performed the first nephrectomy in Chicago.[7] Table I shows the pioneer urologists and their contributions to this field.

## Urology at the Cook County Hospital (1880–1900)

The engine that drove Chicago urology was undoubtedly Cook County Hospital, and the catalyst for this surgical explosion at CCH was undoubtedly Christian Fenger.[8] Fenger, while an innovative surgeon himself, was also a surgical pathologist at Cook County Hospital from 1878 to 1893.[9] He first described a longitudinal incision and transverse closure for ureteral pelvic junction obstruction.[10] Fenger also inspired other notable surgeons such as Nicholas Senn, who

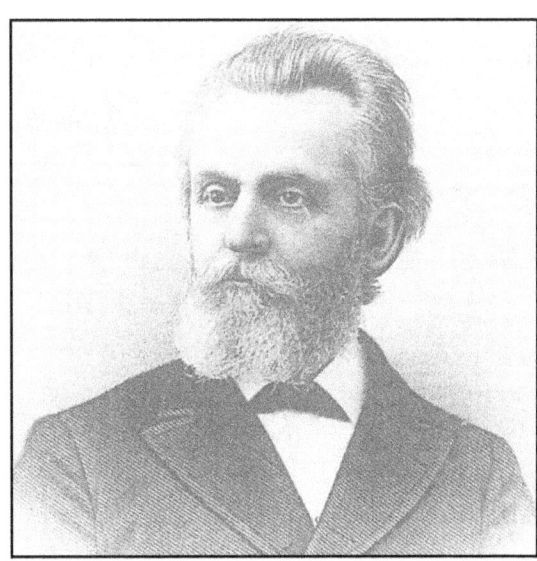

*Figure 18-1 Isaac Newton Danforth (1835-1911) performed first nephrectomy in Chicago.*

### Table I  Pioneers (1833-1880)

| Pioneers | Cook County Hospital Status | Medical School Affiliation | Contribution |
|---|---|---|---|
| Daniel Brainard (1812-1866) | A | Rush | Described Urethral Stricture |
| Edmund Andrews (1824-1904) | A | NU | Chicago's First Urologist |
| Charles G. Smith (1828-1894) | A | NU | Chicago's First Urology Department (1865) |
| Charles Wesley Purdy (1846-1901) | | | Book: Practical Urinalysis and Urinary Diagnosis |
| Isaac Newton Danforth (1835-1911) | A | NU | First Nephrectomy in Chicago |

A: Attending

described TB of the kidney, and J. B. Murphy, who pioneered the perineal prostatectomy as well as many other urologic innovations.

Additional surgeons who performed novel procedures on urologic organs include E. Wyllys Andrew, who performed the first Bottle operation (1882) for hydrocele. Malcolm Harris described ureteral urine collection. Arthur Dean Bevan published his experience treating renal stones, and Alexander Hugh Fergeson reported on vesico-vaginal fistulas.[11]

The pioneers of Chicago urology were products of the Cook County Hospital tradition either as interns or attendings (Table II). They, in turn, inspired and encouraged those who succeeded them to develop the separate specialty of urology.

## Urology Becomes a Separate Specialty (1900–1950)

Prior to 1900, there was no separate urologic specialty. Although most venereal diseases and lower urinary tract pathology was referred to physicians who, in fact, func-

### Table II  Cook County Hospital's Golden Years of the Chicago School of Surgery (1880-1900)

| Surgeons | Cook County Hospital Status | Medical School Affiliation | Contribution |
|---|---|---|---|
| Christian Fenger (1840-1902) | A | Rush | First Ureter-Pelvic-Junction Surgery |
| Nicholas Senn (1844-1908) | I (1868) A | Rush | Described TB of Kidney |
| John B. Murphy (1859-1916) | I (1879) A | Rush | Perineal Prostatectomy |
| E. Wyllys Andrews (1856-1927) | A | | First Bottle Hydrocele Operation |
| Malcolm Harris (1862-1936) | I (1884) A | Rush | Ureteral Urine Collection |
| Alexander Hugh Ferguson (1853-1911) | | | Reported on Vesico-Vaginal Fistula |

A: Attending
I: Intern

tioned as urologists, general surgeons performed most major open urological procedures until a separation of technical skills suggested that urologists be the principal surgeons of the kidney, bladder, and prostate. The years 1900–1950 constitute the transition period.

Most notable during this period was William Belfield (Figure 18–2), known as the father of urology in Chicago. He performed the first suprapubic prostatectomy in 1887 but was also a noted bacteriologist. Early surgeons who took a specific interest in urologic diseases included G. Frank Lydston, who was named "Lecturer on Genitourinary Surgery" at what is now the University of Illinois in 1883. Russell Herrold published on the bacteriology of the urinary tract, and Victor Lespinasse performed the first testicular transplant. Malcolm Harris pioneered segregated urine collections. Daniel Eisendrath wrote a popular textbook on urology that was reprinted several times.

Many of these early urologists received their initial training at CCH under inspirational and aggressively innovate surgeons. These include Felip Kriessl, William Baum, Frank Pfifer, and Harry Culver, who with their training complete went into solo or partnership practice while remaining active in surgical research and academic teaching. Also noteworthy were the contributions of Charles Huggins and Louis Schmidt.

As surgeons became proficient in surgery of the kidney, bladder, and prostate, they began to limit themselves to these anatomic areas and thus became the specialists to whom other physicians referred patients with these specific diseases. Table III summarizes the leading urologists and their contributions that made urology a specialty. The Chicago Urologic Society was founded in 1903, a year after the American Urologic Association. It was only a matter of time before urologists, in an effort to promote proficiency and competence, founded the American Board of Urology to set standards ensuring a high level of urologic practice. The first

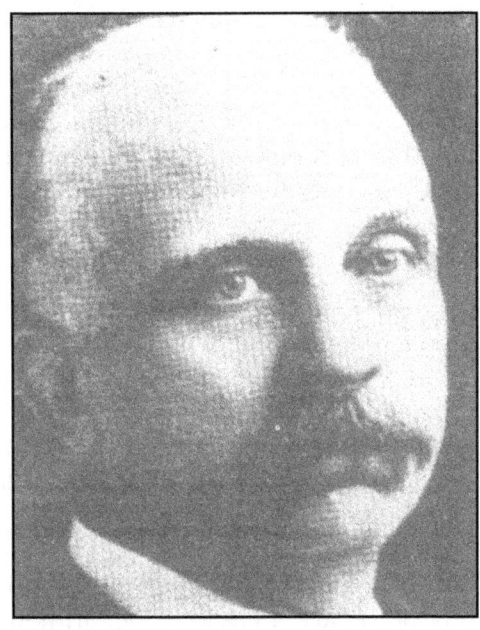

*Figure 18–2* **William Belfield**

**Table III Urology Becomes Separate (1900-1950)**

| Urologists | CCH Status | Medical School | Contribution |
|---|---|---|---|
| William Belfield (1856-1929) | I (1877) A | Rush | Dean of U.S. Urologists |
| G. Frank Lydston (1858-1923) | A | UI | Early Cystoscopic Work |
| Daniel Eisendrath (1867-1939) | I (1891) A | UI-Rush | Textbook on Urology |
| Malcolm Harris (1862-1936) | | | Urine Segregation |
| Victor D. Lespinasse (1878-1946) | I (1903) | NU | First Testicular Implant |
| Russell D. Herrold (1888-1960) | A | UI | Bacteriology of the Urinary Tract |
| Felip Kriessl (1859-1920) | A | | First Urology Chairman at Loyola |
| William Ludwig Baum (1867-1932) | A | St. Lukes | First Use of Cystoscope in Chicago 1891 |
| Frank Pfifer (1886-1978) | A | | |
| Harry Culver (1885-1959) | A | | First Cystoscopy Training Center |
| Charles Huggins | | UC | First Chairman, University of Chicago |
| Louis Ernest Schmidt (1869-1957) | | NU | First GU Department in Alexian Brothers Hospital |

A: Atattending
I: Intern

certifications were issued in 1935,[12] but the certifications were not recognized by the AMA until 1943. The board required two written examinations, letters of recommendation, and submission of an operative log book.

## Contribution of Medical Schools and Residencies

There has been interdependence between urologic surgeons, Chicago medical schools, and urology training programs and residencies. Again, it must be noted that Cook County Hospital was the single most important influence in the development of urologic residencies in Chicago.

### Medical Schools

As medical schools acquired teaching hospitals, they sponsored their own urology residencies, resulting in a reduction from 13 private hospital residencies in the 1940s to five university programs by 2007.

While CCH technically was not a medical school, it had been a teaching institution from the beginning and has been the major teaching hospital for several of Chicago's medical schools, including the University of Illinois, Loyola, Rush, and the Chicago Medical School.

Formal urologic training in Chicago evolved slowly over 130 years. The University of Illinois Medical School, founded in 1882, was the first medical school to have a Urology Department (as mentioned, Cook County Hospital had a Urology Department in 1865) and its pioneer urologist was Theodore Keeton.[13] Dr. Keeton was succeeded with the appointment of G. Frank Lydston as lecturer on genitourinary surgery. Dr Lydston was also an attending at Cook County Hospital.

Daniel Brainard founded Rush Medical College in 1843, and early in its history it attracted urologic practitioners. Its first Urology Department chairman was William Belfield, appointed in 1883. Rush is one of the most noteworthy and typical of medical schools, first founded in Chicago in 1843. It went through many faculty changes and affiliations (its collaboration with the University of Chicago from 1910–1949 being only one), and then the school's dissolution and reconstitution in 1985.

Northwestern University, founded in 1859, appointed Dr. Louis Ernest Schmidt chairman in 1900. In 1911, Loyola opened the Stritch School of Medicine with Dr. Felip Kriessl as the chief urologist. Dr. Charles Huggins became the first urology chairman for the University of Chicago in 1927.

## Residencies

Residencies in urology developed after World War I. The U.S. military had promoted urological specialization, and returning veterans continued the trend. The first urology resident was appointed at Cook County Hospital in 1921.[5] Genitourinary education at CCH was under the supervision of many of the leading urologic surgeons of the time who donated their services and conducted their private practices at a number of hospitals throughout the city, initially Presbyterian, Mt. Sinai, Mercy, St. Luke's, and Michael Reese. Table IV shows the Chicago area medical schools and their hospital-based residency programs.

## Cystoscopy Era (1915–1965)

While urologists were asserting control over the operative intervention of the kidney, bladder, and prostate, there were developments in that heretofore unexplored area of endoscopic procedures. The cystoscope was invented by Max Nitze in 1877, and its use spread in the following 20 years.[14] This, coupled with ureteral catheterization and renal retrograde pylography, allowed visualization of the internal architecture of the kidney. This was to become the undisputed sphere of the urologists, and again, Cook County Hospital pioneered many of these innovations.

Various individuals experimented with the developing endoscopic instruments. These included Drs. Edmund Andrews, Robert Herbst, and William Belfield. William Ludwig Baun and Lydston also pioneered early cystoscopy. The first cystoscopy training center was established at CCH in 1915[15] by Frank Pfifer and Harry Culver. Ureteral manipulation, including retrograde pylography, was advanced in Chicago especially by Dr. Gustav Kolischer, who was a pioneer in the electrocautery of bladder tumors and ureteral catheterization. Others improved the management of benign prostatic hypertrophy by improving the resectoscope. These innovators included Herman Kretschmer and George Baumrucker. William Baker continued this tradition during the World War II period.

### Table IV Chicago Medical Schools

| School | Date School Founded | Urology Department Begun | Chairman | Cook County Hospital Status | Urology Residency Program |
|---|---|---|---|---|---|
| Cook County Hospital | 1833 | 1865 | Charles G. Smith | A | 1921 |
| Rush | 1836 | 1883 | William Belfield | I A | 1975 |
| Northwestern | 1859 | 1900 | Louis Ernest Schmidt | | 1958 |
| U of Illinois | 1882 | 1883 | G. Gordon Lydston | A | 1955 |
| U of Chicago | 1901 | 1927 | Charles Huggins | | 1942 |
| Loyola University | 1911 | 1911 | Filip Kriessl | A | 1985 |
| Chicago Medical School | 1912 | 1968 | Irving Bush | A | 1948 |

A: Attending
I: Intern

## Modern Era (1965–Present)

The modern era of Chicago urology could be characterized as the introduction of newer technology. Because urology is more amenable than general surgery to creative instrumentation, these advances have been more rapid and far-reaching in the former specialty. While surgery is constantly innovating, the Bard-Parker scalpel has been the instrument of choice for 100 years. Newer operative urology procedures included the nerve-sparing radical prostatectomy and techniques to correct impotence and stress urinary incontinence.

The newer technology was more prominent in urology more than any other surgical subspecialty. And again, Chicago and Cook County Hospital took the lead in many areas. During the 1960s these innovations included a fiber optic light source for cystoscopes, which replaced incandescent light. This greatly improved visualization of the prostate and the bladder. Dr. Irving Bush developed prostatic desiccation,[16] a nonoperative form of treatment for benign prostatic hypertrophy, in the 1960s. Ureteroscopy and renoscopy were pioneered at the Cook County Hospital, also by Dr. Bush, in 1970.[17] It was subsequently further developed at the University of Chicago by Dr. Edward Lyon. The first Bruel & Kjaer prostate ultrasound unit was used clinically at CCH in 1972.[18] The Prostate Specific Antigen test was pioneered at Cook County Hospital,[19] in conjunction with Roswell Park Memorial Institute, and percutaneous nephroscopy and stone management were pioneered at CCH in the late 1970s.[20] Bacillus Calmette-Guerin for urologic use was manufactured at Cook County Hospital from the same period.[21] Urologic laparoscopic surgery was developed at Michael Reese Hospital in the 1980s, and lithotripsy was used clinically at Northwestern University by late 1985. Finally, the Da Vinci robotic surgery was performed at the University of Chicago in 2005. Table V summarizes CCH innovations in urological surgery over the years.

The modern era also included changes in the chairmanships of the major

Departments of Urology. In closing, we will mention the chairmen of the division of urology at Cook County Hospital from 1915 to the present (see also Table VI): Frank Pfifer, MD (1915–1935); William Baker, MD (1935–1960, Figure 18–3); Lester Wilkey, MD (1960–1965, Figure 18–4 ); Irving Bush, MD (1965–1975); Patrick Guinan, MD (1975–1985, Figure 18–5); Paul Ray, DO (1985–2008); and Courtney Hollowell, MD (2008–present).

## Conclusion

Cook County Hospital has played an important role in the development of surgery in the United States and indeed the world. The County Hospital has been

**Table V Cook County Hospital Urologic Innovations**

| Innovation | Year | Comment |
| --- | --- | --- |
| Fiber Optic Cystoscopic Light Source | 1966 | Fiber Optic Light Source Introduced |
| Nonoperative Prostatectomy (e.g., Desiccation, Laser Removal) | 1969 | Replacement for TURP |
| Ureteroscopy and Pyeloscopy | 1970 | 1970 CCH, Dr. Irving Bush |
| Transrectal Prostate Ultrasound | 1972 | First Bruel and Kjaer Ultrasound Unit in Chicago |
| PSA Use in Prostate Cancer Diagnosis | 1974 | In Collaboration with Roswell Park Hospital |
| BCG Use in Urologic Cancer | 1976 | CCH Sole Source of BCG |
| Ureteral Lithotripsy | 1980 | Electrohydraulic Lithotripsy |

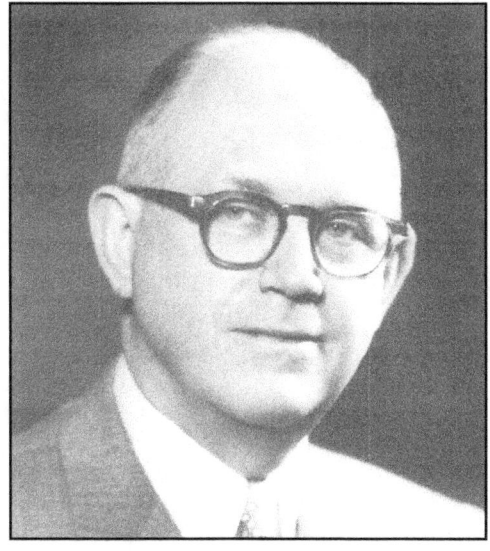

*Figure 18–3  William Baker*

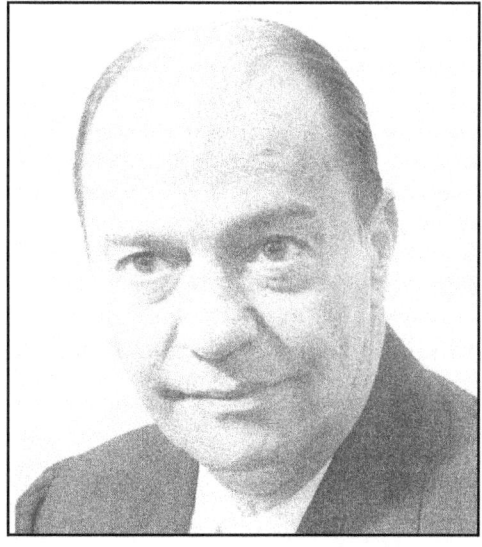

*Figure 18–4  Lester Wilkey*

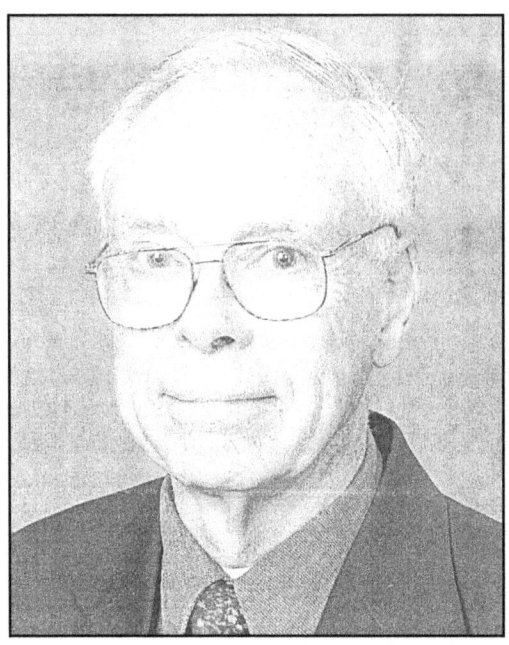

*Figure 18-5 Patrick Guinan*

**Table VI Cook County Hospital Division of Urology Chairmen**

| | | |
|---|---|---|
| 1865 | Charles G. Smith | 1865-1915 |
| 1935 | Frank Pfifer | 1915-1935 |
| 1960 | William Baker | 1935-1960 |
| 1965 | Lester Wilkie | 1960-1965 |
| 1975 | Irving Bush | 1965-1975 |
| 1985 | Patrick Guinan | 1975-1985 |
| 2007 | Paul Ray | 1985-2007 |
| Present | Courtney Hollowell | 2008-Present |

equally instrumental in the development of urologic surgery. Most of the urologic pioneers were associated with the County Hospital either as attending surgeons, residents, or interns. It has been a full and exciting history and will continue to live on in succeeding generations of urological surgeons.

# Referencess

1. Ellis Harold. *A History of Surgery*. Greenwich Medical Media, London, 2001, Belfield, 1886.
2. Haeger, Kurt. *The Illustrated History of Surgery*. Harold Starke Publisher, London 2002.
3. Dankers, Ulrich. Chicago earliest physicians: 1675-1838. *Chicago Medicine*. 102, 40-48, 1999.
4. Johnson, Charles B. *Growth of Cook County*, Chapter 9, World's Largest Hospital. Board of Commissioners of Cook County, IL, 1960.
5. Kiefer, Joseph. History of Urology in Illinois. *IL Med J*. 1970: 56.
6. Barber, K. History of Urology in Chicago. *Chgo Med*. 1961;May 13,pt 1;40. Chgo Med. 1961;May 20,pt 2:36. Chgo Med. 1961;May 27,pt 3; 32.
7. Kretchmer, H. Early History of Urology in Chicago. In: *History of Urology AUA*. Baltimore; Williams and Wilkins: 1933.
8. Rappensburger, JG. *The Old Lady on Harrison Street, Cook County Hospital, International Healthcare Ethics*. Chicago, Ill; Cook County Hospital;1987.
9. Dragstead, Lester. Christian Fenger and the Midwestern School of Surgery. *Bull Guthrie Clin*. 1963;33;13-29.
10. Fenger, Christian. Operation for the relief of valve-formation and stricture of the ureter in hydronephrosis or pyonephrosis. *JAMA*. 1898;22:335.
11. Kretschmer, H. Early History of Urology in Chicago. In: Ed. Ballener E, Prontz W, Hamer H, and Lewis B. *History of Urology*. Baltimore; Williams and Co: 1933.
12. Perlmutter, Alan. *The History of the American Board of Urology*, American Board of Urology.
13. Kiefer, J. History of the Division of Urology of the University of Illinois College of Medicine. *IL Med J*. 1983;Dec:493-505.
14. Rutkow, I. *An Illustrated History*. St. Louis; Mosby:402, 1993.
15. Baker, W. The history, program and present states of cystoscopy at Cook County Hospital. *Proc Inst Med Chgo*. 1958;22:32-36.
16. Bush I, Morelli F, Wilkey J L. Transurethral Desiccation of the Prostate. American Urologic Association, 64th Annual Meeting. San Francisco, May 11-15, 1969: 66.
17. Bush I, Goldberg E, Javadpour N, Chakroborty and Morelli F. Ureteroscopy and renoscopy: A Preliminary Report. *Chgo Med Sch Q*. 1970;30: 46-49.
18. Guinan P, Ray P, and Rubenstein M . Prostatic ultrasound in follow-up of prostatic diseases. *Urology*. 1988; 31:275-278.
19. An evaluation of five tests to diagnose prostate cancer. In: Liss, A. *Prostate Cancer, Part A. Research, Endocrine Treatment, and Histopathology*. New York:Alan Liss; 1987:551-558
20. Bush I, Bush S, Williams S, Bush R B and Guinan P. Further experiences and pitfalls in the performance of electro-hydraulic lithotripsy and high stone manipulation under ureterorenoscopy control in the treatment of renal pelvic and ureteral calursli. American Urologic Association, 75th Annual Meeting , Aug. 1980:196.
21. Guinan P, John T, Sahadevan V, Crispen R, Nagale V, Mclel C, Ablin R. BCG Immunotherapy in Prostate Cancer. In: Crispin R, ed. *Neoplasm Immunity: Solid Tumor Therapy*. Chicago, Ill: The Franklin Press; 1977:127-133.

# 19
# Orthopedic Surgery
## *John A. Elstrom, MD*

- *Introduction*
- *Contributions*
    *John Murphy and Paul Magnuson*
    *John Ridlon*
    *John Lincoln Porter and Henry Bascom Thomas*
    *Edwin Ryerson and Philip Lewin*
    *Kellogg Speed and William Cubbins*
    *James Callahan and Carlo Scuderi*
    *Fred Shapiro*
    *Frank Murphy*
    *Jack Stevens*
    *Ted Hartman*
    *Arsen Pankovich*
    *Robert Hall, Jr.*
    *Mark Gonzalez*

## Introduction

At the end of the 19th century, orthopedic training was largely accomplished by preceptorship, and concerned itself primarily with the prevention or treatment of deformities. Infectious diseases (Potts disease) or developmental processes such as scoliosis or hip dysplasia were the major entities most often treated. Fractures were the sphere of the bone-setter if the fracture was closed or likely the general surgeon if the fracture was open. Since open injuries frequently became infected, amputation was often the treatment of choice. The major advances in orthopedics were either just beginning (as in the case of Buck's traction, the Thomas splint, and tenotomy) or were just around the corner (in the case of roentgenography). In 1875, Hugh Owen Thomas of Liverpool described the Thomas splint used initially in 1865 for treating tuberculosis of the knee and later in the management of lower extremity fractures. The splint was important in the reduction of morbidity and mortality secondary to amputation from gunshot fractures of the femur in WWI. Joseph Lister in Glasgow, Robert Koch in Germany, and Christian Fenger in Chicago were doing work regarding preparation of the skin for surgical procedures, wound sepsis, and steam sterilization of instruments.

American orthopedics was initially under the influence of men who were either not surgeons or physicians not inclined to do surgery. Newton Shaffer of New York City believed that the orthopedist should be treating deformities by mechanical means (traction, bracing, or plaster-of-paris casting). He frequently argued that the orthopedist should have a shop and an apparatus fabricator to accomplish his aims. Prevention of surgery was felt to be the highest aim of treatment and was to be accomplished by the use of traction apparatus.

Shaffer complained:

*Since the Lister method has become so universally accepted, the knife, the saw, the chisel and the osteoclast have become potent factors in the reduction of obstinate osseous deformities as general surgery begins to invade the domain of orthopedic surgery.*

He went on to point out that, the allurements of the operating table are very great and for a time, he had had his own attack of surgical fever which he was happy to say proved self-limiting. He felt that "Listerism" had given license to general surgeons to perform operations for which they were not properly trained. The fallacy of this argument was that many needed operations had yet to be devised. This very ability to create a needed surgical procedure led to the recognition of John B. Murphy as an outstanding surgeon.

## Contributions

### John Murphy and Paul Magnuson

The history of orthopedic surgery at Cook County Hospital would not be complete without a consideration of the contributions of Dr. Murphy to this discipline. This favorite son of Chicago surgery was a product of Rush Medical College and the Cook County Hospital intern class of 1880. After additional training in Europe, he returned to Chicago where he quickly established himself as a rare, gifted surgeon who boldly devised new operative procedures. The observations of P. G. Skillern Jr. of Philadelphia, entitled *A Visit to the Surgical Clinic of John B. Murphy at Mercy Hospital in Chicago,* published in 1915, confirm that Murphy was an accomplished orthopedic operator. After describing the clinic and numerous general surgical procedures that were performed, Skillern describes a multiplicity of orthopedic procedures performed at the three-day clinic including a forequarter amputation for sarcoma of the humerus, tendon transplantation for Volkmann's contraction, an arthrodesis of the knee for tuberculosis, several cases of osteomyelitis, and a club foot operation on a baby.

A fuller treatment of the influence of Murphy on Chicago orthopedics is brilliantly recorded by one of his students and a colleague, Dr. Paul B. Magnuson (Figure 19–1) in *Ring the Night Bell* published in 1960. The title refers to Magnuson's experience as a surgeon on South Halsted Street for the Junction Railway and the Stockyard Company. As he put it,

*We never went to bed without the knowledge that somewhere in Chicago, somebody was working up an attack of appendicitis or a switchman in the stockyards would get his foot smashed by a coupling. Then the telephone bell would ring, and I'd have to haul myself out of a warm bed and do something about it.*

Later on, Magnuson worked with Dr. Edward Martin, a professor of surgery who was interested in "bone work,"' especially femoral fractures. It was

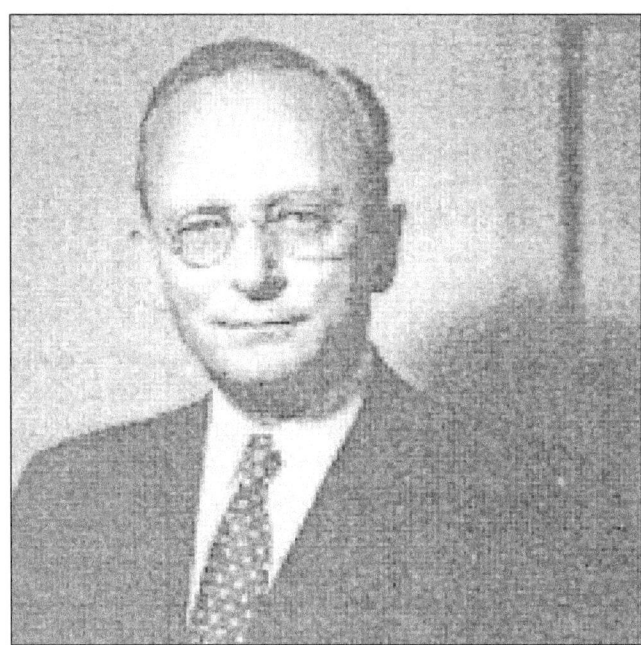

*Figure 19–1 Paul Magnuson*

Martin who told Magnuson of an opportunity to work with Murphy in Chicago. Magnuson describes it as "feeling like a young Roman soldier who had been offered the chance to learn military science under Julius Caesar."

Among the operations Magnuson describes was a patient who underwent a fascial arthroplasty of the knee and threw away his crutches (that he still needed) at one of Murphy's clinics just to put on a good show for his surgeon. From the vantage point of nearly a half-century of dealing with fractured hips, Magnuson commented on the advances in hip surgery from the use of three months of a plaster hip spica with the injured femur internally rotated and a formidable morbidity and mortality to the routine use of internal hip fixation as follows:

> *A major difference in the 1950s was that instead of iron nails, we have nails made of vitalium, a non-irritating, non-electrolytic metal that does not cause softening when it comes in contact with the bone.*

The spica was 1909 therapy: diagnosis, reduction, and fixation without benefit of radiographs.

These are just a few examples of the legacy of such Chicago surgeons as John B. Murphy and Paul Magnuson. Magnuson himself had three major orthopedic procedures associated with his name. Two of these are still useful today. Magnuson's book is fascinating Chicago medical history, even though the only connection he seems to have had with County was through his associate Bill Hendricks. Hendricks was an authority on stab and gunshot wounds of the abdomen and the difficulties they could present in the operating room. This was knowledge he gleaned by spending three nights a week for 15 years at Cook

County Hospital taking care of police cases that came into the emergency room.

## John Ridlon

Dr. John Ridlon was born in Vermont and earned his medical degree from the College of Physicians and Surgeons (New York City) in 1878. He worked with Newton Shaffer as an assistant at St. Luke's Hospital. In 1887, Dr. Ridlon was part of the group of east coast orthopedists that formed the American Orthopedic Association, and he became AOA president in 1895. By 1889, the Association was publishing the transactions of their meetings in what would become the *Journal of Bone and Joint Surgery*. Issues still to be decided at this time concerned whether the orthopedist should accomplish his aims by invasive (general) surgical means, and should he treat fractures.

In 1887, Ridlon went to Liverpool to work with Hugh Owen Thomas. On his return from Liverpool he introduced the first Thomas splint in America, applying it to a patient suffering from tuberculosis of the hip. Evidently, Shaffer ordered the splint removed, and Ridlon refused. As a result, Ridlon was not re-appointed to the hospital staff, and in 1889, he left New York for Chicago.

In 1892, he reported (along with Mr. Robert Jones, the nephew of Hugh Owen Thomas) the use of "The Thomas-Hip Splint in the Treatment of Fractures of the Neck of the Femur." In 1897, Ridlon reported "Further Observations on the use of the Thomas-Hip Splint in Treating Fractures of the Neck of the Femur" in the *Journal of Bone and Joint Surgery*. The patients were kept in this fixed-traction device for six to seven weeks, and then propped up in a chair or at bed rest for another seven weeks. At follow-up (four years later in one instance), there was typically an inch of shortening, but the external rotation deformity had been corrected, and the patient was able to walk without a limp. Knee flexion was limited. All this took place without benefit of radiographic confirmation of the injury (displacement, reduction) or result.

Among Dr. Ridlon's students and colleagues were John Lincoln Porter, Henry Bascom Thomas, Philip Lewin, Elven Berkheiser, and Edwin Ryerson. In 1921, these orthopedic surgeons signed a statement indicating that Professor Adolph Lorenz, the Vienna surgeon who was then holding clinics in New York City, would be "persona non grata" when he arrived in Chicago. They proposed his visit would do more harm than good, avowing that "to invite him to appear before the Cook County Hospital or any other hospital where a well-trained and devoted orthopedic staff was giving its time and attention to taking care of the poor cripples of Cook County is nothing short of an injustice. The public jumps to the conclusion that he is a 'miracle worker' who is able to do things that local surgeons are unable to do." Dr. Ridlon felt that Dr. Lorenz' technique of reduction of the congenitally dislocated hip was especially brutal.

In honor of Dr. Ridlon's 71st birthday, many of his former students and current colleagues unveiled a portrait that they commissioned to celebrate the "Father of Orthopedic Surgery." The celebrants were a "Who's Who" of midwestern orthopedics at that time, from Arthur Steindler at the University of Iowa to Henderson and Meyerding of the Mayo Clinic to Willis Campbell in Memphis.

## John Lincoln Porter and Henry Bascom Thomas

John Lincoln Porter (Figure 19–2) was a professor of orthopedic surgery in the College of Physicians and Surgeons of the University of Illinois and an attending surgeon at Cook County Hospital and St. Luke's Hospital. Among his interests were tuberculous spondylitis and coxitis. In 1905, he gave clinics describing the use of a plaster-of-paris jacket for Pott's disease in an attempt to correct dorsal kyphosis and put the spine at rest. His descriptions of the problems with patient compliance demonstrate the limitations and suffering these treatments imposed.

Henry Bascom Thomas (Figure 19–3) was chief of the Cook County orthopedic service from 1906 to 1919. He subsequently became professor and head of the Orthopedic Department at the University of Illinois. While at the University of Illinois, Thomas published *Some Orthopedic Findings in 98 cases of Hemophilia* where he pointed out that hemorrhages into joints resulted in hemophiliac arthritis, and that Volkmann's contracture developed after spontaneous bleeding into the forearm compartment muscles. He lectured to the New York Academy of Medicine on orthopedic surgery at Cook County Hospital.

Both Drs. Ridlon and H.B. Thomas describe visits to Liverpool where the H.O. Thomas club foot wrench was used to correct malunited distal radial fractures. In one instance, Dr. John B. Murphy was present to wager (10 dollars) successfully that the feat could be accomplished. It is of interest that the same type of device and principle are still in use today to align femoral fracture fragments for closed intramedullary nailing.

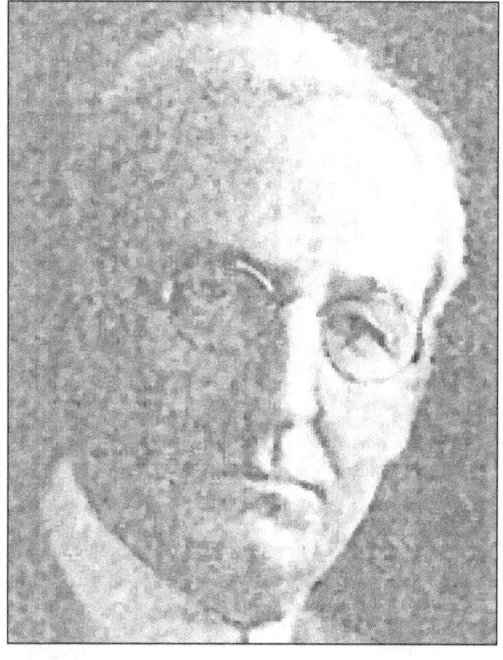

*Figure 19–2 John Lincoln Porter*

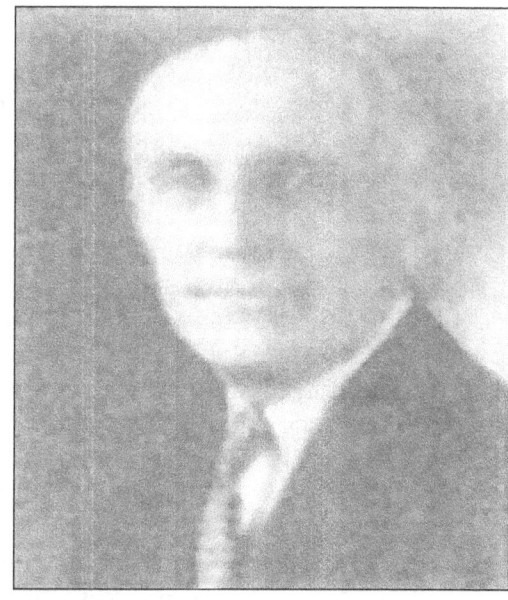

*Figure 19–3 Henry Bascom Thomas*

## Edwin Ryerson and Philip Lewin

In 1933, Edwin W. Ryerson (Figure 19–4) and Philip Lewin were members of the original group of orthopedic surgeons that founded the American Academy of Orthopedic Surgeons at Northwestern Medical School in Chicago. It was their hope that the AAOS would serve as an umbrella society for local orthopedic societies that had begun to spring up all over the country, and also that it would provide an outlet for the clinical and scientific experience of new people entering the specialty. The stated goals were nationwide recognition of orthopedic surgery, the elevation of the standards of education in the field, the systematic study of important orthopedic problems, the free exchange of information and ideas, and assorted guidance and advice on public questions. It was felt that orthopedic surgeons should be well trained and able to treat patients medically as well as surgically.

Edwin W. Ryerson, who was a professor of surgery at Rush Medical College and became head of the Department of Orthopedic Surgery at the University of Illinois until 1919, had an interest in children's orthopedics and was an attending orthopedic surgeon at Children's Memorial Hospital as well as at Cook County Hospital. In 1922, Ryerson and others reported a study of stabilizing operations for the flail or paralytic foot. This study recognized that tendon transplantation in the paralytic foot needed to be supplemented by stabilization of the smaller joints of the foot to prevent or correct varus or valgus deformity. One of Dr. Ryerson's

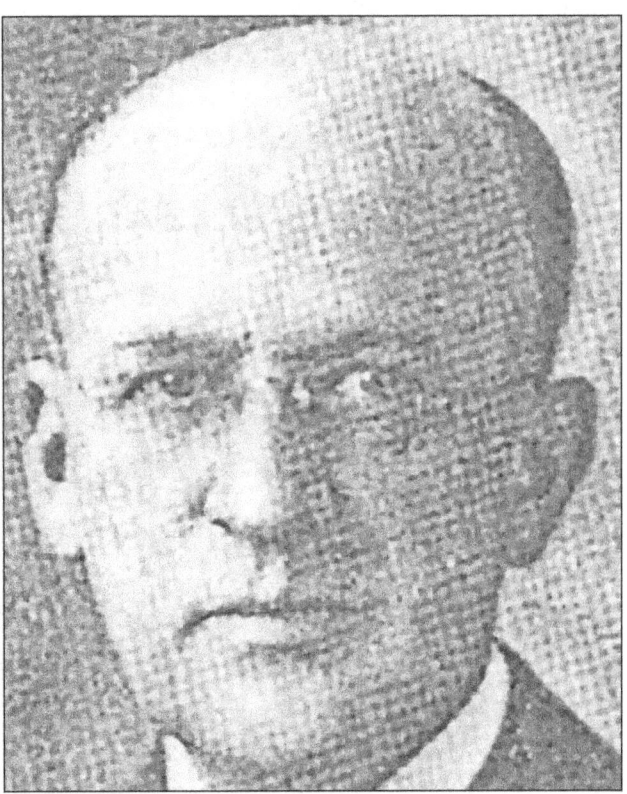

*Figure 19–4  Edwin W. Ryerson*

contributions was a method of triple arthrodesis of the foot.

Dr. Philip Lewin was professor of bone and joint surgery at Northwestern University, in private practice in Evanston, and an attending orthopedic surgeon at County. He wrote several textbooks, among which are *The Foot and Ankle* (4 editions), *The Knee and Related Structures*, and *Orthopedics Surgery for Nurses*.

Both Drs. Ryerson and Lewin were active in the attempts to restore function that had been lost to the "summer plague," poliomyelitis.

In 1935, Frank Ober of Boston, Ryerson and others reported on Graduate Instruction in Orthopedic Surgery in the United States in the *JBJS*. This was a time when most orthopedic surgery was still taught by preceptorship. Sixty-two medical schools were surveyed: 15 had orthopedic departments and of these, nine offered graduate study in orthopedic surgery. These varied from a few months to 24 months (eight months of pathology, eight months at the Children's Hospital, and eight months at Massachusetts General Hospital for Harvard).

## Kellogg Speed and William Cubbins

Two general surgeons who were well known for their affiliation with Cook County Hospital were Drs. Kellogg Speed (Figure 19–5 ) and William Cubbins (Figure 19–6 ). Together they established the County fracture service. They preferred to be called bone and joint surgeons.

Kellogg Speed graduated from Rush Medical College in 1904 after having excelled as one of the great athletes at the University of Chicago in his undergraduate days. He completed an internship at Cook County Hospital and served as an associate in surgery at Rush Medical College until 1908. He was affiliated

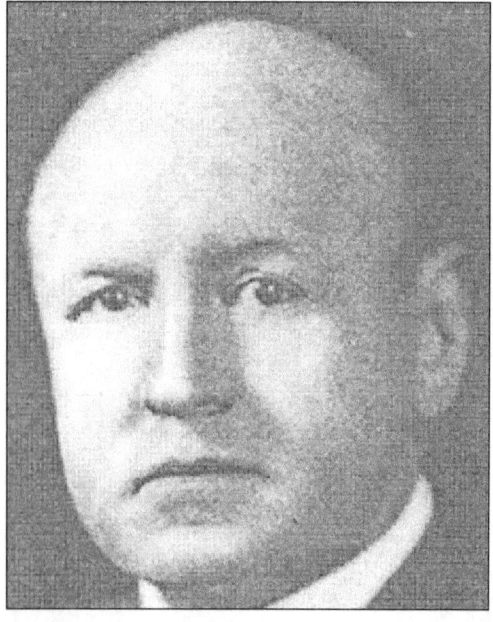

*Figure 19–5  Kellog Speed*

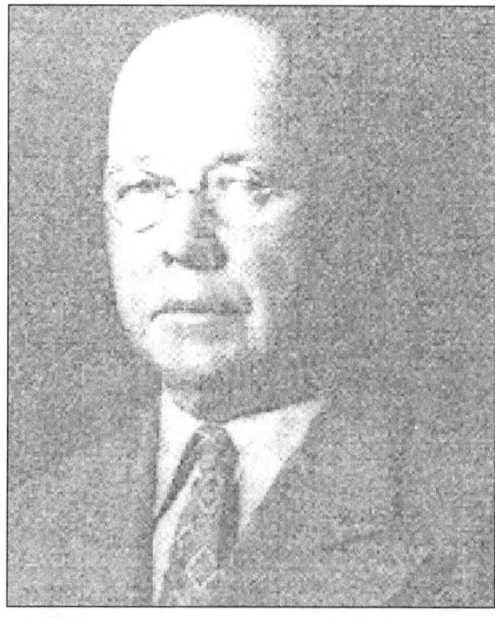

*Figure 19–6  William Cubbins*

with Northwestern University until 1918. From 1912 to 1933, he served as an attending surgeon at Cook County Hospital. His experiences with the County fracture service resulted in his *Textbook of Fractures and Dislocations*, originally published in 1916 and last published in 1942. These experiences led to having first aid equipment installed in police cars and ambulances in Chicago. He admonished those early rescue workers to carry a fracture splint and "splint fractures where they lie."

Dr. Speed saw military service in France in WWI and was a founding member of the American Board of Surgery and the American Board of Orthopedic Surgery. The ABOS was founded in 1934. By 1936, it had established standards for the formal education of orthopedic surgeons and their evaluation by examination. By 1938, three years of concentrated instruction and knowledge of basic science were required.

Dr. Speed was a member of the special committee on fractures of the American Medical Association from 1936 to 1951 and chairman of the committee from 1938 to 1951. He was chairman of the Chicago regional fracture committee of the American College of Surgeons for more than 20 years and a member of the national committee on trauma of the ACS. Dr. Speed was the first president of the American Association for Surgery of Trauma in 1939. His work with Charles Scudder of Boston, who had written his own text, *The Treatment of Fractures*, and numerous other experts resulted in the *Outline of the Treatment of Fractures* in 1922.

Dr. William R. Cubbins was Kellogg Speed's associate in the establishment of the Fracture Service. He was a graduate of Northwestern Medical School and interned at Cook County Hospital. He was an attending at County from 1918 to 1945 and followed Dr. Speed as chief of the fracture service. He was also chairman of the division of bone and joint surgery at Loyola School of Medicine from 1937 to 1945.

In a 1940 *Archives of Surgery* publication entitled "Compound Fractures," by John Reynolds and Chester Zeiss, they noted that the proper technique of debridement and the proper treatment of the wound after debridement were still points of debate. They went on to describe their study on the male fracture ward of Cook County Hospital. The investigators compared two groups of patients, both of which were debrided by removing all foreign material and dead tissue from the wound, one followed by copious irrigation with saline solution and green soap and then again by saline solution, and the other in which iodine and alcohol were introduced into the depths of the wound after it had been debrided. The conclusion was that iodine and alcohol do not sterilize the interior of the wound. They injure the wall of the wound, and bodily defenses now have to handle a layer of dead cells as well as attack the organisms in the wound. Methods used for stabilization at this time included Buck's traction, plaster, and skeletal traction. The wound, however, was closed with the idea of accomplishing a layer-by-layer approximation. Infection rate, in the days before antibiotics, was right around 15 percent. During WWII, contaminated wounds were managed with delayed primary closure. The clinical appearance of the wound following debridement became the most important criterion for determining the feasibility of closure, lack of drainage, erythema, foreign material, and the presence of healthy-appearing tissue to determine whether wound closure was appropriate. This was felt to be one of the major advancements in wound care recognized in WWII.

In the 1930s, Cubbins, Callahan, and Scuderi wrote extensively on fractures and dislocations of the shoulder and humerus, fractures of the neck of the femur, and knee ligament injuries.

### James Callahan and Carlo Scuderi

James J. Callahan (Figure 19–7) interned at Cook County Hospital and was a resident on the fracture service from 1935 to 1939. At the beginning of WWII, he was asked by the Surgeon General to provide instruction to military surgeons in the principles of traumatic surgery and fracture care. He was subsequently a lieutenant colonel and chief of a section at McCloskey Army General Hospital in Temple, Texas. He became chief of the fracture service at Cook County Hospital in 1946 and became chairman of the Department of Orthopedics at Loyola University from 1946 to 1972.

Carlo Scuderi (Figure 19–8) was also a resident on the fracture service and became an attending there from 1947-1969. He had an academic appointment at the University of Illinois in orthopedic surgery and usually moderated the Monday afternoon fracture conferences.

### Fred Shapiro

In the 1950s, Cook County Hospital had an orthopedic residency headed

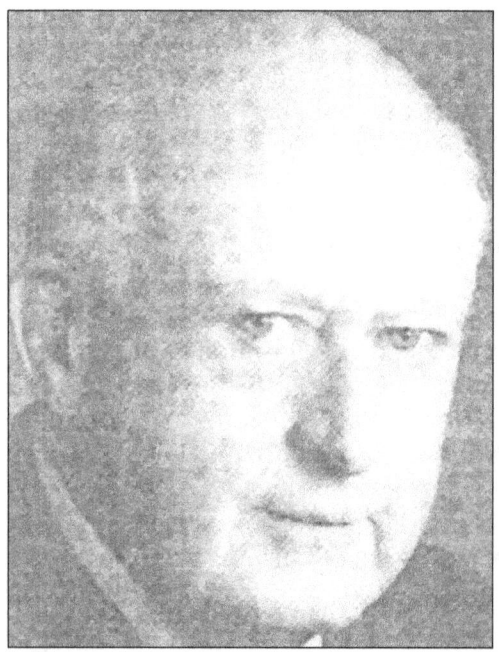

*Figure 19–7 James Callahan*

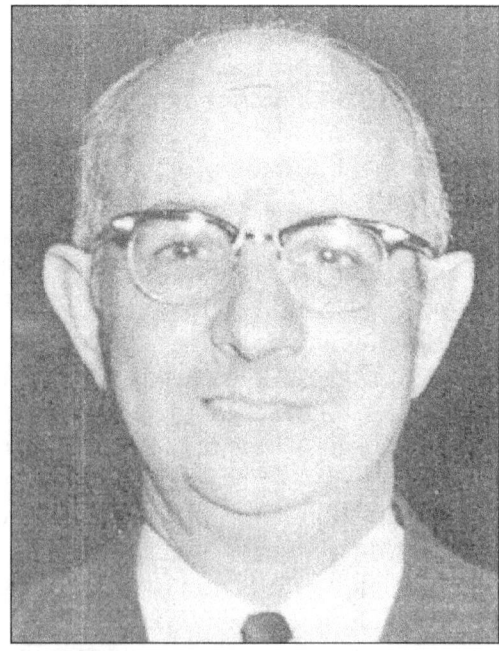

*Figure 19–8 Carlo S. Scuderi*

by Dr. Fred Shapiro (Figure 19–9). Among the residents trained during that time were Drs. William Newman, Allan Murphy, John Gleason, Jerry Loftus, Bill Kelly, Leo Quinn, and Morrie "Red" Stamler. The residency lasted for three years and started with a rotation on pediatrics, included six months of basic science at Northwestern University, then rotations on adult orthopedics and the fracture service. At that time, adult orthopedics was located on Ward 66 in the Children's Hospital, and the fracture service was on Wards 41 and 42 in the main building. The major attending surgeons at that time, in addition to Dr. Shapiro, were Drs. Callahan and Scuderi. Dr. Callahan was assisted by Drs. Arthur Conley and Leo Weinstein and Dr. Scuderi by Dr. John Gleason.

### Frank Murphy

Dr. Frank Murphy (Figure 19–10) was also an attending orthopedist. He saw military service in both world wars, and his sons Allen and Jerry became orthopedic surgeons and attendings at County. Another notable attending at this time was Dr. Elven J. Berkheiser (Figure 19–11). Dr. Berkheiser had been Dr. John Ridlon's assistant and was the preceptor to Dr. Fred Shapiro. He was an attending orthopedic surgeon at County from 1924–1946 and remained a consultant until 1958. Dr. Berkheiser was chief of the orthopedic service at Presbyterian Hospital from 1933–1957, was affiliated with the Municipal Tuberculosis Sanitarium of Chicago, and taught orthopedic surgery at both Rush Medical College and the University of Illinois. He was also on the staff of Children's Memorial from 1919 to 1930 and head of the service from 1925 to 1930. A part of his legacy is the

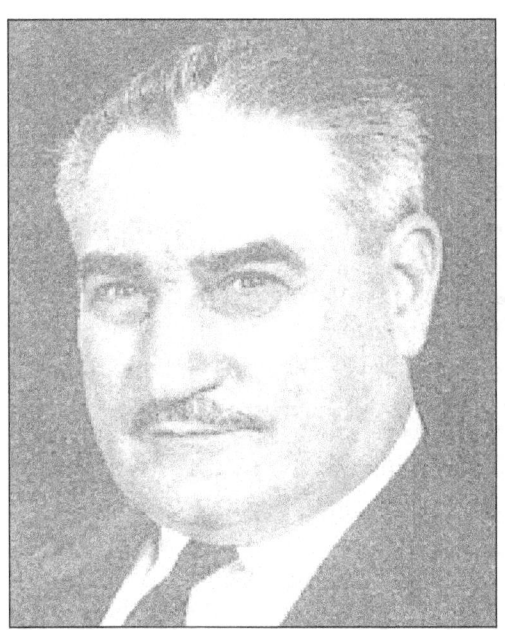

*Figure 19–9  Fred Shapiro*

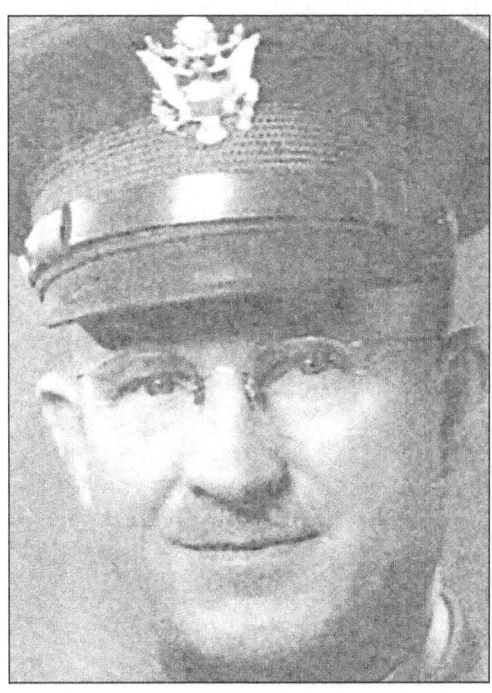

*Figure 19–10  Frank Murphy*

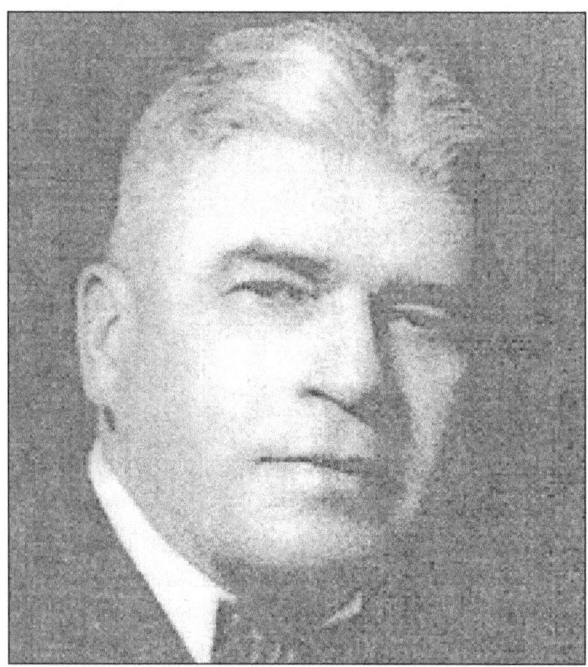

*Figure 19–11  Elven J. Berkheiser*

named lecture in orthopedic surgery at the annual clinical conference of the Chicago Medical Society. Dr. Bill Newman recalls, at this time, that pediatric patients with Pott's disease were treated on a Bradford frame, and it was not unusual to see arthrodesis performed for tuberculosis of the hip and knee. The Thomas wrench was still in vogue for correcting club feet.

One of the major advances after WWII was the arrival of the Kuntscher nail for fractures of the femur. This intermedullary rod had been used by the Germans to fix femur fractures in downed airmen. Sheer fractures of the pelvis were treated in traction for weeks and open book fractures with a pelvic sling. Comminuted open or closed tibial fractures were treated with calcaneal traction. Dr. Scuderi and Brother Angelus from Alexian Brothers wrote a book on how to set up traction. One of the more appreciated innovations, at this time was the development of the cast saw by Dr. Homer Striker of Kalamazoo, Michigan.

Dr. Fred Shapiro, who headed the County residency program in the 1950s and early 1960s, was an orthopedic trauma surgeon who served with the U.S. Marine Corps in some of the major island battles of the South Pacific in WWII. One of his former residents recalls that Shapiro had gone ashore with the landing parties and had actually engaged in combat operations. Another former resident, Dr. Jules Shapiro, recalled that Fred's division was celebrated in a history, Gung Ho, and Fred appeared in the book cover photograph as one of the eight or nine troops who made it through the campaign still standing. He was on the orthopedic residency committee at Northwestern, and along with Dr. James Stack, ran a popular, well-attended Sunday morning trauma conference in the Cook County Children's Hospital amphitheater. Chairmen of many of the surgical departments were often in attendance and the repartee, including many of Dr. Raffensperger's flaming arrows, was always stimulating. During Dr. Shapiro's time, there were four to five residents from Northwestern and one from the U of I in the residency pool at County.

One of the more illustrious residents from the University of Illinois was Jorge Galante, who had come to the United States from Argentina. Later, Dr. Galante went to Göteborg, Sweden, to do postgraduate training with Carl Hirsch in bioengineering. After he returned to the United States, Galante subsequently became chairman of the Department of Orthopedic Surgery and founder of the orthopedic residency program at the resurrected Rush Medical School. He was president of the Orthopedic Research and Education Foundation and won numerous awards including two Kappa Delta awards. Dr. Galante became world-renowned in joint replacement surgery of the hip and knee.

Dr. Riad Barmada was the chief resident in 1964, and he remembers Dr. Shapiro's excellent knowledge of orthopedics and medicine and his meticulous supervision of the residents. Dr. Shapiro made rounds and appeared in the operating room. He never scrubbed but helped the resident find his way through a surgical procedure by watching and providing verbal instruction. In those days, orthopedics occupied the west end of the eighth floor operating suite and had an amphitheatre for visitors. In some rooms, the windows opened up onto the street. It was common, during this time, to find the windows open if the OR became too stifling on a humid summer night or on occasion, to see an attending man in street clothes providing guidance with his hand or tie over his mouth as a mask.

## Jack Stevens

The first full-time chairman of the Department of Orthopedic Surgery at Cook County Hospital was Jack Stevens (Figure 19–12). Stevens was born in Ingleton, Yorkshire, England, and had the most distinguished lineage of any of the orthopedic department chairman. He won scholarships to Christ College, Cambridge, and started his surgical career at the Western Infirmary in Glasgow,

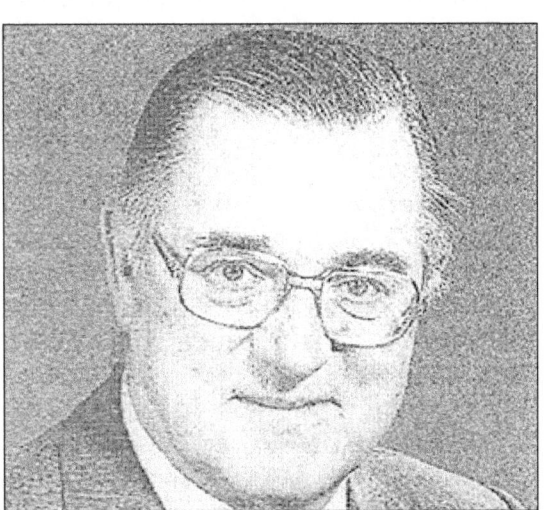

*Figure 19–12 Jack Stevens*

Scotland. In 1957, he was awarded a Commonwealth Fund Fellowship to visit Chicago, where he spent 18 months studying the properties of living and dead bone at what was then known as the U of I Research and Education Hospital with Dr. R. D. Ray, the chairman of the Department. He returned to the Western Infirmary in Glasgow as a senior lecturer and in 1961 was awarded the Robert Jones prize and gold medal of the British Orthopedic Association for his interest in femoral neck fractures.

Stevens returned to Chicago in 1965 to become chairman of the Department of Orthopedics at Cook County Hospital with the responsibility for 13 residents and 264 beds. The change in orthopedic care must have been dramatic. Residents previously had been supervised by the part-time private practice attending force who dropped by the operating room for part of a surgical case. The indications for the procedure were discussed while the surgery was in progress. For Mr. Stevens, this rather casual approach to orthopedic training was an anathema. He rounded and operated with the residents and was a keen observer of resident potential and abilities. He didn't hesitate to make his displeasure with orthopedic management known. The old school of trial and error surgery, best formulated and fortified with a visit to the Karl Meyer Library (an anatomic atlas and *Campbell's Operative Orthopedics*) was swept away by a surgeon whose commitment was first and foremost to making sure the patient got the right operation for his problem, and that his surgery was carried out in a competent manner, even if it meant that Mr. Stevens did the surgery himself.

The misadventures of Dr. Julio Jove, a Northwestern orthopedic resident about to treat a patient with slipped capital femoral epiphysis, were memorable. When a brown material smelling strangely like feces bubbled up through the drapes just after the skin incision was made, a short but acrimonious discussion followed. The procedure and Julio Jove were terminated on the spot. It seems the patient had had a bowel movement as the result of the anesthetic and lack of bowel prep, according to Mr. Stevens.

A 1969 article concerning an unusual fracture-dislocation of the tarsal navicular published by Nasser Eftekhar, Donald Lyddon, and Jack Stevens reflects the state of fracture treatment at that time. The references included Reginald Watson-Jones, *Fractures and Joint Injuries*, 1955; Kellogg Speed, *Fractures and Dislocations*, 1942; R.J. Joplin, *Injuries of the Foot in Fractures and Other Injuries*, edited by E.F. Cave, 1958; DePalma, *The Management of Fractures and Dislocations*, 1959; and Lorenz Böehler, *The Treatment of Fractures*, 1957. The most current reference was Conwell, H.E. and Reynolds F.C., *Management of Fractures Dislocations and Sprains*, 1961.

Stevens went on to become professor of orthopedic surgery at the University of Chicago in 1967. In 1972, he accepted the newly established chair of orthopedic surgery at Newcastle-upon-Tyne. He was president-elect of The British Orthopedic Association from 1981 to 1982 but was prevented by illness from becoming president in 1983. He died in 1995. Jack Stevens was remembered in his obituary for his forthrightness, loyalty, humility, and honesty, all qualities greatly appreciated during his time at Cook County Hospital.

## Ted Hartman

Ted Hartman became chairman of the Department of Orthopedic Surgery in 1969. He had gone to Northwestern Medical School and had his orthopedic training at the University of Michigan with a fellowship under Professor Joseph Trueta at Oxford University. Before coming to Cook County, he was on the orthopedic faculty of the University of Michigan and the Cleveland Clinic. In 1971, he became chairman of the Orthopedic Department at the Texas Tech University Medical School in Lubbock, Texas. Dr. Hartman went on to become the dean of the Medical School. While at County, Dr. Hartman published *The Effect of Limb Elevation in Preventing Venous Thrombosis in Patients with Femoral Neck and Trochanteric Fractures* with Drs. Peter Alter and Robert Freeark, and *The Use of Intra-dural and Extra-dural Corticosteroids for Sciatica* with Dr. Alon Winnie.

Hartman has written an account of his experiences as a 19-year-old Sherman tank driver in the Battle of the Bulge with the 11th Armored Division. The online excerpts of his account, constructed from letters he sent home, are riveting.

This premodern period of orthopedic surgery (following the tenure of Dr. Shapiro and continuing through the early years of Dr. Stevens' tenure) at Cook County Hospital was characterized by very loose supervision and an extremely conservative approach to fracture management. Residents typically rotated through in their fourth year after having spent time in a private hospital with such local authorities as J.J. Fahey, Newton Mead, Edward and Clinton Compere, James K. Stack, J.J. Callahan, or Sam Banks, and they tended to imitate their mentors, both in their areas of expertise and weaknesses.

The main concern was that operative intervention would lead to infection; therefore, fracture management was frequently associated with inadequate stabilization. Early orthopedic implants frequently failed due to lack of uniformity in the metals and the poor holding ability of the screws used to fix a plate to the bone.

Resident supervision in the County ORs consisted of an attending surgeon coming in to watch a resident pin a hip with a Smith-Peterson nail or fix an intertrochanteric fracture with a fixed angle Jewett nail plate. Radiographic control of the reduction and internal fixation was carried out with Polaroid imaging that could be developed on the spot. In the early 1960s, about 300 hip fractures were admitted to CCH annually; the residents found time to operate on approximately half of these patients. The remainder were still treated in traction.

Attending physicians seldom made substantial rounds, and there were frequent cases of infected fractures. These usually were due to the inadequate debridement of open injuries and the lack of stabilization of these injuries, which were often immobilized with a cast (windowed for wound care) or supported in a splint. Also, there was no separate trauma service, so orthopedic injuries were admitted directly to the floor through the emergency room to be worked up and treated, initially, by the intern. The major reference and source of guidance for both the intern and resident was Watson-Jones' *Fractures and Joint Injuries* or *Campbell's Operative Orthopedics*, 4th Edition, published in 1963. For a few years in the early 1960s, between Fred Shapiro and Jack Stevens, a senior resident might have to travel to Carlo Scuderi's Michigan Avenue office for guidance.

## Arsen Pankovich

The premodern period of orthopedic surgery at Cook County definitely ended in 1972 with the appointment of Arsen Pankovich as department chair. By the time of his arrival, the historic surgical amphitheatres, which had long been used for "wet clinics," were closed down and used instead for storage. Arlene Fox, R.N., was in charge of operating room orthopedics. Miss R. was OR supervisor. The recovery room was on the seventh floor with the orthopedic office just below on the sixth. A trip up two flights of occasionally trash-littered stairs was faster than the unbelievably slow elevators.

Pearl Howard came to Cook County Hospital in the early 1960s on a grant from the NIH and was employed initially on the hand and burn unit in the pediatric hospital. She was hired by Jack Stevens when he took over the Orthopedic Department and was the administrative assistant to Drs. Stevens, Hartman, Pankovich, and Hall. Her desk was the entry to the office. From there, she organized the cacophony of salesmen, residents, jangling telephones, typing secretaries, students, and attending staff. Just to her left, three private suites (and a restroom) extended along the south wall of the office and provided a panoramic view of the hospital complex. Ms. Howard was responsible for preparing the numerous journal and textbook publications for submission. She was outstanding, well-thought of and appreciated by everyone. In 1989, she moved to Alabama where she became full-time program coordinator for professional development activities at the Central Alabama Regional Education Inservice Center at Alabama State University in Montgomery.

Dr. Pankovich was born in Banja Luka, Bosnia. He went to medical schools in Sarajevo and Belgrade where he graduated in 1954. Arriving in the United States via a refugee camp in Greece in 1958, Dr. Pankovich served an internship and one-year general surgery residency in New York City. He came to Chicago in 1960 and subsequently became a physiology fellow under Franklin C. McLean, MD, PhD, professor of pathologic physiology in the Department of Physiology at the University of Chicago. Subsequently, he finished an orthopedic residency under Robert Moore at the University. He spent almost two years at the Hospital for Special Surgery in New York City working as an orthopedic research fellow under Drs. Leonhard Korngold and Goran Bauer and studying immunological properties of cartilage and bone. Following his fellowship, he joined the orthopedic faculty at the University of Chicago in 1967 during the tenure of Jack Stevens. The University of Chicago, at this time, was a research center with an interest in bone physiology.

When Stevens left the University of Chicago in 1972, Dr. Pankovich took the position at Cook County Hospital. His chairmanship at CCH was marked by numerous innovations. His correspondences with the medical administration before his acceptance of the position clearly demonstrate his goals and requirements for accepting the position. The three basic departmental functions on which the success of a chairman would be judged were cited as quality patient care, education of all department personnel, and the amount and quality of basic and clinical research. The minimum requirements for this new department were seen as follows:

1. Recruitment of four full-time attending, with the assurance that they could be appointed, if indeed they could be found.
2. Exploring the possibility of a County orthopedic residency to replace the fragmented system of six-month rotations from a number of outside orthopedic programs.
3. The orthopedic service would care for all bone and soft tissue problems above the wrist. In other words, the hand did not extend to the shoulder.
4. There should be a peripheral nerve call rotated daily between neurosurgery, orthopedics, and the hand service.
5. In order to better supervise the administrative and nonmedical personnel of the department, the chairman should have direct control of departmental finances.

In a letter dated March 1972, the then-head of the hospital expressed his agreement with Dr. Pankovich on the status of the residency and pledged the full support of his board in achieving the status of an independent residency in orthopedics for the County Hospital. This was accompanied by the authorization to hire three full-time attending surgeons. As a pleasant addendum to this agreement, Dr. Pankovich was surprised to find that he had also inherited a top-notch cadre of orthopedic operating room personnel in the eighth-floor ORs.

The acquisition of a full-time attending staff resulted in improved resident supervision and more dynamic teaching conferences. Dr. Pankovich had no difficulty in attaining an AMA-approved residency program that trained two residents per year for over 10 years until it came to an end in the early 1980s, when the training pendulum took a swing toward more university-sponsored academic programs. The names and pictures of 16 of these trainees are found in a tribute given to Dr. Pankovich at the time of his departure in 1980. Their names are:

| | |
|---|---|
| Spiros Stamelos, MD | Imad Tarabishy, MD |
| Prabhakar Gadry, MD | Mark Lorenz, MD |
| Richard Pearson, MD | Jorge Prieto, MD |
| Richard Egwele, MD | Clayton Perry, MD |
| Mitchell Goldflies, MD | Dave Mann, MD |
| Mysore Shivaram, MD | Bill Lowry, MD |
| John McClellan, MD | Ken Davenport, MD |
| Chris Dangles, MD | Steve Traina, MD |

In addition, 10 other residents started or finished their training under Dr. Robert Hall, Dr. Pankovich's successor. They were David Butler, Henry Fuentes, Jerry Dzwinyk, David Witham, John Burna, Robert Nelson, Salil Rajmaira, David Phillips, Daniel Edwards, and Thomas Becker.

Dr. Pankovich initiated an orthopedic technologist program that trained five students per year for over 15 years. He also began the microsurgery lab at the Hektoen Institute, which resulted in patients from all over the midwest arriving for upper extremity and digital reimplantation. In 1974, Dr. Boonmee Chunprapaph (Figure 19–13), who had trained for several months sewing jugular veins and arteries of rats, became the first surgeon in the world to successfully replant a four-finger amputation. It was his first clinical case. The result, Dr. Chunprapaph recalls, was a very functional hand with which the patient could feel and grasp.

The first replantation at the County was done on an index finger by a U of I resident, Dr. Edward Abraham. When presented to the Saturday morning University of Illinois orthopedic conference, Dr. Peter Alter pronounced it the work of the "charlatans" at Cook County. Somewhere, the shade of John B. Murphy must have been smiling.

In 1959, the Association for the Study of Internal Fixation (ASIF) began giving courses in Davis, Switzerland, on osteosynthesis of fractures. Early on, Dr. Pankovich recognized the importance of these advances and established an osteosynthesis lab at the Hektoen Institute in the early 1970s where the residents could work to perfect the surgical techniques of compression plating and stabile osteosynthesis. The cumbersome ineffective methods of fracture management that had dominated the English-speaking world were soon abandoned. By 1972, Reginald Watson-Jones and *Fractures and Joint Injuries* came to be surpassed by the *Manual of Internal Fixation Techniques* recommended by the Arbeitsgemeinshaft fur Osteosynthesfragen (AO) and ASIF group. And the names Müller, Allowed, and Willenegger became the guiding lights with regard to fracture stabilization.

In spite of the best efforts of Jack Stevens and Ted Hartman, fracture care at Cook County Hospital was, during their time, largely a matter of almost religious belief. The same ankle fracture could be managed differently on three different orthopedic services. A new approach initiated on the Cook County orthopedic

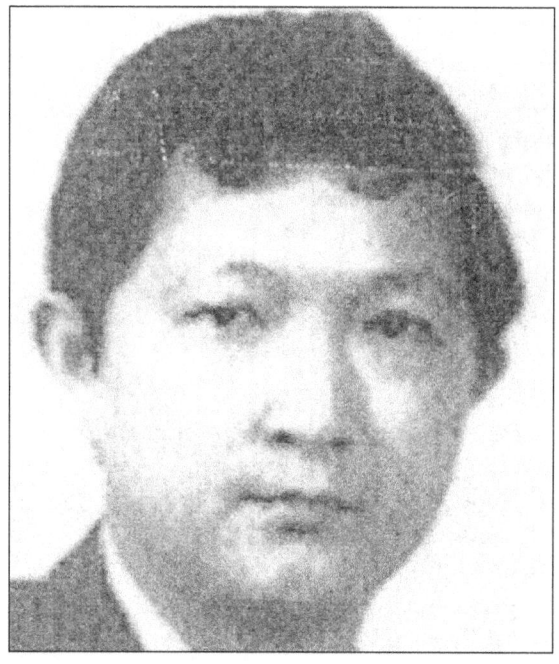

*Figure 19–13*
*Boomee Chunprapaph*

service was stabilization of both the fibular and medial malleolar fractures. The principles of Lauge-Hansen and the Swiss became required knowledge for an orthopedic resident, while the names Potts and Dupuytren became largely remembered for historic interest. Dr. Pankovich extended research in ankle fractures and published several classic papers concerning this particular area of injury. Mysore Shivaram and Dr. Pankovich published a landmark paper on the "Anatomic Basis of Variability in Injuries of the Medial Malleolus and Deltoid Ligament" in *Acta Northup Scand* in 1979.

One of the University of Illinois orthopedic residents, Dr. T. L. Huang, had studied with Dr. Masaki Watanabe in Japan. As a result, in the early 1970s, primitive arthroscopy (largely diagnostic in nature), was started with the operator looking through the lens of the microscope. This was time before arthroscopic surgical intervention existed in any useful form, and diagnostic methods and instrumentation were extremely primitive.

The period from 1972–1980 resulted in a number of visiting professors appearing at County Hospital, including Drs. Enders from Vienna, Willenegger from Bern, Switzerland, Morton Spinner (Mr. Nerve) from New York, and Robert Winquist from Seattle. Winquist's Seattle group was a major contributor to the development of closed intramedullary nailing using C-arm imaging.

Dr. Enders developed the flexible nailing, otherwise known as Enders nails, to fix intertrochanteric and basilar neck femoral fracture. It was accomplished by inserting these rods from just above the knee and driving them up the medullary canal and across the fracture site into the head and neck of the femur. Dr. Pankovich realized that intramedullary nailing of this type could be used to stabilize a wide variety of long-bone fractures such as those of the femur, tibia, and humerus. A number of publications resulted from this innovation. Two residents, Richard Pearson and Mitchell Goldfies, suggested a modification of the bevel on the end of the Enders rods and the orientation of the insertional eyelet to facilitate their use. Thus, the Pearson, Goldfies, and Pankovich (PGP) rods came to be manufactured. Locked intramedullary nailing, developed a few years later, has largely eclipsed this advance in long-bone fracture treatment except in pediatric patients.

Drs. Robert Hall and Mark Gonzalez, Dr. Pankovich's successors in the department, extended flexible intramedullary nailing into the hand where it is still useful. There is even locked IM nailing for that CCH special: the comminuted gunshot fracture of the hand metacarpals (designed by Dr. Hall and manufactured for a time by Smith and Nephew).

Dr. Pankovich was also an early advocate of the use of methyl methacrylate cement as an adjunctive fixation in fractures associated with metastatic disease or significant osteopenia. The innovation created quite a stir when first presented to the reactionary group that gathered on Saturday mornings at the University of Illinois. His experience led to the publication of "Stabilization of Pathologic Fractures with Acrylic Cement" in *Clinical Orthopaedics and Related Research Journal* in 1974 with Asok Ray and J. S. Romine.

Significant publications included "Neglected Rupture of the Achilles Tendon Treated by VY Tedious Flap" in 1975 with Edward Abraham, "Maisonneuve Fracture of the Fibula" in the *Journal of Bone and Joint Surgery* in 1976, and "The Anconeus Approach to the Elbow Joint and Proximal Radius and Ulna" in *JBJS* in 1977.

Dr. Pankovich was among the first to recognize that low-velocity gunshot fractures of the long bones could be treated more expeditiously with open reduction and internal fixation in view of their limited soft-tissue damage. This resulted in the publication of "Extra-Articular Low-Velocity Gunshot Fractures of the Radius and Ulna" in *JBJS* in 1978 with Drs. Elstrom and Egwele.

In the late 1970s, the Orthopedic Trauma Hospital Association was founded by the chairmen of nine major orthopedic trauma centers. This ultimately gave rise to the Orthopedic Trauma Association in 1985, with Dr. Pankovich as an initial member.

When he first came to County, Dr. Pankovich summoned the four chief residents and asked them what they felt the main problem with the residency was from their point of view. "Not enough surgery" was the response. In a year, the number of surgical cases doubled.

Though the Fantus orthopedic clinic could be long and grueling, there was never a shortage of pathology that could be seen nowhere else. Residents in training, with their self-assuredness and often cavalier attitude toward patients and attendings, confirmed John Boswick's classic definition of a surgeon: "seldom right, but never in doubt." One resident would attribute end-stage arthritis in a 20-year-old patient to the fact that he had been playing lots of football. Further inquiry into the patient's history revealed that it wasn't football but hemarthroses due to hemophilia that had caused his knees to degenerate.

Dr. Pankovich saw that the pediatric orthopedic section was run by a strong attending staff competent to teach the residents. Dr. Sharukin Yelda (Figure 19-18) had come to Chicago from George Washington University. He was a close associate of Dr. Mike Tachjian at Children's Memorial Hospital. Svante Rolander came from the University of Göteborg, Sweden, where he was a student of Carl Hirsch and did significant research on the lumbar spine. Dr. Spiros Dallas, who had his training with Robert Salter in Toronto, was an attending at Children's Memorial Hospital. Dr. Edward Abraham, who spent a good deal of his University of Illinois residency with Dr. Pankovich, ultimately became head of the section, and went on to become chairman of the Orthopedic Department at the University of Illinois. He has written extensively on pediatric leg lengthening.

Edward Schaumberg initially ran the foot and back service. He was followed by several outstanding spine surgeons including Drs Don Miskew, Tom Gleason, Steve Mardjetko, and Chris Dewald.

Dr Pankovich was very skeptical of the claims made in the early 1970s by the "touts" for chymopapain injection in lumbar disc disease. For that reason (and lack of a permit from Dr. Robert D. Ray), County patients were not subjected to it. Whatever the case, this was good fortune as chymopapain tended to be overused and did more harm than good.

A typical Cook County surgical ward consisted of a wing extending south from a long corridor that ran parallel to Harrison Street. There was a nurses' station at the entry to the ward. Across from the nurses' station was a post-op observation unit of four to six beds and an examining room for new admissions.

In the case of the hand ward, there was a room for the resident on call to sleep. Near the nurses' station was a restroom and a bath. Beyond the nurses' station, extending for 15-20 beds on each side, was the main ward. Well into the 1970s, it was not unusual to see numerous patients with long-bone fractures in some type of traction.

One of the nice architectural touches at the end of the ward was a sunroom that opened out onto an space behind the main ward. From it, one could see the hospital parking lot, the internal medicine wards, and the Children's Hospital, as well as the relatively low-lying power plant. There were a number of pay phones at the entrance to the ward, and televisions and radios were brought from home. "Boom boxes" were in their infancy. The construction of the building prevented the wards from becoming unduly hot and humid despite the lack of air conditioning. There were fans, however, in the main corridors. The sun porch at the end of the ward was the ideal place to be located unless you were seriously ill. The patients were separated from the rest of the ward by a small barrier, and after lights out, the activities and carryings on might resemble any busy street on the south side of Chicago. One mother, after receiving a report from her son concerning his first night's stay, signed him out immediately. It was not unusual, late at night, to detect the aroma of pot. Other drugs, liquor, gambling, and even "working girls" were available. Any altercations were quickly broken up by the Chicago Police who provided security for the hospital.

In 1990, McGraw-Hill approached Dr. Arsen Pankovich and asked him to prepare a pocket-size *Handbook of Hand Fractures*, which would be a portable reference on fracture management written for the practicing orthopedic surgeon. In 1995, the first edition of the *Handbook* was published. The contributing authors, with a few exceptions, had obtained their trauma-management experience at the Cook County Hospital. This *Handbook* has now gone through three editions, the most recent published in 2006. The number of contributing authors is now 32 with contributions coming from all over the United States and Scotland.

## Robert Hall, Jr.

Dr. Robert F. Hall, Jr., chairman following Dr. Pankovich, grew up in Grand Junction, Colorado, where his father was an orthopedist. He graduated from Northwestern University School of Medicine and had his orthopedic residency at that institution from 1972 to 1976. After a tour in the U.S. Army, during which time he was chief of orthopedic surgery at Reynolds Army Hospital in Fort Sill, Oklahoma, he returned to Cook County Hospital in 1979 where he became chief of the section of hand surgery from 1979 to 1988. He was acting chairman of the division of orthopedic surgery from 1980 to 1985, and became chairman of the division from 1985 to 1998. His 18 years as chairman make him the current record holder.

The Department of Orthopedic Surgery at Cook County Hospital was reported by *U.S. News and World Report* in its July 1993 issue on "Best Hospitals," as being in the top 3 percent in the nation. It was considered a leading center for those who seek the very best care. In 1994, the hospital was ranked 37th in the nation. Among the innovations brought to the department by Dr. Hall were the use of 3.2 mm flexible rods for intramedullary fixation of humeral fractures, the use of blunted rush rods for intramedullary fixation of radius and ulnar fractures, and the use of 0.8 mm blunted intramedullary rods for fixation of metacarpal and phalangeal fractures. During his 18 years as chairman, Dr. Hall appeared in nearly 100 forums, largely related to hand injuries and flexible intramedullary nailing. Dr. Hall had a number of publications concerning intramedullary rodding of diaphyseal fractures of the humerus and tibia, and locked and flexible intramedullary nailing for fracture fixation of the metacarpals and proximal phalanges.

In the 1980s, the attending staff consisted of Fred Pollock, who had trained in the residency program at the University of San Francisco, Jorge Prieto and Allen Mock, who had come to the United States from South Africa, William Dobozi, and Edward Abraham. During the heyday of flexible intramedullary nailing, Drs. Pankovich, Hall, and Dobozi gave a number of instructional courses at the annual meeting of the American Academy of Orthopaedic Surgeons and elsewhere.

Dr. Hall was known for his quick wit and sharp tongue. One of the attending staff was known for his fondness for harness racing and playing the futures market in soy beans. When he complained to Dr. Hall one day about his fortunes in the soy-bean market, Dr. Hall replied that he was doing pretty well in the market by doing just the opposite of the attending. This led to an opening on the attending staff shortly thereafter when the man resigned in a huff.

In 1987, Dr. Hall hired Dr. Mark Gonzalez, who subsequently became his successor as chairman of the division of orthopedics at Cook County Hospital. During the tenure of his chairmanship, the residency was closed down due to the desire of the certifying body to have residency programs more closely affiliated with academic institutions for their research and full-time academic capabilities.

It has been said you can teach a gorilla to operate, but the gorilla will need instruction and practice. Orthopedic surgery is basically a craft; the decision of when and how to apply the technical skills comes with experience, and that comes from the ability to learn by observation and from mistakes. Strangely, to qualify for orthopedic surgical training or practice does not require one to demonstrate manual dexterity or the ability to work in a three-dimensional model; only prospective dental students are required to demonstrate this skill. The conflict between the technical and intellectual is best illustrated by Dr. Pankovich's nameless MD/PhD: "When he goes to the lab they say, he must be a hell of a surgeon because he doesn't know much about research, and when he is in the OR they say, he must be a terrific investigator because he sure as hell doesn't know how to operate."

Dr. Hall is remembered by many of his former residents as an outstanding teacher and surgical technician. He devoted long hours to the residency program and the residents. He was available, in person, 12 hours a day, six days a week. The structure of surgical instruction was felt to be crucial. In a three-month rotation, the first month was given over to demonstration by the attending, the second month to direct supervision of the resident as a surgeon, and by the third month, the resident could manage the set-up and surgery himself with a carefully critiqued postmortem.

Hall is also remembered as having little patience with those who would waste his time. When he was chief of Orthopedic Surgery at Reynolds Army Hospital, a visiting field-grade officer who was passing through brought his daughter into a busy clinic for what he termed a "checkup." Dr. Hall, whose patience was running short by that time, obliged him with a marking pen check to the child's forehead. Needless to say, this did not reflect well with the commanding officer of the post.

Dr. Hall was known as a skillful, expert witness on behalf of the orthopedic community. In the days before the American Academy of Orthopedic Surgery took much interest in the importance of expert testimony, either on behalf or against a defendant orthopedic surgeon, Dr. Hall had an enviable record against the plaintiff's bar. It wasn't until recently that the Academy recognized the importance of providing member expert witnesses with the skills to deal with situations where the standard of care might be defined in any way the plaintiff's attorney and his expert wished to define it. Today, the quality of adverse testimony is reviewed by the Academy, and if it is found to be factually incorrect or fabricated, the expert is subject to severe censure. It is of note that one of Dr. Hall's most frequent adversaries in these courtroom battles was a former attending orthopedic surgeon at the County.

The relationship between the Cook County Hospital and the University of Illinois has been especially close over the years due to the geographic proximity of the institutions. The use of the County by the U of I orthopedic residency program has been even more enhanced by the fact that most of the County orthopedic attending staff have an academic appointment at the University of Illinois. And finally, the last three department chairmen at the University of Illinois had much of their training at Cook County Hospital. Both Dr. Raid Armada and Dr. Edward Abraham were senior residents at the County, and the current chairman of the Department of Orthopedics at the University of Illinois, Dr. Mark Gonzalez, a former U of I resident, was hired by Dr. Hall in 1987 to become chief of the section of hand surgery. Dr. Gonzalez became chairman of the division of orthopedic surgery at County in May 1998. He continues in that position to this day. Problems with funding (paying the vendors of orthopedic materials and implants), managed with difficulty but successfully by his predecessors Drs. Hall and Pankovich, have recently become significant issues for Dr. Gonzalez and the hospital administration.

One of the delightful things about the history of orthopedic surgery at Cook County Hospital is the number of innovations that occurred there and the unexpected opportunities that arose to follow up some of these pioneering operations 15–20 years later.

In the development of the flexible intramedullary Ender's (by this time PGP) rods for nailing tibial fractures, Dr. Arsen Pankovich and his resident Jorge Prieto, worked in the anatomy laboratory to develop the best surgical approach to insert the rods and to provide stability for fracture healing. In the midst of their research, an internal medicine resident broke his tibia playing basketball in the gym at Karl

Meyer Hall. Without any hesitation, research was extended to clinical practice and the first flexible nailing of a fractured tibia was carried out on the medical resident. Previously, the options would have been a cast, an external fixator, or what was known as a Lottes nailing that did not control rotation.

One of the radiology residents, Dr. Mike Hummel, injured himself when he whiffed on an overhead playing tennis and fell backward onto his dorsiflexed wrist. Some weeks later, when the wrist was still too painful to play tennis and was now clicking with motion, he went to see Dr. Mark Gonzalez, who diagnosed carpal instability. The question was what to do about it. Dr. Gonzalez admitted that none of the current procedures was very reliable, but he had just learned of a new reconstructive procedure that made pretty good sense. If Hummel didn't mind, Dr Gonzalez would try this procedure on him. Ten years later, now in private practice, Dr Hummel showed the result to one of Dr Gonzalez' colleagues. He was still playing tennis, had no carpal instability, and has been asymptomatic after the initial phase of rehabilitation.

In 1995, a 20-year-old man fleeing from a drug deal gone bad hopped into a taxi where a couple of bullets were pumped into his arm through the cab window. The taxi driver sped away. The man subsequently got patched up and then went to a bar for a beer. He got on the phone to arrange another deal, ran into the street, and woke up a few hours later in Cook County Hospital with an open tibial fracture. The patient was taken to surgery and his wound debrided. Two days later, he was returned to the OR and had an 18-hole plate applied from the proximal to distal tibial metaphysis with lag screw fixation of the butterfly fragments. He underwent a delayed wound closure and for all practical purposes, would never be seen again. He did, however, carry his original radiographs with him, the staples still visible. This is what came to be termed "fire and forget" by his surgeon, Dr. Robert Hall. This immediate stabilization of an open fracture with internal fixation hardware followed the principles laid down some 20 years earlier at County by Dr. Arsen Pankovich. It did not require patient cooperation for follow-up. Fifteen years later, this same patient showed up in a suburban orthopedic office complaining of some discomfort around the proximal end of the plate. X-rays showed the fracture healed in perfect alignment with no evidence of infection. The patient, who had turned his life around after his near-fatal experience, had been working without interruption or impairment ever since as a construction laborer. Dr. Hall, who had done the initial surgery, had the opportunity to do the follow-up 15 years and 60 miles later in his office.

## Mark Gonzalez

Dr. Mark Gonzalez became chairman of the Department of Orthopedic Surgery at the University of Illinois in March 2007 and became the Riad Barmada Endowed Chair of Orthopedic Surgery in October 2008. He holds a master's degree in engineering and is currently enrolled in the mechanical engineering PhD program. Dr. Gonzalez has had two hand fellowships and one joint replacement fellowship. His publications and research reflect a continuing interest in these areas. Under his leadership, the Cook County Hospital division of orthopedics was voted into the top 50 departments in *U.S. News and World Report* in 2001.

## Acknowledgements

With acknowledgment to Drs. Arsen Pankovich, Sidney Blair and E. Boone Brackett for their help in verifying the historic validity of this chapter.

## Reading List

1. Allard K, Bunch WH. *Orthopaedics at Loyola University, Heritage and Legacy*. Washington, D.C.: Color Press; 1980.
2. Cubbins WR, Callahan JJ, Scuderi CS. Cruciate Ligaments; A Resume of Operative Attacks and Results Obtained, *Am J Surg*. 1934;43:481-485.
3. Cubbins WR, Callahan JJ, Scuderi CS. Cruciate Ligament Injuries. *Surg Gynecol Obstet*. 1937;54:218-225.
4. Directory, Cook County Hospital Interns and Residents Alumni Association (1872-1972) 1972.
5. Gonzalez MH, Hall RF. *Intramedullary Fixation of Metacarpal and Proximal Phalangeal Fractures of the Hand*. Clin Orthop Relat Res. 1996;327:47-54.
6. Panvovich AM, Elstrom JA, Dangles CJ, *Chapter 25. Fractures and Dislocations of the Ankle*. In: Elstrom JA, Virkus WW, Pankovich AM, Eds. *Handbook of Fractures $3^{RD}$ edition*. New York: McGraw-Medical Publishing Division, 2005.
7. Raffensperger JG, Ed. *The Old Lady on Harrison: Cook County Hospital, 1833-1995*. New York: Peter Lang Publishing Group; 1997.
8. Speed K. *A Text-book of fractures and dislocations, with special reference to their pathology, diagnosis and treatment*. Philadelphia and New York; Lea and Febiger; 1916

# 20

# Plastic Surgery

*Raymond L. Warpeha, DDS, MD, PhD, FACS*

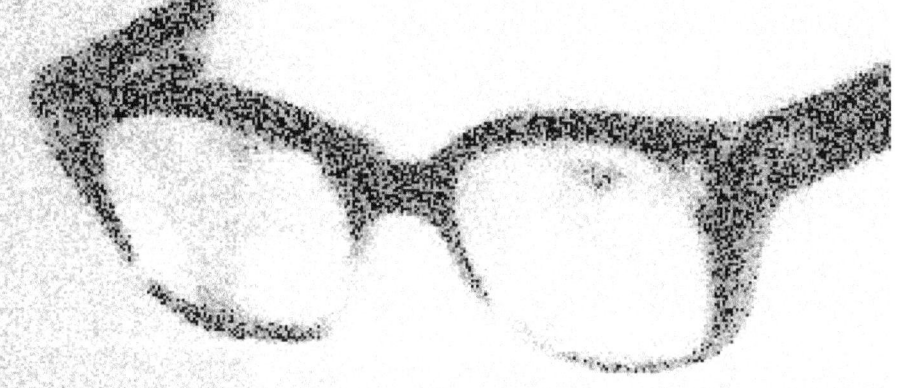

- *Introduction*
- *The Beginning*
- *Orion Harry Stuteville*
- *The Cook County Plastic Surgery Program and*
- *Northwestern University*
- *Loyola University Medical School Affiliation*
- *University of Illinois Affiliation*
- *References*

## Introduction

Since plastic surgical practice cuts across multiple surgical disciplines including burn care, cosmetic and reconstructive surgery, hand surgery, maxillo-facial surgery including facial fractures, and head and neck tumor surgery, it had been established as a subdivision of surgery within the American Board of Surgery when that body was first formed in 1937. This marriage of convenience was dissolved in 1961, when plastic surgery was recognized as an independent surgical specialty by the AMA's Advisory Board of Medical Specialties.[1] That is not to say that there was not any significant activity in the disciplines covered by plastic surgery in the almost 100 years between the founding of Cook County Hospital and the recognition of plastic surgery as an independent surgical specialty. As with the majority of surgical specialties, general surgeons performed whatever surgery eventually would be co-opted by the plastic surgical community, when the specialty gained its independence. The available records show that some of the general surgery attending surgeons at Cook County operated quite well and often in the realm of plastic surgery.

## The Beginning

The contributions of Allen Kanavel, Sumner Koch, and Harvey Allen in the areas of hand and burn surgery are well known and represent significant contributions to the field of what would become plastic surgery. But there were other contributions by County attending surgeons, even in earlier times. Nicholas Senn was clearly a master surgeon with a variety of interests, but of particular interest to this chapter is his book *Pathology and Surgical Treatment of Tumors*, which was published in 1895.[2] This text details the treatment of various head and neck tumors and stresses the necessity of both excision of the lymphatic drainage and total excision of the tumor as most important components of proper surgical therapy. The surgical approaches are presented in detail, but there is less attention to reconstructive activity. In fact, Senn states that, "The surgeon who operates with a view of securing a good cosmetic result is very liable to perform an incomplete operation."[3]

Another of the early surgeons with a flair for head and neck surgery was Dr.

Albert Ochsner, professor and chairman of surgery at the College of Physicians and Surgeons (University of Illinois) from 1900 to 1925. A prolific surgeon and writer of articles and books, he is mostly known for his treatise on the treatment of acute appendicitis. He was also a pioneer in the surgical treatment of thyroid and parathyroid disease on which he published a book in 1910.[4]

Carl Beck is one of the four Beck brothers who contributed much to general, maxilla-facial, and otolaryngological surgery, as well as radiotherapy beginning in the late 1890s and early 20th century. He is most often cited as a great friend of Albert Einstein and as a collaborator of Alexis Carrel in work on organ transplantation and refinement of vascular anastamotic techniques. He was, however, a very competent and busy surgeon with an interest in surgery of the hand as regards technique and reconstructive methods. Beck devised methods for handling damaged tendons and set forth his three stages of repair that he felt would best ensure function could be attained and deformities prevented. Beck offered to help military surgeons in Austria learn his techniques in 1914, which he included in his book, *The Crippled Arm and Hand*, that was ultimately published in 1925. Simply put, the key features were prophylaxis by saving as much tissue as possible; adjusting treatment so that deformities would be minimized; removing scars and obstacles to function; and finally, the building of new parts. These were addressed as well by Dr. Sterling Bunnell in his classic volume on hand surgery some 20 years later after World War II.[5]

Cosmetic surgery was not neglected during these early days, either. Dr. Max Thorek, an attending at County from 1932 until the late 1950s, began his interest in reconstructive surgery in 1916. Thorek conducted an operative clinic at County Hospital twice a week. He was also active in postgraduate teaching with Cook County Graduate School of Medicine. His special field was working with obese women who had failed every medical and dietary attempt to control weight gain. Some 50 years before the advent of bariatric surgery, he undertook body contour surgery to produce weight loss with better function. In one case, he performed a series of operations on a 20 year-old woman who initially weighed 400 pounds. His contouring ultimately reduced her to 200 pounds. Work in this specialized area provided the material for his book, *Plastic Surgery of the Breast and the Abdominal Wall*, published in 1942.[6] *A Surgeon's World*, the autobiography written by Thorek, summarizes the career of this remarkable surgeon.[7]

## Orion Harry Stuteville

An accredited plastic surgery residency was established at Cook County Hospital in 1959 by Dr. Orion H. Stuteville (Figure 20-1) at the request of Dr. Robert J. Freeark who had recently been hired as the first full-time member of the County surgical staff. Although he had been active in teaching since the early 1930s, both as an oral surgeon and later as a plastic surgeon, the history of plastic surgery at County during this period is really the history of Dr. Stuteville's legacy to the residents and fellows he taught and the patients whose care he directed.[1]

"Stutie*," as he was respectfully known, was born in 1901 in a Studebaker

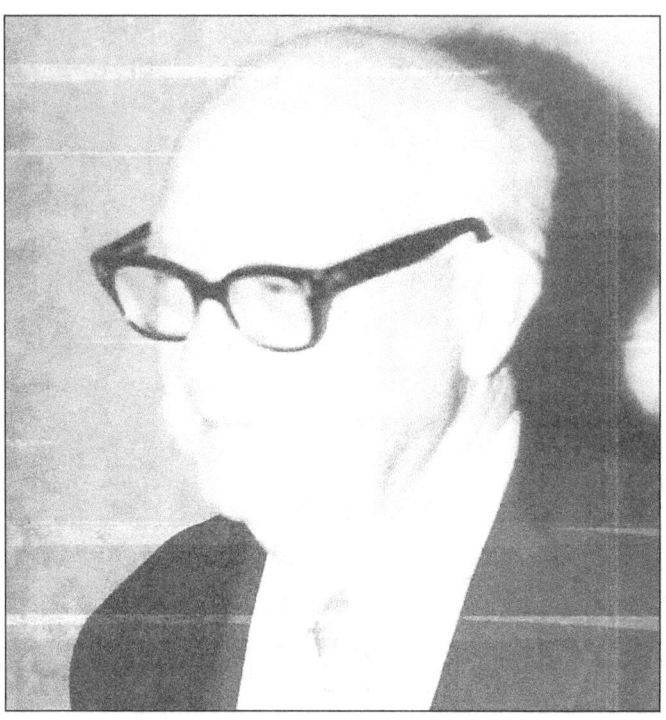

*Figure 20–1*
*Orion Harry Stuteville*

covered wagon under the stars on the Oklahoma plains. His father, the U.S. Indian Agent of the then "Oklahoma Territories," had set out with the family to escort a friendly Native American hunting party to their reservation as required by a government treaty. Mrs. Stuteville went into labor on the trip and delivered a healthy son. The proud and politically correct father asked the tribal chief to name the child. As was the custom, the chief named the baby for the first object that came into his view. In this case, it was the constellation Orion. I asked Stutie how the chief came up with the white man's name for the constellation. His reply was, "The chief was a graduate in astronomy from Harvard?"

Dr. Stuteville grew up up a mud-brick house near Okeene, Oklahoma, and by the age of 12 was plowing fields with a mule and riding point on cattle drives north to the railhead in Kansas. He later won a scholarship to prep school by writing the winning essay in an open competition. Dr. Stuteville subsequently graduated from Oklahoma State University, where he had won the intercollegiate light-heavyweight wrestling championship. He made the Olympic wrestling team that competed in the 1924 Olympics in Paris, but he was prevented from competing due to a chronically dislocating shoulder. In a post-Olympic tournament, he pinned the gold medalist at his weight in one minute, 30 seconds. Stutie always claimed his pursuit of Olympic gold was inspired by his meeting with gold medal winner Jim Thorpe when he was a boy of 12. In those days, professional wrestling was more a display of technique and muscle power, but due to dwindling

---

*All residents referred to him as Steudy, but Stuteville signed his name as Stutie.

audiences, the promoters decided to begin some of the sport's entertainment programs that are familiar to present-day wrestling fans. They recognized what an attractive act an Oklahoma farm boy with a college pedigree would be. Two promoters arrived at the Stuteville home to sign him to a $12,000 annual (a fortune in those days) contract for 12 once monthly bouts. When one of the promoters used profanity in the presence of his mother, Stutie promptly threw him out of the house, literally, and decided to accept a position at Northwestern University as the head wrestling coach for $2,200 a year. During his tenure, the program was successful, and several of the team members ended up as collegiate champions. At Northwestern, as he continued to coach, Stutie enrolled in an anatomy course at the dental school and obtained a DDS degree in 1931. He then pursued another dream: medicine. While practicing dentistry in Evanston, he earned an MD degree, also from Northwestern, and a master's degree in orthodontics as well. Subsequently, he completed a surgical residency at St. Joseph's Hospital. A dental school faculty member at Northwestern from 1933 to 1970, Stuteville served as chairman of maxillo-facial and oral surgery, positions without pay.

Early in WWII, Stutie enlisted in the Army Medical Corps as a one-man head and neck surgery "team" in a front-line medical unit in the North African and Italian campaigns, where he treated hundreds of major facial and neck injuries. One afternoon after the war, while he was watching a TV film presentation of the Allied bombing of the German stronghold of Monte Cassino, Stutie felt a feeling of déjà vu. He actually had been there, and the TV show was using copies of the film he had shot from a hill adjacent to Monte Cassino. It seems that an Air Force officer had been visiting his medical unit the day before the attack and had advised Stutie of the impending aerial assault. He also clued Dr. Stuteville in on the best place to safely view the "fireworks." On his discharge, Stutie had to surrender all the originals of the films he had made, which included the visuals of the Monte Cassino battle.

Dr. Stuteville retired from the practice of surgery in 1975 and took a course in cardiology to better serve as a rural general practitioner in the foothills of the Ozark Mountains of Arkansas. There, he set up a ranching operation, and returned to plowing with a mule and roping calves for branding from his beloved horse, Doll. In order to help the population at large reduce dietary fat, he continued to apply his creative instincts in cross-breeding his buffalo and cattle via artificial insemination to produce "beefalo" and "cattleo."

Throughout his active participation at County, he maintained a busy practice at the Passavant Memorial Hospital, a major teaching affiliate of the Northwestern Medical School. A tireless worker, he also conducted a weekly Sunday teaching conference combined with ward rounds and a tumor clinic at County, in addition to his regularly scheduled operating times. His approach to training was definitely "hands-on" from several different aspects. A favorite trick in the OR was to play " pass the knife" during a case. The resident operator was asked to identify some anatomic structure in the field or perhaps to delineate the possible complications that could occur during the performance of a certain procedural step. If he or she didn't know the correct answer, the knife would pass to the next senior trainee, and so on down the line, until control of the blade reverted to Dr. Stuteville for another round of quizzing. This got everyone, even the interns, into the habit of reading up on all the cases in which they were to scrub. In addition, there were times when Dr. Stuteville's prowess as a wrestler influenced his particular type of hands-on instruction. This usually occurred during preoperative discussions concerning the best approaches for tumor extirpation—removing the patient from his disease—and generally involved an uplifting experience, including Stutie's clenched fists, the trainee's crumpled shirt-front, and a wall. Dr. Stuteville's major areas of expertise included the management of soft tissue injuries of the head and neck, otopharyngeal cancer, lymph node dissection of the neck, and reconstructive techniques in major injuries with tissue loss. Both surgery and plastics residents on his service became comfortable with neck explorations for any type of trauma after their extensive experience with Stutie in performing radical neck dissections. The management and closure of many soft tissue wounds during residency led to a confidence that could only come from the hands-on experience under Stutie and his experienced staff, which included Drs. Stu Landa, Martin Sullivan, Robert Felix, and Drs. Kostrabala and Janda, all accomplished plastic surgeons, and many MD-DDS oral surgeons and plastic surgeons.

Aside from the head and neck and wound management areas, the residents received extensive experience in the metabolic treatment of the acute burn and management of burn scars as a result of their experience with the large patient volume on their rotations through the County Hospital burn unit. One of the largest in the United States, the burn unit was founded In 1964 by Dr. John Boswick, an internationally recognized burn surgeon.

In the early 1960s, with plastic surgery becoming more involved in aesthetic (cosmetic) surgery, the American Board of Plastic Surgery informed Stuteville that to maintain accreditation for his program, it would be necessary to increase the exposure of his trainees to cosmesis. He informed a young resident by the name of Jack Sheen of this requirement. By the time this enterprising young resident finished his training in 1964, he had performed 120 rhinoplasty procedures.[8] Dr. Sheen went on to gain international recognition for his innovative and creative approach to nasal surgery. Dr. Sheen was not the only Stuteville trainee to make a mark in the world of international plastic surgery. Dr. Burt Brent, whose name is synonymous with building human ears for those unfortunate enough to be either born without them or to have acquired or congenital deformities of this part of the body, began his work in the field by using autologous rib cartilage and temporo-parietal tissue of the ear region while a resident under Stutie's mentorship. Brent presented his experience with more than 1,800 ear reconstructions at the October 2008 meeting of the American Society of Plastic Surgeons. Brent also cited what he had learned about plastic surgery from Stuteville in an editorial in the *Journal of Plastic and Reconstructive Surgery*.[9]

> *"Plastic surgery is an art form—an exacting discipline characterized by a special approach to handling tissues, repairing wounds and reconstructing deformities. The aspect that most strikingly distinguishes plastic surgery from all other surgical disciplines is the instantaneous, visual aesthetic result and often the dramatic psychological change*

*which it affords the patient. By virtue of the visual impact the surrounding family is correspondingly affected and plastic surgery thus exerts an effect that extends well beyond the obvious and immediate needs of the patient."*

## The Cook County Plastic Surgery Program and Northwestern University

In 1967, the American Board of Plastic Surgery again advised the County Plastic Surgery Residency about the need for greater exposure to aesthetic surgery. Arrangements were then made for residents to rotate to Northwestern teaching hospitals. With the approval of Dr. John Beal, then chairman of the Department of Surgery at Northwestern, a combined CCH-Northwestern program was established. Beal appointed Stuteville chair of plastic surgery and professor of surgery at the medical school. At the same time, Dr. Herold Griffiths was recruited by Dr. Walter Maddock, chief of surgery at the Wesley Memorial Hospital, a major Northwestern teaching affiliate, as the first full-time plastic surgeon. With the cooperation of Dr. Griffiths, residents from County began to rotate to Wesley, Passavant, Children's, and Lakeside VA Hospitals, all within the Northwestern teaching system.[10]

When Dr. Stuteville retired in the early 1970s, he was succeeded by Dr. Griffiths. By mutual agreement, the combined program separated and the County residents no longer rotated within the Northwestern system. Residents of the NU program still rotated to County for experience on the burn unit.

## Loyola University Medical School Affiliation

From 1970 to 1986, Drs. Conrad Tasche and Bengalore Jayaaram, two of Dr. Stuteville's former residents, served as directors of plastic surgery at County. Dr. Stuteville had retired from County and Northwestern, but at the urging of Dr. Freeark, who assumed the chairmanship of the Loyola Stritch School of Medicine Department of Surgery in 1970, he agreed to establish a a division of plastic surgery with a board-accredited residency program. In due course, this was accomplished with a County affiliation as a major part of the program. From 1972 to 2007 (and during my tenure as chief of plastic surgery at Loyola [Figure 20–2]), 59 Loyola plastic surgery residents experienced junior and senior resident rotations at Cook County Hospital.

## University of Illinois Affiliation

From 1978 to 1986, Dr. Olga Jonasson was the chair of surgery at the County Hospital. One of the very first things she did was to fully integrate the independent County surgical residencies with the University of Illinois. Dr. Tasche was

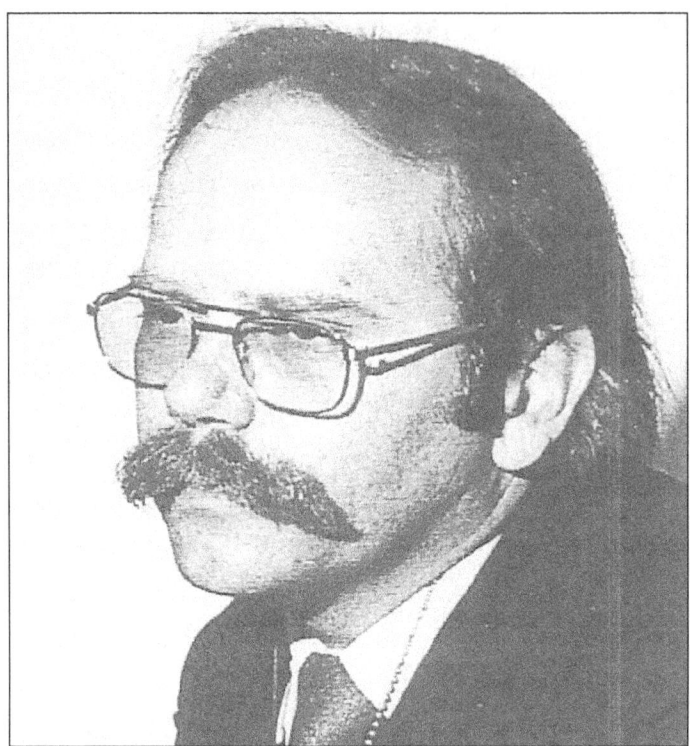

*Figure 20–2*
*Raymond L. Warpeha*

appointed director of medical education at County, as well as the co-coordinator of the internship program. In 1986, Dr. Mimis Cohen from the University of Illinois Department of Surgery was named the chair of plastic surgery at County.[11] At about the same time, sex-change operations, which were being done at the County, were discontinued due to pressure from the County board and the hospital administration.

Under Cohen's leadership, plastic surgery training at the County progressed in all aspects of reconstructive and aesthetic procedures, including such state-of-the-art techniques as micro-surgical free tissue transfer. Others from the University of Illinois plastic surgery team, notably Ai Ramasastri and John Polley, provided excellent clinical and surgical service to patients at County. Dr. Cohen was able to maintain two full-time resident positions while training 40 University of Illinois residents during his tenure (1986-2007). From 1972 to 2007, over 100 plastic surgical residents from the University of Illinois, Loyola University, and the University of Chicago had a significant part of their training at the County Hospital. For his part, Dr. Cohen has been able to focus on the long-term results of cleft lip and palate surgery, and the evaluation of the fascial anatomy of the upper and lower extremities. He has also edited a three-volume textbook entitled *Mastery of Plastic and Reconstructive Surgery* (1994).

It is no fluke that the County Hospital environment, with the leadership of Dr. Stuteville building on the earlier work of such giants as Beck, Senn, and Kanavel, among others, helped to produce such world-renowned surgeons as

Burt Brent and Jack Sheen. Medicine and the public can only benefit from the extensively trained plastic surgeons who can only be produced at places such as Cook County Hospital. It is unfortunate that as with all public hospitals, there are times when political upheavals interfere with the provision of patient care and medical education. One of the more recent outbursts of this type occurred at County in 2007, and resulted in the dissolution of the plastic surgery training program. One can only hope that this is a temporary state of affairs.

## References

1. Aufricht G. Development of plastic surgery in the United States. *Plas Reconstr Surg.* 1945;1:3-25
2. Rutkow IM. *American Surgery; an illustrated history*. Philadelphia, Lippincott & Raven. Publishers. 1998:275-276.
3. Shedd DP, DeLacure MD. *Bull Am Coll Surg.* 1996;Aug:19-24.
4. Griffith BH, Yao JST. *A Centennial History of the Chicago Surgical Society*. Chicago:Chicago Surgical Society;2000.
5. Blair S, Carl Beck MD. Pioneer Hand Surgeon of Chicago, Loyola University of Chicago, D Orthoped Surg Rehabil J;14:68-72
6. Thorek M. *Plastic Surgery of the Breast and Abdominal Wall*.1942.
7. Thorek M. *A Surgeon's World. The autobiography of Max Thorek.* Philadelphia, New York:JB Lippincott;1943
8. Sheen, Jack. Personal communication
9. Brent B. The Reconstruction of Venus. *Plas Reconst Surg.* 2008;121:2170-2171.
10. Griffith, BH. Personal communication
11. Cohen, M. Personal Communication

# 21

# Otolaryngological Surgery

*Kenneth Printen, MD*
*Hugh Hazenfield, MD*

- *The Beginning*
- *Rush Medical College*
- *Department of Otolaryngology*
- *Jack Kerth*
- *Hugh Hazenfield*
- *Acknowledgements*
- *References*

## The Beginning

In the early 1800s, ophthalmology and otorhinolaryngological surgery evolved together. This was apparent in the establishment of institutes such as the New York Eye and Ear Infirmary in 1820, the Pennsylvania Infirmary for Diseases of the Eye and Ear in 1822, and the Chicago Eye and Ear Infirmary in 1858. It soon became evident, however, that there was a vast difference between these two specialties. Each subsequentially developed, with ophthalmology emerging as the first specialty board established in the United States. The American Board of Ophthalmic Surgery Examination was given in May 1916. Later, the board was incorporated, and the name was officially changed to the American Board of Ophthalmology in 1933. In the 1930s, there were residencies training at CCH. The first resident at County was in ophthalmology and ENT, then in pediatrics. The American Board of Otolaryngology, the second certifying board formed in the United States, was established in 1924. Dr. George F. Shambaugh Sr., a noted Chicago otolaryngologist, played an important role in the formation of that board. The history of otolaryngology at Cook County Hospital is unique in at least several ways. In the makeup of the original staff, only the head specialties (eye and ENT) are listed as having a named individual as the specialist in charge of patients with diseases in this area who required surgery.[1] That individual was Dr. James S. Hildreth, a University of Pennsylvania graduate who had studied pathology under Virchow and EENT under DesMarres in Paris, but who was rumored to have been given the County position on the strength of his father-in-law's position as a U.S. Senator,[2] perhaps a foreboding of the well-known "I'm not going to hire anybody who wasn't sent by somebody" attitude that those of us who worked at County much later often encountered when dealing with the administration. In any case, his credentials were sufficient for him to be appointed professor of ophthalmology and otology at the Chicago Medical College, the precursor of the Northwestern University Medical School. This appointment established the beginning of the long association of these two institutions in the realm of otolaryngology.

An altered medical staff arose from some administrative manipulations in the late 1860s, and the new County medical staff listed Dr. Hosmer A. Johnson (Figure 21–1) as a medical consultant. Johnson was one of the pioneers of the specialty of laryngology in the midwest.[3] Dr. Johnson had been the first intern at Mercy Hospital in the early 1850s and served as a professor of material medica

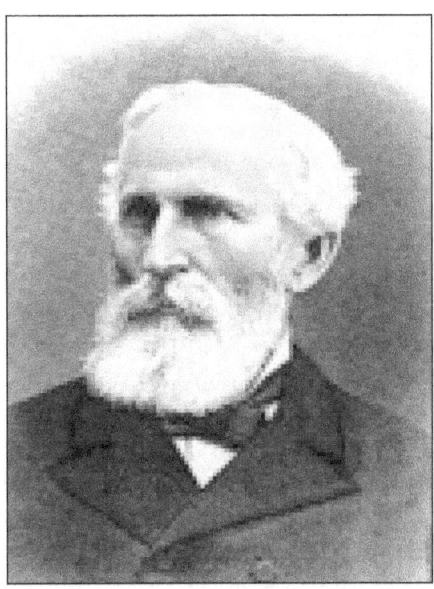

*Figure 21-1  Hosmer A. Johnson*

at Rush, as did his contemporaries, Drs. Ephraim and E. Fletcher Ingals. All of these physicians were active in the foundation of the American Laryngological Association and maintained an affiliation with the County despite busy practices at Rush, the Lind Medical College, and the Chicago Medical College. In addition, they all also emphasized the fact that many of the earliest laryngologists, unlike their counterparts in the other surgical specialties, were not general surgeons with a particular bent for a specific organ system, but rather internists or general practitioners with an interest in chest diseases and secondarily diseases of the ear, nose, and throat.[3] While it is true that Daniel Brainard described a maxillary tumor removal as early as 1864, and Nicholas Senn published a text on treatment of head and neck tumors, many of the prominent general surgeons felt as did Moses Gunn, the mentor of J.B. Murphy, Arthur Dean Bevan, and Albert Ochsner, that "laryngectomy for malignancy was a futile effort and the patients might be better off with a tracheotomy tube for their remaining days."[5] The future development of ENT as a surgical specialty had to wait, like laparoscopy, for the development of new tools. By the1870s, E. Fletcher Ingals was using bronchoscopy to investigate both upper and lower respiratory disease.

As the 1870s drew to a close, the division between the head surgical specialties at County became more clearly defined. Dr. Edward Holmes was recruited to Chicago after studying in Vienna, Paris, and Berlin. He was appointed as the ophthalmologic consultant at County and founded what was to become the Illinois Eye and Ear Infirmary. At about the same time, Dr. Edmund Andrews described an endoscope with a perforated mirror, and the effort to begin improved diagnosis and treatment for ENT disease was afoot. Dr. William Casselberry continued the Northwestern influence at County in otolaryngology as the chairman of laryngology and rhinology at Northwestern from 1896 to 1908. Prior to that, interestingly enough, he was, from 1884 to 1892, like his Rush counterparts, a professor of materia medica and theraputics, and not a surgeon.

## Rush Medical College

The Rush laryngologists continued a close association with the County Hospital until after the Great Chicago Fire of 1871, when the Rush Medical School Building burned to the ground. At that time, the Rush group and the County Hospital grew closer out of necessity and convenience. Unfortunately, this marriage did not last, and the result was the building of the Presbyterian Hospital, which was opened in 1894. While subsequent Rush laryngologists maintained staff privileges at the County, more and more the administrative leadership moved to Northwestern.

By the late 1890s and early 20th century, the otolaryngology service had changed dramatically. The attendings were Drs. Joseph Beck of the famous Chicago surgical family, George Boot, and Stanton Friedberg Sr. Dr. Beck was mainly interested in head and neck tumors and facial plastics, and reconstruction. He was active at County but also maintained a busy practice with his brothers at the family's proprietary hospital on North Clark Street. In addition, he was on the staff of the Illinois Eye and Ear Infirmary. Dr. Karl Meyer was one of the young physicians who spent time with Beck at the North Chicago Hospital (about six months) learning the nuances of ENT. Dr. Friedberg, an 1897 graduate of Rush and former intern at the German American (Grant) Hospital, was an associate of Fletcher Ingals of broncho-esophagology fame, who was appointed to the County staff in 1903 and served as chief of service from 1913 to 1919. He continued the tradition of the laryngologists, and along with Dr. Hektoen, studied the efficacy of tonsillectomy and adenoidectomy in the elimination of the diphtheria carrier state. His son, Stanton Friedberg Jr., was an attending until 1941 and was involved in the first use of sulfa in the treatment of pneumococcal meningitis. By the 1930s, the otolaryngology service based on Ward 21 was a burgeoning operation responsible for the treatment of sinusitis, mastoiditis, head and neck soft tissue infections, and the occasional tumor. Patients were usually treated as outpatients sandwiched in between the 10-15 tonsillectomies per day performed under open drop ether anesthesia on inpatients. The medical staff had increased to three residents, three interns, and six attendings who rotated responsibility for the clinic and the operating room.[6] Before the early 1970s, when family practice became a boarded specialty, interns (especially those who were planning to practice in rural areas without a plethora of specialists) were encouraged to spend elective time, in some instances up to an extra year, on services where they thought they might learn useful skills. Among the most popular of these rotations on the surgical side of the house were ENT (for experience with tonsillectomy and adenoidectomy—T&A, myringotomies, and complex sinus problems), fractures, and Ward 53 (high-risk OB for experience with medical complications of pregnancy and C-sections).

With all the teaching activity on this service, it was always surprising that the student activity was minimal. Mostly, ENT was taught to sophomores by lecture in the Introduction to Clinical Medicine courses or in physical diagnosis by demonstration of the proper use of the otoscope. There was precious little time for elective clerkships. As a matter of fact, during the 1950s and 1960s, the only way for Loyola students to get clinical exposure in otolaryngology was to follow Dr. Myron Hipskind around while he performed his attending duties on the ENT service at County.[7]

## Department of Otolaryngology

By at least the early 1950s, the division of otolaryngology had become officially a service of the Department of Otolaryngology–Maxillofacial Surgery of the Northwestern Medical School. Dr. Howard Ballenger was one of the professors of ENT, as was Thomas Galloway who continued the departmental interest in upper airway problems encountered in the treatment of diphtheria, especially, in his case, as concerned the salutary effects of early tracheostomy and frequent suction on survival of pediatric patients. His co-investigator was none other than Dr. Archibald Hoyne who was active at the County Contagious Disease Hospital on Wolcott Street until the late 1960s. During this general period, the Department of ENT at NU had three chairmen, all of whom were remembered for very different reasons by their residents. Dr. George Shambaugh Jr. was an internationally known ear surgeon who introduced micro-ear surgery into the United States when he brought the first operating microscope to Chicago. This innovation allowed microsurgery to be applied to the performance of stapedectomy and tympanoplasty. Along with his associates Eugene Derlacki and Wiley Harrison, Shambaugh ran an extremely busy service at the Henrotin Hospital on Oak and LaSalle Streets. Dr. Harrison came to County once a week, and all the residents wanted do to surgery just like him. But most couldn't, since Dr. Harrison was tall and skinny with long fingers that allowed him to do things in ear surgery that most people didn't have the physical capability to perform. His great surgical ability was exceeded only by his kindness, character, and personality. He was undoubtedly the most popular attending in the program at the time. For all his innovation in surgery, Dr. Shambaugh was well-known among the house staff for his inability to remember any of his residents' names. Dr. George Allen served for several years (1964–1967) during this period as the acting chair at Northwestern. He was an excellent head and neck surgeon and a man of extreme patience. Much like Dr. Freeark in general surgery, he was there to patiently assist on big cases for as long as it took (within reason, of course). Dr. George Sisson, a noted head and neck surgical oncologist, took over as the chief of service in 1968, and this accession, coupled with the retirement of Dr. Stuteville from the chairmanship of the plastic surgery program in 1970, began a paradigm shift in the care of head and neck tumors away from plastic surgery to otolaryngology at County. Besides the chief of service at NU, who generally made appearances for cases of his particular interest, Northwestern maintained a full-time person in ENT assigned to CCH. During the 1950s and 1960s, it was Dr. Armagan and Dr. Jack Kerth, both of whom were widely respected otolaryngologists.

## Jack Kerth

During his long tenure as chief of service at County, Dr. Kerth brought much of the aura of private practice to Ward 23. While on call, the residents were required—even in the middle of the night—to wear a collared shirt and necktie. Kerth occasionally stopped by off-hours to see what was happening, and it was not good to be caught with an open-necked shirt on the ward. It happened to one of our contributors (Dr. Hazenfield) just once, and that was plenty. Dr. Kerth had a very busy facial cosmetic service, but he always found time to do rounds with the residents and help them on these types of procedures, provided the residents were able to recruit the patients. As a matter of fact, it was on the occasions of staffing these cosmetic procedures that he could be found at his comic best. Dr. Hazenfield recalls that, as a resident, he was able to convince a female patient to undergo a rhytidectomy and blepharoplasties.[8] When the patient was presented, Dr. Kerth and the resident retired outside the room door but within earshot, where Kerth commented, "She's so ugly, she should be shot." The patient couldn't help but hear; still, she opted for the procedures, and was ecstatic with the results and effusive in her praise of the surgeons. Most patients felt the same way, especially during the cold winter months when they could be quite easily moved by suggestions to add facelifts and nose jobs to minor improvements and thereby increase the length of their hospital stay.

Dr. Kerth was followed as chief of service by August (aka, Bob) Stemmer, MD, who was very much a documentation buff. He photographed and took motion pictures of all the interesting and sometimes not-so-interesting cases. As a result of this activity, he was able to establish a video library in the divisional office with these and other professionally produced videotapes of procedures for the residents to watch during their rare moments of downtime while on call. In the mid-1970s, a videotape of the X-rated movie *Deep Throat* made it into the library under the label of "Upper Airway Obstruction and Difficult Intubation." There was a bit of an uproar when one of the female ENT residents inadvertently viewed it, believing it to be a serious educational film.

The more scientific side of the residency was not neglected, and many residents remember the weekly meetings with Dr. Paul Szanto, at the time chairman of one of the largest pathology departments in the world. Residents and staff would go over the weekly examination of gross and microscopic specimens from recent surgical cases. Although Dr. Szanto was reportedly from Budapest, Hungary, he insisted he was really Transylvanian, which provided him with a certain mystique well before the *Rocky Horror Picture Show* became famous.

Most of the ENT patients were still quartered on Ward 23, along with patients from plastics and oral surgery. At that time, the plastic surgery group was still doing gender reassignment surgery, and many of the male-to-female transformations were placed in the four-bed rooms with other female patients from the ENT or oral service, depending on the status of their sexual reassignment. One female patient from Winnetka on the ENT service who was recovering from a rhytidectomy and blepharoplasties complained that she couldn't get any sleep because of a sex re-assignment patient who showed off her new anatomy to everyone all night long. With the head specialties combined on one huge ward, there was always a plethora of facial fractures and head and neck tumor patients in various stages of reconstruction wandering around the floor. One of the ENT correspondents recalls trying to get his wife to quit smoking by taking her to the ward to see a post-op patient with a mandibulectomy and radical neck, whom he claimed was a heavy smoker. The truth was the patient wasn't a smoker, but it didn't matter because the wife didn't quit smoking for another five years, anyway.[9]

## Hugh Hazenfield

When Dr. Stemmer left the County in 1975 for private practice in San Francisco, he was succeeded by Dr. Hugh Hazenfield, a product of the Northwestern program. During his tenure, several other attendings worked with him, namely John Gorny, Cheng Wang, Norman Markus, and Francisco Belizario. About this time, otolaryngologic care really became committed to the team approach, which included County residents, Northwestern residents, attending surgeons, nurses, a speech pathologist, and occasional chaplains of differing faiths. Candy Addis, known for blazing red hair, was the primary speech pathologist. The team made weekly rounds face-to-face with all the patients. These were enlightening sessions for all involved, even the patients. It is an experience that some feel must be guarded from possible extinction at the hands of the electronic medical record. Just like there was a team on the ward, most of the surgical specialties were privileged to have a dedicated team in the operating room. Audrey Avant (scrub tech) and Juanita Witalka (circulating nurse) ran the Otolaryngology operating theater. They had done it for so long that many times, if the attending had to leave the OR for any reason, these two were able to guide a resident through even intricate head and neck tumor cases. Many times, a resident would be overheard asking Mrs. Avant for a specific instrument, only to be handed a different one, while she intoned, "I know this is not what you asked for, but it's what you need." While the rule of "see one, do one, teach one" was not uniformly applied, it was pretty close, and sometimes even if you hadn't seen one, you'd have to make up how to do the procedure. However, it seemed that in a real pinch, there was always a more-senior resident, attending, or night surgeon available with advice on how to handle the situation.

In mid 1979, Dr. Hazenfield left CCH for a practice opportunity, first at Chicago's Michael Reese Hospital and later in Hawaii. He was replaced at County as chief of service by Dr. Bill Powell, in whose lab at the University of Chicago Dr. Hazenfield had worked as a resident. Shortly after Dr. Powell became chairman of the County Hospital division of otolaryngology/head and neck surgery, the clinic and operative numbers substantially increased due to a University of Illinois ENT residency rotation facilitated by the new head of the County Department of Surgery, Dr. Olga Jonasson. This resident complement was in addition to the longstanding ENT resident rotation from Northwestern.

Dr. Powell believed the healthy competition between the services was fruitful for both residency programs as well as the County service.[10] During the 20-year tenure of Bill Powell, the following attending staff made significant contributions to the teaching and patient care activities: Arthur Curtis, Robert Berktold, Nick Lygizos, Vito Grabauskas, John Danielson, and Stuart Morgenstein. In 1998, the Cook County ENT service was listed in the top 50 programs nationwide by *US News and World Report*. Bill Powell retired at the close of 1998. In 1999, Dr. Robert Kern from the Northwestern ENT program, was appointed as chair of the County program. He was accompanied by his Northwestern colleague David Conley and joined as well in 2003 by Dr. Urgeet Patel, who assumed a full-time position after completion of fellowships in head and neck surgery and microsurgical techniques. By June of 2006, Dr. Kern was appointed chief of ENT at Northwestern, and Dr. Patel became the chair of the County department. Both of the residency programs continued to flourish with a population of 1,200 to 1,400 clinic patients annually and 700-800 operative cases per year. Attending full-time surgeons are David Conley and Sarah McDonald, as well as Dr. Patel, with additional staff members Robert Berktold, Nick Lygizos, and Alan Micco.

## Acknowledglments

The editors would like to acknowledge the assistance of Drs. Hugh Hazenfield, Joseph O'Grady, Charles Weingarten, and Ms. Louise Rzeszewski, RN, in providing some of the more intimate details of the otolaryngology program, especially as it existed from the 1950s forward.

## References

1. Quinne W E. Early History of the Cook County Hospital to 1870. In: Quinne W E. History of Medicine and Surgery and Physicians and Surgeons of Chicago. (endorsed by the Council of the Chicago Medical Society), Chicago: The Biographical Publishing Corporation; 1922.
2. Friedberg SE. The Memorable Life of Hosmer A. Johnson, Early Midwestern Laryngologist. Ann. Otol. Rhinol Laryngol. 1983;93:470-472
3. Friedberg SE. History of Laryngology in Early Chicago and Rush Medical College. Ann Otol. 1979;88;136-141.
4. Raffensperger JG. The Old Lady on Harrison Street. New York: Peter Lang Publishing; 1977:174.
5. Ibid.
6. Raffensperger, John G. " The Old Lady on Harrison Street." Peter Lang Publishing, New York,1977, p 174.
7. Hipskind M. Reminiscences of Otorhinolaryngology from Loyola University and Hines Veterans Hospital. Proc Inst Med Chgo. 1982;35:51-52.
8. Dr. Hugh Hazenfield, MD, Personal Communication.
9. Dr. Joseph O'Grady, MD, Personal Communication.

# 22

# Oral and Maxillofacial Surgery

*John M. Sisto, MD*
*James L. Stone, MD*

Although a general dental clinic was established at Cook County Hospital in 1906 under T.H. Conley, the beginning of oral surgery services came in 1927 when the Cook County Board of Commissioners opened the Children's Dental Clinic to serve the indigent children of Chicago under the age of 16. Working with the Cook County Department of Public Health, this clinic performed diagnoses, preventive dentistry, extraction, dental X-rays, and operative dentistry (oral surgery). Referral of difficult children came from the Board of Health Clinics, Board of Education, Audy Home, County Jail, and parochial schools. Concurrently and by necessity, adult dentistry services at CCH were expanded as well. Following World War II until the early 1970s, the CCH general dentistry staff also provided ancillary forensic dentistry services for the Cook County coroner, the FBI, and Sheriff's Police in the dental identification of missing and deceased persons.

By 1933, an oral surgery section was in place at CCH staffed by attending members William H. Logan and Joseph E. Schaefer, both with dental and medical degrees. Residents were accepted for training who had completed at least one year of previous postgraduate oral surgery in an approved, usually Chicago-area, dental school. In the 1940s and 1950s, the oral surgery residency lasted 16 months to include rotations in anesthesia, the outpatient clinic, and junior and senior rotations in major dental surgery. Approximately 400 patients a year were admitted to the oral surgery service, and the clinic had 15,000 visits a year.

From 1959 through 1966, Orion H. Stuteville headed the CCH oral, plastic, and ENT services, although the designated chair rotated among Kenneth Lewis, Stewart Landa, and Joseph Kostrubala, all of whom had dental and medical degrees. In particular, Orion Stuteville (1902–1994) had a most remarkable career and became a legend in the Chicago area and at CCH. Born in a covered wagon in Oklahoma, he became an American collegiate wrestling champion and a member of the 1924 Olympic team. As a wrestling coach at Northwestern, he was attracted to anatomy and physiology courses, and graduated from its Dental School in 1931. After several years of dental and orthodontic practice in Evanston, Illinois, he obtained an MD degree from Northwestern (1939) and interned at St. Joseph Hospital in Chicago. He next served in the Army during World War II (1942–1946) and attained the rank of major. From 1933 until 1979, he was on the faculty of Northwestern Dental School and served as chairman from 1952 to 1970. He was also professor of plastic surgery at Northwstern (1950–1979) and directed that residency program for 17 years. Similar positions were held at Loyola Medical School (1946–1950 and 1970–1975). "Stutie," as he was affectionately known, taught about 40 hours a week for most of his professional life. He steadfastly refused to accept any salary for teaching. For many years, he additionally devoted his Sunday mornings to teaching oral surgery and plastic surgery residents at CCH until his surgical retirement from that institution in 1975. However, he delivered a final lecture to the CCH oral surgeons during 1985. Stuteville's steady, sound, practical, and dominant influence on multiple generations of Chicago area oral, maxillofacial, plastic, and reconstructive surgeons was profound. The Stuteville Surgical Society was formed in 1968 by his former residents, and in 1984, he received Northwestern University's highest honor, the Alumni Medal.

In March of 1966, the oral and maxillofacial surgery (OMFS) division was finally formed within the Department of Surgery at CCH with Walter Dalitsch acting chair until Daniel M. Laskin became chairman (1967–1972), the first nonplastic surgeon to head OMFS at CCH. Under Dan Laskin in 1968, the training program first obtained formal certification. Felix R. Lawrence followed as chairman (1972–1984), and upgraded and consolidated the dental services into OMFS (three-year postgraduate resident program), and adult and pediatric general dentistry (one-year postgraduate resident program). The OMFS service is most supportive in regularly rotating first-year residents through many of the CCH surgical and nonsurgical patient care areas.

In 1985, John M. Sisto, a product of the CCH program, was appointed chair and provided steady leadership until his recent retirement in January 2011. Salvatore Termini presently directs the OMFS service and is ably assisted by Henry Fung, James Babiuk, and George Panos. Currently, more than 400 major surgeries are performed yearly, and the service sees greater than 15,000 outpatients a year. The County Hospital Alumni Oral Surgeons (CHAOS) continues to meet yearly in Chicago to socialize and share fond memories.

# 23

# Ophthalmological Surgery

*Philip Dray, MD*
*Alexander Constantaras, MD*

- *The Beginning and Dr. Ted Zekman*
- *The Era of Marcel Frankel*
- *The Era of Alex Constantaras*
- *The Era of Alan Axelrod*
- *Days of Philip Dray and the New CCH*

## The Beginning and Dr. Ted Zekman

The division of ophthalmology functioned as a consult service and eye surgery service for over seven decades. All of the division's functions (surgery, inpatient, and outpatient) were initially located in the old hospital at 1835 W. Harrison. Eventually, outpatient functions were moved to the then "new" Fantus Clinic in the 1950s. The earliest living memory of the division of ophthalmology recalls it as a service primarily supervised by voluntary part-time private practitioners without full-time faculty. While there were residents in training, most of their day-to-day direct supervision—surgical and medical—was performed by a more-senior resident.

The late Ted Zekman was the chairman of ophthalmology beginning in the 1940s until he stepped down in 1968. Zekman was a beloved chairman with his own busy private practice, as was the norm for most staff in all areas at County. Zekman appointed residents, attended staff meetings, and participated in hospital affairs. Teaching during the Zekman era came primarily from the voluntary attendings.

## The Era of Marcel Frankel

In 1968, Marcel Frankel became the first-full time salaried chairman of the ophthalmology division. Frankel, a neuro-ophthalmologist at the University of Chicago, was the only salaried physician. Volunteers during the 1960s included Ted Shapira, Graham Dobbie, Chester Black, Martin Urist, Eugene Folk, Paul Steinberg, Paul Sarnat, Maurice Rabb, Sam Pollack, Gholam Peyman, Alan Putterman, and Lee Trachtenberg. Ward 24 functioned as the inpatient unit, and the outpatient service was on the second floor of the Fantus Clinic. Inpatient surgery was performed on the Ward, often two operations at the same time in the same room. In the early 1970s, the inpatient ward was moved to a remodeled and modern, four-unit west, and inpatient surgery moved to the main OR on the eighth floor. As one of his first administrative actions, Frankel selected Alex Constantaras (a future chairman) as his first resident. Alex joined the training program on January 1, 1969, after returning from Vietnam. In the 1960s and 1970s the three-year training program consisted of the experience at County combined with four-month rotations to Oak Forest Hospital and St. Joseph's Hospital for clinic and surgical experience. The retina training was provided by Howard Wilder and Charley Vygantas at St. Joe. Additionally, a multiple-week basic science course had to be taken in Maine, Philadelphia, or New York. Some elective rotations were individually arranged at Northwestern or the University of Illinois. Constantaras completed his residency in December of 1972 and was offered a salaried position to stay on with Frankel at County. Constantaras opted for a half-time position so as to develop his own private practice.

## The Era of Alex Constantaras

In the winter of 1972, Frankel left for his private practice and work at the University of Chicago. The then-chairman of surgery, Jerry Moss, offered the chairmanship to Constantaras, and he stayed as chair until 1979. Formalizing the education and training with paid faculty began under his leadership with the creation of four half-time salaried positions. These were filled by Bill Kearns, Dimitri Perros, Gary Morris, and Miltos Moschandrew.

## The Era of Alan Axelrod

Alan Axelrod, a cornea and external disease specialist, became chairman in 1979 and ushered in an era of intense faculty supervision, subspecialty support, didactics, and standardized surgical training. The Oak Forest rotation was discontinued because of lack of faculty supervision. The St. Joseph rotation was strengthened with the participation of George Wyhinny and Gary Morris. The beginnings of a regular "in-house" didactic program was developed, and residents no longer took time off to go to the multiple-week didactic course. Subspecialists were added to the training program and participated for varying periods of time. Included in this program were:

Donna Johnson in strabismus;
Neal Lucchese in pediatrics;
Motilal Raichand, Tim Green, Jill Johnson, Carla Territo, John Gieser,
  Susan-Anderson Nelson, and Richard Ahuja in retina;
Linda Lippa and Joan Whelchel in ophthalmic pathology;
Mark Baskin and Dan Ritacca in plastics;
Mildred Olivier in glaucoma;
Andy Berman and Jeff Nichols in neuro-ophthalmology;
Norbert Becker in uveitis;
Gary Rubin in general; and
Dave Greenberg in cataract.

The ophthalmology OR was moved to the eighth floor of the pediatrics building with a dedicated room five days a week. Axelrod oversaw the transition of cataract surgery from large wound intracapsular technique without intraocular lenses to extracapsular procedures with intraocular lenses, and finally to phacoemulsification small-wound surgery. Early on, patients were still admitted regularly to four-unit West for a four- or five-day stay in the hospital for routine cataract surgery. But with ophthalmic surgical procedures evolving to nearly strictly outpatient, Axelrod oversaw the closure of the dedicated ophthalmology ward of four-unit West and the return to a shared area in the large open ward area of Ward 30. The outpatient clinic received its first argon laser, Neodymium YAG laser, and diode laser. In the first group of residents selected to join the training program Axelrod selected Philip Dray (a future chairman). After finishing the program in 1984, Dray joined the faculty part-time. In 1988, Dray became full-time, and in 1997 Axelrod appointed Dray as the program director overseeing the training program of nine residents. The St. Joseph Hospital rotation was discontinued because of diminishing volume, and the residents returned to Oak Forest Hospital with full-time faculty supervision.

## Days of Philip Dray and the New CCH

Axelrod retired in 2002, and Philip Dray was appointed acting chair and then chairman in 2004. Dray oversaw the addition of new subspecialists: Lisa Thompson in pediatrics, Tom Patrianakos in glaucoma, Surendar Dwarakanathan in cornea plastics, and the return of Dan Ritacca in plastics. The new hospital was opened in 2001, and the eye clinic moved to a new outpatient facility within the new hospital in 2002. Dray oversaw the move to the new facility with the addition of digital photography, ocular coherence tomography, nerve fiber layer analysis, and ultrasound to the diagnostic area of the clinic. Dray appointed Rick Ahuja as program director in 2004 and oversaw the expansion of the didactic program to lectures on average of four days a week, grand rounds, journal club, and a division of ophthalmology-sponsored board review course. The program has received a five-year accreditation from the Accreditation Council for Graduate Medical Education (ACGME), and the current board pass rate is 100 percent for the past five years. All subspecialty services in ophthalmology are provided, and currently the ophthalmology service has 10 attendings (four full time, nine residents, three technicians) and sees over 33,000 patients a year, providing more than 800 major surgical procedures, 2,000 laser procedures, and 500 minor procedures each year. The program selects the brightest residents from the best medical schools around the country and offers medical-student ophthalmology experience to the six local schools as well as other medical schools throughout the United States.

The ophthalmology program is proud to have given society scores of ophthalmologists in the past 70 years. The service that County provides to patients is unmatched anywhere, and the training that is given to our select group of residents is unique and sought-after by top students from top medical schools. The division of ophthalmology has become a powerhouse of training and excellence known for turning out hard-working, capable residents who perform outstanding work and contribute to society.

# 24

# Colon and Rectal Surgery

*Herand Abcarian, MD, FACS*

- *Introduction*
- *The Beginning—Drs. Theodore (Ted) Lescher and Durand Smith*
- *The Procto Room*
- *Colon and Rectal Surgery Training Program*
- *The Abcarian Era*
- *Flexible Colonoscopy and Surgical Stapling*
- *Expansion of the Colon and Rectal Surgery Program*

## Introduction

I began my internship at Cook County Hospital in July 1966. At that time, Colon and Rectal Surgery (CRS) as a specialty and service did not exist at County. Many then, as today, were not aware that colon and rectal surgery is a primary independent board within the American Board of Medical Specialties, established as such about a decade prior to the American Board of Surgery.

At that time, all colorectal surgical cases were admitted and treated on the general surgical services. However, there was not much enthusiasm and interest among the many volunteer attendings in surgery for colorectal, and especially anorectal, cases. The attendings interested in teaching residents and interns how to perform hemorrhoidectomy or fistulotomy were few and far between, and the knowledge of the anorectal anatomy and technical expertise were woefully inadequate. The large volume of anorectal abscess fistulas and gangrenous hemorrhoids requiring urgent surgery were relegated to nights as the regular operating room day schedules were too full to accommodate these cases. Needless to say, all emergencies operated on at night were supervised only by the chief residents who helped get the anorectal emergencies done and out of the way. This way, the patient could be discharged expeditiously, because in the 1960s, the inpatient census of each of the six surgical services averaged 60-65 patients.

In 1968, concern for mixing infected "dirty" cases with clean pre- and postoperative patients resulted in housing all common infected cases admitted on an urgent or emergency basis on a second floor unit on the Harrison Street side of the hospital called 2 Unit East (2UE). The patients were predominantly composed of anorectal abscesses including Fournier's gangrene, breast abscesses, and diabetic wet gangrene of the lower extremities. This unit was affectionately called "the sewer." No single service was charged with running the area, and each of the six surgical services cared for their share of admissions.

## The Beginning—Drs. Theodore (Ted) Lescher and Durand Smith

Organization of CRS at County under a special service must be credited to the work of two volunteer attendings. Theodore ( Ted ) Lescher, MD, a colorectal surgeon trained at Mayo Clinic, had returned to his hometown of Chicago in 1967 and joined Durand Smith, MD (Figure 24–1), a prominent colorectal surgeon practicing at the Wesley Pavilion of Northwestern University. He was approached by the chief of surgery at County, Robert J. Freeark, MD, who knew Ted from Northwestern and asked if he would like to organize a CRS unit with the hopes of starting a residency program. Ted asked Freeark if he could get Dr. Smith involved because of his senior status at the American Society of Colon and Rectal Surgeons, and Freeark agreed.

## The Procto Room

Dr. Freeark assigned 24 beds on 4 Unit East to allow consolidation of anorectal cases scattered throughout the six general surgical services, plus all rectal cancers. An unused storage space next to 4 UE was converted to the "Procto Room" where proctosigmodioscopies for all surgical services were done on a daily basis. Colorectal surgery was assigned two clinic sessions on Monday and Thursday mornings at the Fantus Clinic. Soon afterward, the clinics were overflowing with 35-40 patients in each session.

## Colon and Rectal Surgery Training Program

In order to apply to the residency review committee (RRC) for colon and rectal surgery for an approved colorectal surgery residency, patient data needed to be collected for a 12-month period. Dr. Lescher undertook this task and collected

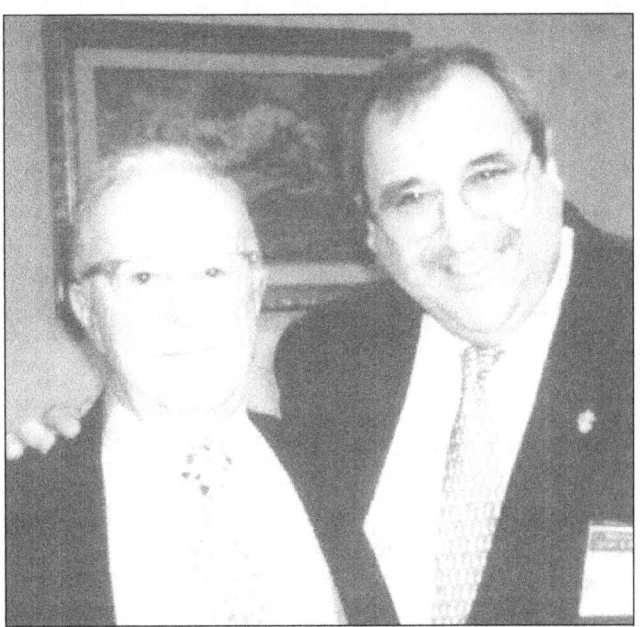

*Figure 24–1 Durand Smith (left) with Herand Abcarian*

the data from July 1, 1968 to June 30, 1969. In addition to Drs. Smith and Lescher, there were three other volunteer attendings on the CRS teaching service: Drs. Clyde Phillips, Francis Banish, and Joseph Cannon. All of these men had busy private practices with a slant toward colon and rectal surgery. No longer were the anorectal procedures relegated to night surgery. They were scheduled and performed under the supervision of the five volunteer attendings during normal operating room hours.

After submitting the performance data to the RRC, Dr. Smith invited Patrick Hanley, MD, the chair of CRS at Oschner Clinic in New Orleans and the secretary of the American Board of Colon and Rectal Surgery, for a site visit to inspect the fledgling CRS program. The RRC of CRS and ABCRS approved the Cook County Hospital colon and rectal surgery residency program in 1970, in time for the first resident, John F. Bartizal Jr., to start his residency on July 1, 1970. I followed John as the second resident trained by this young residency program and completed my training on June 30, 1972.

Because of the impending departure of Dr. Lescher for Ft. Lauderdale in 1971, Dr. Smith was named as the program director of our residency at its inception. I was asked by the chief of surgery, Dr. Frank Folk, to stay on as an attending in general surgery as well as colon and rectal surgery beginning July 1, 1972. I was thrilled, especially when Dr. Smith asked me to help him in his private office during his frequent visits to Sun City, Arizona, where he was in the process of building a retirement home.

## The Abcarian Era

By September 1972, when I sat for my CRS board exams in New Orleans, Dr. Folk had left for Loyola University, and County had a new chief of surgery, Dr. Gerald S. Moss. The board examination results were due in six weeks, but two weeks after the examination, I was called to a meeting with Drs. Moss and Smith. They asked me if I would consider running the CRS program at County as section chief and program director. Dr. Smith then informed me that he had called the ABCRS office and found out that I had indeed passed my boards in CRS (a requirement for the program director). He also informed me that he was leaving for Arizona the following week and wanted me to take over his private practice as well as the CRS program at County. Thus began my 23-year tenure as the program director of the CRS residency and section chief of colon and rectal surgery at County (Figure 24–2).

## Flexible Colonoscopy and Intestinal Stapling

The 1970s was the beginning of a meteoric rise in the field of colon and rectal surgery, fueled by the introduction of flexible colonoscopy followed by intestinal stapling devices. County purchased one of the earliest Olympus Colonoscopes sold in the United States, and Dr. Smith and I went to watch and learn from Dr. Eddy in Long Island, New York, in April 1972 while I was still a resident. Colonoscopy became a routine procedure, and the Procto room at County was expanded to accommodate flexible endoscopy of the upper and lower gastrointestinal tract in a new surgical endoscopy unit. Colonoscopies were done by the colon and rectal surgery service and EGDs by the general surgery attendings. Surgical stapling, especially the circular anastamotic staplers, heralded a new era in restoring gastrointestinal continuity and revolutionized techniques for both low and ultra low colorectal anastomosis.

During the first five years of the fellowship program, one resident was trained each year. However, with the increase in the volume of patients, as well as the expansion of the curriculum in colorectal surgery including sphincter-sparing surgery for ulcerative colitis and low rectal cancers, an application to the RRC resulted in approval for the CRS residency to train two residents each year. The CRS service was also relocated to Ward 43, which had a capacity of 35 beds.

In 1988, when I was appointed as the interim head of the Department of Surgery at the University of Illinois by Dean Gerald S. Moss, the CRS residency was expanded to include UIC Medical Center, and CRS became a bona fide division within the Department of Surgery

## Expansion of the Colon and Rectal Surgery Program

In the late 1990s, the CRS residency expanded to Advocate Lutheran General Hospital (LGH) where CR residents are trained under the watchful eyes of Drs. M. Lela Prasad, John Park, and Slavi Maricek. The training program is considered one of the premier colorectal residencies in the United States, and currently three residents are trained yearly, spending four months in each of the three sites (County, UIC, and LGH).

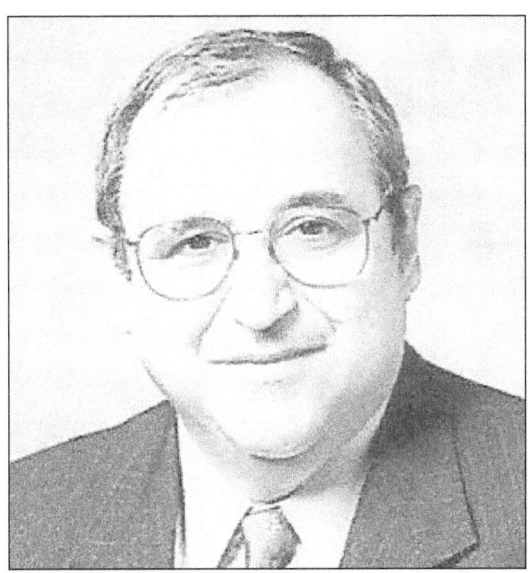

*Figure 24–2* **Herand Abcarian**

# Section V

*Remembrances*

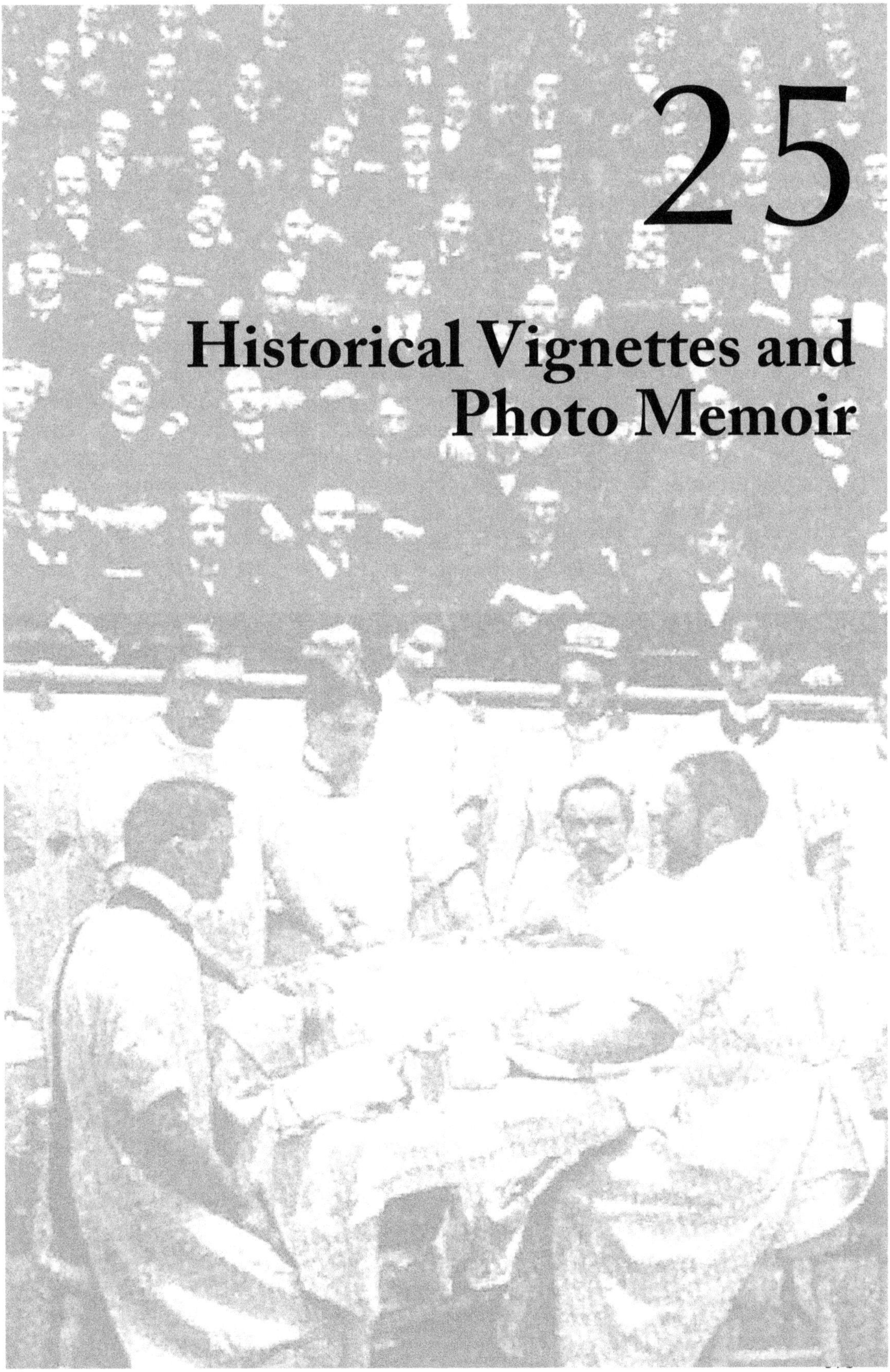

# 25

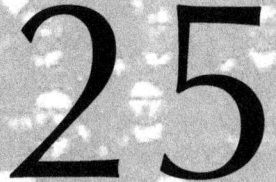

# Historical Vignettes and Photo Memoir

HISTORICAL VIGNETTES AND PHOTO MEMOIR

*Section V*
- *Introduction*
- *Karl Meyer, the Man and the Legend*
- *Other Notable Stars*
- *Only at the County*
- *See One, Do One, Teach One*
- *Quotable Quotes*
- *The Human Side of Being a Surgical Resident*

The editors would like to take this opportunity to thank all those individuals who took the time to share some of their favorite remembrances of County with the rest of us. The amazing thing to us was that once people found out what we were doing, we received stories not only from surgical alumni, but from nurses, wives, and people who had rotated through County as students, interns, or affiliated residents. We made every effort to corroborate the stories by calling contemporaries of the writers, so we are reasonably certain that all the tales are true. Even in the cases where we might have thought the story to be apocryphal, we all agreed that given the individual and the circumstances as presented, the story stood a good chance of being authentic.

For continuity and ease of reading, these 169 vignettes are divided into six categories. We hope you will enjoy reading them as much as we enjoyed putting them together. Happy memories.

*—The Editors*

## Karl Meyer, The Man and the Legend

Dr. Meyer was operating on a young woman who had previously been operated on elsewhere and had persistent drainage and evidence of bowel obstruction. We were operating in one of the smaller operating rooms, and in the gallery were three men in shirt sleeves observing what was going on. When the patient was draped, Dr. Meyer said in a whisper, "I think we are going to find a sponge in here. Under no circumstances are you to talk or show any emotional changes. Those fellows are 'West Side Boys.' A slip of the tongue could be disastrous." Dr. Meyer very quickly found the sponge, said nothing, and began putting in laps, taking them out, sponging, and discarding sponges. Then in the confusion of the sponge count, he removed all the sponges and laps, picked up a reddened ileum, and said to the men, "Here are some adhesions, which we have broken up. She should do well." He proceeded to suture her up with the calmness of a father at a Christmas dinner.
*—Carlo Scuderi, MD, Cook County Hospital Intern's and Resident's Alumni Association Newsletter, July 1980*

He (Dr. Meyer) was fond of telling the story of the night he was walking from the old University Hospital to the County Hospital when he was held up at gunpoint by two thugs who took his wallet and money. One of them, who was looking through the wallet for more money, suddenly exclaimed, "Hey, Joe, its Dr. Karl Meyer." They returned the wallet and money, apologized, and fled.
—Sam Hyman, MD, Cook County Hospital Intern's and Resident's Alumni Association Newsletter, July 1980

Dr. Meyer and Dr. McNealy were the usual stars of the Saturday operative clinics generally put on for the benefit of the County postgraduate school. The Friday before, the chief surgical resident would go to the warden's area on the second floor with his assistants to present the case to the chief. One Friday in 1951, Bill Hobbins started the presentation on Saturdays patient by saying, "This man is rather old. He's 70." Dr. Meyer broke in brusquely, "I'm 65!!" We were all more sensitive about age evaluations after that.
—Frank Folk, MD, Private Communication

The Saturday afternoon gastrectomy was generally scouted out by the chief resident after it had been located by one of the juniors. Dr. Milloy remembers that the chief preferred gastric ulcers for the clinic since they were usually large and impressive to palpate when the fresh specimen was passed around the members of the audience. They were also easy to describe to the audience once the abdomen was opened. Dr. Philip Sheridan remembers one occasion when Dr. Tom Sheridan was the first assistant. Dr. Meyer made the incision and reached inside while speaking about peptic ulcer disease. Unfortunately, there was no gastric ulcer to be palpated. Totally nonplused, the chief lapsed into a discussion of the value of palpating the whole abdomen during a laparotomy. As luck would have it, a cecal mass was discovered, and the lecture changed gears to a discussion of the treatment of undiagnosed colon masses, much to the relief of the house staff who had selected the patient.
—Frank Milloy, MD, and Philip Sheridan Sr., MD, Private Communication

Dr. Meyer's aversion to smoking was legendary. According to Dr. John Howser, however, an early resident who admitted to swallowing a lighted cigarette when Dr. Meyer stepped into an elevator with him, Meyer did not have the same aversion to the house staff having overnight visitors. The 11 p.m. full dinner in the interns' dining room (the third floor area in the main building, which later became the trauma unit) used to look like a coeducational college dining room. After all, who ever heard of one getting cancer of the lung from being over-hospitable?
—John Howser, MD, Cook County Hospital Intern's and Resident's Alumni Association Newsletter, July 1980

When the interns' quarters were on the third floor of the hospital, there were occasional female guests who were spirited in despite the published prohibition against such activity. One night, Dr. Meyer was doing a walk-through, opened a door, and came across a couple in one of the beds. One of the partners was smoking a cigarette. Meyer stood at the doorway and said, "You get rid of those cigarettes right now!" He then turned on his heel and walked away.
—David Berger, MD, Personal Communication

During his time as the chief of surgery, Dr. Meyer was personally involved in resident discipline. Dr. Louis Boshes, who became one of the greats in Chicago neurology, recalled, "Your attending calls you on Thursday for cases for his Friday surgery class in the eighth floor east amphitheatre. 'I want one gastric resection, one third-degree burn, one carcinoma of the transverse colon, and a thyroid or two for my Friday afternoon class.' 'Yes, Sir,' you vow. What does he get? This all depends on the morbidity and mortality figures on your ward. Maybe you give him an abscess of the knee or an uninvolved appendix. What do you get? A trip down to Dr. Meyer's office. What do you say? 'Dr. Meyer, have you seen our morbidity and mortality records?' Answer: 'I will.' You are not called back."
—Louis Boshes, MD, Cook County Hospital Intern's and Resident's Alumni Association Newsletter, December, 1980

One resident remembers that on his return from military service, Dr. Meyer was most gracious and allowed him to resume his residency immediately. His first service as a resident and his last as an intern had been neurosurgery. After two weeks, the neurosurgery resident (there was only one) quit. The surgery resident was immediately in charge, with "burr hole" privileges and 24/7 on call for the remainder of the first three months of his residency. Aware that residents on some services with only one assigned resident were allowed to share call with another service, he decided to ask Dr. Meyer if this was a possibility. He told Dr. Meyer his situation, and without looking up from his desk, the chief responded, " We don't have any GD crybabies here. Get out!" The resident dutifully took his call.
—Marvin Tiesenga, MD, Personnel Communication

Another ex-resident remembers a less volatile Dr. Meyer. "After spending seven years at Cook County Hospital, my last day came, and I thought I would stop and say goodbye to Dr. Karl Meyer. The conversation went like this: 'Dr. Meyer, this is my last day, and I wanted to stop by and say good-bye.' Dr. Meyer asked 'Where are you going?' I said 'To Dubuque, Iowa.' Meyer said, 'I think we have a man there.' He reached into a desk drawer and pulled out the intern alumni directory. 'Yes, there's a man out there by the name of Ott.' I said 'That's me and good-bye.'"
So much for personal attention, interest, and encouragement.
—Roger A. Ott Sr., MD, Personal Communication

In Democratic Party circles Dr. Meyer was highly regarded. At one time he was even considered as a candidate for governor, which he declined. But he did have enough power to have a special signal put up along the main train line through his hometown in downstate Gilman, where he maintained a farm. Dr. Meyer had a key to the signal, so whenever he wanted to come back to Chicago by train, he simply threw the signal, stopped the crack Mid-Continental Express train, and rode comfortably back to Chicago. Never has it come to my knowledge before or since that a civilian not in the railroad business had that power.
—Carlo Scuderi, MD, Cook County Hospital Intern's and Resident's Alumni Association Newsletter, July, 1980

While many of the residents remembered the farm as a place where special outings took place, one of the house staff from the early 1960s had a more personal view of the farm. "Dr. Meyer's farm had a sizable number of dairy cattle, and during WWII, he was interested in obtaining automatic milking machines for them. He went to my parents' hardware store/implement dealership in Chebanse to check on this equipment. My mother, who was tending the shop at the time, explained that the machines were available for purchase but there would be a nine-month wait for the delivery. At this point, Dr. Meyer asked if he could talk to my father. When dad was located, Dr. Meyer repeated his request for the milking machines. to which my father replied, 'What did Mame (my mother) say?' 'She said there would be a nine-month wait for delivery,' came the reply. 'Well, if that's what she said then that's what it is,' my father responded. Dr. Meyer asked, 'Do you know who I am?' My father replied, 'Yes, I do, but the wait will still be nine months.' And so it was, but from that point on, my father did all the plumbing and electrical work, as well as a good amount of farm equipment sales for Dr. Meyer's farm. Additionally, I believe that I am the only former County intern to have been consistently kicked out of Dr. Meyer's farm pond by the man himself for unauthorized swimming."
—Raymond Dieter, MD, Personal Communication

I arrived at the County Hospital in the mid-1950s fresh out of my residency in surgery at Harvard, and as the only salaried member of the Loyola University Surgery Department was given privileges at Mercy Hospital and also assigned to County as associate for Dr. John Keeley, the chief of surgery at the medical school and attending surgeon on Ward 46. My wife and I were in the process of transforming our house into a home with our own decorative impressions when someone suggested that we look at the modestly priced art at the Hanzel Galleries on Michigan Avenue. We did so, and we found some nice pieces to our liking both visually and financially. One day, while browsing at the gallery, I found it set up for an auction of the high-end art, which the gallery also sold. The first row of seats was clearly marked as reserved; when I asked for whom, the reply was, "Why, for Dr. Karl Meyer, of course." I had met Dr. Meyer on several occasions but really never knew him well at all during my 14 years in Chicago. However, just knowing that he was held in such esteem in the art world, at least locally, added a new dimension to the man I knew as a leading surgeon and medical administrator in Chicago.

—Harold B. Haley, MD, Personal Communication

The Meyer-McNealy Service was most sought after by the interns. Dr. Meyer was the better surgeon, but Dr. McNealy was the better teacher. He had the carriage and dignity of General Douglas MacArthur and the dashing good looks of the French movie star Maurice Chevalier.

—John Raffensperger, MD, *The Old Lady on Harrison Street*, 1997, p. 99

One night, I admitted a young man who had just returned from Mexico. I thought his abdominal pain was from something he had eaten. Dr. Meyer and I took him to surgery the next morning, and as a diseased appendix popped out of the incision, Meyer said, "Doesn't look like Mexican food to me."

—James Kennedy, MD, Personal Communication

A few months after I finished at County and was establishing a practice in the south suburbs, I was called to see a lady with an acute bowel obstruction. Examination revealed an incarcerated femoral hernia, and I advised the family and the referring physician. It happened that the patient's son was a Cook County Commissioner, and he proceeded to call Dr. Karl Meyer for a second opinion. Dr. Meyer came out, examined the patient, and confirmed my diagnosis. In fact, he stated that, "Dr. Duke can do this procedure as well as I can," or words to that effect. While the OR was being set up, I escorted Dr. Meyer to his car. On the way he said, "I know you'll do a good job. By the way, charge them a nice fee. These politicians always expect me to work for nothing." You can imagine the boost this episode was for my fledgling practice.

—Sidney Duke, MD, Personal Communication

Dr. Meyer was innovative in his use of sulfa and other antibiotics in contaminated wounds. I remember the day he was doing an appendectomy and asked the scrub nurse for sulphur crysrals. She said the OR didn't have any. He told her to get some, and she replied, "Doctor, they don't make them any more." Dr. Meyer was visibly disappointed with medical progress at this time.

—James Kennedy, MD, Personal Communication

When I got near the end of my two-year internship, I stood in line on a Friday afternoon to see Dr. Meyer in his office. I had been on service for three months, had assisted him at a number of operations, and hoped he would remember me, but I knew he was bad with names. I introduced myself and said I would like a surgical residency. He said, "We're filled up for July, but fill out an application

tomorrow and don't forget to leave a picture." I said, "Thank you" and left after 30 seconds. This was my job interview for how I was going to spend the next four years of my life.
—Frank Milloy, MD, Personal Communication

Not all the personal remembrances of Dr. Meyer are so gruff. Several alumni remember summertime picnics at the Meyer farm near Gilman, Illinois (between Chicago and Champaign, now just off I-57). There, we'd spend an afternoon of food and festivities around KAM Lake, enjoy a viewing of some of the horse barns and their occupants, all capped off by mint juleps in authentic silver mint julep cups.
—Frank Folk, MD, and Frank Banich, MD, Personal Communications

In the early days of the 20th century, certainly before the Second World War, communication means were limited, and many times, groups of surgeons from the same state or ones who had come to know each other well from the American College of Surgeons or the American Surgical Association, would tour the country by train, stopping in various cities to watch noted surgeons perform newly described operations or to listen to lectures about new discoveries in physiology, biochemistry, or other basic science applications to clinical medicine. Dr. Meyer's frequent companions were George Crile, the Mayo brothers, Frank Lahey, and Alton Ochsner.
—James Kennedy, MD, Personal Communication

Dr. Meyer had many friends in Chicago who were powerful in the social and political system. He was a good friend of Virginia Marmaduke, a newspaper woman, who was influential in Chicago politics. His early connections were with the political powers of the Old First Ward John "Hinky Dink" Kenna, "Bathhouse" John Coughlin, and the Eberly sisters. It was rumored that he advanced so far politically as to be considered a potential candidate for governor. While he was considering the move, his rival in the top strata of surgeons, both as an operator and teacher, Dr. Raymond McNealy, counseled him, "Karl, you are a surgeon. Tell them to go to hell," which he did, I am sure, with tremendous grace and political finesse.
—Carlo Scuderi, MD, Cook County Hospital Intern's and Resident's Alumni Association Newsletter, July, 1980

## Other Notable Stars

Foster McMillan was a fine surgeon and teacher from the 1940s through the 1960s, who looked the part. He carried his private-practice attitude to Cook County. It is said that once in his private practice on the near North side, a well-to-do patient asked what he could do for the doctor. The patient was told, "Uhm, a car, a Cadillac."

—*Frank Folk, MD, Personal Correspondence*


At the beginning of the 1960s, the need for a full-time MD chairman of the Anesthesia Department was recognized and acted upon. Dr. Vincent Collins was recruited from Belleview in New York City, and another County legend was born. A long-time attending vividly remembers his first encounter with Dr. Collins. "I was a rotating UIC resident trying to enter the operating room from a stairwell leading up from the seventh floor. Little did I realize that I was stumbling head-long into a rite of passage at the County Hospital operating rooms. Dr. Collins' face was calm as I started through the door; however, there was a sudden change in appearance from a calm and sober demeanor to howling rage and clenched-tooth anger. He had looked at my feet and didn't like what he saw. Collins bellowed, 'Get the hell out of here until you get white shoes.' My laughing fellow residents had purposely not mentioned Dr. Collins' interest in white shoes so that I could learn first-hand about their importance. Needless to say, I made a quick exit and obtained white shoes. They would eventually become crusted with blood, body fluids, and other unrecognizable debris from the OR. Most residents wore them in and out of the OR until they fell apart."

—*Philip Donahue, MD, Personal Communication*


Dr. Collins entered a world that had been dominated by excellent nurse anesthetists, including Gloria Blado and Rosie Hamberger, to name just two. His success in building an excellent MD anesthesia service and residency while integrating the NAs and their long-standing training program speak volumes about his organizational capability and dedication. However, there were many instances when he came away with the short straw when dealing with the surgical residents. One morning, at the end of his shift as night surgeon, Bill Dippel, likely one of the best natural surgeons to ever have been trained at County, was scrubbing so that he could finish the last case admitted on his watch. This was a gentleman admitted to male medicine in shock with a tender, distended abdomen and a diagnosis of myocardial infarction made by the admitting intern because of the shock. After a night of IV fluids, he was finally stabilized, urinating, and taken to the operating room. During the patient preparation time, Dr. Collins and a group of visitors appeared in the room. Dr. Collins picked up the chart, read it, and then asked Dr. Dippel, "Why are you operating on an acute MI?" Dippel, who by this time was gowned and gloved, replied, "Wrong diagnosis." Dr. Collins asked, "Says who?" Dippel retorted, "Says me." At that, Dr. Collins ordered the nurse anesthetist not to put the patient to sleep. Dippel picked up two syringes off the nurse's tray (anectine and pentothal), injected them into the patient's IV, and while he was painting the abdomen, asked, "If you won't put him to sleep, will you please breathe for him?" During the flurry to intubate, Bill finished the draping, made the incision, and copious amounts of black bowel flopped onto the abdomen. He stared across the ether screen at Dr. Collins and intoned, "Myocardial infarction, my ass," whereupon Dr. Collins and his entourage retreated silently from the OR. Moral of the story: Don't mess with the night surgeon.

—*Thomas Murphy, MD, Personal Communication*

Dr. Collins was perhaps second only to Dr. Meyer in his zeal to stamp out human use of tobacco. Since he was around more often than Dr. Meyer, he also had more chances to encounter smoking residents. One of the long-serving urology attending recalls being assigned to a surgical service where the senior resident was an inveterate cigar smoker. One day, while they were in the ICU tending to a patient, the resident had a cigar firmly anchored in the side of his mouth. Dr. Collins appeared and launched into his customary tirade, at which point the resident said over his shoulder, ""It's alright. The cigar's not lit." Dr. Collins exited speechless.

—*Patrick Guinan, MD, Personal Communication*

On another occasion, a surgical resident was cutting through the seventh floor ICU on his way to the stairway up to the eighth floor operating room changing room with a cigar, clearly lit, in his mouth. Dr. Collins leaped from behind a bedside screen with an exultant air of "gotcha," and proceeded to call down the names of Drs. Meyer and Freeark, among others, who would hear of this transgression and be convinced at the very least to suspend the wayward resident. At about this time, the automatic doors on the west side of the ICU just next to Dr. Meyer's apartment opened and Leo, Dr. Meyer's chauffeur, appeared with the chief's two large black standard poodles in tow. They proceeded across the whole length of the ICU corridor and out the east doors to the doctors' elevator for their afternoon constitutional. The resident suggested to Dr. Collins that perhaps he should direct his energies at keeping animals out of the ICU rather than worrying about the dangers of an occasional puff of random cigar smoke and exited the west door to go to the OR. Nothing further was ever heard of the incident.

—*Ken Printen, MD, Personal Experience*

While on the subject of smoking within the confines of the County, one of the surgical attending recalls an attending surgeon of the 1940s-1960s, Dr. Arkel Vaughan, making ward rounds with a lit cigar in his mouth. He told the concerned patients not to worry since the cigar ashes were sterile and even if they did fall on an incision, they would not cause infection but would likely enhance healing.

—*Philip Sheridan Sr., MD, Personal Communication*

Dr. Meyer's dogs were a matter of concern, not only to the medical staff but also on occasion to the patients and their families. Early in the beginning of the cardiac surgery program (late 1950s to mid-1960s), a young man aged 20 or so underwent triple valve (aortic, mitral, and tricuspid) replacement. Since the operation took about seven hours, the patient was taken to the intensive care unit for recovery and the parents brought to the main hallway of the unit. As you may remember, the doctors' elevator was on one side of the unit and Dr. Meyer's apartment on the other side. As the operating surgeon, I was helping the parents into gowns and masks, all the while cautioning them about the possibility of infection in their son. Dr. Meyer came off the elevator and walked his two dogs right through the unit hallway to his apartment. Fortunately, the young man did very well, and the parents' threat to notify all the local and national newspapers if their son developed an infection was replaced by a very nice letter to the *Tribune* describing the fine care their son received at Cook County Hospital.
—Milton Weinberg, MD, Personal Communication

One day, while at the scrub sink with Dr. Manny Lichtenstein, he said, "I bet you wonder why you have to scrub for 10 minutes and I only have to scrub for five. Want to know why?" He proceeded to explain that when he knew he was to operate the next morning, he didn't volunteer to do dirty dishes the night before, never took out the garbage, and never petted the dog. Furthermore, on the morning of surgery, he never went to the toilet. "So," he explained, "my hands are cleaner than yours in the first place."
—David Berger, MD, Personal Communication

Several of the surgical alumni remembered operating on Ward 63 with Dr. Henri Conte, one of the associates on the service. He was an excellent surgeon, a fine operating room teacher, and also very diligent about covering his operating periods. This was important, since Ward 63 was a male ward where the most-senior resident was either in the end of his second year or in the third year, usually did not have independent operating privileges, and as such was dependent on his associate or attending to show up or at least call the OR supervisor to allow the resident to begin surgery. Dr. Conte had not trained at County, and the rumor was that he had trained in Paris. Wherever it was, he was known to prefer retro-colic BII reconstructions for gastric resections used quite often in the treatment of persistent peptic ulcers on the male wards at County. This was in definite contradistinction to Dr. Meyer and nearly all the others surgical attending, who felt that the theoretical advantages of that operation were far outweighed by the better exposure and relative simplicity of the anti-colic reconstruction. Ken Printen recalls, "For the first three weeks of my rotation on Ward 63, Dr. Conte's participation was predictable: a call on the night prior to surgery to discuss the patient and his pathology (always a peptic ulcer), performance of a retro-colic BII operation with a running commentary on the hazards and benefits of the procedure, and a call to inquire about the patient either on the evening of surgery or the next day. The fourth-week session began with the typical phone call for a typical ulcer patient, but at the end of the presentation, Dr. Conte said he would be late, but would call the OR supervisor (Miss R) to let me get started. 'By the way,' he said, 'You know how to do the retro-colic operation and why some people do it, so do this one anti-colic like all the rest of us do. At least now if you get some of those doctors from Minnesota on the Board Exam, you'll know the right answers to their questions on gastric resections.' I never did another retro-colic operation for ulcer disease in 45 years of practice.

—Ken Printen, MD, Personal Experience

Dr. William Requarth of Decatur, Illinois, was a University of Illinois student, a St. Luke's intern, a researcher for Dr. Cole at the U of I, and a surgical resident at Cook County before he joined the Navy in early 1941. Even though he wasn't a County intern, he got the residency through the good graces of Dr. Sumner Koch, so he spent considerable time on Dr. Koch's hand and burn service on Ward 46. He was at Pearl Harbor, and because he knew how to fly, went through the Navy flight school, qualified as a carrier pilot, and was a flight surgeon when the flight surgeons actually flew. He went to England to study high-altitude oxygen use and physiology. Requarth flew Mosquito bombers over France, was transferred to carrier duty in the Pacific, and actually flew torpedo bombers on combat missions. After the war, he returned to County, finished his residency, spent a few years working for Dr. Cole and serving as one of the County night surgeons, and authored his classic text on the acute abdomen before going into private practice in downstate Decatur. He continued to fly a stunt plane for some time and was a founding member of the Illinois Surgical Society, as well as the Karl Meyer and the Warren Cole Societies.

—John Raffensperger, MD, Personal Communication

Several attendings recall a memorable attending of staunch religious convictions who on several occasions had the team kneel in the operating room in prayer for the patient on the operating room table, sometimes before the procedure and sometimes after the operation was completed, in thanksgiving for the Lord having provided such a challenging case from which everyone was able learn so much. It's hard to tell whether the preoperative prayers had a measurable effect, and it seemed that the results of the postoperative prayers were very much operator-dependent.

—Frank Folk, MD, and James Kennedy, MD, Personal Communication

While OB-Gyn is not covered in this treatise, the following example will bring back the remembrance of the dedication with which the volunteer attendings provided their care to the patients on their service. As interns on the labor line in the early 1960s, we delivered close to 60 babies a day in what could only be considered hectic circumstances. One night, we had an obese primipara with ruptured membranes, dilated to about four or five cm, and who seemed to have

ceased her desultory labor. The resident (Ron Lorenzini, I think) examined the patient and decided that she should be given IV Pitocin to move the labor along. This necessitated a call to the attending on call for the labor line, who agreed that this was a reasonable course of action and said he would be in to examine the patient. In my own simple mind, I figured that since by now it was close to 3 a.m., this meant we would have to wait until 7:30 or 8:00 to get the requisite exam, with a loss of valuable time and increased exposure to infection to begin the drip. About one hour later, a distinguished gentleman in a white shirt and tie appeared and asked to see the patient and the resident. After a few minutes with the patient and the resident, he took off his suit coat, pulled the screen around the bed, and performed the exam, which agreed in every detail with ours and with the same recommendations. Soon he left, saying that he had a hysterectomy to do at Highland Park Hospital at 7:30. I found out later that Dr. Phil Stein (the attending) lived in Highland Park and made the trip to County in suit and tie in the middle of the night to see the patient for whom he would never be paid. I gained life-long respect for the volunteer attendings who staffed the County.
—Ken Printen, MD, Personal Experience

Dr. Collins was not the only anesthesia legend of his time. Dr. Alon Winnie, an intern in the class of 1958-59, fell victim to polio during his internship and spent a long time in the Contagious Disease Hospital on the County grounds. He was constantly monitored by members of his Northwestern Medical School class and of his internship group. He survived the acute phase of the disease but was slow to come off the Moerch respirator. One night, in the midst of a kegger in the condemned tenements across Ogden Avenue from the Hospital, there was a party in Bill Kelly's (one of the chief orthopedic residents) apartment. A group of Winnie's mates decided to spur him toward ventilator independence by invading his hospital room and making a great show of disconnecting the single-piston respirator. They explained to Winnie that the tapper on the keg at the party had failed and they needed the ventilator to power the tapping apparatus. Al was stronger than anyone thought. He survived this incident to become chief of anesthesia at County and the University of Illinois College of Medicine at Chicago.
—Michael J. Fitzgerald, MD, Personal Communication

Dr. John B. O'Donohue Sr. was a noted Chicago surgeon who practiced mostly at Mercy but was a long-time faithful County attending who had definite ideas about how most everything should be done. Most of his time at County was spent in the OR or the Monday-afternoon resident conferences, but on occasion, he would make ward rounds, at which time all the wounds would be examined and all the dressings changed. When he made ward rounds, his senior resident at the time, Dr. George Simonian, had the intern decked out in gown, mask, gloves, and booties, as if in the OR, much to the amusement of the patients who were used to much more casual house staff attire for dressing changes.
—Frank Folk, MD, Personal Communication

Character-building was very much a part of the residency training at County, and it presented itself in a multiplicity of forms, as the following example demonstrates. Dr. Bill Norcross, the night warden, supervised night surgical activities and was considered a mentor by many of the surgical residents. I was once awakened at midnight on my night off and commanded to meet him at his table in the Greek's. When I arrived, he reminded me that I had recently berated one of the OR scrub nurses for not having the proper instruments available. He then told me the story of a squadron of flies who flew over a farm and noticed a large pile of fresh cow manure in the barnyard with a pitchfork stuck in the middle of it. They swarmed down and gorged themselves on manure, and then one by one, climbed to the top of the pitchfork and attempted to fly away. However, they were so heavy that as they tried to take off, each crashed to the ground and was killed. Norcross asked me if I knew the moral of the story. When I indicated that I didn't, he said, "Don't fly off the handle when you're full of s—t." I have never forgotten that story and through the years have passed it on to many students, residents, and colleagues.
—David M. Berger, MD, Personal Communication


Dr. Moerch, whose single-piston respirator was rumored to be able to ventilate a stone, was well known for his reading the litany of the patient's data before beginning an anesthetic. No matter how terrible the data was in terms of hypotension, pulse rate, and the like his response was always the same: "Wonderful, wonderful." Then the patient would be put to sleep. The doctor was an avid sailor, and he elected to sail his boat across the Atlantic to Denmark and Scandinavia. Unfortunately, the boat ran into difficulties, and Moerch had to be rescued by the U.S. Coast Guard. He was undoubtedly comforted by the two-word telegram from Dr. Winnie: "Wonderful, wonderful."
—Michael J. Fitzgerald, MD, Personal Communication


Shoes seem to have some type of fixation for those in the operating room hierarchy with even a modicum of authority, real or imagined. An order came down to Miss Gaukroger (OR Supervisor before Miss R.) that all personnel were required to wear conductive shoes in the OR. Frank Jirka, a nephew of Chicago Mayor Anton Cermak and a urology resident at the time, appeared with ordinary looking shoes. Miss G. was preparing to throw him out of the OR when he raised his pant legs to show that he was a bilateral below-knee amputee with prostheses. He explained these rendered him conductive and proceeded to suggest that, if she insisted, he could insert a chain in his rectum and drag it along the floor to dissipate any static electricity he might be building up. She never bothered him again.
—Raymond Firfer, MD, Personal Communication


Dr. George Blaha was, for many years, involved in the administration of the County Hospital, especially in the supervision of the internship program as the assistant DME to Dr. Ole Nelson and later DME in his own right. Like his mentor, it does not seem that he was overly involved in the care and treatment of patients. Quite by accident, while discussing some formatting issues for this book with John Glavin, a noted Chicago author of fiction, I mentioned that the book we were discussing would involve Cook County Hospital. He asked if I knew of a Dr. Blaha at that hospital. When I said I did, he related the following story. As a sophomore in high school in the mid- to late 1940s, the writer had attended St. Phillip's, about a mile and a half west of County on Jackson Boulevard. As with most school playgrounds of the day, equipment was rudimentary and grass absent. At recess one day, the boys were playing a pick-up football game, and Glavin went long for a pass. Unfortunately, the pass was too long, but with youthful exuberance, Glavin tracked the ball. He turned to see how close he was to the chicken-wire fence that surrounded the field just in time to run face first into the barrier. He suffered impressive enough cuts to be offered the gym coach's handkerchief, told to go to the County Hospital, and was given a quarter for carfare. He was also assured that his parents (mother most likely) would be notified to meet him at the hospital. About a half-hour later, Glavin showed up in the County ER, met up with his mother, and endured the customary wait to see the doctor, probably at the Surgical Dispensary. The doctor was a tall, good-looking young man who put the anxious teenager at ease with his quiet, confident manner. Glavin clearly remembers the physician was Dr. George Blaha. The results of the 20-odd sutures were excellent, even when viewed by me 50 years later. What was more amazing to me was the incontrovertible evidence that Dr. Blaha had actually treated a real live patient.

—Ken Printen, MD, Personal Experience

Dr. Alfred J. Kobak Sr., was a well-known OB/GYN attending during the period from the 1940s to the 1960s. One of his areas of interest was the use of hypnosis in the delivery process, which he would demonstrate in lectures to the residents, interns, and nursing students, usually using one of the nursing students as a demonstration model. Most volunteers could be hypnotized, but the student nurses were dubious about the efficacy of this technique when real labor began. The interns, medical students, and residents, however, were quite interested in the possibilities of this addition to their armamentarium, at least until it was explained to them that, for the most part, people under hypnosis could not be made to do anything they would not usually do when they were awake.

—Janice M. Jenkins, RN, Personal Communication

Dr. Roscoe Giles, a native of Brooklyn, New York, the first black physician appointed to the attending surgery staff, was a graduate of the Cornell College of Medicine. He could not get an internship in New York City, so he came to Chicago and the Provident Hospital where he thought he had been promised a position. It turns out that he had not, so he went to work as a busboy at the Tip

Top Inn at 72 W. Adams. One night, a kitchen worker was stabbed in the neck during a fight, and Giles stopped the bleeding, found some cotton thread and a needle, and sewed the wound up. The cashier and her husband, a Cook County Hospital physician, helped Dr. Giles out, and after passing the Illinois state board exam, he was able to begin his internship at the Provident Hospital. After he was in practice for a while, he was appointed to the surgical staff of County and the faculty of the Chicago Medical School with the help of Drs. Leo Zimmerman and Raymond McNealy.
—*Chicago Medicine, vol. 94, no. 12, pp.11-20, June 21,1991*

In the late 1960s, when Dr. Constantine Tatooles was the chairman of cardiothoracic surgery at County, he convinced the then hospital director, Dr. Bob Freeark, to set the hospital charges for open heart procedures at $2,000. The volume, especially of pediatric cases, increased just as Tatooles had suspected, since a number of ethnic charitable societies undertook this opportunity to raise the necessary funding to bring patients from Europe to County for the surgery.
—*Constantine J. Tatooles, MD, Personal Communication*

Dr. Roger Vaughan, a full-time night warden and chief night surgeon, was from an immensely wealthy family who owned a chain of seed stores in the city. Each midnight, he walked across Harrison Street to the Greek's to eat his supper. One night, Nick Gaso, one of the owners, was eating soup. Dr. Vaughan asked, "Nick! How's the soup tonight?" "It's so good that I could eat 10 bowls of it.," came the reply. Dr. Vaughan took out five dollars and said to the waiter, "I'll bet five dollars he can't and I'll pay for them. Bring him nine more bowels of soup." Laboriously, Nick ate eight more bowls. Dr. Vaughan said, "I lose the bet. I'm sure he can do it, so I'll take the last bowl myself."
—*William C. Beck, MD, Proc. Inst. Med. Chgo. Vol. 40, 1987, p.137*

In the late 1940s and early 1950s, the oral boards in surgery were given on the wards at County, and the surgical residents served as guides for the examinees, getting them to the right place and the right set of examiners. One of the alumni remembers taking an examinee to be quizzed by Harvey Allen, the noted hand and burn surgeon of that time. After a few questions about techniques for hand surgery, Dr. Allen asked the examinee if he knew the tensile strength of 3/0 black silk, which, at the time, was favored in tendon repairs of the hand and wrist. Aside from a profusion of sweat and a rather terrified look, there was no response from the young physician. The exam proceeded, and several weeks later, Dr. Allen and the resident-guide were doing a hand case. The resident asked Dr. Allen, "What is the tensile strength of this 3/0 silk?" "How should I know, and what do you want to know for?" came the reply from Allen. The resident's reply was as unclear as the board examinee's had been, and aside from a flutter in Miss Hamburger's pulse rate, the case proceeded to its conclusion.
—*Philip Sheridan Sr., MD, Personal Communication*

For many years, Dr. Orion Stuteville was in charge of the plastic/head and neck tumor service at County. In those days, head and neck tumors were not segmented to any particular specialty, and like hand surgery, were operated on a variety of individuals from different specialties with an interest in these lesions. One of the most challenging of these lesions was carcinoma of the upper third of the esophagus. There was a patient on Ward 21 in the late 1960s who had just such a carcinoma that eroded into the larynx. In the finest of Stutevillean tumor management, the patient was "separated from his disease" by undergoing a combined resection of the larynx, upper third of the esophagus, and a radical neck, followed by a course of radiation therapy to the neck. His permanent tracheostomy was brought out through his sternum for which he periodically underwent dilatation and cautery for bleeding granulation tissue. He was fed by a permanent gastrostomy, and except for minor inconveniences, was doing well. He was readily recognizable by his magic message pad around his neck with which he would gladly communicate with his doctors and nurses, his large Dave Garroway plastic glasses, and his generally cheerful demeanor. One day when the patient was in the hospital for some minor tracheostomy problem, Stutie noticed him while on rounds, and recalled that the patient was now several years postresection. He wondered what they collectively thought about restoring gastrointestinal continuity. As it turns out, several of the general surgery residents on the service had been speculating about that very thing. Stutie walked over to the bed and said good morning to the patient, lifted up the top sheet, and examined the abdomen and genitalia. He said, "He'll do." Then he asked if any of us had read the Israeli literature on management of CA of the upper third of the esophagus. We hadn't, but we did that afternoon and found that one of the methods used in that area of the Middle East was to skin the penis, invert the resultant tube graft, and interpose it between the ends of the esophagus. We had our doubts, but on the appointed day, Stutie skinned the penis, applied a split thickness skin graft, and splinted the penis while the residents prepared the esophagus. The tube graft fit nicely in place, and the patient made an uneventful recovery. Reports and patient sightings up to a year post-op indicated that the patient continued to do well on a carefully selected soft diet: clear proof of the value of separating the patient from his disease, even under unusual circumstances.

—David M. Berger, MD, Personal Communication


The Richter scissors is named after which one of the following Chicago surgeons?
   a) Harry Richter Sr.
   b) Harry Richter Jr.
   c) Harry Richter III
   d) None of the above

The answer is d). The scissors were named after instrument maker Bruno Richter, who was a neighbor of Dr. Willis Potts in Oak Park. Incidentally, the Potts clamp used in the correction of Tetralogy of Fallot was designed and built for his neighbor by Mr. Richter.

—Daniel Deziel, MD, Personnel Communication

## Only at County

The early 1970s were the last years that operations were performed with daylight illumination in the eighth floor operating rooms. After that, air conditioning was installed, the windows were sealed, and the view obliterated. I will never forget the thrill of seeing the sunrise in the east at 5:00 a.m. on one August morning in 1971 as we finished a long, hard case. The chief resident and the juniors had just finished suturing multiple gunshot perforations of the stomach and small intestine, cleaned out the belly, and closed the incision. These wounds, without a doubt, would have killed the patient without the operation. Just then, the darkness of night exploded into a sunrise, and it was almost as though a heavenly presence had manifested itself. Many (if not all) experienced surgeons feel that the presence of a good Lord is often quite apparent in the operating room. We were all elated, forgot how tired we were, and instinctively knew that what we had done was good.
—*Philip Donohue, MD, Personal Communication*

Dr. Bill Norcross, who finished the County surgical program in 1959, stayed on after the completion of his training as an attending surgeon and night warden for a number of years, much after the manner of Dr. Roger Vaughan. Unlike Dr. Vaughan, who never scrubbed and rarely saw the patients, Dr. Norcross mostly sat at the Greek's, drinking coffee and waiting for the chief resident (night surgeon) to call if he needed help with a case, at which point he would scrub in as first assistant. If he felt that the resident didn't know when he needed help, he would go up to the OR and look over the ether screen to provide words of encouragement like "stop the bleeding" or "make the incision bigger." If this failed to produce the required result, he would scrub in and gradually assume control. One night, a relatively new chief resident was exploring a trauma patient with abdominal bleeding and found that the patient had a ruptured spleen. He called Norcross, who after a few minutes of watching him struggle, scrubbed in and edged the junior resident out of the first assistant spot. While encouraging the medical student to pull harder on the Mayo retractor that was elevating the lower left ribs, he slid his left hand into the abdomen, pulled out the spleen, placed several lap pads in the vacated left upper quadrant, turned on his heel, and told the chief resident to stop the bleeding. Luckily, the resident was up to that task, and the patient survived all aspects of his traumatic injuries that night.
—*Edwin Carey, MD, Personal Communication*

One of the surgical residents of the 1960s, who later had a distinguished career as a plastic surgeon in a downstate Illinois community, was obsessed with operator speed in the OR. One night, when he was the night surgeon, a thin, youngish gentleman presented with acute onset severe abdominal pain and free air under the diaphragm on plain abdominal X-rays. This was to be the perfect patient for the world speed record in patching a perforated duodenal ulcer, which was held

to be somewhere under 10 minutes, skin to skin. To make sure that not a second was wasted, the patient was anesthetized, shaved, prepped and draped, and the timing clock, usually reserved for timing cardiac pump runs, was set. When all was in readiness, the resident placed his left hand over the bottom of the sternum, checked the timing apparatus, and asked for the scalpel. While watching the sweep second hand of the clock get to 12, he made a rapid sweeping incision with the scalpel, which was followed by a loud yell and admonition to "get Norcross" and call "the Bake." A quick look at the abdominal site confirmed that the blood on the field came primarily from the surgeon's index finger. He was held for examination and later repair of a lacerated digital nerve, and closure of his traumatic finger laceration. The junior resident patched the perforated peptic ulcer without further incident, but not in world-record time.
—David M. Berger, MD, and James Kennedy, MD, Personal Communication

One of the residents remembers watching the west side of Chicago burn the night of Dr. Martin Luther King Jr.'s assassination. He asked his diverse house staff whether they thought he was prejudiced. A large black intern named Lowry responded, " Hell no, Charlie. You treat us all like shit!"
—Charles Humphrey, MD, Personal Communication to Dr. Folk

Six uniforms were allotted for the 18 months of service as an intern, laundry included. The fringes of your trousers in your senior year out-styled the best tailored fringe of Pierre Cardin's jeans of today, maybe even those of Jordasch.
—Louis Boshes, MD, Cook County Hospital Intern's and Resident's Alumni Association Newsletter, December, 1980

In the late 1960s, intern George Savas was told to tidy up Ward 60 at the end of his rotation on June 30th and be sure all the post-ops had their sutures out. He proceeded to take out all retention sutures as well, sending two patients back to the OR to repair their dehiscences later that evening.
—David M. Berger, MD, Personal Communication

While the wet operative clinics of the postgraduate school were monopolized early on by Drs. Meyer and McNealy, attendings of all the surgical services got their chance to shine before what was usually a very appreciative audience. One of the orthopedic/fracture attendings was a theatrical teacher who kept the attendees amused with vivid descriptions of the fractures and their complications. At one of these sessions, he had a patient with a fresh Colles' fracture. He rapidly injected local anesthetic into the hematoma, explaining the rationale of the procedure as he skillfully reduced the fracture. Responding to the enthusiastic reception of this maneuver by the audience, he reproduced the fracture and then re-reduced it before applying the cast. The patient, who of course had been awake for the whole performance, chimed in with her appreciation for this painless procedure.
—Frank Folk, MD, Personal Communication

The power of the night surgeon was legendary, but sometimes, guile had to be employed as well. One day, a visitor from the hills of West Virginia was admitted with an acute onset of abdominal pain, board-like rigidity, and free air under the diaphragm on plain abdominal X-rays. The night surgeon, Dave Yocum, an excellent surgeon, was called in to see the patient. He walked into the room, examined the patient, and explained that he would need an operation on his stomach, or "you are going to die." The patient said, "Ain't nobody cutting on me, Doc." Dave turned and asked me, as the junior resident, to call down to the carpenter shop and have someone come up and "measure this guy for a coffin." Then he turned to walk out of the room. The patient recovered and said, "Doc, come here and let me sign the paper for the operation." The permit was signed, the ulcer patched, and the patient's life saved, thanks to Dave's psychological and surgical expertise.
—Frank Milloy, MD, Personal Communication


One specific night, which was very busy, all of the more senior residents and even most of the interns were in the operating room when an abdominal stab wound came in. I called the senior resident after I had evaluated the patient, and he indicated that I should get hold of Dr. Baker, which I did. Dr. Baker said to get the patient ready for the OR. So I took the patient to the operating room where I was expecting to assist him. It was that night that I did my first splenectomy. Dr. Baker was absolutely great and made me feel like I was the best surgeon on the face of the earth. Dr. Frank Banich was another of those great County teachers who made you feel that you were a real part of the system and not just a cog.
—Jerome F. Wall, MD, Personal Communication


I was taking my night on emergency call for OB in May of 1955 when a 14-year-old patient, who spoke only Spanish, presented with acute abdominal pain. She had eaten pinto beans for lunch, and with the wide communication gap that existed, got a diagnosis of pinto bean poisoning. Luckily for her, one of the experienced ER nurses felt her rigid abdomen, got the history that the girl might be pregnant, and also got 0/0 for a blood pressure. The nurse yelled for the OB resident who pushed the girl into the elevator and up to the eighth floor OR, screaming for help. The intern on anesthesia did not want to give an anesthetic to an underage patient with no permit, IV, or blood pressure, but the OB resident got nursing to help open an OR pack, splashed some tincture of iodine on the abdomen, and made a lower abdominal incision. With his gloved hand, he reached in and grabbed the involved tube. Someone manned the suction and appropriate clamps were placed. Fortunately, the pressure began to rise, an IV was started, and blood obtained and transfused. She survived, but the resident still had to survive the weekly OB conference later that week. The staff asked him to tell the story, which he did. But when he said, "I make ze incision and she no bleed, so I say 'Manuel what a great surgeon I am.'" The room exploded with laughter. I don't remember anything bad that happened, either to the patient or the resident, as a result of this adventure.
—F.R. Brueckmann, MD, Personal Communication

One afternoon in the late 1950s, there was a commotion at the big scheduling board in the main OR. It seems Miss R. and a chief resident were having a discussion about the propriety and possibility of adding a patient who desperately needed an emergency esophagectomy as a life-saving procedure. As the resident became more and more agitated, Miss R. held her ground and quietly suggested that it would be appropriate before scheduling to at least consult by phone with an attending. As the discussion continued, a small knot of interested residents, nurses, and medical students collected. In the midst of the argument, Mrs. Purvinas, one of the OR head nurses who was responsible for the room in which the operation would be done, quietly edged her way through the crowd and tugged on the sleeve of the resident's white coat. When he finally took a breath and turned to her, she said, "Doctor. It's not an emergency any more. The patient just expired." The discussion stopped and the knot of people disbanded without any rancor.
—Ken Printen, MD, and Mrs. Jane Schwab, RN, Formerly Scrub Nurse
8th floor OR, Personal Experience

When friends asked about where they should go after an auto accident or some other emergency, my standard answer was, "If you know your doctor or your hospital, go there; if not, go to County." This advice was based on my confidence that the care given would be first rate, although the amenities were sometimes lacking. One January night on call, I went to see a new admission on Ward 45. The patient was comatose, having been brought in by police from the Union Station. My roommate, George Gould, stopped by to see a new patient on Ward 55. He said, "You've got a man of quality here." I asked, "How can you tell?" "Because he has clean feet," came the learned answer. The man had no identification, but in his pocket was a room key to the Edgewater Beach Hotel. We called the room at the hotel, and a man answered. He told us that he was sharing the room with his boss. They were from Louisville and in town for an insurance convention. They had gone to a bar on South Wabash. "I left him sitting at the bar when I went to the john; when I returned, he was gone. The bartender didn't know where he went." He came to the hospital and identified his friend. As the patient gradually recovered, he recalled that while he was sitting alone, someone came up and offered to buy him a drink. He remembered nothing after that. How he got from the bar to the Union Station remained a mystery, although it was clear that he had been drugged and robbed. When he awakened, he sat up and looked around from his bed in the double middle aisle of the ward surrounded by bedraggled men. "Where am I?" "You're in the Cook County Hospital," came the reply. "I've heard about this place but never thought I'd end up here," he answered. So without the benefit of my advice, he had done the right thing: He came to County!!
—Frank Folk, MD, Personal Communication

Pay-to-play has received quite a bit of notoriety in recent years but is not new to the County Hospital, at least not since the 1890s when the commissioners were caught selling attending-physician positions for the princely sum of $1,000, the price charged to Dr. Christian Fenger for his position on the County staff. There was also a longstanding tradition of being paid for playing as recalled by several of the house staff of the early 1960s.

Tom Murphy and I had a patient die on Ward 61 after we took out what proved to be a normal appendix. Naturally, we wanted to get a post to see what the cause of death was. The patient had no family, so I asked for a four-day post, which meant that if no one claimed the body in four days, an autopsy could be performed on medical grounds. Each day I went to the admitting office to check if anyone had called for the body. No one did, until the last moment on the fourth day when a long-lost relative sent a telegram from somewhere denying the post. I smelled a rat and went to one of the medical administrators in a major snit. He told me to just cool it and said "that this was just the system working itself out." Public aid would pay for the burial, and the undertaker would see to it that everyone involved in the disposition of the departed from the admitting clerk through the administrator to the alderman of the patient's ward would receive their customary $25 cut.

—James Kennedy, MD, Personal Communication

Paying-for-playing had a different spin on the fracture wards where a particular law firm employed an "ambulance chasing" attorney to get information from the ward clerks on accident victims. Minions of this connected firm would visit the hospitalized patients, claiming to be County attorneys, and get the patients to sign with the firm to settle the claim, usually well below what could have been garnered from a settlement awarded at trial. The patient would get what was many times more money than he or she had ever seen, and the rest was kicked back to the ward clerks, the attorneys, and other hospital administrative personnel. In the early 1960s, several interns threw the contract attorney off the ward and told the patients on admission never to sign anything. This worked for a while until the surgical resident on the service, Ed Quartetti, told the interns that if they really wanted to get surgical residencies at County, they should cool it with the fake County attorneys. This was punctuated several days later by a foray onto the ward by the senior attorney in the connected practice and several of the hospital administrators, looking for the involved interns, who, as luck would have it, were off the ward at the time.

—Raymond Dieter, MD, and James Kennedy, MD, Personal Communication

There always seemed to be a lack of operating room time in which to complete our thoracic surgery elective caseload. Being the conscientious fellow I was, each Sunday morning I would begin calling the operating room at 5 a.m. to see if any cases were underway. If not, I would select either a lung or an esophagus case to book for 8 a.m. This, of course, would then entail calling Dr. Bill Warren at home on a Sunday morning and cajoling him into foregoing a day of rest in lieu of a day in the OR to do an elective lobectomy or esophagectomy. He never refused. What a great mentor!

—Francis Podbielski, MD, Personal Communication

One of the omnipresent figures of the County medical administrative system from the 1950s to the 1980s was Dr. George Blaha, a member of the intern class of 1940. He completed a medical residency and then stayed on the staff, first as assistant medical director to Dr. Ole Nelson and later as the medical director. It was largely his job to assign the interns and to keep an eye out for their general welfare. He was a non-stop cigarette chain smoker who was quite involved in Democratic politics as they related to the hospital. One alum recalls that Dr. Blaha took him to a Democratic fundraiser at McCormick Place in October of 1965 and admonished him to take an active part in the dinner conversation, voicing approval of the Democratic initiatives in health care whenever asked. When the intern told him he was a Republican, the reply was predictable. "Since you're working at Cook County Hospital, if you want to keep your job, tonight you're a Democrat."
—LeRoy Smith, MD, Personal Communication

There was always a lot of spirited discussion when differences of opinion surfaced about diagnosis, treatment, or adherence to protocol, which was generally settled by the fact that the resident had a long white coat, while many times the intern had no coat at all. One notable exception recalled by many individuals occurred in the 1960s when a burly intern with a notoriously short temper, Joe Flynn, took exception with the opinions of a sharp-tongued and sarcastic surgical resident. He promptly cold-cocked him in the ER. It didn't stop Dr. Flynn from getting an OB residency at County.
—David M. Berger, MD, and a number of others, Personal Communication

One Christmas Eve, I was the emergency urology resident on call, and a rather belligerent patient needed an operation. The intern mentioned that the patient wanted Dr. Karl Meyer to perform the procedure. The patient was taken to the OR, and the intern announced my arrival by saying, "Here comes Karl Meyer." As I walked through the OR door, I said, "I'm here. I'm Karl Meyer." The patient turned his head toward me and said, "You've grown quite a bit."
—John Zumerchik, MD, Personal Communication

The emergency room was a fertile field for remembrances. One alumnus remembered having a patient catch fire in the ER while restrained on a gurney. He was promptly transferred to the burn unit and had a satisfactory outcome. The same resident remembered a patient walking out of the ER restrained to the stretcher, which was on his back.
—Jeffery Friedman, MD, Personal Communication

Another resident remembers sitting on the chest of a wild drunk with a huge scalp laceration just to control him and sew it up. The next day, the patient had to be discharged early because he was preaching a sermon that morning.
—William Briney, MD, Personal Communication

John Dillinger's body lay in state, sort of, in the Cook County morgue. The lines were five blocks long in each direction to the morgue, like for a couple of days.
—*Louis Boshes, MD, Cook County Hospital Intern's and Resident's Alumni Association Newsletter, December 1980*


One night I had a patient with a stab wound of the chest with tamponade. He was in shock and on his way out. I grabbed a large needle (probably 12 gauge) and emptied the pericardial cavity. This allowed him to wake up, look at me, and say, "I'm going to get you, you bald-headed bastard."
—*James Kennedy, MD, Personal Communication*


We had a trauma victim with a knife stuck up to the hilt into her forehead. She was drunk but still coherent. As she was transported from the trauma unit on the third floor to the eighth floor OR, the visitors riding up to see their family members looked at her in shock. She said a bit blearily, "What're you looking at? This is just my Halloween costume." I never suspected such tragedy could also be the source of such clever humor.
—*William Lindsey, MD, Personal Communication*


One night in the ER, we recovered one of the original BIC pens from a male patient's colon. Seems he had inserted it per rectum a year or two previously. After it was retrieved, it still wrote in brilliant green ink.
—*Don R. Read, MD, Personal Communication*


I remember taking calls from the Greek's and using their "in house" to answer the pages.
—*Carlotta Hill, MD, Personal Communication*


At one time, it was the custom to award a diligent intern the opportunity to do a cholecystectomy before ending his rotation on the surgical service. This was especially true if the intern was planning on applying for the surgical residency. While I was an intern on Ward 60, Dale Snyder, the senior resident, told me that if a patient was admitted to the ward that night with a "hot" gallbladder, I could do the case the following morning. As it happened, such a patient was admitted late in the evening. I decided that she could wait until morning for surgery, so I put a tube in her stomach, started an IV and antibiotics, and put her out on the sun porch, out of the way of marauding senior residents. As luck would have it, the night surgeon, Myles Cunningham, and his assistant Neil Woodward, were in the midst of a slow night, so they came to Ward 60 to see if there were any cases to do. My patient with the IV and NG tube on the sun porch immediately caught their eye. Myles examined her and, despite my objections and plaintive

explanation that this was to be my case for the morning, he ordered that she be in the OR in 45 minutes. His demeanor did not improve when I told him that he would have to roll the bed over me to get the patient to the OR. Neil Woodward, who was a friend of mine, privately conferred with Dr. Cunningham and told him that I was a former U.S. collegiate boxing champion and maybe he should not mess with me. I was, of course, nothing of the sort, but it was enough for the night surgeon to contemplate. He did not operate on my patient, but I did, first thing in the morning.
—*David Berger, MD, Personal Communication*


I remember getting shot at by a patient in the emergency room. He missed.
—*David Johnson, MD, Personal Communication*


I was the triage doctor at the desk in the ER when a patient brought a prescription to me to correct. The pharmacy wouldn't fill it because it didn't have a Drug Enforcement Agency (DEA) number on it. Unfortunately, the patient had signed my name to the fake prescription. The security guards hauled him off to the back room for a "talking to."
—*Don R. Read, MD, Personal Communication*


I was a resident on the hand service (1973) and was debriding a gunshot wound of the forearm in the trauma unit. It was early morning and I had been up all night. I became aware of another presence in the area, and when I looked up, I found that I was surrounded by a visiting group of officials from communist China, complete with their trademark grey uniforms and red stars on their caps. It was disorienting, and with my lack of sleep, I wondered if we had just lost World War III without my knowing it.
—*Henry Bernstein, MD, Personal Communication*


As a second-year medical student at the University of Illinois, I witnessed my first autopsy in the morgue at County. The case was a 13-year-old Hispanic boy who had a cardiac arrest shortly after being admitted to the ER. The history, as far as we could tell, was that of a high fever for several days accompanied by abdominal pain for which his mother gave him aspirin and enemas. When the abdominal cavity was opened, there was an audible release of noxious gas, which was awash with pus and contained a huge phlegmon of necrotic material in the right lower quadrant just above his gangrenous perforated appendix. To this day, I can still visualize this boy's abdomen. It was a learning experience that has stayed with me for life, and had a profound effect on me in my practice of surgery.
—*Elliot Goldin, MD, Personal Communication*

The demand that "All ward house staff drop everything to make afternoon staff rounds" did not usually produce a flurry of activity on any service but the burn unit. When asked one afternoon where the overflow burn patient that we were taking care of was, the intern stated that he had left him in the bath tub while he came to make rounds. We found him in the tub, under water, very blue, and very dead.
—Charles Humphrey, MD, Personal Communication

One day I was on duty in the ER and a DOA came in. It was a part of our duty to check the body, pronounce the death, and then sign the death certificate. On this occasion, there had been a police chase on the Eisenhower Expressway with exchange of gunfire required to apprehend the suspects, who were drug dealers. My wife picked me up after my shift and was excited to tell me that she witnessed the shoot-out. When I told her that I not only was aware of the incident but had pronounced the desperado dead from multiple gunshots, both her story and excitement became visibly deflated.
—George M. Miks, MD, Personal Communication

Someone called the general information number at County and got misinformation, so Dr. Meyer decided that one of the surgical residents would sit at the second floor desk every night just to answer the phone calls. Bill Hagstrom, one of the senior surgical residents, loved to call the desk and harass the resident, pretending he was Dr. Meyer. One night, Jimmy Yao was on the phone, and when a caller identified himself as Dr. Meyer, Jimmy answered, "Go to hell." Within minutes, Dr. Meyer was on the second floor demanding to know who was on the desk. Jimmy just replied, "No speak English. No speak English."
—James Kennedy, MD, Personal Communication

In the trauma unit triage area, we were working on a stab-wound victim when another patient was wheeled in and placed at the other end of the room, four stretchers away. Our patient sat bolt upright and yelled, "That's the guy who stabbed me." We had to forcibly restrain both patients to keep the fight from restarting.
—Ron Read, MD, Personal Communication

The hiding, moving, and misidentifying of preoperative patients to save them from being taken to surgery by unfavored attendings or ruthless night surgeons who were having a slow night or just wanted to aggravate one of their residency mates, was a time-honored skill that was honed to a fine art at County. According to Dr. Louis Boshes, "you change the ribbons (service assignments) so that a certain attending will not examine that patient for fear that he will operate on him. You either lock your patients in the linen closet or take them to the ward next door during surgical rounds. Complaints by the attending man are referred to Dr. Meyer's office. You are not called for an explanation." More recent residents remember

hiding patients from the night surgeons by sending them to X-ray or putting them on a gurney for a scenic trip around the hospital conducted by the junior medical students assigned to the service. As an alternative, fresh dressings not covering any incisions could be used to camouflage a bogus operative site, since they were clear evidence that a procedure had already been performed.
—*Louis Boshes, MD, Cook County Intern's and Resident's Alumni Association Newsletter, December, 1980; and Richard Mladick, MD, and Lawrence Gibson, MD, Personal Communications*

At County, many things were not always as they appeared. While rotating in plastic surgery (Ward 23), we took care of some patients undergoing sexual re-assignment operations. One of my young interns became attracted to a very pretty woman visitor on the ward and finally got a date with her. While they were sharing a romantic moment, he found out that "she" was in fact a man. The intern stated, later on, that he had never run away from someone so fast in his life.
—*Fereydoon Majouri, MD, Personal Communication*

I remember wearing short pants for a whole year because no matter where I was in the hospital, the air conditioning never worked.
—*David Jansen, MD, Personal Communication*

When a group of us residents had been at County for two to three years, we started a poker game on the sixth floor of the hospital in a room used for the stand-by resident's sleeping quarters. The usual group was myself, Mel Goodman (OB), Alex Varga (OB), Layton Kest (GU), Arnie Kaplan (surgery), and Alan Tufti (ortho). We were mostly broke, getting either $12.50 or $25.00 a month, so we played for five-, 10-, or 25-cent bets. No wild cards. No food or drinks. Only poker. One day we had our usual group assembled, and for some reason, we put a white mattress cover from an adjoining bedroom on the table. Layton Kest was losing, but he couldn't pay, so he wrote the names of the other five players on the mattress cover so he could keep a running tab of how much he owed the other players. When the maid cleaned up the room, she took exception to all the scribbling on the bed linen and carted it down to Dr. Blaha's office to show him how dissolute the residents were. He knew about the poker games but didn't want to make a big thing out of it, so he called the five of us down to his office, minus, of course, Dr. Kest, since his name wasn't on the tally sheet. He suggested in no uncertain terms that we should cease this terrible thing we were doing in the hospital. That was the end of the regular poker game.
—*William Marshall, MD, Personal Communication*

While the poker game noted above was mostly for dimes and quarters, a substantially more expensive game was begun and became well entrenched during the early 1960s. By this time, the interns were making $125 a month and residents at all levels got the princely sum of $140 a month. The seats were occupied by various players depending on service assignments, moonlighting schedules, and the occasional time-outs for two years of military service. Some of the regular attendees were Boone Brackett, Joe Carey, Ed Montgomery, Ron Manicom, Al Lerner, Ken Printen, E. Barrett Smith, and "One-Eyed" Jim Brown, a noted urology resident of his time. The play was fast and furious, and at times, the bets far exceeded the players' cash on hand so that adequate funding had to either be pledged or guaranteed by a third party, many times by phone. One night, Ron Manicom, who was a native of west Texas, was embroiled in a betting war in a hand where the bet to him to stay was in the neighborhood of $500, which he couldn't cover. He asked for and got a time out to call his father in Texas to cover his bet. This gentleman wanted to hear the betting sequence and also to know what his son was holding, so I was chosen to convey the information. When I told the father the progression of the betting and ended by telling him that his son was holding a full house with queens over, the reply was short and crisp, "See. Hell. Tell him to raise another $500 and I'll cover him." The information was passed on to the two bettors. The raise was made and seen. The result: A full house, kings up still beats a full house, queens up, every time.

—*Ken Printen, MD, Personal Experience*

One cannot leave the topic of County poker games without including the following story by one of the most avid of the players. One evening, we were playing poker in our usual spot in Karl Meyer Hall, and the betting kind of got out of hand. Pretty soon, everyone had dropped out except for Joe Carey and me. The bet was well over what either of us had, so we ended up betting the value of my powder-blue Mustang against the value of Joe's sailboat, the *Mary Lou*. When I showed my hand, Joe pushed his cards in and said, "Boone, you just won the *Mary Lou*." Some weeks later on an evening when I was on call and sitting at the Greek's having a cup of coffee with Bill Norcross, Joe Carey walked in with a briefcase, put it on the table, opened it, and paid off the bet. So I never did get to sail the *Mary Lou*.

—*E. Boone Brackett, MD, Personal Communication*

Traveling from Oak Park to Cook County Hospital for my first day's work as an intern in 1963, I was wearing "street clothes." While waiting for the train at the Oak Park stop, a man posing as a Chicago transit officer pulled a gun and was just starting to ask for our money when the train pulled in. The doors opened and I jumped into the car as quickly as possible. The doors closed and I was whisked off to the hospital. Needless to say, from then on, at the advice of the hospital personnel, I wore my "whites" to work every day thereafter.

—*George M. Miks, MD, Personal Communication*

As a senior resident, I asked a junior resident to get a dermatology consult for a patient with an unusual skin rash. The next day on rounds, the junior reported that the derm resident had said the rash was due to bed-bug bites. The patient angrily retorted, " That can't be true. I haven't slept in a bed in months!"
—*Don Read, MD, Personal Communication*


In the middle of my two-year internship, the Korean War broke out. Around October of 1950, a number of us who were in the Naval Reserve received orders to report to Fort Sam Houston, Texas. We had been assigned to the Army. This was disturbing to us and of great concern to the hospital administrators. We brought this news to Dr. Ole Nelson, Dr. Meyer's right hand man in the day-to-day administrative affairs and the specific manager of all things related to the internship. He got on the phone to Admiral A.A. (Alphabet) Agnew, Commanding Officer of the Great Lakes Naval Base. He explained to the admiral that it was true we had completed our one year of required internship, but Nelson had a big hospital to run, and "By, God," we were needed there. Our orders were cancelled. All of us initiated our individual requests for delay in reporting. A year later, my new orders came to report to Camp LeJeune, North Carolina, for field medical training with the Marines. My request for the Naval establishment had been granted. When called to military service, the attitude was often somewhat resentful and with a tendency to look down on the service docs and their practice of medicine. In short order, we learned how dedicated these career professionals were and how fortunate we were that while we were in school and training, they covered for us and allowed us to lead relatively normal lives. Now it was our turn to step up to the plate.
—*Frank Folk, MD, Personal Communication*


There was a man brought up from Hammond, Indiana, after suffering amputations of his nose, ears, and you can guess what else, apparently at the hands of a very angry man—rumored to be a surgeon—who found this patient in bed with his wife. We patched him up and sent him to psyche for safekeeping, on the grounds that the wounds were self-inflicted. Where else but County?
—*Donald Dexter, MD, Personal Communication*


I remember delivering a baby in the back seat of a car just outside the hospital ER and doing mouth-to-mouth to suck out the meconium from the baby's respiratory tract.
—*David Jensen, MD, Personal Communication*


The Cook County Blood Bank was one of the first in the United States and has always been associated with a lot of stories worth remembering and retelling.

When the blood bank became active during and just after the Second World

War, there was no lab technician to type and cross the blood for night blood transfusions. Since the OB department used a lot of blood transfusions at night, the OB residents did all the typing and cross-matching for the blood bank. We did a very good and accurate job.
—Philip C. Williams, MD, Personal Communication


The maintenance of a positive blood balance in the blood bank was essential, since without it, the chief residents of all the surgical services were prohibited from doing any elective surgery. So it was necessary to improvise.

The delivery room residents kept the blood bank usable, because for every patient with a bloody show prior to delivery, the boyfriend, husband, and as many other family and friends available on site were sent to the blood bank to donate, since the patient in labor might need a transfusion. At the end of my six months on the labor-line, I had a 150,000 cc. credit in the bank.
—Evan F. Evans, MD, Personal Communication


An alternative to the donation of real blood was to donate $10 so that the money could be used to pay a donor. Since the blood bank had the disturbing habit of erasing all blood balances to zero at the beginning of each calendar quarter, it made little sense for the chief resident on the service to turn in all the money at the time it was paid by the patient or his or her relatives, especially the $20 most individuals were asked to contribute to have their inguinal hernias repaired. The net result was that most of the chiefs built up a monetary reserve that could be used in the name of those patients without friends or family who required blood to be set aside for potential use in elective cases. In my own case, I gave $1,500 in "blood money" to Lloyd Henry when I stopped being a chief resident and became an attending.
—Ken Printen, MD, Personal Experience


The blood bank was not without its own cast of memorable performers. Red, the supervisor, was an excellent photographer, and could always be counted on to come to the OR to take a shot or two of interesting or unexpected findings at surgery. There was also the street-wise but acerbic night technician who was not only technically superb but doled out pearls of conventional wisdom free of charge. One of the residents remembered taking a tube of blood for type and cross-match from a patient who was bleeding from a duodenal ulcer and was being taken to the OR for an emergency gastrectomy. "I need two units right away, with two more made up and on hold," was the resident's request. "Who's the night surgeon?" asked the tech. The resident identified him, to which the tech replied, "You'd better take four now and I'll make up another four. He's pretty slow and not so good either."
—David Berger, MD, Personal Communication

Long before he was professor and head of plastic surgery at the Loyola University Stritch School of Medicine, Juan Angelats was coming off an "intern of the year" performance in the late 1960s. As a junior resident to John Bartizal, Juan had an intern fresh from the Far East by the name of Wang whose command of English was less than ideal. They had a patient who required an elective colectomy, and were going through the work-up with Angelats reminding the intern to get a CBC and chest X-ray on the patient. The patient arrived in the OR the next morning with the CBC but no chest X-ray, and anesthesia cancelled the case. Once again, Juan and the intern went over the patient with stress on the requirement for a chest X-ray. The next day, the patient went to the OR again, and again was rejected for lack of a chest film. This time, it was Dr. Bartizal who communicated with Angelats. He, in turn, attempted to make himself understood to the intern, who was adamant that he indeed had ordered a chest X-ray, not once but twice. When a review of the chart failed to reveal any evidence of a chest X-ray report, the junior resident and the intern went to the radiology department where the intern proudly found not one but two reports as well as the films, both bearing Dr. Wang's name, not the patient's. The patient was returned to the OR the following day with his own X-ray and received his colectomy.
—*Juan Angelats, MD, Personal Communication*

Dr. Leander Riba, one of the stalwarts of the urology attending staff, was very hard of hearing. When he scrubbed to help our chief resident, John Zumerchik, John would often do the case, muttering under his breath, "Look out Riba" or "Get your (blank) hands out of my way." Once the case was over, John would rush to find his dead, chewed-up cigar butt that was squirreled away, either in the cysto room or the OR, depending on where we were operating.
—*Kent Borkovec, MD, Personal Communication*

On Ward 60, one of the medical services, each new intern had a special mission. There was an elderly woman patient, who though she took up a bed, had no reason to be in the hospital. She had been in that bed for several years. All attempts to discharge her to home or a nursing facility were unsuccessful. She had an obscure medical condition. The attending MD had fractured her shoulder in a failed chiropractic manipulation, and didn't want to be sued.
—*Frank Folk, MD, Personal Communication*

Ed Dobie introduced me to urology and emphasized utilization of urethral catheters in three different patients before discarding them.
—*Jerrold Widran, MD, Personal Communication*

I remember that the elevator operators used to sell clothing and shoes on the elevators while the visitors and patients were being transported upstairs. The clothes were hung in neat rows on the handrails, and the elevator men would yell at people who leaned against them.

—*William Lindsey, MD, Personal Communication*

One of the great wonders of County was the tunnel system that allowed one to get throughout the whole of the County block from Harrison Street to Polk, and Wolcott to Wood Streets, without seeing the light of day or having to step even once in slush and snow. As medical students, we were always amazed at how adept the house staff was at negotiating these subterranean byways, popping up in exactly the place they needed to be on the first floor of the hospital.

—*Matthew Hyser, MD, Personal Communication*

During the early to mid 1960s, there was a surgical resident known much more for his surgical aggressiveness and desire to accumulate more cases than for his clinical expertise. One night when he was on the ER rotation, a woman was wheeled past him on a gurney, and the one lower extremity, which was protruding from the knee down out from under the blanket, was a deep purple. The resident shouted out, "Get that woman to surgery stat. She needs a venous embolectomy ASAP." The surgeon had spoken, so the patient was admitted to the next surgery ward up in the rotation, where the intern on call pulled down the blanket and found the patient to be purple from the costal margins to the soles of the feet, bilaterally. The vital signs, besides a negligible systolic pressure, were a temp of 105, a pulse of 120, and a history of a febrile illness in a family member that included hospitalization for temperature with headaches. The intern had the patient transferred to the Old Contagious Disease Hospital across Wolcott Avenue from Karl Meyer Hall, where the diagnosis of meningococcal meningitis was confirmed. The patient recovered and was discharged with both legs.

—*M. Craig Champion, MD, Personal Communication*

While writing about the practice of medicine at County during the Great Depression, Dr. William Beck, a former night surgeon in the Vaughan regime, remembered a family with an unemployed father that decided this was a good time to redecorate their home. The father, a painter by trade, was not displeased by this prospect and sipped wine as he painted everything in sight, including the bathroom. Nothing escaped his decoration, including the toilet seat. His daughter came home from work, and not recognizing her father's zeal, sat on the toilet but found herself unable to get up. Naturally, a plumber was called to solve the dilemma. He unscrewed the toilet seat and called for a police ambulance, which took the young lady to County. She was placed prone and modestly covered with a sheet. The intern was completely lost on how to deal with the situation, so he called the attending night surgeon, Dr. James J. Callahan, who in later years,

when he directed all his efforts to fracture management, would become an international figure in the field of orthopedic surgery. The intern removed the sheet and asked the surgeon whether he had ever seen anything like this. "Yes," replied Callahan quietly, "but never in a frame."
—William C. Beck, MD, Proc. Inst. Med. Chgo. Vol 40, 1987, p.138


The Greek's, a favorite eating establishment and watering hole for medical students, house staff, nurses, nursing students, and just about any type of allied health personnel known to man, was located directly across Harrison Street from the front door of the County Hospital. One summer evening in 1961, two County interns were sitting at a table in the Monkey Room, named for its frescos of monkeys depicting various medical and nursing activities. An orthopedic resident and his date for the evening, a striking senior nursing student who one of the interns had met while working on R-3 (the neurosurgery service), entered and occupied one side of a booth across the aisle. The intern from neurosurgery clearly was interested in visiting with the nursing student and observed that since the couple was sitting on the same side of the booth, the two interns could sit opposite them. He suggested this to his friend and also suggested that while he sat opposite the nursing student, his friend could sit opposite the resident and engage him in conversation about how to best apply for an ortho residency (which programs were best, and which attendings should be courted for recommendations). The friend, Dr. David Robbin, agreed, even though he was firmly committed to a career in ophthalmology, which he later pursued. The interns stepped across the aisle and struck up their respective conversations, which were successful in obtaining a raft of information about orthopedic training for Dr. Robbin and a date with the nursing student for his friend. This chance encounter resulted in the nurse and her intern ultimately eloping some 49 years ago. They are still married. The payback for Dr. Robbin was unlimited home-cooked dinners for him and girlfriends of his choice at the newlywed's house on Okinawa where both doctors were stationed in the military during the 1963-64 time period.
—Ken Printen, MD, Personal Experience


A patient was brought up from the ER to the neurosurgery ward where I was on duty. The patient presented with a screw through the calvarium into the grey matter. It was a Sunday afternoon, and I was the junior resident on call for neuro. Like any County surgeon I was in complete control. I didn't have a screwdriver, so I borrowed a dime from a visitor and screwed it out, layer returning the dime to the visitor. The patient did fine. The next day, Dr. Raimondi told me to never do that again. I was never sure whether he meant borrowing money from a visitor or screwing out the screw.
—Joseph O'Grady, MD, Personal Communication

## See One, Do One, Teach One
See one (preferably), do one (absolutely),
teach one (or write it up and stay out of the way)

One Friday evening in August of 1961, I was the intern on R-3 neurosurgery with Tom Murphy, at that time a general surgery R-2 but the most senior resident on the neurosurgery service. It was a typical summertime Friday night, with lots of folks getting hit on the head with beer bottles, becoming a bit unconscious, and being transported to County, where we saw to it that they got their mandatory carotid angios. In the midst of this, we got a call from one of the male fracture wards about a normally chipper old gentleman with a fractured humerus and long-arm cast who had fallen out of bed and was now densely comatose. I went to see him, confirmed the nurse's observations, put him on a gurney, and took him down for angios. Since we were so busy that night, we did the bilateral angios at one sitting and surprisingly found no shift of the pineal. We figured this meant the patient had bilateral subdurals, so Tom called the OR to schedule the case for bilateral burr holes under local and the night surgeon (Bob Eberle) for coverage. That done, I pushed the patient to OR and found Dr. Eberle waiting in white with a cap and mask. He helped me get the patient on the table, and by the time I had the patient prepped and draped, Murphy had arrived and was scrubbed, gowned, and gloved. We did the case under local, and as we hoped, found subdural hematomas on both sides, which we drained. Even more amazingly, the patient woke up while I was putting the dressing on post-operatively. The night surgeon had not scrubbed but did give us encouragement each time we found the predicted subdural. While Tom was typing the OP report, Eberle helped me get the patient on the gurney. As we were doing that, I commented that I thought he was going to help us do the operation. His response was a bit of night surgeon wisdom I never forgot, " I could see that you guys seemed to know what you were doing and were doing pretty well. Besides, I never rotated through neurosurgery." Moral of the story: Don't try to fix what's not broken, even if it requires that you actively do nothing.

—Ken Printen, MD, Personal Experience

I was a resident on Ward 34 fractures in 1957 when this guy came in with his distal femur sticking out of the back of his leg and a cold, pulseless lower leg. This was just after the Korean War, when vascular surgery was in its infancy. I called Joe Hincamp, who was the night surgeon. We reduced the dislocation, in a torrent of blood. Joe then applied a Potts clamp and sutured the artery. There was a prompt return of the dorsalis pedis pulse. We splinted the leg in 90 degrees of flexion and later extended it. A year later, he was fine. This was a good example of the sort of stuff we could do at night with minimal attending supervision.
—Raffensperger, JC, and Hincamp, J.,"Compound Dislocation of the Knee with Popliteal Artery Injury." Archives of Surgery, 1959, pp799-800.
—John Raffensperger, MD, Personal Communication

One Saturday morning, Dr. McNealy was performing a thyroidectomy for the postgraduate class, and I was the third assistant, crowded in between him and the anesthesiologist, holding a retractor to expose the upper part of the thyroid. Obviously, I was not doing it very well because at one point, McNealy stepped back and with hand outstretched, dramatically and loudly said, "Are you for me or against me in this operation?" much to the amusement of the audience.
—Frank Milloy, MD, Personal Communication

Speaking of thyroidectomies, I remember Nick Capos, one of Dr. Meyer's associates, standing behind me as I was doing one of my first thyroids. He kept whispering instructions in my ear. After one admonition to "Cut," I did, and the contents of the jugular vein filled the field. He then said, "Now, take care of it." I also learned a lot from him about how "money surgeons" thought. I was asked how I would manage a case of acute diverticulitis just when the one-, two-, or three-stage approach was quite a controversial topic. Capos opined, "Well, I know what they're writing at the universities, but if this were my banker's wife and I needed a loan, I'd do the tried and true."
—Charles Humphrey, MD, Personal Communication

In the early 1960s, there was a patient with a uretero-cutaneous fistula on the general surgical service on whom both the general surgeons and the urologists wanted to operate. An agreement was reached that if the urologists could slip a catheter up the ureter to serve as a splint, then no operation was necessary. The urologists tried to get a catheter up but couldn't, so they taped the catheter to the abdomen under a dressing, took X-rays, left a Foley in the bladder to drain urine, and transferred the patient to the urology ward where he was later operated.
—John Zumerchik, MD, Personal Communication

I had the privilege of working with Dr. Milloy just before his retirement. He staffed a case of a 23-year-old patient who required a median sternotomy and thymectomy for myasthenia gravis. I was somewhat uncertain of myself, and after the mediastinum was open, Dr. Milloy appeared in the room, looked over the ether screen—coffee in hand—and said, "Oh, Frank, it looks like it's going well. Did you read up on the case? If you have any trouble, I'll be in the coffee room." In the days of surgical giants, you did not rely on "surgical simulation" to get the job done. You just did it.
—Francis Podbielski, MD, Personal Communication

It was not uncommon for the night surgeon, responsible for all the cases done on his watch, to stretch out and catch a few winks between cases on the red couch in the OR dictating room. One night, while I was enjoying such a cat nap, my

junior resident, Jim Monks, expertly repaired a perforated peptic ulcer that we had examined together earlier in the evening. As I woke up, I saw a patient on a cart go by the door of the dictation room door toward recovery. "Who was that patient?" I asked Jim. "That was the case you just did," he replied.
—David Berger, MD, Personal Communication


In 1970, Bob Freeark and I made a movie for the American College of Surgeon's meeting. The case was that of a retrograde jejeuno-gastric intusussception. Freeark entitled the movie "Eating Your Guts Out."
—Charles M. Brown, MD, Personal Communication


Ken Printen was my senior resident on general surgery during my internship year in 1967–68. He talked me through my first and last-ever hernia surgery. Then he squirted me with the irrigation syringe during the closure. Must have been some kind of initiation rite.
—Gary Waters, MD, Personal Communication


I remember Dr. Gonzales requiring us to wear loupes to do hand cases. But if Dr. Hall was covering, he would yell at us for having them on and insisted we remove them.
—David Butler, MD, Personal Communication


Several surgical residents who morphed into plastic surgeons remember nurses swatting flies with sterile towels in the OR, as well as the cancellation of the elective OR schedule because of too many flying insects in the OR.
—Jeffery D. Friedman, MD, and David Jansen, MD, Personal Communication


I went to Cleveland with Bob Freeark to present my first paper to a surgical society (the Central Surgical Society). The paper was titled The Partially Severed Artery. We hadn't written the paper yet so Bob just told me to cram some papers in an envelope and give it to the Society secretary as I went up to give the talk. After the presentation, he said, "We better write the paper." The next day, with the paper written and typed, he told me to hand it in, get the old envelope back, and say "We made a few changes!" Bob Freeark. What a guy. No one was cooler.
—Jack Saletta, MD, Personal Communication


My first encounter with Dr. Irving Bush as the new chairman of urology was as his assistant in a transurethral resection of the prostate (TURP). When he wanted me to insert my finger in the rectum of the patient to serve as a guide while he did the procedure, I refused. This definitely started our relationship out on the wrong foot.
—Mel Simon, MD, Personal Communication

I was granted independent operating privileges by Drs. Freeark and Stevens one-half the way through my second year of the Northwestern orthopedic program. This probably would not even be considered today, but it worked well in 1966.
—Donald W. Lydden Jr., MD, Personal Communication


There was a patient or Ward 60 with an empyema for whom I could never seem to get OR time to do a thoracotomy and decortication. After two weeks in the hospital with spiking temperatures to 104 degrees, the intern and I armed ourselves with 20 mgms of morphine, local anesthetic, a scalpel, and a suction device. I did my first and only bedside thoracotomy and decortication (no telemetry, of course). Ultimately, the joke was on me as it was a tuberculous empyema. I still remain PPD negative, a miracle given my experiences at County. Its place as a legendary training center in American surgery is richly deserved.
—Francis Podbielski, MD, Personal Communication


Sometime in 1979 I saw a 20-year-old male in the ER in shock with a stab wound in the precordium. I paged Dr. Jack Roberts, the chief resident in thoracic-cardiovascular surgery, and took the patient directly to the OR. County was not routinely doing open-heart surgery at that time, and try as we might, we could not get the sterna saw to work. We had to use the Leubke knife and mallet to do the sternotomy. We fixed the right ventricular laceration, and the patient went home on post-op day four. The next week's resident's conference was more heavily populated with attendings than residents, and no resident brought a case with slides. So rather than stare at each other in silence, I grabbed some chalk and an eraser, went to the blackboard, and presented the case. It nicely filled the hour.
—James Gianfrancisco, MD, Personal Communication


While on the subject of performing stressful operations, I recall doing Dr. Olga Jonasson's carpal tunnel release when she was chief of surgery at County.
—Salil Rajmaira, MD, Personal Communication


I was on call as a junior resident when Dr. Bob Freeark walked into the urology emergency examining room as I was checking out a patient with obvious urinary retention and extravasation. He said, " I will cystotomize this patient myself if you aren't going to do anything." Without wasting a second, I wheeled the patient to the OR and did the suprapubic cystotomy myself.
—Mel Simon, MD, Personal Communication


Dr. David M. Berger vividly remembers his first "do one" as it pertains to endoscopic pediatric esophageal foreign body removal. It was in the middle of the

night, with instructions being given on the phone by John Raffensperger, likely from the call room at the Hines VA Hospital.
—*David M. Berger, MD, Personal Communication*


The first patient admitted to the trauma unit was a 13-year-old boy named Reynaldo Coleman who fell from a 12th story window. He had bilateral talar fracture dislocations compounded through the soles of both feet and bilateral compound fractures of the femurs at the knees. In addition, he had hemoptysis, hypoxia, and clouded consciousness. He underwent tracheotomy with improvement in his overall status, then thoracotomy that revealed no aortic transaction, and exploratory laparotomy that revealed a ruptured spleen for which he got a splenectomy and appendectomy. Several days later, he underwent bilateral burr holes for subdural hematomas, and was ultimately discharged from the hospital. Surgeons involved were John Raffensperger attending and Mike Fitzgerald resident.
—*Michael Fitzgerald, MD, Personal Communication*


One Friday afternoon in late summer 1968, I and my attending, Dr. David Movitz, were scrubbing for what was scheduled as an exploratory laparotomy but was, as everyone in the OR knew, an abdominal hysterectomy. The fifth that I had scheduled for that week. In the midst of our scrub-time small talk, Dr. Abraham F. Lash burst into the scrub room, demanding to know if I realized this was the fifth hysterectomy I had scheduled electively for that week. I said that I was and then looked at my attending for moral support, but Dr. Movitz, who was a nonconfrontational person, kept looking straight ahead and continued washing his hands without comment. Caught red-handed, as it were, I reminded Dr. Lash that I had been his junior resident for three months on Ward 40 some years previously, and he had been the one who taught me how to do hysterectomies. This didn't make him any less angry, though he did acknowledge the fact of his mentorship, and added that "You're good at it, but what really makes me angry is, where do you find all these women to operate for fibroids?" The answer, which I didn't give him until six weeks later, when I was an attending, was quite simple. In the old Fantus Clinic, the surgery and gyn clinics were on the same floors but in different wings. So we just sent our medical students to visit with the gyn patients in the hall, and if it turned out they were there to be evaluated for "fireballs," the students shuttled them into the surgery clinic from where they were worked up and admitted for surgery.
—*Ken Printen, MD, Personal Experience*


Dr. Abcarian was doing a periodic proctoscopy and fulguration of polyps on a patient who had undergone a colectomy and ileorectal anastamosis for familial polyposis. When he hit the cautery to burn a polyp, there was a loud explosion as flame came rushing out of the scope. That's when I learned that the first rule of proctology is "Stand to the Side."
—*Don Read, MD, Personal Communication*

In the mid-1960s, one of the more aggressive interns on general surgery convinced his resident that he was well experienced with the placement of chest tubes. Therefore, when the next patient who needed a chest tube for pneumothorax showed up on the ward, the intern, with the help of a willing medical student, was turned loose to place the tube. It turned out that his experience was vastly overstated, but as a result of his dead-eye tube placement, he was able to first-assist for the first time on a splenectomy performed by the junior resident.
—David M. Berger, MD, Personal Communication


Long before Dr. Hernand Abcarian was a world-famous colon and rectal surgeon, he arrived from Iran as a bright but sometimes bewildered intern on Ward 60, the Illinois surgical ward staffed mostly by former Rush staff men who had migrated to the university faculty when Rush closed in the 1940s. Abcarian was the intern on the service of an attending who enjoyed less-than-favored status among the senior residents, so the service was slow and the cases usually limited to hernias, leg amputations, and decubitus ulcers. The trickle-down of even these cases to the intern was not up to Dr. Abcarian's expectations. Finally, a 90-year-old blind man was admitted with vague lower abdominal pain and bilateral nonincarcerated inguinal hernias, a hungry surgical intern's dream. Work-up for any other pathology proved negative, so in due course, the attending was called to examine the patient and agreed that he and his intern should repair both hernias on the next available operating day. On the appointed day, the patient was taken to the operating room, and some four-and-a-half hours later, a visibly shaken Dr. Abcarian returned to the ward with a tale of huge scrotal hernias, extensive dissection to remove the sacs, and a huge dressing around the scrotum that he had been instructed to change twice a day and keep the attending informed about patient progress. This course of action was dutifully carried out for the next week with little change in patient status except for an exponential increase in appetite and a change in character of the Penrose drain wound output from sero-sanguinous to dirty brown. The chief resident suggested removal of the drains and the intern complied. When the drains were pulled, a long strip of mummifying but unmistakable gonadal tissue exited from each of the scrotal drain incisions. When Abcarian relayed this information to the attending, there was a notable hesitation before the usual questions about his overall status. Since the patient was eating, had no more lower abdominal pain, and was afebrile, the advice from the Michigan Avenue office was to proceed with plans for nursing home placement ASAP. This was accomplished without delay and the patient discharged as improved.
—Hernand Abcarian, MD, and Ken Printen, MD, Personal Communication


Dr. Gerry Moss, one of the past chairmen of surgery at County, used to tell the following story on himself. In the days before bariatric surgery, he was doing a laparotomy on a 500-pound man for whom they had to put two OR tables together. The surgeons made a midline incision and kept going deeper and deeper into the fat until they finally saw the blue sheets that had been placed on the OR

table. Clearly, the surgeons had missed the abdomen completely. Nonplused, they turned the patient over and closed the wounds in his back. On the second try, they successfully entered the abdominal cavity.
—*Don R. Read, MD, Personal Communication*


I operated on a patient with a ruptured ectopic pregnancy who had no palpable pulse or blood pressure at the express insistence of Dr. Augusta Webster, the chief of OB/GYN, who was scrubbed as first assistant. The anesthesiologist refused to give any anesthetic, but we proceeded, and though she had no recorded blood pressure until 20 minutes post-op, she made a complete recovery. This proves the adage that it is better to operate on people who are young and basically healthy rather than those who are old and baseline sick.
—*William Jones, MD, Personal Communication*


One night in the intern year of 1962-63, things were rather slowly, and the night surgeon, Ed Quartetti, in a fit of desperation, made rounds on his ward to see if there were any patients in need of surgical intervention who could be helped that night. Surprisingly, he found three men who were in need of lower extremity amputations. He told his intern, a small-town country boy from Iowa, to get them ready for surgery. The plan would be that Quartetti would do the first one, the intern would do the second, and the operator for the third would depend on how the first two went and whether time was of the essence. The first amputation went smoothly, according to plan. Before beginning the second one, the intern protested that he was already set on going back to the University of Iowa for an internal medicine residency, and that the needs of medical education might be better served by letting an intern or junior resident who was going into surgery or orthopedics do the case. His reasoning fell on deaf ears, so he did the case with Quartetti as the first assistant. While they were closing the skin and putting on the posterior splint, the anesthesiologist, Dr. Manny Guererro, who had done a year of surgery and a year of pathology in preparation for an orthopedic residency, leaned over the ether screen and said, "You know, I haven't done a leg amputation for a year and I don't want to get rusty. How about if I do the next one?" This was agreeable to all parties, so Manny did the third case with the intern as first assistant and Quartetti as the anesthesiologist. The patients all did well. The intern returned to Iowa for his medicine residency and 45 years of practice in Iowa City, Manny stayed in anesthesia and practiced for 40 years in Rock Island, Illinois, and Ed Quartetti finished the surgery residency in June of 1963. Not quite a case of "see one, do one, teach one," but close enough for government work.
—*M. Craig Champion, MD, Personal Communication*


The plastic surgery service in the 1950s and 1960s was more known for its expertise with head and neck tumors and reconstructive surgery than for its efforts in the field of cosmesis. When breast augmentation and reduction became more mainstream, Bill Hagstrom, one of the fellows on the service, went on a personal crusade to visit the Cicero strip clubs at least once a week to explain the benefits of this type of surgery to the performers. This resulted in a marked increase in volume on the plastics service and a greater appreciation for the finer aspects of this type of dancing on the part of the aficionados, who frequented these clubs.

—*Name withheld by Request*


In the late 1950s and early 1960s, the Loyola student surgical rotations included time on both the urology and orthopedic services. Part of the urology time was spent in the Fantus Clinic learning the ancient art of urethral dilatation for a variety of conditions mostly related to long forgotten episodes of STDs, usually gonorrhea. One afternoon with Dr. Gene McEnery, the first-year GU resident as our leader, several of us Loyola students were passing Van Buren sounds for the good of mankind. We worked side by side in little cubicles separated from our classmates and other patients by draw curtains. Usually, the procedures were completed quickly and quietly with a maximum of K-Y jelly and a minimum of force exerted on the sound. However, that afternoon, the patient next to my cubicle seemed to be having a difficult time of it and was making a lot of noise. Finally, after what seemed an eternity, a pudgy little bald man edged out from behind the curtains, clad in boxer shorts with a bit of blood on the front and a sweat-soaked t-shirt. He was followed by my classmate, fully clad but equally sweaty. The patient was quite chatty and thanked his sounder for what to him had been the best treatment he had undergone for his stricture in 20 years. The student, Ray Burrell, who would later become the chief of OB/GYN at the Marshfield Clinic, responded lamely and asked the man to get dressed while he checked with the resident. Ray explained the case to Dr. McEnery, who had some trouble suppressing a grin, and then asked Ray to show him the sound he had used. The instrument was produced, then the resident picked up a Van Buren sound and asked if anyone could see a difference between the two instruments. Even to our eyes, it was apparent that the Van Buren was smooth and tapered at its business end, while the follower for the filiform that Ray had used was finely threaded to connect to the filiform. The patient was called in and asked how he felt. Fine was the answer. His abdomen was nontender, so he was given the admonition to drink a lot of water and not worry about the little bit of blood he would likely pass with urination for the next several days, since it should clear. If it didn't, he was to return to the clinic. He didn't call or come back, but to be completely sure he would be okay, we had written down his name and checked the obits in the Chicago papers for the next two weeks. His name never appeared.

—*Ken Printen, MD, Personal Experience*


One day in the fall of 1973, as a hard-working and eager senior medical student on the trauma unit, I had the opportunity to assist Dr. Bob Lowe in the performance of his first-ever Whipple procedure for a gunshot wound of the pancreas. After the case, Bob took us to the Greek's for lunch, and I changed my interest in medical neurology to surgery and have never looked back.

—*James L. Stone, MD, Personal Communication*

In the early 1960s, the concept of a total abdominal colectomy with or without anastamosis for massive lower GI bleeding of causes not demonstrable at laparotomy was quite the new thing. One night, the runner called his night surgeon to report that he a case of massive lower GI bleeding that required several units of blood and showed no signs of resolving his problem in the face of a diminishing hemoglobin. The instructions came back to get the patient to the OR with all possible haste. This was done, and the patient underwent the standard colectomy with anastamosis and without incident. The patient was stable in the recovery room but shortly after arrival was noted to be exhibiting signs of massive lower GI bleeding once again. The first-year resident was called and confirmed the presence of bleeding. After the perineum was cleaned up and the linen changed, he spread the patient's legs and elevated the knees. To everyone's amazement, a large profusely bleeding hemorrhoid immediately popped into view and was treated with the appropriate suturing and removal. The patient suffered no further bleeding and was discharged as improved.

—*Edwin J. Carey, MD, Personal Communication*

## Quotable Quotes

"All I want is license plate #105." An often-heard response from Dr. Frank Milloy when asked what he most wanted in post-residency years. Dr. Meyer had #106.
—*Submitted by Dr. Frank Folk*

"If you take 100 patients to the OR at County and trim their toenails, two of them would not come back." Dr. Bob Freeark at the tumor board in response to a boastful surgeon citing his superior results with neurosurgical procedures.
—*Submitted by Dr. Jim Kenned*

"You can bullshit other people, but don't bullshit yourself." Dr Manuel Lichtenstein's comment on a surgeon's self-assessment of clinical skills.
—*Submitted by Dr. Frank Folk*

"You just have one stitch down there." Dr. Phillip Williams' consistent response when asked by new mothers about the size of their episiotomies. (The one stitch was almost always the whole length of a 2/0 chromic suture).
—*Submitted by Dr. Ken Printen*

"Only insecure surgeons yell at scrub nurses." Dr. Bob Baker discussing OR decorum with the residents.
—*Submitted by Dr. Jim Kennedy*

"Save lives and stamp out disease." The motto of Dr. Tom Murphy.
—*Submitted by Dr. Floyd Okada*


"You know, in this case, it would be nice to get longitudinal sections of the spinal cord. Lichtenstein, be sure to take down his name and address." Dr. George B. Hassin, attending neurologist to his resident Dr. Ben Lichtenstein after examining a patient with unusual manifestations of Tabes Dorsalis on Ward 4.
—*Submitted by Dr. Zigmond Lebensohn in the Alumni Newsletter, Dec., 1987*


"Give more blood." Dr. George Holmes; advice on treatment of persistent hemothorax after the sun went down.
—*Submitted by Dr. David Berger*


There were several references to the camaraderie among attending and the fact that though there were often differences of opinion about specifics of case management, there were few instances of outright criticism of peers in the circle of attendings. The comments were more circuitous like this quote ascribed to Manny Lichtenstein given in answer to a resident's question about the opinion of one of the lesser lights in the program. Pointing at the concrete floor, he said," See that floor? Think you can grow corn on it?"
—*Submitted by Dr. Frank Folk*


"Oozers are losers."
—*Attributed to both Dr. Jimmy Yao and Dr. Joe Carey by a large number of 1960s residents*


"I don't care what they say." Attributed to Dr. William Shoemaker, MD, when discussing the opinions of other attendings about surgical treatment of diseases that did not square with his own ideas.
—*Submitted by Dr. Joe Carey*


"These are the Golden Days, and this is the Club Car of the Gravy Train." Words of encouragement to the internship class of 1949 from senior intern Ed Hayes, MD.
—*Submitted by Frank Folk, MD*


"The assistant is supposed to assist." Words of encouragement to a bewildered resident from Dr. Manny Lichtenstein.
—*Submitted by Dr. Bill Briney*

"You can always cut more off." The mantra of many of the attendings in the fledgling days of vascular surgery, usually following a sympathectomy and a fem-pop bypass ( the original Baker's Triad).
 —*Submitted by several of the residents of the 1967*


"What do you do when you don't know? Raise the hood and look." A bit of Dr. George Holmes' philosophy on the reason for exploratory thoracotomy.
 —*Submitted by Dr. Bill Briney*


"DOCTOR." In a piercing nasal whine before any verbal communication with a surgical resident. Miss Ruth Gressitt, RN Supervisor, Children's OR.
 —*Name withheld by Request*


"Lay it all out." Advice from Dr. Manny Lichtenstein on how to make sure the pathology was identified completely.
 —*Submitted by Dr. Joe Carey*


Dr. Lichtenstein used the following comment to preface one of his published papers: "For those who understand, no explanation is required. For those who do not understand, no explanation will suffice."
 —*Submitted by Dr. David Berger*


"We need to separate the patient from his disease." The guiding principal of Head and Neck Tumor surgery according to Orion Stuteville, DDS, MD.
 —*Submitted by Dr. Ken Printen*


"Modern, aggressive surgery has made the hospital a hotel for the temporary care of the vivisected. All that the surgeon cares for is a room for his patient to occupy during the three or four weeks while recovering from his or her incisions. The patient then may then go home and get well or live a life of invalidism, as it happens."
 —*Bayard Holmes, as quoted by Dr. Norman Barnsby in "Medical Chaos and Crime," New York: Kennerly, 1910*


"...the very serious crimes that are committed by absolutely ignorant men must be prevented by the men who have force and character." Comments by Albert Ochsner, MD, on the lack of ethical behavior of the nontrained would-be surgeons in many cities in the early 20th century.
 —*Discussion, 63rd annual meeting of the AMA, JAMA 1912;59:1677*

"We had attendings who really cared, residents who were very good (mostly), interns who worked, and memories that I will never forget, even if I wanted to. I learned my science, art, and craft at Cook County Hospital."
—Submitted by Dr. Alfred J. Kobak, Jr. (No one said it better.)

"If you are going to get hurt, do it in Illinois." Comments by Senator Charles Percy, Speaking of the Cook County Hospital's initiatives in trauma management (Congressional Record., Oct.14, 1972, S 18315, United States Senate).
—Submitted by Dr. David Boyd

"Don't get emotional, sonny." Quote attributed to Dr. Jimmy Yao as a useful tool to tone down arguments, usually about patient care.
—Submitted by Dr. David Berger

## The Human Side of Being a Surgical Resident

In the late 1940s and 1950s, an intern's pay was $15 per month plus room, board, and laundry. Not much, but there were other desirable programs that paid nothing. In any case, the pay was hardly adequate for a single intern, but what about the small number who were foolish enough to be married? When my entrepreneurial father-in-law asked me about my intern's salary, I honestly told him, "Fifteen dollars a month." He pretended to believe me. When his accountant did our taxes the next spring, he no longer had to pretend. He knew. Two years later on my being appointed to the surgical residency, he showed that he was proud of me. He again dared to ask, "How much are you making now?" "Thirty dollars a month," I honestly replied. An uncomfortable pause followed. Then generously, he said, "Well, I guess you can't beat a hundred percent increase." For the moment, he handled the bad news quite well, and we had no further discussions about income. However, he died within six months. I think the bad news killed him.
—Frank Folk, MD, Personal Communication

In the 1960s, at various times, Ed Carey, Jimmy Yao, and Ken Printen intermittently shared the same suite of rooms on the 15th floor of Karl Meyer Hall next to the apartment occupied by the hospital warden, Fred Hertwig and his wife. The suite became the repository and swap shop for discarded whites, mostly clothes but shoes as well, and the occasional other items of apparel that departing residents did not feel they would need again. One of the alums recalled an occasion on which he needed a suit-coat and tie for a special occasion on the weekend, but he didn't have either in his wardrobe. He proceeded to the 15th floor, knocked on the door, and was invited to browse through the collection of what now was called "flashy trash" for the appropriate items. Suitably attired, he was able to cut a dashing presence at his social engagement.

—Miguel Teresi, MD, Personal Communication

I met my wife, Sumiko Tsukamura, MD, on internal medicine and married her October 12, 1968. We were allowed to move to adjoining rooms in Karl Meyer Hall so we could share the bathroom.

—Gene Hamilton, MD, Personal Communication

The fatal stabbing of one of our interns—I think on Ward 24—by a crazy, irate patient, was perhaps the worst thing that happened. His family were refugees from Poland who had worked hard to see to it that he became a doctor (he had been accepted to the medicine residency at the Mayo Clinic). I think he was Dick Brinkley's intern.

—Donald Dexter, MD, Personal Communication

One afternoon, while working on neurosurgery as an intern, I was informed of a tragedy on Ward 24. I ran over, and lying on the floor was intern Bruno Epstein with a stab wound in the epigastric area of the abdomen. He had been stabbed by a disgruntled Chinese patient who had a recent hernia repair. Two residents, Bill Cahill and Don Dexter, were attending to him, but to no avail. At the end of the year, during the annual intern and resident dinner, I was awarded the First Annual Bruno Epstein Achievement Award as intern of the year. It came with a nice plaque and a check for $125.

—Roger A. Ott, MD, Personal Communication

Most of the married interns and residents had wives who worked. Only one of the female interns was married, to a doctor. Besides local apartments, housing was available through the Medical Center District, which had bought up condemned local buildings in anticipation of new development. Our third-floor walk-up rented for $20 per month, unheated. We had an oil heater, but the oil tank was in the basement, so that meant lugging the full oil can up four flights during the Chicago winter. One space heater didn't quite make the four rooms cozy, and it was drafty, but it was home. The apartment was in a rough neighborhood, with frequent fighting in the streets and adjacent buildings. One night, after coming home from being on call, my wife told me of a shooting in a nearby house: lots of excitement, complete with sirens and police activity. Another night, a chain gang of men stole a load of cement bags from a stack on Paulina Street and threw them into a nearby truck. This was a rather common West Side activity in those days. The utility meter reader nervously asked my wife about the place directly across the street on the northeast corner of Paulina and Polk. "They sent me into the back where the meter was. Do you know, they had stiffs (dead bodies) there?"

We did know. It was the site of the Illinois Demonstrators Association, which provided cadavers for the medical schools. Knowing they were not murderers was reassuring, but the odor in hot weather was a pungent reminder of who the occupants were.

Our third-floor apartment had a rickety back porch that faced east and gave a marvelous view of the downtown Chicago skyline. Being one of the marrieds, it fell to us to hold occasional parties out there with a dozen or more fellow house staff and their dates (I cringe when I read about the deadly porch fallings these days). Our friends referred to that porch as the "West Side Tip-Top Tap," pirating the name of the roof-top bar at Michigan Avenue's Allerton Hotel, one of our occasional date sites. Another favorite place for an outing was Don the Beachcomber's downtown. We referred to it as the CPIT, the cheapest place in town. You could buy a round of drinks (usually Mai Tais) and nurse one for hours. The original Pizzeria Uno (long before there was a Due) on Wabash was another favorite, for much the same reason: good food and an overwhelming tolerance of minimal purchasers.

—Frank Folk, MD, Personal Communication

Sunday dinners at Karl Meyer Hall were always special for the interns and residents and their families. After not seeing much of the doctors all week, the moms would dress up the children and meet the dads for a lovely free dinner together. Remember, in those days, the interns were paid $25 a month. I did this with my children for several years. After a morning church service, we drove down the Congress Expressway to meet Dad. Once we asked if we could see his room on the seventh floor. Dr. John Boswick shared a bathroom with him in what was grand;y called a suite. He and his family were good friends of ours. June Boswick often brought her children, as did Evelyn Norcross, the wife of Dr. Bill Norcross. All of these doctors were at the dinner table, and they explained to us that they could be expelled if they ever let a woman into the men's call rooms, so we never went. After one dinner, I remember saying good-bye as my husband walked across the street to the hospital to do two leg amputations on a hot, humid summer afternoon with no air conditioning, But they could open the windows in the operating rooms.

—Mrs. Ardythe (Marv ) Tiesenga, Personal Communication

The nurses' residence at the northwest corner of Wolcott and Polk Streets, immediately next door to Karl Meyer Hall, was, for most of the County house staff, much like the great city of Minas Tirith in *The Lord of the Rings,* assailable but largely impenetrable. It followed the grand design of the early 20th century nurses' residences such as St. Luke's and Michael Reese, with grandiose entryways and vast second-floor parlors with sofas, over-stuffed chairs, patrolling house mothers, and, many times for added protection in the later evening hours, a smattering of off- and on-duty Chicago police officers. In early 1962, when nursing students were still forbidden to marry before graduation from the County

Nursing School, one of the senior students was hospitalized in the nurses' infirmary on the 15th floor of the residence with a high fever and a viral infection. Her soon–to-be-husband was a County intern who thought it might cheer her up if he stopped by to visit. Accordingly, he borrowed a clean, long white coat from one of his resident friends (interns, of course, wore short white coats, if they had coats at all), put on a white shirt with necktie, and a pair of dress slacks, traded his grey-brown white bucks for a pair of loafers, and marched up the stairs of the nurses' residence with his stethoscope prominently displayed in the side pocket of his lab coat. When the elevator came, he stepped in. When it stopped on the second floor, the policeman on duty, after surveying the occupants of the car, asked him what he thought he was doing. He replied, "I'm the resident on Dr. Afermow's (director of the nurses' infirmary) service, and I have to check on a nursing student with a high fever and a virus infection." Satisfied, the officer let the car pass, and when the doors opened on the top floor, the nurses on duty, who knew both the doctor and his lady, kindly showed him the way to her room. After appropriate time for consultation and consolation on her sickness, the intern left in the same way he had entered, stopping to thank the officer on the second floor and reassuring him that the student nurse seemed to be suffering from nothing serious.

—Ken Printen, MD, Personal Experience

In the early 1960s, one intern's wife was lucky enough to land a job as a substitute teacher in the Chicago school system, and since her husband had to use the car to get to the hospital, she took public transportation to her teaching assignments, which were likely to be at different locations in the inner city each day. She developed a liking for the *Sun-Times* newspaper since it allowed her to carry her pistol unnoticed from place to place. Being a west Texas lady, she knew how to use the weapon but never had the occasion, although she may have been close the time that her husband, who occupied one of the seats in the high-stakes house-staff poker game, had to tell her that he had a bad night and had lost both their checks in the card game.

—E. Boone Brackett, MD, Personal Communication

John Raffensperger has written about the "Old Lady of Harrison Street" where no one was refused hospitalization and everyone got state-of-the-art treatment, whether medical or surgical. Attending physicians from the faculties of nearly all the medical schools of Chicago who were able to pass the County qualifying exams trained the resident physicians, who lined up to learn from the likes of John Keeley, Morris Friedell, Robert Schmitz, and innumerable others who were supervised under the aegis of Karl Meyer's close supervision to become the next generation of "Captains of the Art." Financial and professional pressures were as stringent then as they are now, but not one of the staff of doctors who served as attending or associate, to my knowledge, drew a salary. They were true volunteers. Let's take a step back. Let's re-invigorate the philosophy that was best seen in the "County way" of thinking that has been seemingly lost. Let us give back to

Medicine what has been lost: its heritage to heal the sick. We must take this step back in order to take the next step forward in our profession of medicine.
—*Edwin S. Sinaiko, MD, Personal Communication*

The Greek's, of course, was the restaurant directly across Harrison Street from the hospital. The joint was always jumping, and the owners were very kind to the interns and residents. Many times, they would give you a free meal if you were a little behind on your check. Or if you needed a loan, it was the place. There was a Greek's when my father was at County in the 1920s, and it was an institution.
—*Howard Traisman, intern, 1946, quoted by Dr. John Raffensperger in* The Old Lady on Harrison Street, *1997, p. 203*

## Photo Memoir

For a collection of historic photographs of Cook County Hospital and a memoir of the people mentioned in this book, visit the website, *A History of Surgery at Cook County Hospital: Photo Memoir* by James S.T. Yao, MD, at www.cchphotomemoir.com.

# *Appendices*

# List of Surgical Residents at Cook County Hospital

This is an alphabetical list by decades of residents that we obtained from the sheets returned in response to our call for information. Spellings are as we received them. Identifying residents from the 1930s through 1960s is difficult because of the turmoil of WWII and Korea in the late 40s and early 50s, and then the pretty much universal physician draft for Vietnam which actually began in the mid-1950s until the 1960s. My criteria for inclusion in a group was that if I knew them as a resident when I was an intern or resident they fit in the 50s or 60s, if they finished before I was an intern in 1961, they fell into the 1930s –50s category.

—Ken Printen

**1930s–1940s**

Robert J. Baker
George Bard
Barkley Bell
Richard Bodie
John Boswick
Eugene Broccolo
William Cahill
Leo Cigerroa
--- Cohen
Donald Dexter
Birney Dibble
Edward Donohue
Sidney Duke
Robert Freeark
Frank Folk
Al Fortman
William Frymark, Sr.
Aaron R. Grossman
Edward Goldberg
Jay Gubler
Joseph Hincamp
William Hobbins
John Howser
James Kane, Sr.
Arnold Kaplan
Jack Kerrigan
--- Kligensmith
James Long
W.S. (Sam) Lorimer

Carl Lum
--- Markovin
William Marshall
Robert Mason
William Mayer
Gordon McCoy
Frank Milloy
Kathy Mogan
William Moss
Everett Nicholas
Bill Norcross
John B. O'Donohue, Jr.
Arthur Poppins
--- Posey Brothers
John Raffensperger
William Reed
William Requarth
Harry Richter(?)
Eli Samet
Thomas Samuels
Bud Shannon
--- Sannan
--- Shropshire
Philip Sheridan, Sr.
Thomas Sheridan
Irving(Bud) Stein
--- Tanov
Marvin Tiesinga

## 1950s and 1960s

Hernand Abcarian
Joseph Amato
James Andre
James Apostol
Francis Banich
John Bartizal
Robert Bass
David Berger
Ed Beheler
David Boyd
William Briney
Brown Brooks
Charles Brown
Edwin Carey
James Carey
Joseph Carey
Roy Cooksey
Richard Corley
Frank Descourouez
William Dippel
Robert Eberle
Rostram Fardin
Mike Fitzgerald
Leonard Gravier
William Hagstrom
Ernestine Hambrick
Irving Harris
Lloyd Henry
Arthur Howell
Charles Jackson
James Kennedy
Harry King
L.K. Kho
Edwin Kissell
Leo Lim
Bernard Lininger
Arthur Lurie
Takayoshi Matsuda
Alan Middelpunkt
Richard Mladick
James Monks
David Monson
Thomas Murphy
Tassos Nassos
Paul O'Brien

Floyd Okada
Roger Ott, Sr.
Kenneth Printen
Max Raminofsky
Hernan Reyes
Philip Ruffalo
Jack Saletta
Edward Saltzstein
Harvey Saunders
Siroos Shirazi
Dale Snyder
Harry Springer
Leon Starkman
David Stern
Conrad Tasche
Philip Taxman
Miguel Teresi
Robert Vanecko
Raymond Warpeha
Sherwin Weiss
Frederick Wentzel
Theodore Will
James ST Yao

## 1970s

Juan Angelats
Samuel Appavu
John Barrett
Leonard Block
Cyril Chrabot
James BeBord
Donna Camara
Bernardo Duarte
Mohammed Eftaiha
Festus Enumah
Larry Ferguson
James Gianfrancisco
Makund Godbole
Harris Goldberg
George Hrycelak
Bruce Irvine
Joseph Janik
Mohammed Jawad
Manohar Jethani
Mazin Kaheeb

Sarath Kumar
Serat Kumar
J. Lakhsmanan
William Lindsey
Bob Lowe
---Mostafi
Jon Nicosia
Colarthur Palani
Leela Prasad
Jay Radakrishnan
Don Read
Cesar Romero
Robert Rose
Alfred Rossi
Sam Sadow
Robert Schoenwald
James Schuler
Sushil Sethi
Peter Smiley
Vernon Strand
Joseph Thornton
Niauha Udenye
Helen Wiedemer
Nabil Yamut

## 1980s

Robert Aki
Robert Andrews
William Barnes
Eric Bass
Juan Bonilla
Keith Bowman
Susan Briley
Robert Buras
Jerome Cahill
James Dogholty(sp)
Guy Edelman
Richard Fantus
Jeffery Friedman
William Frymark
Patrick Gartland
Loretto Glynn
Robin Graham
Pat Graham

Victor Guerriero
David Jackson
Richard Keen
William Kiener
Michael Kikta
Paul Klazura
Leonard Lapkin
Al Mitsos
Gosel Mohammed
Thomas Nelson
Timothy Nypaver
Alfonso Oliva
--- Pisarelli
Daniel Resnick
Philip Rosett
Thomas Rossi
Jeffery Schwartz
Mindy Statter
--- Vishwanath
John Weiland

## 1990s

Ros Bareni
Steven Bonomo
Lawrence Gibson
Timothy LeSeye
Howard Posson

## 2000s

Mitchell Cohen
Nadav Dujovny
Nadine(Duhan)Floyd
Anthony Kim
Jennifer Manders
John Meyers
Fred Starr
John Tope, Jr.
Herbert Trace
Fabian Udeku
David Yocum
Norman Young
Warren Yenn

# County Ortho Residents

## 1950s and 60s
### (Dr. Fred Shapiro, MD Chief)

Dr. William Newman, MD
Dr. Allen Murphy, MD
Dr. John Gleason, MD
Dr. Jerry Loftus, MD
Dr. William Kelly, MD
Dr. Leo Quinn
Dr. Morris Stamler

## 1970 to 1980
### (Dr. Arsen Pankovich, MD Chief)

Dr. Spiros Stamelos, MD
Dr. Prabhakar Gadry, MD
Dr. Richard Pearson, MD
Dr. Richard Egwele, MD
Dr. Mitchell Goldflies, MD
Dr. Mysore Shivarem, MD
Dr. John McClellan, MD
Dr. Christopher Dangles, MD
Dr. Imed Tarabishy, MD
Dr. Mark Lorenz, MD
Dr. Jorge Prieto, MD
Dr. Clayton Perry, MD
Dr. David Mann, MD
Dr. William Lowery, MD
Dr. Kenneth Davenport, MD
Dr. Steven Traina, MD

## 1980s
### (Dr. William Hall, MD Chief)

Dr. David Butler, MD
Dr. Henry Fuentes, MD
Dr. Jerry Dzwinyk, MD
Dr. David Witham, MD
Dr. John Burna, MD
Dr. Robert Nelson, MD
Dr. Salil Rajmaira, MD
Dr. David Phillips, MD
Dr. Daniel Edwards, MD
Dr. Thomas Becker, MD

# Compendium of Cook County Hospital Trauma Unit (CCHTU) Published Literature

The following is a compendium of selected literature published by CCHTU leadership professionals during their active period and important related experiences. This list was compiled from MEDLINE searches and through acquisitions of several curricula vitae. It is not intended as an exhaustive listing of all CCHTU related works. We have excluded textbook contributions, published abstracts and presentations, of which there are many. These publications are listed chronologically and generally organized by first, prominent contributor or last author.

## Robert J. Baker[1-22]

1. Baker RJ, Dippel WF, Freeark RJ, Strohl, EL. The surgical significance of trauma to the pancreas. *Arch Surg*. Jun 1963;86:1038-1043.
2. Baker RJ, Shoemaker WC, Suzuki F, Freeark RJ, Strohl EL. Low molecular weight dextran therapy in surgical shock, part i. control group and shock patients resuscitated prior to low molecular weight dextran therapy. *Arch Surg*. Aug 1964;89:373-379.
3. Baker RJ, St Ville JM, Suzuki F, Shoemaker WC. Evaluation of red cell equilibration in hemorrhagic shock. *Arch Surg*. Apr 1965;90:538-544.
4. Baker RJ, Taxman P, Freeark RJ. An assessment of the management of nonpenetrating liver injuries. *Arch Surg*. Jul 1966;93(1):84-91.
5. Baker RJ. Nonpenetrating liver injuries. JAMA. Aug29 1966; 197:72.
6. Baker RJ, Bass RT, Zajtchuk R, Strohl EL. External pancreatic fistula following abdominal injury. *Arch Surg*. Oct 1967;95(4):556-566.
7. Baker RJ, Shoemaker WC. Changing concepts in treatment of hypovolemic shock. *Med Clin North Am*. Jan 1967;51(1):83-96.
8. Baker RJ. Hidden injuries to the liver. *Hospital Med*. May 1968; 4:32-42.
9. Baker RJ, Zajtchuk R, Shoemaker WC, Strohl EL. Physiological studies onexternal pancreatic secretion in man. *Bull Soc Int Chir*. Mar-Apr 1968;27(2):81-88.
10. Love L, Greenfield GB, Braun TW, Moncada R, Freeark RJ, Baker RJ. Arteriography of splenic trauma. *Radiology*. Jul 1968;91(1):96-102.
11. Baker RJ, Shoemaker WC. Changing concepts in treatment of hypovolemic shock. *Ariz Med*. Feb 1969;26(2):140-148.
12. Matsuda T, Taube RR, Dern RJ, Elwyn DH, Baker RJ, Shoemaker WC. Red cell survival of 42 day acid-citrate-dextrose (ACD)-adenine preserved blood after transfusion into traumatized patients. *J Lab Clin Med*. Jul 1969;74(1):42-46.
13. Taube RR, Matsuda T, Baker RJ, Dern RJ, Elwyn DH, Shoemaker WC. Use of a double erythrocyte label technique to measure red cell survival of ACD and ACD-adenine preserved blood in trauma patients. *J Lab Clin Med*. Mar 1969;73(3):425-431.

14. Zajtchuk R, Amato JC, Shoemaker WC, Baker RJ. The relationship between blood glucose levels and external pancreatic secretion in man. *J Trauma.* Jul 1969;9(7):629-637.
15. Baker RJ, Boyd DR, Condon RE. Priority of management of patients with multiple injuries. *Surg Clin North Am.* Feb 1970;50(1):3-11.
16. Baker RJ, Lowe RJ, Boyd DR. Immediate transfusion reaction: fact and fancy. *IMJ Ill Med J.* Apr 1973;143(4):349-352.
17. Baker RJ. Newer Techniques in evaluation of injured patients. *Surg Clin North Am.* Feb    1975;55(1):31-42.
18. Baker RJ. Newer technique in evaluation of injured patients. *Surg Clin N Am.* Feb 1975;55:31-42.
19. Baker RJ. Emergency medical services categorization and regionalization: An accomplished fact. (Editorial.) *Arch Surg.* Oct 1978;113:1133-1134.
20. Baker RJ. The impact of emergency medicine on surgical care. (Editorial.) *Curr Surg.*Jul/Aug 1982;39:223-225.
21. Stone JL, Lowe RJ, Jonasson O, Baker RJ, Barrett J, Oldershaw J, Crowell RM, Stein RJ. Acute subdural hematoma: Direct admission to a trauma center yields improved results. J Trauma. May 1986; 26(5):445-450.
22. Baker RJ. Coagulopathy in the Trauma Victim. In: Hurst, J.M. (ed.). *Common Problems in Trauma.* Chicago: Year Book Medical Publishers; 1987:343-349.
23. Kagan RJ, Baker RJ. The impact of the volume of neurotrauma experience on morality after head injury. *Am Surg.* Jun 1994;60(6):394-400.

## John Barrett[1-29]

1. Dawidson I, Barrett J, Miller E, Litwin MS. Effect of intravascular cellular aggregate dissolution in postoperative patients. *Ann Surg.* Dec 1975;182(6):776-781.
2. Browns K, Bhat R, Jonasson O, Vidyasagar D. Thoracoabdominal gunshot wound with survival of a 36-week fetus. *JAMA.* May 30 1977;237(22):2409-2410.
3. Barrett J, Sheaff C, Abuabara S, Jonasson O. Splenic preservation in adults after blunt and penetrating trauma. *Am J Surg.* Mar 1983;145(3):313-317.
4. Barrett J, Sheaff C, Smith S, Jonasson O. Correlation of spontaneous microaggregate formation with the severity of trauma in man. *J Trauma.* May 1983;23(5):389-394.
5. Merlotti GJ, Marcet E, Sheaff CM, Dunn R, Barrett JA. Use of peritoneal lavage to evaluate abdominal penetration. *J Trauma.* Mar 1985;25(3):228-231.
6. Gunnar WP, Merlotti GJ, Barrett J, Jonasson O. Resuscitation from hemorrhagic shock. Alterations of the intracranial pressure after normal saline, 3% saline and dextran-40. *Ann Surg.* Dec 1986;204(6):686-692.
7. Pasch AR, Bishara RA, Schuler JJ, et al. Results of venous reconstruction after civilian vascular trauma. *Arch Surg.* May 1986;121(5):607-611.
8. Barrett J. Emergency thoracotomy. Care of the patient in the ER. *AORN J.* Dec 1987;46(6):1077, 1080-1074.

9. Jonasson O, Barrett JA. Transfer of unstable patients: dumping or duty? *JAMA*. Mar 20 1987;257(11):1519.
10. Meyer J, Walsh J, Schuler J, et al. The early fate of venous repair after civilian vascular trauma. A clinical, hemodynamic, and venographic assessment. *Ann Surg*. Oct 1987;206(4):458-464.
11. Meyer JP, Barrett JA, Schuler JJ, Flanigan DP. Mandatory vs selective exploration for penetrating neck trauma. A prospective assessment. *Arch Surg*. May 1987;122(5):592-597.
12. Rogers F, Baumgartner N, Nolan P, Robin A, Lange D, Barrett J. Repair of traumatic splenic injuries by splenorrhaphy with polyglycolic acid mesh. *Curr Surg*. Mar-Apr 1987;44(2):112-113.
13. Samelson SL, Robin AP, Merlotti GJ, Lange DA, Barrett JA. A new method of rapid fluid resuscitation during thoracotomy performed in the emergency room. *Surg Gynecol Obstet*. Aug 1987;165(2):175-176.
14. Gunnar W, Jonasson O, Merlotti G, Stone J, Barrett J. Head injury and hemorrhagic shock: studies of the blood brain barrier and intracranial pressure after resuscitation with normal saline solution, 3% saline solution, and dextran-40. *Surgery*. Apr 1988;103(4):398-407.
15. Lange DA, Zaret P, Merlotti GJ, Robin AP, Sheaff C, Barrett JA. The use of absorbable mesh in splenic trauma. *J Trauma*. Mar 1988;28(3):269-275.
16. Merlotti GJ, Dillon BC, Lange DA, Robin AP, Barrett JA. Peritoneal lavage in penetrating thoraco-abdominal trauma. *J Trauma*. Jan 1988;28(1):17-23.
17. Meyer JP, Goldfaden D, Barrett J, et al. Subclavian and innominate artery trauma: a recent experience with nine patients. *J Cardiovasc Surg (Torino)*. May-Jun 1988;29(3):283-289.
18. Meyer JP, Walsh J, Barrett J, et al. Analysis of 18 recent cases of penetrating injuries to the common and internal carotid arteries. *Am J Surg*. Aug 1988;156(2):96-99.
19. Orsay CP, Merlotti G, Abcarian H, Pearl RK, Nanda M, Barrett J. Colorectal trauma. *Dis Colon Rectum*. Mar 1989;32(3):188-190.
20. Robin AP, Andrews JR, Lange DA, Roberts RR, Moskal M, Barrett JA. Selective management of anterior abdominal stab wounds. *J Trauma*. Dec 1989;29(12):1684-1689.
21. Jimenez E, Martin M, Krukenkamp I, Barrett J. Subxiphoid pericardiotomy versus echocardiography: a prospective evaluation of the diagnosis of occult penetrating cardiac injury. *Surgery*. Oct 1990;108(4):676-679; discussion 679-680.
22. Soyka JM, Martin M, Sloan EP, Himmelman RG, Batesky D, Barrett JA. Diagnostic peritoneal lavage: is an isolated WBC count greater than or equal to 500/mm3 predictive of intra-abdominal injury requiring celiotomy in blunt trauma patients? *J Trauma*. Jul 1990;30(7):874-879.
23. Himmelman RG, Martin M, Gilkey S, Barrett JA. Triple-contrast CT scans in penetrating back and flank trauma. *J Trauma*. Jun 1991;31(6):852-855.
24. Rogers FB, Baumgartner NE, Robin AP, Barrett JA. Absorbable mesh splenorrhaphy for severe splenic injuries: functional studies in an animal model and an additional patient series. *J Trauma*. Feb 1991;31(2):200-204.

25. Drugas D, Duarte B, Robin A, Barrett J. Salmonella typhi splenic abscess in an intravenous drug abuser following splenorrhaphy: case report. *J Trauma*. Jul 1992;33(1):143-144.
26. Bannon MP, O'Neill CM, Martin M, Ilstrup DM, Fish NM, Barrett J. Central venous oxygen saturation, arterial base deficit, and lactate concentration in trauma patients. *Am Surg*. Aug 1995;61(8):738-745.
27. Stone JL, Lichtor T, Fitzgerald LF, Barrett JA, Reyes HM. Demographics of civilian cranial gunshot wounds: devastation related to escalating semiautomatic usage. *J Trauma*. Jun 1995;38(6):851-854.
28. Cohen M, Morales R, Jr., Fildes J, Barrett J. Staged reconstruction after gunshot wounds to the abdomen. *Plast Reconstr Surg*. Jul 2001;108(1):83-92.
29. Bokhari F, Nagy K, Roberts R, et al. The ultrasound screen for penetrating truncal trauma. *Am Surg*. Apr 2004;70(4):316-321.

## David R. Boyd[1-78]

1. Boyd DR. General Principles . Estimation of Blood Loss and Suggested Therapy. In: Condon RE, Nyhus LM, eds. *Manual of Surgical Therapeutics*. Boston: Little, Brown and Company; 1969:1-65.
2. Baker RJ, Boyd DR, Condon RE. Priority of management of patients with multiple injuries. *Surg Clin North Am*. Feb 1970;50(1):3-11.
3. Boyd DR, Folk FA. The resuscitation and initial management of the severely injured. *J Occup Med*. Jul 1970;12(7):262-266.
4. Boyd DR, Folk FA, Condon RE, Nyhus LM, Baker RJ. Predictive value of serum osmolality in shock following major trauma. *Surg Forum*. 1970;21:32-33.
5. Boyd DR. Computerized trauma registry. *J Trauma*. 1971 1971;11:449-450.
6. Boyd DR. Open wounds. *Emerg Med*. 1971;3:100-105, 107, 109, 113-114, 119-120.
7. Boyd DR, Addis HC. Solute aberrations in traumatic shock. *Rev Surg*. Nov-Dec 1971;28(6):449-451.
8. Boyd DR, Addis HM, Chilimindris C, Lowe RJ, Folk FA, Baker RJ. Utilization of osmometry in critically ill surgical patients. *Arch Surg*. Apr 1971;102(4):363-372.
9. Boyd DR, Baker RJ. Osmometry: a new bedside laboratory aid for the management of surgical patients. *Surg Clin North Am*. Feb 1971;51(1):241-250.
10. Boyd DR, Rappaport DM, Marbarger JP, Baker RJ, Nyhus LM. Computerized trauma registry: a new method for categorizing physical injuries. *Aerosp Med*. Jun 1971;42(6):607-615.
11. Boyd DR, Rappaport DM, Marbarger JP, Baker RJ, Nyhus LM. Computerized trauma registry: a method for a comprehensive investigation of a major health problem. Paper presented at: San Diego Biomedical Symposium, 1971; San Diego, California.
12. Brown RS, Boyd DR, Matsuda T, Lowe RJ. Temporary internal vascular shunt for retrohepatic vena cava injury. *J Trauma*. Sep 1971;11(9):736-737.

13. Chilimindris C, Boyd DR, Carlson LE, Folk FA, Baker RJ, Freeark RJ. A critical review of management of right colon injuries. *J Trauma.* Aug 1971;11(8):651-660.
14. Flashner BA, Boyd DR. The critically injured patient: a an for the organization of a statewide system of trauma facilities. *IMJ Ill Med J.* Mar 1971;139(3):256-265.
15. Flashner BA, Boyd DR. The critically injured patient: a plan for the organization of a statewide system of trauma facilities. *IMJ Ill Med J.* Mar 1971;139(3):256-265.
16. Nadeau N, Weisz GM, Boyd DR, Folk FA. Hyperalimentation intraveineuse. [Intravenous hyperalimentation]. *Union Med Can.* Dec 1971;100(12):2357-2361.
17. Shoemaker WC, Boyd DR, Corley RS, Reinhard JM, Dreiling DA, Kark AE. Sequential hemodynamic events after trauma to the unanesthetized patient. *Surg Gynecol Obstet.* Apr 1971;132(4):651-656.
18. Shoemaker WC, Boyd DR, Kim SI, Brown RS, Dreiling DA, Kark AE. Sequential oxygen transport and acid-base changes after trauma to the unanesthetized patient. *Surg Gynecol Obstet.* Jun 1971;132(6):1033-1038.
19. Weisz GM, Boyd DR. [Resuscitation and evaluation of the multiple-injured patient]. *Harefuah.* Nov 15 1971;81(10):506-509.
20. Bombeck CT, Boyd DR, Nyhus LM. Esophageal trauma. *Surg Clin North Am.* Feb 1972;52(1):219-230.
21. Boyd DR. Monitoring patients with posttraumatic pulmonary insufficiency. *Surg Clin North Am.* Feb 1972;52(1):31-46.
22. Boyd DR, General Principles. In: Condon RE, Nyhus LM, eds. *Manual of Surgical Therapeutics.* 2nd ed. Boston: Little, Brown and Company; 1972:1-11.
23. Boyd DR. Initial care and management of open wounds. *Emergency Room Care, Twenty-Third Hahnemann Symposium.* New York, NY, USA; 1972.
24. Boyd DR. What we had was a nonsystem. *Med Opinion.* 1972;1:26-27.
25. Boyd DR. A total emergency medical service system for Illinois. *IMJ Ill Med J.* Nov 1972;142(5):486-488.
26. Boyd DR, Flashner BA, Nyhus LM, Phillips CW. Clinical and epidemiologic characteristics of non-surviving trauma victims in an urban environment. *J Natl Med Assoc.* Jan 1972;64(1):1-7.
27. Boyd DR,. The evaluation and management of trauma: abdominal injury. In: Condon RE, Nyhus LM, eds. *Manual of Surgical Therapeutics.* 2nd ed. Boston: Little, Brown and Co.; 1972:27-36.
28. Boyd DR, Mains KD, Flashner BA. Status report: Illinois statewide trauma care system. *IMJ Ill Med J.* Jan 1972;141(1):56-62.
29. Mains KD, Boyd DR. A new health professional: the trauma coordinator. *Ill Med J.* 1972;42:158-160.
30. Boyd DR. A systems approach to improve trauma patient care. *S Afr J Surg.* Dec 1973;11(4):163-175.
31. Boyd DR. A symposium on The Illinois Trauma Program: a systems approach to the care of the critically injured. Introduction: a controlled systems approach to trauma patient care. *J Trauma.* Apr 1973;13(4):275-276.

32. Boyd DR. Resection of the distal end of the ulna. Case report: 13-year post-trauma study. *IMJ Ill Med J*. Jan 1973;143(1):45-46.
33. Boyd DR. Cardiopulmonary resuscitation. In: Schneewind JH, ed. *Medical and Surgical Emergencies*. 3rd ed. Chicago: Yearbook Medical Publishers; 1973:25-31.
34. Boyd DR. Trauma care: no longer a matter of chance. *Medical Dimensions*. 1973;2(6):33-34.
35. Boyd DR, Dunea MM, Flashner BA. The Illinois plan for a statewide system of trauma centers. *J Trauma*. Jan 1973;13(1):24-31.
36. Boyd DR, Lowe RJ, Baker RJ, Nyhus LM. Trauma Registry. New computer method for multifactorial evaluation of a major health problem. *JAMA*. Jan 22 1973;223(4):422-428.
37. Boyd DR, Lowe RJ, Sheaff LC, Hoecker C, Rappaport DM. A profile of the trauma registry. *J Trauma*. Apr 1973;13(4):316-320.
38. Boyd DR, Mains KD, Flashner BA. A systems approach to statewide emergency medical care. *J Trauma*. Apr 1973;13(4):276-284.
39. Boyd DR, Mains KD, Romano TL, Nyhus LM. New health specialists for trauma patient care. *J Trauma*. Apr 1973;13(4):295-300.
40. Boyd DR, McGrady MK, Anderson CE, Pizzano WA. An ambulance strategy for Illinois. *IMJ Ill Med J*. Nov 1973;144(5):487-492.
41. Boyd DR, Pizzano WA. Illinois Emergency Medical Service System. Status report II (July, 1973). *IMJ Ill Med J*. Sep 1973;144(3):210-216 passim.
42. Weisz GM, Boyd DR. Psyche-trauma-psyche: surgeons' observations of psychiatric conditions in trauma patients. *Isr Ann Psychiatr Relat Discip*. Jun 1973;11(2):91-98.
43. Bartizal JF, Boyd DR, Folk FA, Smith D, Lescher TC, Freeark RJ. A critical review of management of 392 colonic and rectal injuries. *Dis Colon Rectum*. May-Jun 1974;17(3):313-318.
44. Boyd DR. Current concepts in the initial therapy of shock. In: Finders JC, ed. *Emergency Medical Care*. Vol 1. New York: International Medical Books; 1974:3-20.
45. Boyd DR. New health professionals in an emergency medical system: the Illinois experience. In: Finders JC, ed. *Emergency Medical Care*. Vol 1. New York: International Medical Books; 1974:281-191.
46. Boyd DR, Pizzano WA, Silverstone PA, Romano TL. Categorization of hospital emergency medical capabilities in Illinois: A statewide experience. *IMJ Ill Med J*. Jul 1974;146(1):33-38.
47. Heller RF, Rahimtoola SH, Ehsani A, Boyd, DR et al. Cardiac complications. Results of penetrating chest wounds involving the heart. *Arch Intern Med*. Sep 1974;134(3):491-496.
48. Pizzano WA, Romano TL, Nance JC, Boyd DR. Illinois emergency medical service system: status report III (July, 1974). *IMJ Ill Med J*. Aug 1974;146(2):125-129 passim.
49. Boyd DR. Program guidelines for emergency medical services systems. In: Department of Health EaW, ed. Washington, D.C.; 1975.
50. Boyd DR, Pizzano WA, Romano TL, Van Stiegmann G, Nyhus LM. Regionalization of trauma patient care: the Illinois experience. *Surg Annu*. 1975;7:25-52.

51. Boyd DR, Reardon JD. Federal involvement in EMS. *J Emerg Nurs.* Jul-Aug 1975;1(4):26-27.
52. Boyd DR, Sato T. Emergency Medical Research. *Annual Meeting of the Japanese Society for Emergency and Trauma.* Anjo-city, Aichi-ken, Japan; 1975.
53. Boyd DR. Emergency medical service systems development: a national initiative. *IEEE Trans Vehicular Tech.* 1976;25(4):104-115.
54. Boyd DR. Papers presented and published for the *Bicentennial Emergency Medical Services and Traumatology Conference.* Baltimore, Maryland; May 10-12, 1976.
    - The increasing role of the helicopter in EMS.
    - Integration of the six critical care groups in a regional categorization scheme.
    - National emergency facilities categorization revisited;Boyd DR. Outlying coronary care units in a regional EMS system.
    - Organization and regionalization of trauma patient care; Boyd DR. Transportation care of the critically ill and injured.
    - Evaluation methodology for determining regional impact of facility categorization for critical trauma patients.
    - Emergency medical services progress report for the United States of America with future program projection.
    - The multiply injured patient.
55. Boyd DR. *White House Conference on Emergency Medical Services Systems.* (DHEW Report),5 January 1976; Washington, D.C.
56. Boyd DR. Efforts to improve emergency medical services: the Illinois experience. *JACEP.* May 1977;6(5):209-217.
57. Boyd DR. Modern concepts in the care of the critically injured; Categories of Trauma-Hemorrhage Assessment and Treatment. In: McCredie JA, ed. *Basic Surgery.* New York: MacMillian Publishing Co., Inc.; 1977:167-180.
58. Boyd DR. A systems approach to EMS. *Emerg Med Serv.* Nov-Dec 1977;6(6):93-104.
59. Boyd DR, Romano T. Prehospital mobile ICU paramedics in the USA--a national experience. *Intensive Care Med.* 1977;3(3).
60. Edlich RF, Krome RL, Crampton R, Boyd DR, Jelenko C, 3rd, Poliafico F. Emergency medical support plan for the President of the United States and VIPs. *JACEP.* Oct 1977;6(10):462-464.
61. Boyd DR, Micik SH, Lambrew CT, Romano T. Medical control and accountability of emergency medical services (EMS) systems. *IEEE Trans Vehicular Tech.* 1979;28(4):249.
62. Boyd DR. Trauma--a controllable disease in the 1980's (Fourth Annual Stone Lecture, American Trauma Society). *J Trauma.* Jan 1980;20(1):14-24.
63. Whittier FC, Boyd DR, Warren J. The role of the Emergency Medical Services in organ donation. *Proc Clin Dial Transplant Forum.* 1980;10:155-159.
64. Edlich RF, Rodeheaver GT, Halfacre SE, Tobiasen JA, Boyd DR. Systems conceptualization of burn care on a regional basis. *Top Emerg Med.* Oct 1981;3(3):7-15.

65. Boyd DR. Emergency Medical Services Systems. In: Pascarelli EF, ed. *Hospital-Based Ambulatory Care*. Norwalk: Appleton-Century-Crofts; 1982:113-140.
66. Boyd DR. The conceptual development of EMS systems in the Unites States, Part II. *Emerg Med Serv*. Mar-Apr 1982;11(2):26, 28-30, 32-23 passim.
67. Boyd DR. Contributor; In: Cowley RA, Dunham CM, eds. *Shock Trauma--Critical Care Manual*. Baltimore: University Park Press; 1982.
68. Boyd DR. The history of emergency medical services (EMS) systems in the United States of America. In: Boyd DR, Edlich RF, Micik SH, eds. *Systems Approach to Emergency Medical Care*. Norwalk: Appleton-Century-Crofts; 1983:1-82.
69. Boyd DR, Cowley RA. Comprehensive regional trauma/emergency medical services (EMS) delivery systems: the United States experience. *World J Surg*. Jan 1983;7(1):149-157.
70. Boyd DR, Cowley RA. Systems approach to the care of the trauma patient. In: Boyd DR, Edlich RF, Micik SH, eds. *Systems Approach to Emergency Medical Care*. Norwalk: Appleton-Century-Crofts; 1983:432-508.
71. Boyd DR, Edlich RF, Micik SH. Medical control and accountability. In: . ed. *Systems Approach to Emergency Medical Care*. Norwalk: Appleton-Century-Crofts; 1983:103-117.
72. Boyd DR, Morgan RF, Crowley RA. Traumatology and the regionalization of trauma care. *Curr Concepts Trauma Care*. 1983;6(1):16-20.
73. El Serwi B, Boyd DR. Emergency Medical Services in Egypt The Problem and Solution. *Zagazig University Medical Journal*. December 1983 1983;6(4).
74. Boyd DR. Trauma center (update). *The World Book Encyclopedia*; 1984.
75. Whittier FC, Boyd DR. Emergency medical services and organ donation. *Emergency*. 1984.
76. Boyd DR. Trauma registries revisited. *J Trauma*. Mar 1985;25(3):186-187.
77. Boyd DR. EMS systems development in the United States. In: Schwartz GR, Safar P, Stone JH, Storey PB, Wagner DK, eds. *Principles and Practive of Emergency Medicine*. Vol 2. 2 ed. Philadelphia: W. B. Saunders Co.; 1986:553-565.
78. Poirier LR, Brown B. Etude exploratoire sur l'implantation regionale d'un systeme de soins d'urgence integres selon le modele de Boyd en Montegregie. Comité régional de la sécurité routière des DSC de la Montérégie . In: LeMoyne DdscdlHC, ed. Vol 1. Montérégie, administrative region in the southwestern corner of Quebec 1989.

## John Fildes[1-5]

1. Fildes J, Bannon MP, Barrett J. Soft-tissue infections after trauma. *Surg Clin North Am*. Apr 1991;71(2):371-384.
2. Fildes J, Seymour M, Gilke S, Wey C, Nagy K, Barrett j. Abdominal trauma assessment in pregnancy: comparison of computed tomography (CT) and diagnostic peritoneal lavage (DPL). *J Trauma*. 1994;36:150.
3. Fildes JJ, Betlej TM, Barrett JA. Buckshot colic: case report and review of the literature. *J Trauma*. Dec 1995;39(6):1181-1184.

4. Fildes JJ, Betlej TM, Manglano R, Martin M, Rogers F, Barrett JA. Limiting cardiac evaluation in patients with suspected myocardial contusion. *Am Surg.* Sep 1995;61(9):832-835.
5. Fabian TC, Richardson JD, Croce MA, et al. Prospective study of blunt aortic injury: multicenter trial of the American Association for the Surgery of Trauma. *J Trauma.* 1997;42 374-383.

## Robert J. Freeark[1-19]

1. Freeark RJ, Kane JM, Folk FA, Baker RJ. Traumatic Disruption of the Head of the Pancreas. Arch Surg. Jul 1965; 91:5-13.
2. Freeark RJ, Corley RD, Norcross WJ, Baker RJ. Unusual aspects of pancreatoduodenal trauma. *J Trauma.* Jul 1966;6(4):482-492.
3. Freeark RJ, Corley RD, Norcross WJ, Strohl EL. Intramural hematoma of the duodenum. *Arch Surg.* Apr 1966;92(4):463-475.
4. Freeark RJ, Fardin R. Venographic study of the lower extremity in patients with fracture of the hip. *Surg Forum.* 1966;17:444-446.
5. Freeark RJ, Norcross WJ, Corley RD. Operation for obstructing duodenal hematoma. *Surg Clin North Am.* Feb 1966;46(1):85-87.
6. Freeark RJ, Boswick J, Fardin R. Posttraumatic venous thrombosis. *Arch Surg.* Oct 1967;95(4):567-575.
7. Yao ST, Carey JS, Shoemaker WC, Weinberg M, Freeark RJ. Hemodynamics and therapy of acute hemopericardium from stab wounds of the heart. *J Trauma.* Sep 1967;7(5):783-792.
8. Freeark RJ, Love L, Baker RJ. The role of aortography in the management of blunt abdominal trauma. *J Trauma.* Jul 1968;8(4):557-571.
9. Freeark RJ, Shoemaker WC, Baker RJ. Aortography in blunt abdominal trauma. *Arch Surg.* May 1968;96(5):705-711.
10. Printen KJ, Freeark RJ, Shoemaker WC. Conservative management of penetrating abdominal wounds. *Arch Surg.* Jun 1968;96(6):899-901.
11. Stevens J, Fardin R, Freeark RJ. Lower extremity thrombophlebitis in patients with femoral neck fractures. A venographic investigation and a review of the early and late significance of the findings. *J Trauma.* Jul 1968;8(4):527-534.
12. Freeark RJ. Role of angiography in the management of multiple injuries. *Surg Gynecol Obstet.* Apr 1969;128(4):761-771.
13. Folk FA, Freeark RJ. Reoperations for pancreatic pseudocyst. *Arch Surg.* Apr 1970;100(4):430-437.
14. Hartman JT, Altner PC, Freeark RJ. The effect of limb elevation in preventing venous thrombosis. A venographic study. *J Bone Joint Surg Am.* Dec 1970;52(8):1618-1622.

15. Freeark RJ. The surgeon's role in the staffing of hospital emergency departments. *J Trauma.* Apr 1973;13(4):300-306.
16. Freeark RJ. Penetrating wounds of the abdomen. *N Engl J Med.* Jul 25 1974;291(4):185-188.

17. Mains DB, Freeark RJ. Report on compound dislocation of the elbow with entrapment of the brachial artery. *Clin Orthop Relat Res*. Jan-Feb 1975(106):180-185.
18. Freeark RJ. 1982 A.A.S.T. Presidential Address: The Trauma Center: its Hospitals, Head Injuries and Heroes. *J Trauma*. March 1983; 23(3):173-179.
19. Freeark RJ. The Accident Hospital, Scudder Oration on Trauma, *ACS Bulletin*. Oct 1986:l71(10).

## Robert J. Lowe[1-12]

1. Lowe RJ, Boyd DR, Folk FA, Baker RJ. The negative laparotomy for abdominal trauma. *J Trauma*. Oct 1972;12(10):853-861.
2. Lowe RJ, Boyd DR, Phillips CW. Management of complex fluid and electrolyte derangements in critically ill surgical patients. *J Natl Med Assoc*. Mar 1972;64(2):122-130.
3. Lowe RJ, Baker RJ. Organization and function of trauma care units. *J Trauma*. Apr 1973;13(4):285-290.
4. Lowe RJ, Romano TL, Boyd DR. Initial care of critically injured. *IMJ Ill Med J*. May 1973;141(5):474-478.
5. Lowe RJ, Moss GS. Pulmonary failure after trauma. *Surg Annu*. 1976;8:63-89.
6. Lowe RJ, Moss GS, Jilek J, Levine HD. Crystalloid vs colloid in the etiology of pulmonary failure after trauma: a randomized trial in man. *Surgery*. Jun 1977;81(6):676-683.
7. Lowe RJ, Saletta JD, Moss GS. Pancreatoduodenectomy for penetrating pancreatic trauma. *J Trauma*. Sep 1977;17(9):732-741.
8. Lowe RJ, Saletta JD, Read DR, Radhakrishnan J, Moss GS. Should laparotomy be mandatory or selective in gunshot wounds of the abdomen? *J Trauma*. Dec 1977;17(12):903-907.
9. Shuck JM, Lowe RJ. Intestinal disruption due to blunt abdominal trauma. *Am J Surg*. Dec 1978;136(6):668-673.
10. Lowe RJ, Moss GS, Jilek J, Levine HD. Crystalloid versus colloid in the etiology of pulmonary failure after trauma--a randomized trial in man. *Crit Care Med*. Mar 1979;7(3):107-112.
11. Meyer J, Abuabara S, Barrett J, Lowe R. A bullet in the appendix. *J Trauma*. May 1982;22(5):424-425.
12. Stone JL, Lowe RJ, Barrett J, et al. Inner-urban acute subdural hematoma- A plea for the regionalization of severe injury. Chicago Surgical Society, Dec 2,1983. Proc Inst Med Chgo 1984; 37:33-36,
13. Stone JL, Lowe RJ, Jonasson O, et al. Acute subdural hematoma: direct admission to a trauma center yields improved results. *J Trauma*. May 1986;26(5):445-450.

## Kimberly Ormsby Nagy[1-43]

1. Nagy KK, Duarte B. Post-traumatic inferior vena caval thrombosis: case report. *J Trauma*. Feb 1990;30(2):218-221.
2. Nagy KK, Gunnar WP, Soyka JM, et al. Metabolic acidosis associated with hypertonic saline resuscitation in a head-injured hemorrhagic shock model. *Surg Forum*. 1990;41:45-46.
3. Duarte B, Nagy KK, Cintron J. Perforated duodenal diverticulum. *Br J Surg*. Sep 1992;79(9):877-881.
4. Nagy KK, Davis J, Duda J, Fildes J, Roberts R, Barrett J. A comparison of pentastarch and lactated Ringer's solution in the resuscitation of patients with hemorrhagic shock. *Circ Shock*. Aug 1993;40(4):289-294.
5. Fildes J, Seymour M, Gilke S, Wey C, Nagy K, Barrett J. Abdominal trauma assessment in pregnancy: comparison of computed tomography (CT) and diagnostic peritoneal lavage (DPL). *J Trauma*. 1994;36:150.
6. Nagy KK, Massad M, Fildes J, Reyes H. Missile embolization revisited - a rationale for selective management. *Am Surg*. Dec 1994;60(12):975-979.
7. Nagy KK, Fildes JJ, Sloan EP, et al. Aspiration of free blood from the peritoneal cavity does not mandate immediate laparotomy. *Am Surg*. Sep 1995;61(9):790-795.
8. Nagy KK, Lohmann C, Kim DO, Barrett J. Role of echocardiography in the diagnosis of occult penetrating cardiac injury. *J Trauma*. Jun 1995;38(6):859-862.
9. Nagy KK, Fildes JJ, Mahr C, et al. Experience with three prosthetic materials in temporary abdominal wall closure. *Am Surg*. May 1996;62(5):331-335.
10. Nagy KK, Gilkey SH, Roberts RR, Fildes JJ, Barrett J. Computed tomography screens stable patients at risk for penetrating cardiac injury. *Acad Emerg Med*. Nov 1996;3(11):1024-1027.
11. Fabian TC, Richardson JD, Croce MA, et al. Prospective study of blunt aortic injury: multicenter trial of the American Association for the Surgery of Trauma. *J Trauma*. 1997;42 374-383.
12. Mahr CC, Fildes JJ, Becker EJ, et al. Recovery rate of candidiasis in trauma patients with unresolved sepsis. *Complic Surg*. 1997;16.
13. Nagy KK, Brenneman FD, Krosner SM, et al. Routine preoperative "one-shot" intravenous pyelography is not indicated in all patients with penetrating abdominal trauma. *J Am Coll Surg*. Dec 1997;185(6):530-533.
14. Nagy KK, Krosner SM, Joseph KT, Roberts RR, Smith RF, Barrett J. A method of determining peritoneal penetration in gunshot wounds to the abdomen. *J Trauma*. Aug 1997;43(2):242-245; discussion 245-246.
15. Nagy KK, Sloan EP, Barrett J. Diaspirin cross-linked hemoglobin: a promising new oxygen carrying resuscitation fluid. *Curr Surg*. 1997;54:285-289.
16. Harrison JM, Nagy KM, Fareed JMDP, et al. The effects of hyperthermic resuscitative fluid on coagulation in hypothermic canines. *JTrauma-Inj Infec Crit Care*. 1998;45(6):1116.
17. Bokhari F, Nagy K, Roberts R, et al. Complications of angiographic embolization for traumatic hemobilia. *J Trauma*. Nov 1999;47(5):977-978.

18. Nagy K, Roberts R, Joseph K, An G, Barrett J. Evisceration after abdominal stab wounds: is laparotomy required? *J Trauma*. Oct 1999;47(4):622-624; discussion 624-626.
19. Nagy KK, Joseph KT, Krosner SM, et al. The utility of head computed tomography after minimal head injury. *J Trauma*. Feb 1999;46(2):268-270.
20. Nagy KK, Perez F, Fildes JJ, Barrett J. Optimal prosthetic for acute replacement of the abdominal wall. *J Trauma*. Sep 1999;47(3):529-532.
21. Kim SS, Roberts RR, Nagy KK, et al. Hemosuccus pancreaticus after penetrating trauma to the abdomen. *J Trauma*. Nov 2000;49(5):948-950.
22. Nagy K, Fabian T, Rodman G, Fulda G, Rodriguez A, Mirvis S. Guidelines for the diagnosis and management of blunt aortic injury: an EAST Practice Management Guidelines Work Group. *J Trauma*. Jun 2000;48(6):1128-1143.
23. Nagy KK, Roberts RR, Joseph KT, et al. Experience with over 2500 diagnostic peritoneal lavages. *Injury*. Sep 2000;31(7):479-482.
24. Nagy KK, Smith RF, Roberts RR, et al. Prognosis of penetrating trauma in elderly patients: a comparison with younger patients. *J Trauma*. Aug 2000;49(2):190-193; discussion 193-194.
25. Wiley D, Sheaff C, Nagy K, Reiman H, Jr., Leslie C, Barrett J. Hyperthermic resuscitation is safe and effective after hemorrhagic shock in dogs. *J Trauma*. Jun 2000;48(6):1052-1056; discussion 1056-1057.
26. Asensio JA, Chahwan S, Forno W, et al. Penetrating esophageal injuries: multicenter study of the American Association for the Surgery of Trauma. *J Trauma*. Feb 2001;50(2):289-296.
27. Cushman JG, Agarwal N, Fabian TC, et al. Practice management guidelines for the management of mild traumatic brain injury: the EAST practice management guidelines work group. *J Trauma*. Nov 2001;51(5):1016-1026.
28. D'Amours SK, Simons RK, Scudamore CH, Nagy AG, Brown DR. Major intrahepatic bile duct injuries detected after laparotomy: selective nonoperative management. *J Trauma*. Mar 2001;50(3):480-484.
29. Demetriades D, Murray JA, Chan L, et al. Penetrating colon injuries requiring resection: diversion or primary anastomosis? An AAST prospective multicenter study. *J Trauma*. May 2001;50(5):765-775.
30. Nagy KK, Krosner SM, Roberts RR, Joseph KT, Smith RF, Barrett J. Determining which patients require evaluation for blunt cardiac injury following blunt chest trauma. *World J Surg*. Jan 2001;25(1):108-111.
31. Bokhari F, Brakenridge S, Nagy K, et al. Prospective evaluation of the sensitivity of physical examination in chest trauma. *J Trauma*. Dec 2002;53(6):1135-1138.
32. Demetriades D, Murray JA, Chan LS, et al. Handsewn versus stapled anastomosis in penetrating colon injuries requiring resection: a multicenter study. *J Trauma*. Jan 2002;52(1):117-121.
33. Hoff WS, Holevar M, Nagy KK, et al. Practice management guidelines for the evaluation of blunt abdominal trauma: the East practice management guidelines work group. *J Trauma*. Sep 2002;53(3):602-615.
34. Nagy KK, Roberts RR, Smith RF, et al. Trans-mediastinal gunshot wounds: are "stable" patients really stable? *World J Surg*. Oct 2002;26(10):1247-1250.

35. Brakenridge SC, Nagy KK, Joseph KT, An GC, Bokhari F, Barrett J. Detection of intra-abdominal injury using diagnostic peritoneal lavage after shotgun wound to the abdomen. *J Trauma*. Feb 2003;54(2):329-331.
36. An G, Walter RJ, Nagy K. Closure of abdominal wall defects using acellular dermal matrix. *J Trauma*. Jun 2004;56(6):1266-1275.
37. Bokhari F, Nagy K, Roberts R, et al. The ultrasound screen for penetrating truncal trauma. *Am Surg*. Apr 2004;70(4):316-321.
38. Maxwell RA, Campbell DJ, Fabian TC, et al. Use of presumptive antibiotics following tube thoracostomy for traumatic hemopneumothorax in the prevention of empyema and pneumonia--a multi-center trial. *J Trauma*. Oct 2004;57(4):742-748; discussion 748-749.
39. Dennis AJ, Valentino DJ, Walter RJ, et al. Acute effects of TASER X26 discharges in a swine model. *J Trauma*. Sep 2007;63(3):581-590.
40. Karmy-Jones R, Jurkovich GJ, Velmahos GC, et al. Practice patterns and outcomes of retrievable vena cava filters in trauma patients: an AAST multicenter study. *J Trauma*. Jan 2007;62(1):17-24; discussion 24-15.
41. Valentino DJ, Walter RJ, Dennis AJ, et al. Neuromuscular effects of stun device discharges. *J Surg Res*. Nov 2007;143(1):78-87.
42. Valentino DJ, Walter RJ, Nagy K, et al. Repeated thoracic discharges from a stun device. *J Trauma*. May 2007;62(5):1134-1142.
43. Walter RJ, Dennis AJ, Valentino DJ, et al. TASER X26 discharges in swine produce potentially fatal ventricular arrhythmias. *Acad Emerg Med*. Jan 2008;15(1):66-73.

## Max L. Ramenofsky[1]

1. Ramenofsky ML. Standards of care for the critically injured pediatric patient. *J Trauma*. 22(11):921-923, November, 1982)

## Roxane R. Roberts[1-2]

1. Roberts R, Martin M, Farkas L, Bonilla J, Barrett J. Diagnostic peritoneal lavage: the Cook County Hospital experience. *Can J Surg*. Oct 1991;34(5):427-429.
2. Kim SS, Roberts RR, Nagy KK, et al. Hemosuccus pancreaticus after penetrating trauma to the abdomen. *J Trauma*. Nov 2000;49(5):948-950.

## Teresa Romano[1-15]

1. Romano T. Trauma nurse specialist. *Am J Nurs*. Jun 1973;73(6):1008-1011.
2. Romano T, Boyd DR. Illinois Trauma Program. *Am J Nurs*. Jun 1973;73(6):1004-1007.
3. Romano T. Trauma nursing in Illinois. *Hospitals*. May 16 1973;47(10):147-154.

4. Romano T, Boyd DR. Illinois Trauma Program. *Am J Nurs*. Jun 1973;73(6):1004-1007.
5. Romano T. The LP/VN's role in trauma nursing. *J Pract Nurs*. Mar 1974;24(3):28-30.
6. Romano T. Initial evaluation of the multiple injury patient. *Emerg Med Serv*. Jul-Aug 1976;5(4):24, 26, 28-30.
7. Romano T. Trauma Notebook. 2. Cardiac tamponade. *J Emerg Nurs*. Jan-Feb 1976;2(1):35.
8. Romano TL, Boyd DR. In-hospital emergency care. In: Zschoche DA, ed. *Mosby's Comprehensive Review of Critical Care*. 1 ed. St. Louis: CV Mosby Co.; 1976:115-134.
9. Romano T. Tension pneumothorax. *J Emerg Nurs*. Mar-Apr 1977;3(2):47.
10. Romano T. Flail chest. *J Emerg Nurs*. Jan-Feb 1977;3(1):37.
11. Barber J, Romano T. Trauma notebook. Oxygen. *J Emerg Nurs*. May-Jun 1978;4(3):53-54.
12. Budassi SA, Romano T. Trauma Notebook No. 9. Cardioversion: synchronous electrical countershock. *J Emerg Nurs*. Jan-Feb 1978;4(1):29-30.
13. Romano T. Trauma notebook 14: Hemorrhagic shock - compensatory hormonal mechanisms in hemorrhagic shock. *J Emerg Nurs*. Sep-Oct 1978;4(5):58.
14. Romano T. Trauma notebook 13: Stress ulcer - stress ulcer as a complication of major trauma. *J Emerg Nurs*. Sep-Oct 1978;4(5):57.
15. Romano T, Boyd DR. In-hospital emergency care of the critically injured. In: Zschoche DA, ed. *Mosby's Comprehensive Review of Critical Care*. St. Louis: CV Mosby Co.; 1981:169-190.

## John D Saletta[1-8]

1. Saletta JD, Freeark RJ. The partially severed artery. *Arch Surg*. Aug 1968;97(2):198-205.
2. Monson DO, Saletta JD, Freeark RJ. Carotid vertebral trauma. *J Trauma*. Dec 1969;9(12):987-999.
3. Saletta JD, Freeark RJ. Occult vascular injuries of the extremities. *J Occup Med*. Aug 1970;12(8):304-307.
4. Saletta JD, Freeark RJ. Injuries to the profunda femoris artery. *J Trauma*. Sep 1972;12(9):778-785.
5. Saletta JD, Folk FA, Freeark RJ. Trauma to the neck region. *Surg Clin North Am*. Feb 1973;53(1):73-86.
6. Moss GS, Saletta JD. Traumatic shock in man. *N Engl J Med*. Mar 28 1974;290(13):724-726.
7. Saletta JD, Lowe RJ, Lim LT, Thornton J, Delk S, Moss GS. Penetrating trauma of the neck. *J Trauma*. Jul 1976;16(7):579-587.
8. Lim LT, Saletta JD, Flanigan DP. Subclavian and innominate artery trauma. A five-year experience with 17 patients. *Surgery*. Dec 1979;86(6):890-897.

## Norma J Shoemaker[1]

1. Shoemaker WC, Carey JS, Yao ST, et al. Hemodynamic alterations in acute cardiac tamponade after penetrating injuries of the heart. *Surgery.* May 1970;67(5):754-764.

## William C Shoemaker[1-48]

1. Brown RS, Carey JS, Mohr PA, Monson DO, Shoemaker WC. Comparative evaluation of sympathomimetic amines in clinical shock. *Circulation.* Aug 1966;34(2):260-271.
2. Yao ST, Shoemaker WC. Plasma and whole blood viscosity changes in shock and after dextran infusion. *Ann Surg.* Dec 1966;164(6):973-984.
3. Brown RS, Mohr PA, Carey JS, Shoemaker WC. Cardiovascular changes after cranial cerebral injury and increased intracranial pressure. *Surg Gynecol Obstet.* Dec 1967;125(6):1205-1211.
4. Carey JS, Brown RS, Mohr PA, Monson DO, Yao ST, Shoemaker WC. Cardiovascular function in shock. Responses to volume loading and isoproterenol infusion. *Circulation.* Feb 1967;35(2):327-338.
5. Carey JS, Yao ST, Kho LK, Tasche C, Shoemaker WC. Cardiovascular responses to acute hemopericardium, compression by balloon tamponade, and acute coronary artery occlusion. *J Thorac Cardiovasc Surg.* Jul 1967;54(1):65-80.
6. Shoemaker WC. Principles of therapy in shock from hemorrhage, trauma, and sepsis. *Mod Treat.* Mar 1967;4(2):256-276.
7. Shoemaker WC, Baker RJ. Evaluation and treatment of the patient in shock from trauma. *Surg Clin North Am.* Feb 1967;47(1):3-16.
8. Shoemaker WC, Printen KJ, Amato JJ, Monson DO, Carey JS, O'Connor K. Hemodynamic patterns after acute anesthetized and unanesthetized trauma. Evaluation of the sequence of changes in cardiac output and derived calculations. *Arch Surg.* Sep 1967;95(3):492-499.
9. Long DM, Kim SI, Shoemaker WC. Vascular responses in the lung following trauma and shock. *J Trauma.* Sep 1968;8(5):715-723.
10. Shoemaker WC. Emergency management of acute injury and shock. *Med Times.* Jun 1968;96(6):598-607.
11. Shoemaker WC, Elwyn DH, Rosen AL. Development and goals of a trauma and shock research center. *J Mt Sinai Hosp N Y.* Sep-Oct 1968;35(5):451-472.
12. Yao ST, Vanecko RM, Printen K, Shoemaker WC. Penetrating wounds of the heart: a review of 80 cases. *Ann Surg.* Jul 1968;168(1):67-78.
13. Carey JS, Mohr PA, Brown RS, Shoemaker WC. Cardiovascular function in hemorrhage, trauma and sepsis: determinants of cardiac output and cardiac work. *Ann Surg.* Dec 1969;170(6):910-921.
14. Guinan PD, Bayley BC, Metzger WI, Shoemaker WC, Bush IM. The case against "the case against the catheter": initial report. *J Urol.* Jun 1969;101(6):909-913.

15. Brown RS, Mohr PA, Shoemaker WC. Effect of cerebral hypotension on the neural regulation of the cardiovascular system. *Surg Gynecol Obstet.* Sep 1970;131(3):436-440.
16. Kukral JC, Shoemaker WC. The metabolic sequelae of burn trauma. *Surg Clin North Am.* Dec 1970;50(6):1211-1216.
17. Shoemaker WC, Carey JS, Yao ST, et al. Hemodynamic alterations in acute cardiac tamponade after penetrating injuries of the heart. *Surgery.* May 1970;67(5):754-764.
18. Shoemaker WC, Kark AE. Role of physiologic monitoring in the intensive care unit. *Surg Annu.* 1970;2(0):61-81.
19. Kim SI, Shoemaker WC. Development of pulmonary hemodynamic and functional changes after operative and accidental trauma. *Surg Gynecol Obstet.* Oct 1971;133(4):617-620.
20. Shoemaker WC. Physiologic mechanisms in clinical shock. *Adv Exp Med Biol.* Oct 1971;23(0):57-75.
21. Shoemaker WC. Cardiorespiratory patterns in complicated and uncomplicated septic shock: physiologic alterations and their therapeutic implications. *Ann Surg.* Jul 1971;174(1):119-125.
22. Shoemaker WC. Sequential hemodynamic patterns in various causes of shock. *Surg Gynecol Obstet.* Mar 1971;132(3):411-423.
23. Shoemaker WC, Boyd DR, Corley RS, Reinhard JM, Dreiling DA, Kark AE. Sequential hemodynamic events after trauma to the unanesthetized patient. *Surg Gynecol Obstet.* Apr 1971;132(4):651-656.
24. Shoemaker WC, Boyd DR, Kim SI, Brown RS, Dreiling DA, Kark AE. Sequential oxygen transport and acid-base changes after trauma to the unanesthetized patient. *Surg Gynecol Obstet.* Jun 1971;132(6):1033-1038.
25. Taube RR, Matsuda T, Shoemaker WC. Changes in red cell mass after trauma measured by double red cell label technic. *Ann Surg.* Jul 1971;174(1):61-67.
26. Matsuda T, Shoemaker WC. Effectiveness of transfusions in postoperative patients as measured by 24-hour red cell survival. *Ann Surg.* Apr 1972;175(4):577-580.
27. Shoemaker WC. Priorities of resuscitation and subsequent therapy after trauma. *N Y State J Med.* Aug 1 1972;72(15):1948-1954.
28. Yao ST, Vanecko RM, Corley RD, Stuteville OH, Shoemaker WC. Gunshot wounds of the face. *J Trauma.* Jun 1972;12(6):523-528.
29. Baek SM, Brown RS, Shoemaker WC. Cardiac tamponade following wound tract injection. *J Trauma.* Jan 1973;13(1):85-87.
30. Brown RS, Shoemaker WC. Sequential hemodynamic changes in patients with head injury: evidence for an early hemodynamic defect. *Ann Surg.* Feb 1973;177(2):187-192.
31. Bryan-Brown CW, Shoemaker WC. Acute respiratory failure after trauma and surgery. *Semin Drug Treat.* Winter 1973;3(3):269-288.
32. Shoemaker WC. Editorial: Multiple injuries and multiple organ failure. *Crit Care Med.* May-Jun 1973;1(3):157.
33. Shoemaker WC. Seminars in drug treatment. Introduction. *Semin Drug Treat.* Winter 1973;3(3):209-210.

34. Shoemaker WC. Pathophysiologic basis of therapy for shock and trauma syndromes: use of sequential cardiorespiratory measurements to describe natural histories and evaluate possible mechanisms. *Semin Drug Treat.* Winter 1973;3(3):211-229.
35. Shoemaker WC, Bryan-Brown CW. Resuscitation and immediate care of the critically ill and injured patient. *Semin Drug Treat.* Winter 1973;3(3):249-267.
36. Shoemaker WC, Bryan-Brown CW, Elwyn DH. Therapy of nutritional failure. *Semin Drug Treat.* Winter 1973;3(3):301-313.
37. Shoemaker WC, Carey JS, Yao ST, Mohr PA, Printen KJ, Kark AE. Hemodynamic monitoring for physiologic evaluation, diagnosis, and therapy of acute hemopericardial tamponade from penetrating wounds. *J Trauma.* Jan 1973;13(1):36-44.
38. Shoemaker WC, Monson DO. The effect of whole blood and plasma expanders on volume-flow relationships in critically ill patients. *Surg Gynecol Obstet.* Sep 1973;137(3):453-457.
39. Shoemaker WC, Reinhard JM. Tissue perfusion defects in shock and trauma states. *Surg Gynecol Obstet.* Dec 1973;137(6):980-986.
40. Shoemaker WC, Vladeck BC, Bassin R, et al. Burn pathophysiology in man. I. Sequential hemodynamic alterations. *J Surg Res.* Jan 1973;14(1):64-73.
41. Vladeck BC, Bassin R, Kim SI, Shoemaker WC. Burn pathophysiology in man. II. Sequential oxygen transport and acid-base alterations. *J Surg Res.* Jan 1973;14(1):74-79.
42. Brown RS, Kim SI, Shoemaker WC. Hemodynamic mechanisms in the development of pulmonary venous admixture (shunting). *J Surg Res.* Sep 1974;17(3):192-199.
43. Baek SM, Makabali GG, Bryan-Brown CW, Kusek JM, Shoemaker WC. Plasma expansion in surgical patients with high central venous pressure (CVP); the relationship of blood volume to hematocrit, CVP, pulmonary wedge pressure, and cardiorespiratory changes. *Surgery.* Sep 1975;78(3):304-315.
44. Corley RD, Norcross WJ, Shoemaker WC. Traumatic injuries to the duodenum: a report of 98 patients. *Ann Surg.* Jan 1975;181(1):92-98.
45. Shoemaker WC. Algorithm for resuscitation: a systematic plan for immediate care of the injured or postoperative patient. *Crit Care Med.* May-Jun 1975;3(3):127-130.
46. Shoemaker WC. Algorithm for early recognition and management of cardiac tamponade. *Crit Care Med.* Mar-Apr 1975;3(2):59-63.
47. Shoemaker WC. Interdisciplinary medicine: accommodation or integration? *Crit Care Med.* Jan-Feb 1975;3(1):1-4.
48. Walkinshaw M, Shoemaker WC. Use of volume loading to obtain preferred levels of PEEP. A preliminary study. *Crit Care Med.* Feb 1980;8(2):81-86.

# The Greek's

## UNIVERSITY INN RESTAURANT & CONFECTIONARY
## 1824 West Harrison Street, Chicago, Illinois

No attempt to tell the history of Cook County Hospital would be complete without at least a brief mention of our place of refuge to sip a beer or drink a coke in peace and step out of the chaos that was County, if only for a few minutes.

Ask anyone who had ever worked at or visited the old Cook County Hospital before 1990, "Where was *The Greek's* located?" and you would immediately be told, "On Harrison Street, directly across from the main entrance to the Hospital."

Now ask, "What was *The Greek's*?" Depending on who was being asked, this question could evoke a variety of responses. *The Greek's* was an institution unique unto itself.

For starters, the building itself was singular. It was the only structure remaining in what had formerly been a block of long gone bustling commercial buildings. It was the last vestige of a vibrant mostly southern European immigrant community. Today that building is gone as well, but the stories and memories generated within that building still remain and are recounted whenever old County interns and residents have the opportunity to congregate and remember the time when they were young, freshly minted doctors with a world to conquer and an unlimited supply of patients who needed curing.

The original "Greeks" were two immigrant brothers, our uncles, Gus and Nick Maggos, who left Greece in the early 1900s to find their fortune in America. Working their way up the ranks from dishwashers, to bus boys, and then to cooks, they soon were operating a small snack shop in the old Illinois Central Railroad Station at Randolph and Michigan. In the middle 1920s, (no one recalls the exact date) the brothers moved their snack shop to a small store that was available on Harrison Street across from Cook County Hospital.

Fortune visited them when Dr. Karl A. Meyer, the dynamic driving force of the Hospital across the street, stopped in to check out his new neighbors. An immediate and strong lifetime bond was formed between our uncles and Dr. Meyer that developed into something that ultimately surpassed all of their fondest dreams. At that time medical schools and adjacent hospitals were solely dedicated to their respective tasks, and those tasks did not include general dining facilities. After thoroughly checking out the store, its owners and food, Dr. Meyer suggested to his medical staff that they might find the little snack shop across the street convenient for a fast meal. This accomplished several things for the always-thinking Dr. Meyer. The staff did not have to venture out of the area to eat, he knew where they were when he needed them, and he was able to save money for the hospital by not having to expend funds to build a food facility within the building. The little snack shop soon became an extension of the Hospital. A telephone was eventually installed from the hospital switchboard to reach the doctors when they were needed in the hospital.

Other workers at the Hospital soon discovered what the medical staff was doing across the street and decided to join them. As they crowded into the small store a conflict arose as to who would occupy the space. Again, Dr. Meyer came to the rescue. He spoke to the brothers and convinced them that they had to expand. They did and, expansion number one was undertaken. As time went by, visitors to the hospital also started to stop in. They, however, had other purposes in mind. Besides taking carry-outs with them for their visits to patients, they were looking for other things to bring besides food. During WWII, the nearby YMCA was taken over by the Army to house soldiers. Once more, there was added pressure to feed still more people. This prompted several more expansions and finally drove the brothers to buy the entire building. As a result, *The Greek's* became a dining and shopping oasis in the midst of a vast, rapidly growing, medically oriented neighborhood. Years later, as part of a beautification program, the buildings located across from Cook County Hospital were to be demolished to allow for the creation of a park. Because of a grandfathered contract between *The Greek's* and the County Hospital, instigated by Dr. Meyer, the building could remain standing as long as it contained the restaurant and was owned and operated by the Maggos Family.

*The Greek's* had two entrances. The corner double door led through a vestibule into a forerunner of today's mini-mart. Upon entering, one passed by a long glass-fronted counter. Below the glass case was a vast assortment of cigars and cigarettes. On top, and next to the vestibule, was the chrome multi-buttoned cash register. It stood as a guard station with a family member on duty to make sure that no one left without paying. Walking farther into the space one saw a floral display for flowers to be purchased and taken across the street to cheer up patient rooms. Nearby were the fruit bins with apples, oranges, and bananas, as well as other choices. Of course, a large candy case was conspicuous for the sweet-tooth inclined as well. Finally, one could also find the souvenir dolls, trinkets and requisite get-well cards on display to make sure that anyone visiting patients would not go empty handed. For those hungry workers from across the street there was a large serpentine counter and cafeteria at the rear portion of this large front area. The food operation was open 24 hours daily, and no one could remember if there was ever a key for the front door.

A single nondescript side door led into another world. In the center of the building there was a bar and more-formal dining facilities. One could enter into this area through the front door, but typically anyone who came into this section was considered family. They viewed the side door as entrance into a semi-private club. That was where the doctors, nurses, medical-detail salesmen, politicians and visiting dignitaries could be found. At the far end of the building, next to and through the lounge area, was the true inner sanctum and private den for those in favor. This was where the infamous "Monkey Room" was located. Jungle murals with palm trees and swinging monkeys decorated the painted walls, hence, the name. If the front part of the store was a forerunner of the "mini mart", then the Monkey Room surely was a pattern for today's club scene. There was no bouncer at the entrance to the "club", but if there was not a nod of approval from one of the family members scattered throughout the store it was almost impossible to gain entrance to that hallowed ground.

What was so special? Interns and residents could sit with their professors over a beer and gain more insight about medicine casually in a one-on-one session than they ever learned making rounds or in a classroom. Distraught family members might be consoled there after the loss of a loved one. Nurses and doctors were introduced and later married as a result of meeting in the Monkey Room. One cannot even contemplate how many political arrangements were hatched sitting around a corner table in the dim smoke-filled room (remember, even doctors smoked then). Medical-detail salesmen were always good for a freeloaded drink, and wise doctors and staff knew how to play that game. Doubtless a great movie or two could be written about things that took place amongst the swinging monkeys. George Dunne, then the President of the Cook County Board and the titular head of the hospital, enjoyed stopping by for a meal and a drink or two. He often found *The Greek's* to be a first-hand source of information about hospital operations and their needs. For example, the aftermath of having a conversation with Dr. Tatooles, then head of the CardioThoracic Department, was the construction of a eighth floor level skyway bridge. Dunne heard of inefficiencies in their unit because of having their operating suites on the eighth floors of two separate buildings. The interconnecting bridge saved time and improved patient care.

The store was also a philanthropic haven to the many frequenters. Lowly interns and residents who barely managed to exist while they toiled never were refused a meal because of lack of funds. It was normal business to allow them to run up large tabs. The untold story remains as to how many of the future doctors had also received "silent scholarships" from the Maggos family. It numbered in the hundreds. Lore has it that not a bill or obligation ever went unpaid.

And speaking of family, the two immigrant brothers married well, had large families and saw some of their offspring become professionals. Fortunately, a few others kept the family tradition alive by working their way up the ranks within the store. The brothers never learned to drive, shared a two-flat residence that was located near their church, and at the end of the Harrison streetcar line so that a car was unnecessary. Many hours were spent at the store but time was found for philanthropic endeavors at their beloved church. As time passed and the old proud brothers went to their rewards, their children continued to run *The Greek's* in the same traditions and care started by their fathers. Urban growth and eminent domain eventually put an end to that old institution, but ask around. *The Greek's* surely is as much a part of Chicago's medical history as was the beloved Cook County Hospital.

*—October 2011*
*James E. Tatooles*
*Constantine J. Tatooles. MD*
*Chief of Cardio-Thoracic Surgery*
*Cook County Hospital 1969–1981*

# About the Editors

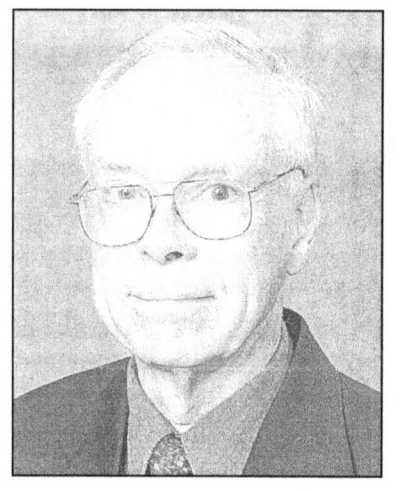

### Patrick D. Guinan, MD, MPH

Patrick Guinan is a Clinical Associate Professor in the Department of Urology of the University of Illinois, College of Medicine in Chicago. He completed his internship at Cook County hospital in 1962 and finished the Urology Residency at CCH in 1969. In 1975, He received a Master's Degree in Public Health from Columbia University, New York. He served as Chairman of the Division of Urology at Cook County Hospital from 1975 to 1985 and at University of Illinois at Chicago from 1978 to 1985. He was Director of Urology of the City of Chicago, Department of health from 1970 to 1975. He is currently Chairman of the Board of the Hetkoen Institute.

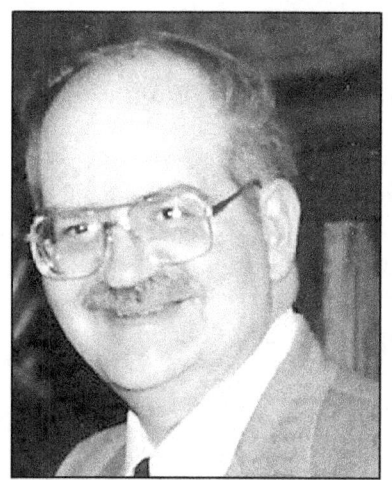

### Kenneth J. Printen, MD

Ken Printen completed his internship at Cook County Hospital from 1961 to 1962 and was drafted for military service in Asia region from 1962 to 1964. He then returned to CCH and finished the surgical residency in 1968. He joined the University of Iowa, College of Medicine and rose to the rank of Professor of Surgery (1969 to 1987). He returned to Chicago and became Chief of Department of Surgery, St. Francis Hospital. Since 1987, he was on the teaching staffs at Loyola, Northwestern, Chicago Medical School, and the University of Illinois Metro Residency. Dr. Printen maintained his affiliation with the Army Reserve and retired as a Brigadier General in 1984.

## ABOUT THE EDITORS

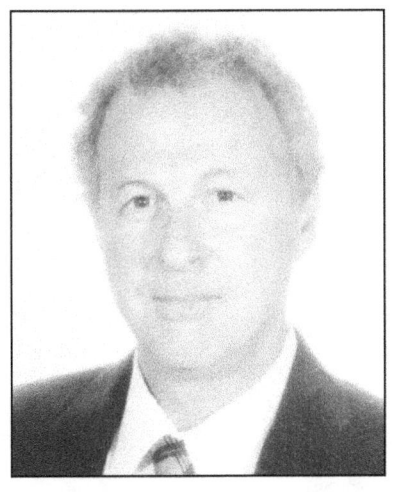

### James L. Stone, MD

James Stone was a senior medical student on the Trauma Unit in 1973 and stimulated to become a Surgical Intern at Cook County Hospital in 1974–1975, followed by Surgical Residency (1975–1976) and a Cook County-University of Illinois (UIC) Neurosurgery Residency from 1976 to 1980. He stayed on as full-time academic faculty in Neurosurgery at UIC based at CCH and attained Associate Professor and Chairman of the Neurosurgical Division at CCH in 1987. In 1992, he was appointed Professor of Neurological Surgery at Loyola, and later Rush, bringing both these residency programs to CCH until his retirement from CCH in late 2003. He acted as Interim Head at CCH in 2004 until he rejoined UIC as Professor of Neurosurgery and Neurology. Dr. Stone remains active in the clinical practice of neurosurgery and neurophysiology at UIC, Advocate Illinois Masonic, and Evanston Hospitals, and also maintains a voluntary appointment in neurosurgery at Stroger Cook County Hospital.

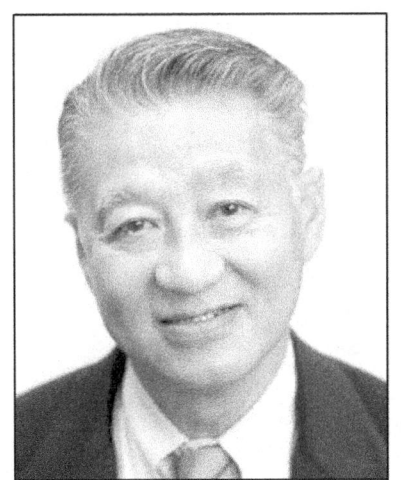

### James S. T. Yao, MD, PhD

Dr. Yao completed a rotating internship at Cook County Hospital in 1961–62 and stayed on for General Surgical Residency training from 1962 to 1967. He then went to St. Mary's Hospital Medical School to further his training in vascular surgery. At the same time, he received a PhD in vascular physiology from the University of London. He returned to Chicago in 1973 and joined the staff as Attending Surgeon at Wesley Memorial Hospital (Now NMH) and on the faculty of Feinberg School of Medicine, Northwestern University. He was appointed Magerstadt Professor of Surgery in 1985 and served as Chief of Division of Vascular Surgery from 1988 to 1997 and Chairman of Department of Surgery 1997 to 2000. After 35 years of service, Dr. Yao is now retired as an Emeritus Professor of Surgery at Northwestern.

www.ingramcontent.com/pod-product-compliance
Lightning Source LLC
Chambersburg PA
CBHW080404300426
44113CB00015B/2396